RHEUMATIC DISEASE
IN THE
ADULT AND CHILD:

Occupational Therapy and Rehabilitation

EDITION 3

RHEUMATIC DISEASE
In The
Adult And Child:

Occupational Therapy and Rehabilitation

EDITION 3

**JEANNE LYNN MELVIN,
O.T.R., M.S.Ed., F.A.O.T.A.**

**Founder and Director
Arthritis and Health Resource Center
Wellesley, Massachusetts**

Illustrated by Lois R. Barnes

F.A. DAVIS COMPANY • **Philadelphia**

Printed in the United States of America

Last digit indicates print number: 10 9 8 7 6 5 4 3 2 1

Library of Congress Cataloging-in-Publication Data

Melvin, Jeanne L.
    Rheumatic disease: occupational therapy and rehabilitation   /
Jeanne Lynn Melvin; illustrated by Lois R. Barnes.—Ed. 3.
        p.   cm.
    Includes bibliographies and index.
    ISBN 0-8036-6137-1
    1. Rheumatism—Patients—Rehabilitation.   2. Occupational therapy.
I. Title.
    [DNLM: 1. Arthritis—rehabilitation.   2. Occupational Therapy.
3. Rheumatism—rehabilitation.   WE 344 M531r]
RC927.M43   1989
616.7′2306—dc 19
DNLM/DLC
for Library of Congress   88-38279
                                                                                      CIP

TO MY FATHER, EARL MELVIN,
FOR HIS LOVE AND SUPPORT

AND

TO MY PATIENTS, WHO,
THROUGH THEIR DETERMINATION AND STRUGGLES,
HAVE TAUGHT AND INSPIRED ME

Preface

Arthritis affects every aspect of a person's life ... how one works, moves, sleeps, relates to others, and, most important, how one feels about oneself—self-esteem and confidence. Fortunately, this connection works in both directions; how a person feels, thinks, works, and moves also affects one's arthritis. Health professionals face the challenge of finding ways of helping people with rheumatic disorders to take action to improve their health through rehabilitative, medical, surgical, and lifestyle processes.

This book was created to bring together, in a single source, the knowledge created by the clinical interface among the fields of rheumatology, rehabilitation, psychology, orthopedic surgery, and pediatrics, which can empower therapists to help patients to take action. But before therapists can help, they need to believe the knowledge can make a difference. Thus, this book emphasizes how this information can make a difference.

It is hoped that this text will further the development of the team approach to patient care by presenting the medical and surgical information from a rehabilitation frame of reference and by communicating to other professionals the role of occupational therapy in the treatment of rheumatic diseases.

This book was designed from the perspective of the clinician. Thus, information is organized according to the way in which problems or issues are presented in the clinic. The first chapter provides an overview of the therapy for arthritis that is common to all the rheumatic diseases, including juvenile arthritis. It is brief in order to provide a gestalt of treatment. The reader is then referred to subsequent chapters for detailed treatment information.

The chapter on drug therapy, now Chapter 3, has been moved to the beginning of the book because the majority of persons with arthritis are treated with medication, and it is critical that therapists be knowledgeable about the effects and side effects of medications in relation to treatment and patient education. This is especially important in therapy where fast-acting medications can influence objective assessments and slow-acting medications can alter longitudinal assessments. The chapter on patient education is also included in Part I as a "basic" because patient instruction is critical to the empowerment process and successful treatment.

Part II, on major rheumatic diseases, has been generally reorganized, in accord with the incidence of the various diseases. A chapter on fibromyalgia, Chapter 5, has been added not only because this condition is extremely common but also because its symptoms can be confused with those of other rheumatic conditions such as rheumatoid arthritis, lupus, carpal tunnel syndrome, and tendinitis. Fibromyalgia provides a model for occupational therapy and rehabilitation in a wide range of chronic fatigue syndromes. Throughout Part II, the treatment for each disease is organized around the common clinical symptoms or by the body areas affected, thereby allowing easy reference for treatment of specific symptoms. These chapters are also purposefully brief in order to facilitate quick review in a clinic setting. All of the chapters have been revised to indicate when treatment of children is similar to or different from that of adults.

Part III, on arthritis in children and adolescents, is new to this edition. This section presents the first publication of a comprehensive biomechanical-developmental approach to children with arthritis. Developed by Marcy Atwood, at Children's Hospital of Los Angeles, this approach has evolved from the occupational behavior approach to pediatric therapy developed at the University of Southern California, School of Occupational Therapy. Chapter 14 defines the nature of juvenile rheumatoid arthritis (JRA) and the biomechanics of joint involvement and outlines treatment options. This chapter includes the first publication of an extensive review of hand involvement in both JRA alone and in comparison with the adult RA hand. Chapters 15 and 16 provide the foundation for integrating the developmental assessment and treatment of children and adolescents with arthritis. Then, to pull all of the theory and process into a unified whole, Marcy Atwood presents in-depth case studies of three different types of arthritis affecting children of different ages. This chapter clearly illustrates the practical implementation of this integrative approach to assessment and treatment.

Part IV concerns evaluation and relates standard evaluation methods to patients with joint disease. Texts that define the standard range-of-motion and strength assessments, for example, relate the procedure only to normal joint anatomy. Assessment of damaged joints requires special considerations.

Chapter 19, on hand pathodynamics and assessment, which was expanded in the second edition, has been updated to reflect the growing knowledge about these processes. Systematic, comprehensive hand assessments can result in the early detection and prevention of many deformities, especially when conducted by therapists knowledgeable in both arthritis pathodynamics and hand rehabilitation. The comprehensive hand assessment process described in this chapter is the result of eight years of development and refinement.

The chapter on the assessment of activities of daily living, Chapter 22, has been expanded to include assessment of the workplace to identify the need for joint protection instruction in industry. This material is also being published here for the first time.

Part V covers five basic occupational therapy modalities as they apply to joint involvement: orthotic treatment, joint protection and energy conservation techniques, assistive equipment, functional activities, and a general discussion of range of motion and strengthening. This material is not intended to teach basic occupational therapy methods but to review the unique aspects of these activities as they apply to joint disease. The chapter on orthotic treatment, Chapter 23, has been extensively revised and expanded. At the request of many therapists, I have included a section on my personal approach to the treatment of specific hand conditions. In Chapter 25, on assistive devices, the information on problem-solving equipment needs has been expanded to cover analysis by activity as well as by site of joint involvement. Also, a new section on resources for services and equipment has been added to Chapter 25.

In Part VI, the seven chapters on surgical rehabilitation are organized around joint involvement. Each chapter reviews the progression of joint destruction, the indications and options for surgical intervention, the rationale for selecting specific surgeries, and an outline for postoperative management. The chapter on the hip, Chapter 33, has been expanded to cover the cementless total hip prostheses, and a new section on postoperative precautions has been added. The descriptions of joint pathodynamics in the surgical chapters differ from the ones in the medical chapters. Readers will find them a helpful supplement to understanding the biomechanical factors affecting joint function.

For therapists new to the field of rheumatology, I recommend reading Part I, "The Basics," and the chapters on osteoarthritis, fibromyalgia, rheumatoid arthritis, and juvenile rheumatoid arthritis. Osteoarthritis occurs in persons with rheumatic diseases with the same incidence as it occurs in the general population. Therefore, it is safe to assume that everyone over 60 years old with another primary rheumatic disease will have some osteoarthritis that can influence joint function. It is very helpful to be able to detect and separate the impact of osteoarthritis from another primary disease, such as rheumatoid arthritis. Understanding the detection and treatment of fibromyalgia is critical in current practice because this condition can be triggered by any disease or condition that causes severe fatigue. The symptoms of fibromyalgia can be misconstrued as symptoms of a primary disease such as rheumatoid arthritis or systemic lupus erythematosus. Chapter 6, on rheumatoid arthritis, provides a model, or prototype, for treating inflammatory arthritis of the peripheral joints.

Practitioners well versed in the treatment of adult arthritis are encouraged to read the chapter on juvenile rheumatoid arthritis (Chapter 14) even if they are not treating children. Many concepts about the pathodynamics and treatment of joint involvement are very clear and easy to focus on in the treatment of children and are quite applicable to adult care. For example, the role of muscle spasm is pronounced in juvenile rheumatoid arthritis. This information is most applicable to adults when spasm is present. Having worked primarily with adults for a number of years, I have found the pediatric rheumatology literature quite illuminating on many points that are quite muddy in the adult literature, and vice versa—the adult literature clear and precise where the pediatric literature is vague. It is hoped that the inclusion of a pediatric section in this edition will encourage communication and learning between practitioners of adult and pediatric rehabilitation.

J.L.M.

Acknowledgments

Only with the help of many people was it possible to write, revise, and update 35 chapters that cover the relationship between rheumatology, rehabilitation, pediatrics, and orthopedic surgery.

First, this new edition would not be possible were it not for the Arthritis Health Professions Association and the Arthritis Foundation, which supported the research and writing of the first edition with a two-year Allied Health Professions Fellowship in Rheumatology. I continue to be indebted to these organizations for their contribution to my education, making my work possible.

Second, the consulting physicians have provided the essential medical and surgical expertise to keep me true to the word of their specialties. Their help has been invaluable in providing a current, state-of-the art perspective on clinical practice and in separating fact from fiction in the literature. Dr. Kenneth Nies has played a special role in this book, as he has provided the medical review of it through all three editions. It is his clear, pragmatic approach to rheumatology that has guided the medical philosophy put forth in this text. His continued participation has greatly contributed to the continuity of style and message through the interminable revisions. Dr. Edward Nalebuff has been extremely helpful in critically reviewing the extensive sections on hand assessment, dysfunction, and surgery. He has an extraordinary ability to review, analyze, and organize complex processes into comprehensible functional forms. This talent shows both when he reconstructs a rheumatoid hand and in his numerous contributions to the classification of rheumatic hand disorders. We have worked together for more than ten years; his teachings and guidance have contributed to the organization and presentation of the hand-related text. Dr. Clement Sledge has also had a strong influence on this text; his philosophy and approach to orthopedic surgery has guided the chapters in this area and the new material on surgery for arthritis in children. I am indebted to both Dr. Nalebuff and Dr. Sledge for their support through review of the current as well as the previous edition of this book. Their participation contributed to the continuity of style and format and greatly facilitated the revision process. Dr. Bram Bernstein has helped develop one of the best treatment programs for children with arthritis in the country. His pragmatic approach and extensive reviews were invaluable in helping me wade through the conflict and controversy of juvenile rheumatoid arthritis terminology and classification and in making Chapter 14 possible.

Marcy Atwood, O.T.R., has made it possible to present the extensive information on evaluation and treatment of children in a cohesive, educational format. Her clinical expertise and ability to organize and integrate the developmental and psychosocial treatment made it possible to present a comprehensive approach to treating children. She did a superb job, and it was a real pleasure to work with her.

I am also deeply grateful to the following persons for their careful reviews of the pediatric chapters and constructive suggestions relevant to their clinical specialties. Susan Simon, R.P.T., Children's Hospital of Los Angeles, kept us true to physical therapy; and Bruce Wood, D.P.M., Brigham and Women's Hospital of Boston, kept us true to podiatric medicine.

I would like to express special thanks to Dr. Don Goldenberg for his review of the fibromyalgia chapter and his support of the programs at my center, which has allowed us to develop one of the first fibromyalgia rehabilitation programs in the country, thus making the material in this part of the text possible.

The surgery chapters needed extensive revision and updating, especially on inpatient therapy protocols. This was made possible by Victoria Gall, M.S., R.P.T., Coordinator, Arthritis Rehabilitation Program at the Brigham and Women's Hospital. She also provided a particularly helpful review of the spinal and lower extremity surgery chapters. Lynn Yasuda, M.S., O.T.R., Education Coordinator, Rancho Los Amigos Hospital, provided a critical review of the hand surgery chapter and shared with me a number of helpful resources. Their assistance was invaluable and deeply appreciated.

The following therapists also provided valuable feedback by reviewing specific chapters related to their area of clinical expertise: Joy Cordery, O.T.R.; Dena Slonager, M.S., O.T.R.; Virgil Mathowietz, Ed.D., O.T.R.; Beverly Bingham, O.T.R.; and Cynthia Phillips, M.S., O.T.R. I am very appreciative of the time and thoughtfulness they put into their reviews. Alice Shafer, M.S., O.T.R., created an excellent table that summarizes the properties of orthotic materials, making it possible to present this information. I am also indebted to the following individuals who were generous in granting me permission to use tables or photographs that enhanced the text and made my work easier: Jerry Jacobs, M.D.; Helen Schweidler Marx, O.T.R.; Edward Nalebuff, M.D.; Andrea Kovalesky, R.N., M.S.; and Cynthia Garris, O.T.R. Also, the occupational therapy and physical therapy departments at Children's Hospital of Los Angeles were very helpful in identifying resources and sharing information and protocols.

I would also like to thank Dr. Adrian Flatt, who, through his classic text, *Care of the Rheumatoid Hand,* served as a guide and teacher. His work made my contribution to hand management possible.

I was fortunate to work with two talented women, Lisa Poniatowski and Maureen Kirby, who assisted with editing, word processing, and organizing the 1355 new references and sources that were ultimately added to this edition. I am appreciative not only for their superb skills but also for their enthusiasm for the project, willingness to work long hours and weekends, and most of all, their buoyant good humor through it all.

Heartfelt appreciation also goes to the staff at the Arthritis and Health Resource Center for their understanding, flexibility, and loyalty during the two years of writing.

I am also very fortunate to be able to work with an excellent publishing house, whose editorial and production staff have been very supportive and have literally made this book what it is today.

Last, but not least, I am grateful to my husband, Jerome Small, whose encouragement, support, and humor made a year and a half of three-day computer weekends bearable and almost fun.

Contributor

Marcy Atwood, M.A., O.T.R.
Specialist in Pediatric Rheumatology, Children's Hospital of Los Angeles;
Co-Director, Options Program, Hope School, Buena Park, California.

Consultants

MEDICAL

Kenneth M. Nies, M.D.
Clinical Professor of Medicine, University of California, Los Angeles; Rheumatologist in private practice, Torrance, California.

HAND SURGERY

Edward A. Nalebuff, M.D.
Professor of Orthopaedic Surgery, Tufts University School of Medicine; Chief, Hand Surgical Service, New England Baptist Hospital; Orthopedic Staff, Brigham and Women's Hospital, Boston, Massachusetts.

ORTHOPEDIC SURGERY

Clement B. Sledge, M.D.
John B. and Buckminster Brown Professor of Orthopaedic Surgery, Harvard Medical School; Chairman, Department of Orthopedic Surgery, Brigham and Women's Hospital, Boston, Massachusetts.

PEDIATRIC RHEUMATOLOGY

Bram Bernstein, M.D.
Professor of Clinical Pediatrics, University of Southern California; Head, Division of Rheumatology, Children's Hospital of Los Angeles, Los Angeles, California.

Contents

Abbreviations

ADL	Activities of daily living
AS	Ankylosing spondylitis
CMC	Carpometacarpal
CTS	Carpal tunnel syndrome
DIP	Distal interphalangeal
DM	Dermatomyositis
DMD	Disease-modifying drug
FDP	Flexor digitorum profundus
FDS	Flexor digitorum superficialis
IP	Interphalangeal
JRA	Juvenile rheumatoid arthritis
MCP	Metacarpophalangeal
MTP	Metatarsophalangeal
NSAID	Nonsteroidal anti-inflammatory drug
OA	Osteoarthritis
PA	Psoriatic arthritis
PIP	Proximal interphalangeal
PM	Polymyositis
PMR	Polymyalgia rheumatica
RA	Rheumatoid arthritis
ROM	Range of motion
SLE	Systemic lupus erythematosus
SS	Systemic sclerosis
TM	Temporomandibular
THR	Total hip replacement

PART I

THE BASICS

Chapter 1 provides an overview—the broad picture—of the full range of treatment that should be considered in the rehabilitation of adults and children with arthritis. It is designed to give a gestalt. Treatment applications for specific conditions are covered in Parts II and III.

Chapter 2 reviews drug therapy from the therapist's perspective. Special emphasis is placed on how medications can affect objective assessment and rehabilitation and importance of patient education. Medications frequently make it possible for patients to participate successfully in rehabil-itation. Understanding medications and how they are used can increase the therapist's options for effective treatment.

Finally, Chapter 3 provides a brief definition of a holistic approach to treatment and the use of patient education as a means of empowerment. In order for education to empower it must fill a specific need; it must be helpful in some concrete way. Understanding the psychological and medical contingencies described in this chapter can help the therapist prepare the needs assessment essential for an effective learning–teaching experience.

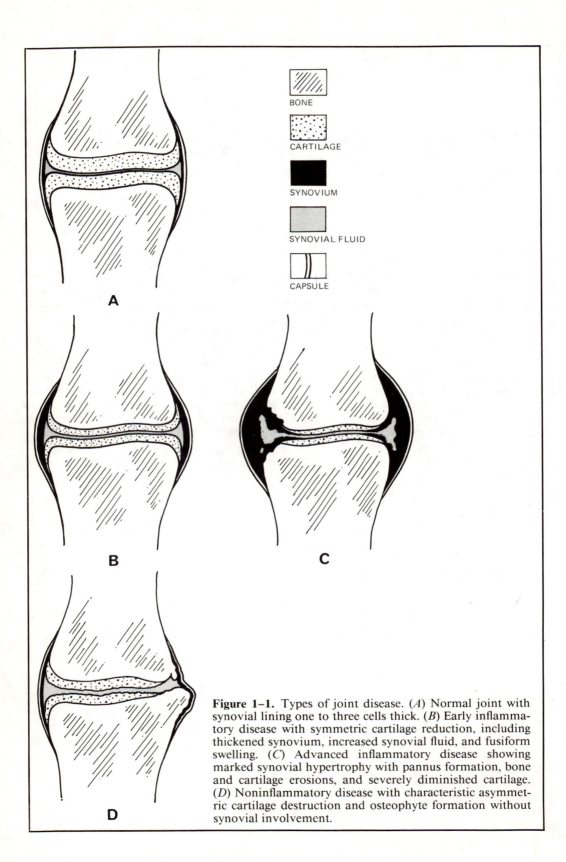

BONE

CARTILAGE

SYNOVIUM

SYNOVIAL FLUID

CAPSULE

Figure 1–1. Types of joint disease. (*A*) Normal joint with synovial lining one to three cells thick. (*B*) Early inflammatory disease with symmetric cartilage reduction, including thickened synovium, increased synovial fluid, and fusiform swelling. (*C*) Advanced inflammatory disease showing marked synovial hypertrophy with pannus formation, bone and cartilage erosions, and severely diminished cartilage. (*D*) Noninflammatory disease with characteristic asymmetric cartilage destruction and osteophyte formation without synovial involvement.

Chapter 1

Overview of Therapy for Joint Disease

THERAPY FOR JOINT DISEASE
INFLAMMATORY JOINT DISEASE
    Primary Occupational Therapy Goals and Suggested Modalities
    for Adults and Children
NONINFLAMMATORY JOINT DISEASE
    Primary Occupational Therapy Goals and Suggested Modalities

There are over one hundred conditions in which joint disease can be a significant feature. The common denominator of joint involvement characterizes these conditions as the rheumatic diseases. Joint involvement, be it localized to a single joint or in combination with a systemic disease, universally interferes with a person's functional ability. Thus effective patient care involves treating both the disease and the person.

Treatment for joint disease is accomplished through control of inflammation, removal of irritating causal factors, and protection of joint structures during periods of exacerbation. From this point, treatment must be directed toward the person and toward relief or control of pain, improvement of functional ability, psychological adjustment to functional loss, and development of health behaviors with regard to nutrition, rest, and exercise.

The physical, personal, familial, social, and vocational consequences of chronic joint disease are so extensive that skilled assistance is beyond the scope of any one professional. Consultation and cooperation among various health care workers become an integral part of treatment.

The rehabilitative approaches described and advocated in this book are based on the premise that effective treatment of joint disease is *experimental* in all phases. There are no absolute answers in therapy; no treatment can be applied with complete certainty as to outcome. There is no treatment without disadvantages as well as advantages and *no treatment that cannot be improved.* There are many successful treatment methods yet to be developed by therapists.

THERAPY FOR JOINT DISEASE

The goals of therapy vary depending on the chronicity of the disease and the responsiveness of the patient to medication. In the beginning stages of rheumatoid arthritis (RA)—particularly the first 2 years—there is a high incidence of sustained remission. It is estimated that 20 to 40 percent of all people diagnosed with RA have only one or two episodes of arthritis and then go into "spontaneous" remission. Spontaneous is a term used when the reason for the remission is not understood. Some clinicians report that the incidence of spontaneous remission may be as high as 80 percent when the diagnosis is made early (within the first 2 months of the disease).[1] It is unclear whether these patients actually develop RA and then, through some unknown process, are able to mobilize their immune system to control the inflammation or whether they have developed an unidentified, short-term, more benign inflammatory condition. It is likely that both of these factors, as well as several other unknown factors, play a role in the development of sustained remissions.[1] In this discussion, RA is used as an example because it is the most common condition treated by therapists and because there is the most information about the natural course of the disease. However, it is possible to have spontaneous remissions in all of the major rheumatic diseases, including osteoarthritis.

The remissions seen in patients diagnosed with RA may last for several years or may be indefinite. The initial episodes of inflammation vary in intensity and duration. They may be mild, lasting several weeks with no residual limitation, or they may be quite severe, lasting as long as a year. If proper therapy is not received, these patients may, despite complete remission of the disease, have to live with deformities incurred during the initial episodes.

Other patients—an estimated 20 to 30 percent—have a variable or intermittent course of RA, with alternating periods of remission and exacerbation. For others, the condition is slowly or rapidly progressive. Fortunately, most of these patients are responsive to antirheumatic medications. It is really a small percentage of patients—3 to 5 percent—with adult RA that have a severe progressive disease that is not responsive to current medications.[1] For children with all types of **juvenile rheumatoid arthritis (JRA)** approximately 10 percent become severely disabled, and approximately 5 percent have an arthritis that is progressive and unresponsive to medications.

In addition to spontaneous remissions, it is possible for some of the stronger antirheumatic medications—such as gold, hydroxychloroquine (Plaquenil), penicillamine, and methotrexate—to induce a nearly complete remission of symptoms. So in the early stages of the disease there is considerable opportunity for the patient to experience sustained remissions. (See Chapter 3, Drug Therapy.)

When a therapist is working with a patient early in the course of the disease (within the first 2 years), *the overriding goal of therapy should be to preserve the integrity of the musculoskeletal system during periods of exacerbation so that the patient will have optimal functioning during periods of remission or in the event of a spontaneous remission throughout his or her life.*[2]

Occupational and physical therapy should be initiated early in the course of the disease (during the first 6 months for outpatients and during the first few days of hospitalization for acutely ill patients) so that treatment can be preventive rather than adaptive in nature.

Many therapists work in facilities in which physicians do not refer patients to rehabilitation until the patient develops significant limitations. In these facilities it is the responsibility of the therapist to make physicians aware of the preventive role of therapy and the value of early patient education. Many of the deformities that occur in arthritis can be avoided, because they are often the result of the patient having inadequate information about the disease and lacking instruction regarding appropriate or effective exercise and positioning techniques. Throughout this text there will be an emphasis on early treatment and the procedures that are most effective for preventing deformity or limitations. Preventive therapy is one of the most rewarding and satisfying aspects of rheumatological rehabilitation, for the therapist as well as for the patient.

Joint disease can take two forms: inflammatory or noninflammatory (which includes osteoarthritis and traumatic arthritis). Figure 1–1 compares these two forms of joint involvement with a normal joint. Inflammatory joint disease is described as having phases. It may start as acute and then diminish to subacute. If it persists over time it is referred to as **chronic-active.**[3]

Rehabilitative therapy for each phase of joint disease is symptomatic and preventive in nature; that is, it is directed toward reducing the signs and symptoms of arthritis and preventing limitations related to specific joints. The principles of rehabilitation are the same whether the disease occurs in a single joint or in association with a major rheumatic disease.[4] For example, rehabilitative therapy for synovitis of the wrist is the same whether it is restricted to only that joint or whether it occurs in conjunction with rheumatoid arthritis, psoriatic arthritis, juvenile rheumatoid arthritis, or any other rheumatic disease.[4] In many instances, it is not possible to ascribe a specific diagnostic label until a clear pattern of joint involvement is established. This may take as long as 6 months. But when medical or rehabilitative treatment is symptomatic, the lack of a definite diagnosis does not alter the course of therapy. However, critical to the treatment process is an understanding of how to reduce the symptoms of arthritis and how to preserve the specific joint structures from the effects of chronic arthritis.

To understand the consequences of chronic arthritis of specific joints in adults it is necessary to be familiar with only three rheumatic diseases. These diseases have characteristic patterns of joint involvement and therefore provide a prototype or model for understanding the consequences of chronic arthritis in specific joints. These diseases are **rheumatoid arthritis (RA),** a chronic inflammatory joint disease of the peripheral joints and the cervical spine; **ankylosing spondylitis (AS),** a chronic inflammatory joint disease of the axial joints; and **osteoarthritis (OA)** (degenerative joint disease), a noninflammatory disease of any joint. This means, for example, that the rehabilitative treatment for chronic synovitis of the peripheral joints in any disease is the same as for RA. A case in point is **psoriatic arthritis (PA),** a condition that may result in inflammatory arthritis of both peripheral and axial joints. Consequently, rehabilitative treatment for the peripheral joints is the same as for RA, and the treatment of the axial joints is the same as for AS. For children, treatment of polyarticular JRA provides the prototype for management of all subtypes of JRA. To treat seropositive polyarticular-onset JRA, the subtype that is like adult RA, you need to know how to treat both JRA and adult RA. Similarly, to treat children with other major rheumatic diseases, such as **systemic lupus erythematosus (SLE), progressive systemic sclerosis (PSS),** and AS, you need to know the protocols for both JRA and the adult form of the disease.

Because the treatment for arthritis is symptomatic and common to all of the rheumatic diseases, it is reviewed separately in this chapter. The following overview is purposely brief to provide a gestalt of treatment for easy reference. The specific application of treatment of a person with a major rheumatic disease is discussed in Part II and in Part III.

INFLAMMATORY JOINT DISEASE

The major inflammatory rheumatic diseases essentially begin with joint inflammation. Sometimes the joint involvement is so prominent that other systemic symptoms pale by comparison, and it appears that the only manifestation is arthritis. It is important to keep in mind that all of these diseases are systemic in nature; that is, they involve all of the body's systems and affect every cell in the body. The **systemic** or constitutional **symptoms** include malaise, weakness, fatigue, depression, decreased libido, and anorexia. When the constitutional symptoms become more acute, low-grade fever occurs and can be accompanied by myalgia, arthralgias, and stiffness. Consequently, when people with RA, PA, AS, and SLE have a flare-up, they often feel as if they have influenza. Generalized morning stiffness is a consequence of both systemic and articular involvement.

The primary site of inflammation is in the **synovial membrane,** which lines joint capsules, tendon sheaths, and bursae throughout the body. It is believed that the synovial lining (or membrane) performs two functions. First, it contributes to the production of synovial fluid, which coats the articular surfaces and aids lubrication by synthesizing a major component of the fluid, hyaluronic acid.[5] Second, it provides for removal of the synovial fluid from the joint. When the synovial lining becomes inflamed, these two functions become impaired.[5] An excess of joint fluid is produced, the drainage mechanism becomes inadequate, and the fluid becomes trapped within the capsule (an **effusion**), resulting in characteristic fusiform-shaped swelling.

If the inflammation is prolonged, the synovial cells begin to proliferate, increasing the thickness of the membrane from the normal 1 to 4 cells to possibly 20 or more.[5] The inflammatory process directly infiltrates and damages the capsule, supporting ligaments, cartilage, and subchondral bone.[1,6]

Both the effusion and thickened synovium result in an increase in **intra-articular pressure** that places the joint capsule and supporting structures on tension or stretch. Joint motion away from neutral further increases intra-articular pressure. In addition to the tissue damage caused by direct inflammatory infiltration, this mechanical stress makes the joint structures extremely vulnerable to overstretching (lengthening) during functional use.[5] (All forms of exercise should take into account the tension to which joint structures are subjected during active synovitis.)

If the synovitis is severe, chronic synovial granulation tissue **(pannus)** can develop in the joint, furthering the inflammatory process and causing erosive changes in the cartilage and subchondral bone. All deformities, joint destruction, and pathological anatomy encountered in severe inflammatory arthritis are the result of the way in which hypertrophied synovial tissue affects its surroundings.[5] A single (limited) acute bout of synovitis usually does not result in residual deformity.

Pain appears to result from the force exerted by increased intra-articular pressure on the innervated capsule and on the attachment of the capsule to the sensitive bone (periosteum) and possible pressure on small areas of exposed bone within the confines of the capsule. Evidence for this theory is often demonstrated by patients with mild synovitis who perceive pain only when compression or motion further increases the intra-articular pressure and patients with severe synovitis who often feel pain at rest.[5] (See section on evaluation of pain and synovitis in Chapter 19.)

Pain and stretch of the joint capsule are also believed to be responsible for secondary changes such as **protective muscle spasm.** The natural protective response of the body in the presence of pain is excitation of the flexors and inhibition of the extensors. Protective spasm is most frequently seen in the flexor and adductor muscles and in the spinal muscles.[6-9]

The terminology for describing the various phases of inflammation varies considerably across the country. In the past, publications have referred to four phases of arthritis: acute, subacute, chronic-active, and chronic-inactive, the last referring to the end-stage, or "burned-out," phase of arthritis.[3,10] These terms can be helpful in describing joint status or relating therapy to severity of inflammation. However, most physicians do not recognize these categories and instead refer to synovitis as **acute, chronic, active,** or **inactive.** (The term *inactive* is used, but technically it is a misnomer, inasmuch as synovitis by definition is active.) Sometimes the term **controlled** is used to describe a low-grade synovitis kept in check by medication. Probably no single classification prevails because the terminology cannot be applied equally to all patients. Acute inflammation for one patient may be considered moderate or subacute for another. Some patients *never* develop hot, red, exquisitely tender joints even at the height of an exacerbation.

The symptoms are the same for all phases of inflammatory joint disease (acute, subacute, and chronic-active); that is, the classic pattern of joint inflammation (pain, tenderness, swelling, warmth, and limited range of motion) is present. The symptoms are the most severe in the **acute phase.** When the symptoms diminish, the patient is entering the **subacute phase** of the disease. If the symptoms continue at a low-grade inflammatory level for an extended period, the disease is in the **chronic-active phase.**[3]

The subacute and chronic-active phases seem very similar. The main difference is that the chronic-active phase is a stable condition. In this phase, individuals usually feel better than in the acute or subacute phase, have adjusted somewhat to the pain, and are more active. Thus therapy can be more vigorous in the chronic-active phase.[3]

For most patients, especially those with recent onset, the illness of systemic arthritis is accompanied by fear, anxiety, irritability, and depression. For children, the anxiety and fear are often acute and are characteristic manifestations of the disease.

Primary Occupational Therapy Goals and Suggested Modalities for Adults and Children

The following is an outline of basic treatment for both isolated and multiple inflammatory joint involvement. The reader is referred to specific chapters for detailed discussions and references.

I. ACUTE AND SUBACUTE PHASES

A. Reduce pain and inflammation
1. Local rest to specific joints—immobilization reduces stress to the joint and enhances the ability of the synovium to reduce inflammation. This can be accomplished with orthoses or positioning; for example, wrist/hand resting orthoses (see Chapter 23); posterior leg or ankle orthoses; soft neck collars; proper support for back and neck while sitting in bed (see Chapter 28).
2. **Bedrest** is extremely effective in reducing both inflammation and associated pain because it affects the person in three profound ways. First, it reduces the demand on the immune and other body systems, so the body can concentrate resources on healing (i.e., controlling inflammation). Second, it reduces mechanical stress to the joints (local rest). Third, it has the potential for emotional rest from the psychological strain of daily activities, as long as this is not supplanted by guilt and self-recrimination for creating a perceived hardship on the patient's family. For inpatients it is essential that the medical, nursing, and rehabilitation programs are coordinated so that the patient can get adequate rest.
3. **Joint protection techniques (JPT)** offer another method for reducing stress and inflammation. For hospitalized patients, JPT instructions may be limited to appropriate transfer and ambulation methods (see Chapter 24). When there is severe synovitis, joint protection instruction is minimal because the patient is in too much pain to participate in activities. As the inflammation becomes less acute and the patient starts feeling better and becomes more active,

joint protection methods and use of assistive equipment play a more important role in reducing pain and ultimately inflammation in the involved joints.
4. Application of **thermal modalities:** ice compresses, heating pads, or hot packs relieve pain secondary to joint inflammation and reduce protective muscle spasm. For acute joint inflammation and tenosynovitis, ice compresses are usually the most beneficial.[11] As the swelling decreases, ice becomes less effective and heat may help more. *Generally, the hotter the joint, the more responsive it is to ice.*[2] Acute tenosynovitis may present with neither heat nor pain; the only symptoms may be swelling and decreased tendon excursion.[2] For tenosynovitis, ice, or cold, is the most effective modality for reducing swelling.[11–16] For children with severe muscle spasm, contrast hot–cold compresses or baths may be the most effective intervention for reducing swelling and/or spasm.[17]
5. Conscious deep muscle **relaxation** or meditation practiced at least 15 minutes twice a day is effective for reducing tension on the joint, decreasing pain, and improving sleep. It generally reduces fear, anxiety, and the impact of psychological stress on the immune system.[18] This should be instituted as early as possible in the patient's program. Children can be taught relaxation techniques (similar to those taught adults) as early as age 9. Conscious muscle relaxation may be combined with meditation and imagery/visualization for healing.

B. Maintain **range of motion (ROM)** and joint integrity
1. *Gentle* passive or active ROM to the point of discomfort—not pain—(without stretch) two times per day. (Stretch is not recommended for children or adults when there is severe intra-articu-

lar swelling because swelling in itself causes the supportive joint structures to be stretched (see Chapter 27, Exercise Treatment). The patient may be able to do effective active self-ranging of the neck, elbows, hands, knees, and ankles but may require *gentle* passive ranging of the shoulders and hips (passive ranging allows the most muscle relaxation).[3] For children, active ROM without muscle substitution and assistance should be encouraged through activities. The flexor, adductor, internal rotator, and supinator muscles are the most prone to developing contractures, and therefore their lengthening and relaxation need emphasis in the ROM program.

2. Proper **positioning** for lying or sitting. This includes a mattress with firm support and a soft top layer (foam), small head pillow or cervical pillow, no knee pillows, and the hospital bed *must not be elevated* at the patient's knees (see Chapter 28). For subacute involvement, proper positioning during leisure activities becomes more important; for example, while reading (especially reading in bed), watching television, or doing homework. Proper positioning includes back and neck support to achieve straight alignment. For knee and ankle involvement, elevation of the feet must be provided, with knees extended and supported. For the fingers, a relaxed open functional position is recommended (see Chapter 28). For patients with hip involvement or on prolonged bedrest, **lying prone** to tolerance is an important adjunct to maintaining hip ROM. For some patients, lumbar rolls are indicated to support the lower back (see Chapter 28 for guidelines for prone positioning).

3. Use of **resting** hand, ankle, or leg **orthoses.** Posterior ankle orthoses are the most effective method for preventing ankle plantar flexion contractures. Footboards are helpful for keeping bedcovers elevated so that they do not pull the feet into plantar flexion and for self-ranging of the ankle, by providing a surface to push the foot against. But they are not sufficient for preventing foot-drop contractures, especially in the nonambulatory patient.

4. Deep breathing and postural exercises to maintain thoracic and scapular joint mobility.

5. Exercises to maintain jaw mobility are indicated for patients with temporomandibular joint involvement.

C. Maintain **strength** and **endurance**

1. Performance of activities of daily living to tolerance. This is particularly important for counteracting the debilitating effects of bedrest. But in achieving this goal it is critical not to fatigue patients, especially children. It is important to acknowledge their endurance level and to encourage activities in positions that avoid joint stress and muscular substitutions. All resistive exercises and activities should be avoided at this stage. (For the inflamed hand, this could include cutting food.) The rationale for doing self-care activities should be part of the patient education program.

2. For adults, isometric exercises for muscles associated with involved joints should be included in the program as long as they can tolerate them without undue joint pain and fatigue. Exercising muscles around noninvolved joints is often well tolerated and very helpful for maintaining strength and endurance. It is critical to consider the effects of exercise on muscular guarding and flexor/adductor spasm. For children (and some adults) it is appropriate only to exercise the extensor/abductor muscles. In the subacute phase, isometric exercise is *to maintain strength and to prevent deconditioning* rather

than actually to strengthen the muscle. For this purpose one to three *full* contractions per muscle group once a day *may* be sufficient for maintaining strength. (See Chapter 27 for muscle strength and endurance rationale.)

3. An appropriate amount of **rest** is critical during all phases of active disease. At least 10 to 12 hours of sleep are recommended in a 24-hour period. This concept needs more reinforcement in the subacute and chronic phases, when the patient is more active, than in the acute phase.

4. Initiation of work simplification and energy conservation as the inflammation decreases.

D. Provide **emotional support**
1. Offer patients an opportunity to express their feelings. If adults or older children have fears or resistance toward a certain treatment, ask what they would need to make the treatment more comfortable or acceptable to them. Acknowledge that they are the experts about their bodies and their needs.
2. Try to provide as much patient control in each session or treatment as possible. When there are alternatives, let the patients choose their preference in orthotics, relaxation techniques, exercise methods, play activities, time of therapy, and so forth. This can go a long way in facilitating compliance.
3. Encourage questions and use patient education as a means for empowering patients to have greater control over their health.

E. Engage children in age-appropriate activity
1. Use play or crafts that interest children to enhance developmental, emotional, and physical status. The activity should be short term, should provide immediate gratification and success, should be intrinsically motivating, and should be graded for the child's endurance and physical needs.

2. Discover the type of positive reinforcer that motivates each particular child and parent. Incorporate positive reinforcement in all therapeutic activities.

F. **Patient education**
1. Assess the patients' and parents' levels of understanding. Find out what they know about the illness; for example, "What do you think is causing the pain in your knee?" Some people believe it is an infection or from drinking too much milk (calcium). The answers to this simple question can amaze you.
2. Next find out what they would like to know. Some adults do not want any explanations; they just want to be told what to do. Extensive explanation can actually cause them more stress.
3. Ask them how they learn best. Some people prefer to read about it. Others may want a family member present so that they will not have to explain it to others. Still others simply want a demonstration. (See Chapter 2 concerning patient education.)
4. In this phase education needs to be simple and focused on what the patients and parents need to know about reducing inflammation and preventing contractures and complications.

II. CHRONIC-ACTIVE PHASE
The treatment protocol is the same as outlined for the subacute phase, but the emphasis is different because clients are able to perform more activities than in the acute and subacute phases. However, they are stiff and have synovitis, thus making the supporting joint structures vulnerable to deformity. In this phase JPT, *assistive equipment, exercise, and orthotics* are the most important treatment modalities for maintaining joint integrity. (See Chapters 23, 24, and 25.) If serial casting is needed to correct contractures in children, they should be applied during this phase. (See Chapter 14.)
A. In addition to a strength maintenance program, exercises to *improve* muscle strength and to *increase*

ROM can now be started. For children, activities can be positioned to increase range slightly. (The type and amount of exercise recommended are discussed in detail in Chapter 27.)

B. **Stress management** training (with or without biofeedback instrumentation) can be added to the program, incorporating earlier instruction in relaxation training. This type of training can be particularly valuable for helping patients develop a sense of control over their lives and bodies, reducing fatigue, pain, and depression as well as improving ability for sleeping.[18–21]

C. For the feet and subtalar joints, **foot orthotics** and appropriate footwear can be helpful in reducing joint stress, pain, and inflammation in the affected joints. These should be incorporated into the patient's program before subluxation occurs, as a measure to reduce or to prevent deforming forces. (Foot orthotics are described in Chapter 24, Joint Protection and Energy Conservation Instruction.) Also, a foot ROM program is essential for preventing muscle and joint contractures secondary to protective spasm of the long toe flexors or tightness of the long extensors (from overuse to avoid metatarsophalangeal [MTP] pressure). (See sections on feet and ankle joint involvement in Chapters 6 and 14, on RA and JRA.)

D. **Vocational counseling.** All of the concepts of joint protection and energy conservation need to be applied in the work setting as well as in the home. A vocational assessment that facilitates this process is described in Chapter 22.

E. For older children and adolescents, the following treatment goals need to be included in their program.
  1. Increase **independent living skills** by:
     a. Encouraging responsibility for follow-through with treatment such as self-care, exercise, and craft projects.
     b. Developing problem-solving and decision-making skills through activities such as cooking, budgeting, and so forth.
  2. Encourage normal daily routines that integrate a balance of work, rest, and play by:
     a. Reviewing typical schedule of hospital and home.
     b. Allowing patients to develop the plan or schedule.
     c. Integrating exercises and play into the daily schedule.
  3. Maintain/increase self-esteem by:
     a. Engaging patients in activities in which they can experience success, especially physical activities.
     b. Reinforcing their progress with frequent feedback about positive gains.
     c. Ending each evaluation and treatment session by focusing on *ability,* not *disability.*

NONINFLAMMATORY JOINT DISEASE

Technically this category includes OA and the variants of OA in which the primary etiological event is not inflammation. For example, it is possible to have severe progressive OA without any inflammation, whereas with RA or other forms of inflammatory arthritis this is not possible. The majority of people in the general population with OA *do not* have pain or inflammation. However, this fact may have little meaning in the occupational therapy, physical therapy, or rheumatology clinic, in which the majority of patients with OA have secondary inflammation and are often quite disabled by it.[22] To encourage more accurate understanding of OA, many clinicians advocate using the term **osteoarthrosis,** because the suffix denotes a joint affection caused by trophic degeneration rather than by inflammation. This is clearly a more accurate description of the early process.[23,24]

The inflammation associated with OA can present quite differently from that associated with RA. For example, it can be mild, with the only symptom being aching at rest or pain with functional use (joint compression)—swelling, warmth, and redness are often absent. However, the inflammation can be severe, with all of the cardinal signs and symptoms of inflammation present.[24]

The end results of prolonged inflammation are also different for OA and RA. In RA the severe joint deformities are due in part to every structure inside and outside the joint—tendons, ligaments, muscles, skin, fascia—being affected by the disease. The joint deformities seen in SLE also exemplify this fact, because they are solely due to soft tissue damage. In OA the capsule and joint ligaments are weakened, but the tissues external to the joint retain basic integrity. Deformity in OA is due more to cartilage degeneration and hypertrophy and secondary ligamentous laxity.

The **stiffness** associated with OA is due to a **gel phenomenon**, as if the fluid in the joint and capsule gels during static positioning, producing a sense of stiffness. It is localized to affected joints. When it occurs in the morning upon arising, it is referred to as "AM stiffness" or "stiffness in the morning." This is not the same as "morning stiffness," which is a generalized stiffness associated with systemic disease.

In the absence of inflammation, OA is characterized by (1) minimal stiffness after prolonged rest or positioning (severe stiffness is probably due to a low-grade inflammatory process); (2) bony hypertrophy; (3) crepitus as a result of irregularities in the cartilage surface; (4) deformity; (5) muscle weakness and disuse atrophy secondary to altered biomechanics resulting from deformity; and (6) possibly pain upon weight bearing and aching during cold weather. When inflammation is present, the following may also be found: (1) marked stiffness after static positioning, (2) joint tenderness, (3) pain at rest or severe pain on weight bearing, (3) frequently redness and swelling, and (4) muscle spasm secondary to pain. The person with OA may also have poor endurance secondary to inactivity (deconditioning) or to a coexistent systemic condition.

In hand joints with OA pain appears directly related to inflammation. It is fairly safe to assume that if a person has pain or aching at rest, inflammation is present, even if there is no swelling, warmth, or redness.[2] In the larger weight-bearing joints such as the hip or knee, pain also can result from pressure on the subchondral bone.

There has been extensive research over the past decade to understand the biochemical, physiological, and histological properties of cartilage. Numerous factors—mechanical, endocrine, genetic, and immunological—have been identified as influential in the inflammatory process. But the reason that some people develop inflammation and others do not or that a person may develop inflammation at a given point in the course of the disease is not known. Many clinicians believe the initiating event is irritation of the synovium by debris created by the degenerative process. In some instances it appears related to mucoidal cyst formation and often disappears after the cyst solidifies. Possibly capsular action over roughened or irregular osteophyte formation creates sufficient irritation to touch off inflammation.

Once inflammation is present, treatment needs to be directed toward improving the person's overall health and fitness. Psychological attitude, fitness exercise, nutrition, and rest all play critical roles in controlling, arresting, or reversing OA.

Primary Occupational Therapy Goals and Suggested Modalities

The following is an outline of treatment for both isolated and multiple joint involvement. A joint may stay in the noninflammatory stage forever or may have episodic or chronic inflammation. For treatment of osteoarthritis in specific joints, see Chapter 4.

I. NONINFLAMMATORY STAGE
  A. Reduce stiffness
    1. Educate the patient about the gel phenomenon that causes stiffness.
    2. Instruct the patient in limbering exercises for involved joints to reduce AM stiffness and stiffness after prolonged static positioning such as riding in a car or handwriting.
    3. Instruct in optimal or proper sitting alignment for specific work or leisure activities that encourage stiffness.

4. When AM stiffness of the neck or back is a concern, sleeping posture and type of mattress and pillow used can contribute to stiffness, and appropriate changes can reduce stiffness. For example, sleeping prone can cause severe strain to cervical joints; sagging mattresses can contribute to lumbar stiffness.
5. Educate the patient regarding use of heat to decrease stiffness. This includes use of thermoelastic gloves, knee warmers, use of turtleneck shirts or collars to protect neck from drafts.

B. Reduce or eliminate aggravating factors that stress the joint—postural, functional, or mechanical

1. Educate the patient about the effect habitual postural stress can have on the joints, and the value of a total body fitness program for improving posture, overall strength, and endurance, thus altering or eliminating habitual loading forces on the joint.
2. Educate the patient about the value of maintaining optimal **weight**. For example, every time a person takes a step, a force four times the body weight is applied per square inch in the hip joint. So, for every pound a patient loses, he or she reduces the force on the hip by 4 pounds per square inch.
3. Analyze **functional activities** that stress the involved joints, and instruct in joint protection. This should also include asymptomatic joints—true preventive therapy. For example, if a person has bilateral OA of the carpometacarpal (CMC) joints and the right hand is symptomatic, doing a stressful task with the left hand is not a solution, because this is likely to bring on symptoms in the left hand.
4. Provide awareness training to help patients become aware of how they use their joints. Follow through with joint-protection training, relaxation training, or

assistive devices as needed to reduce stress on the joint.
5. For cervical OA, relaxation training can be especially effective in reducing muscular compression as a stress force on the facet joints.

C. Maintain ROM

1. In the noninflammatory stage, concentric loss of ROM is due to bony hypertrophy and osteophytes. People use all available ROM during daily activities. Therefore, specific ROM exercises are not indicated at this stage (unless muscle spasm is restricting motion).

II. INFLAMMATORY STAGE

All treatment outlined for the noninflammatory stage is appropriate for this stage. In addition, the following treatments may be beneficial.

A. Reduce pain and inflammation by reducing stress to the joint

1. Use orthotic immobilization for the thumb and occasionally the DIP joints.
2. Instruct in joint protection.
3. Instruct in the use of a cane or other ambulation aid to reduce stress to the hips.
4. For OA of the first MTP, foot orthotics with a metatarsal pad are indicated at the first sign of involvement as a means of reducing weight-bearing forces. However, most people do not seek treatment for the foot until pain and inflammation occur.

B. Reduce pain or inflammation directly

1. Use medications (see Chapter 3).
2. Provide physical therapy.
   a. Transcutaneous electrical nerve stimulation (TENS) for spinal pain.
   b. Phonophoresis or iontophoresis (application of hydrocortisone cream using ultrasound).
   c. Thermal modalities.

C. Maintain or improve ROM

1. In the presence of severe inflammation in the lower extremities and spine, joint contractures can

develop secondary to soft tissue involvement.

    a. If patients are not using the joint through its available ROM during the day, specific ROM exercises should be given. If the patient's ROM limitations are due to bony block, ROM exercises will not help.

    b. Proper positioning during bedrest, leisure, and work may help minimize soft tissue sequelae.

D. Maintain and improve muscle strength

    1. This is critical throughout the disease course. In the presence of inflammation, patients often need guidance from a therapist to develop an exercise routine they can handle.

    2. Generally the inflammation can be controlled by medication to the point that the person can participate in isometric exercise or at least active exercise without resistance.

    3. *Exercises must be done in a pain-free manner to strengthen the muscles.*

E. Emotional support

The emotional issues are different in OA and RA. Generally, people with OA feel healthy except for the joint pain or stiffness. They are also not at risk for life-threatening disease or drug complications. The greatest emotional toll comes from diminished functional ability, which creates an ever-narrowing circle of life experiences and pleasure. This feeds an ongoing cycle of depression, inactivity, weakness, and pain. In the elderly with other medical problems, such as diabetes or heart disease, OA often means another source of limitation, furthering preexisting depression.

Occupational therapy should focus on helping the patient become aware of the progressive narrowing of his or her life-style and methods or opportunities for expanding his or her circle of experience. Any activity that is expansive, that engages the patient in a wider circle of life, is psychotherapeutic for depression associated with illness. (See Chapter 2.)

REFERENCES

1. Harris, ED: Rheumatoid arthritis: The clinical spectrum. In Kelley, WM, et al (eds): Textbook of Rheumatology, ed 2. WB Saunders, Philadelphia, 1985.
2. Melvin, JL: Rheumatic Disease—Occupational Therapy and Rehabilitation, ed 2. FA Davis, Philadelphia, 1983.
3. Kendall, PH: Exercise for arthritis. In Licht, S (ed): Therapeutic Exercise, ed 2. Elizabeth Licht, New Haven, 1965.
4. Melvin, JL: Rheumatic Disease—Occupational Therapy and Rehabilitation. FA Davis, Philadelphia, 1977.
5. Harris, ED: Biology of the joint. In Kelly, WM, et al (eds): Textbook of Rheumatology, ed 2. WB Saunders, Philadelphia, 1985.
6. Vasey, JR, and Crozier, LW: Neuromuscular approach to knee joint problems. Physiotherapy 66(6):193, 1980.
7. Sherrington, CS: The Integrative Action of the Nervous System. Yale University Press, New Haven, 1906. (This is the original source on pain reflex inhibition and excitation.)
8. de Andrade, JR, et al: Joint distention and reflex muscle inhibition in the knee. J Bone Joint Surg 47A:313, 1965.
9. Cohen, LA, and Cohen, ML: Arthrokinetic reflex of the knee. Am J Physiol 184:433, 1956.
10. Manual for Allied Health Professionals. Arthritis Foundation, New York, 1973.
11. Smith, WS: The application of cold and heat in the treatment of athletic injuries. In Michlovitz, SL (ed): Thermal Agents in Rehabilitation. FA Davis, Philadelphia, 1986.
12. Lehmann, JF, Warren, CG, and Scham, SM: Therapeutic heat and cold. Clin Orthop 99:207, 1974 (review article).
13. Kabet, H: Proprioceptive facilitation in therapeutic exercise. In Licht, S (ed): Therapeutic Exercise, ed 2. Elizabeth Licht, New Haven, 1965.
14. Mead, S, and Knott, M: Ice therapy in joint restriction spasticity, and certain types of pain. Gen Pract, February, 1961, p 16.
15. Michlovitz, SL (ed): Thermal Agents in Rehabilitation. FA Davis, Philadelphia, 1986. (This is the most current and thorough review on this topic.)

16. Lehmann, JF (ed): Therapeutic Heat and Cold, ed 3. Williams & Wilkins, Baltimore, 1982.
17. Knox, S: Director of Occupational Therapy, Children's Hospital of Los Angeles. Personal communication, June 1978.
18. Achterberg, J, McGraw, and Lawlis, GF: Rheumatoid arthritis: A study of relaxation and temperature biofeedback training as an adjunctive therapy. Biofeedback Self Regul 6(2):207, 1981.
19. Goldwag, EM (ed): Inner Balance: The Power of Holistic Healing. Prentice-Hall, Englewood Cliffs, NJ, 1979.
20. Grezesiak, RC: Relaxation techniques in treatment of chronic pain. Arch Phys Med Rehab 58:270, June 1977.
21. Olton, DS, and Noonber, AR: Biofeedback: Clinical Applications in Behavioral Medicine. Prentice-Hall, Englewood Cliffs, NJ, 1980. (This book contains a chapter on the treatment of Raynaud's disease.)
22. Huskinsson, EC, Dieppe, PA, Tucker, AK, and Cannell, LB: Another look at osteoarthritis. Ann Rheum Dis 38:423–428, 1979.
23. Bland, JH, and Stulberg, SD: Osteoarthritis: Pathology and clinical patterns. In Kelley, WM, et al: Textbook of Rheumatology, ed 2. WB Saunders, Philadelphia, 1985.
24. Altman, RD, and Gray, R: Inflammation in osteoarthritis. Clin Rheum Dis 11(2):353–365, 1985.

Navarro, AH: Physical Therapy in the Management of Rhematoid Arthritis. Clin Rheum Prac 1(3):125–130, 1983.
President's Committee on Employment of the Handicapped: Impact of Musculo-Skeletal Problems on Employment. National Rehabilitation Information Center, Catholic University of America, Washington, DC, 1984.
Sliwa, JL: Occupational Therapy Assessment and Management. In Ehrlich, GE (ed): Rehabilitation Management of Rheumatic Conditions, ed 2. Williams & Wilkins, Baltimore, 1986, pp 232–256.

Audiovisual

Bluestone, R, and Rosenberg, M: Low Back Pain: Solving the Clinical Challenge. Network for Continuing Medical Education, Secaucus, NJ, 1985.
Golding, DN: Physical Therapy in the Management of Rheumatic Disorders. Medcom Products, Garden Grove, CA, 1983.
Jasso, M: Age-Related Physical Therapy Programs. Arthritis Foundation, Atlanta, GA, 1984.
National Institutes of Health: An Occupatonal Therapy Case Study: Sarah, a Person with Rheumatoid Arthritis. National Institutes of Health, Bethesda, MD, 1983.

ADDITIONAL SOURCES

Books

Ehrlich, GE (ed): Rehabilitation Management of Rheumatic Conditions, ed 2. Williams & Wilkins, Baltimore, 1986.
Kottke, FJ, Stillwell, GK, and Lehmann, JF: Krusen's Handbook of Physical Medicine and Rehabilitation, ed 3. WB Saunders, Philadelphia, 1982.
Pigg, JS, Driscoll, PW, and Caniff, R: Rheumatology Nursing: A Problem-Oriented Approach. John Wiley & Sons, New York, 1985.
Riggs, GK, and Gall, EP (eds): Rheumatic Diseases: Rehabilitation and Management. Butterworths, Boston, 1984.

Brown, D: A Community Model for Arthritis Rehabilitation. Canadian J OT 50(4):115–118, 1984.
Banwell, BF: Physical Therapy in Arthritis Management. In Ehrlich, GE (ed): Rehabilitation Management of Rheumatic Conditions, ed 2. Williams & Wilkins, Baltimore, 1986, pp 264–284.
Basmajian, JV: Clinical Use of Biofeedback in Rehabilitation. Psychosomatics 23(1):67–69, 73, 1982.
Columbia Hospital: Rheumatic Disease Program: Physical Therapy Materials and Occupational Therapy Materials. Columbia Hospital, Rheumatic Disease Program, Milwaukee, 1983.
Erfling, JL: The Role of the Social Worker in the Rehabilitation of Rheumatic Disease Patients. In Ehrlich, GE (ed): Rehabilitation Management of Rheumatic Conditions, ed 2. Williams & Wilkins, Baltimore, 1986, pp 189–197.
Gloag, D: Rehabilitation in Rheumatic Diseases. Br Med J (Clin Res Ed) 290(6462):132–136, 1985.
Griffin, JE, Karselis, TC, and Currier, DP: Physical Agents for Physical Therapists, ed 2. Charles C Thomas, Springfield, IL, 1982.
Jagger, M, and Zmood, D: Hydrotherapy by Physiotherapists in a Community Health Centre. Aust Fam Physician (Sydney) 13(12):878, 880–881, 1984.
Kiviniemi, P: The Illness Process in Rheumatic Diseases. Scand J Rheumatol (Suppl) (Stockholm) 53:5–14, 1984.
Lewis, CB: Aging: The Health Care Challenge. An Interdisciplinary Approch to Assessment and Rehabilitative Management of the Elderly. FA Davis, Philadelphia, 1985.

Pain Management

Bonica, JJ, et al: Advances in Pain Research and Therapy: Recent Advances in the Management of Pain, Vols 1–7. Raven Press, New York, 1976–1984.
Brena, SF, and Chapman, SL: Management of Patients with Chronic Pain. SP Medical and Scientific Books, New York, 1983.
Chapman, CR, and Bonica, JJ: Acute Pain. The Upjohn Company, 1983.
Dudley, HF, and Huskisson, EC: Pain Patterns in the Rheumatic Disorders. Br Med J 4:213–216, 1972.
Fagerhaugh, SY, and Strauss, A: How to Manage Your Patient's Pain and How Not To. Nursing '80, February 1980.
Fordyce, WE: Behavioral Methods for Chronic Pain and Illness. CV Mosby, St Louis, 1976.
Johnson, BG: Biofeedback, Transcutaneous Electrical Nerve Stimulation, Acupuncture, and Hypnosis.

Rheumatic Diseases, Rehabilitation and Management. Butterworths, Boston, 1984.

McCaffery, M: Nursing Management of Patient with Pain. JB Lippincott, Philadelphia, 1981.

Mannheimer, C, and Carlsson, CA: The Effect of Transcutaneous Electrical Nerve Stimulation (TENS) on Joint Pain in Patients with Rheumatoid Arthritis. Scand J Rheum 7:13–16, 1978.

Meinhart, NT, and McCaffery, M: Pain: A Nursing Approach to Assessment and Analysis. Appleton-Century-Crofts, Norwalk, CT, 1983.

Mooney, NE: Coping with Chronic Pain in Rheumatoid Arthritis: Patient Behaviors and Nursing Interventions. Orthopedic Nursing 3:21–25, 1982.

Swerdlow, M: The Therapy of Pain. JB Lippincott, Philadelphia, 1981.

Chapter 2

Psychological Considerations in Patient Education and Treatment

HOLISTIC THERAPY AND PATIENT EMPOWERMENT—THE ROLE OF OCCUPATIONAL THERAPY

It is my belief that patient education about disease, treatment, and health is a critical part of the occupational therapist's role and treatment—as it is of all health care professionals who treat people with chronic illness.

A holistic approach to health care is not a specific treatment; it is a philosophy of health. "What" and "how" we teach patients during an occupational therapy (OT) session can have major impact on how they perceive their illness, their sense of control, and, ultimately, their ability to move beyond fear, denial, and anger to develop a

16

positive, self-enhancing approach to illness and life. Any knowledge that helps a person achieve, or move toward, greater health is empowering. It is the process of **empowerment** through patient education that can allow therapists to practice holistic OT within traditional medical settings.

In order for the therapist to empower a patient, the therapist must be able to *feel* the power of the knowledge he or she is sharing. The therapist must have a clear understanding of how the information can lead the patient to an integrated holistic approach, in which all aspects of the individual's life are moving the person toward greater health. Naturally, the effectiveness of this approach depends on how skilled the therapist is in determining a patient's readiness for learning, as well as the therapist's ability to communicate the material effectively and to assess the learning.

The concept of **holistic health** is simply the application of systems theory to one's life and health.[1] It is based on the belief that each part of our being is a system within a larger system and that when one aspect of life is out of balance it influences the functioning of all other aspects of the system. Consequently, all aspects of the larger system can influence the part that is out of balance. In practical terms, at one level this means that arthritis influences or has an impact on every aspect of a person's life: the way the individual feels about himself or herself and others, how the person works, sleeps, eats, relaxes. But this concept has a two-way aspect; that is, every aspect of a person's life can influence the arthritis. A holistic approach to treatment of arthritis at a very basic level is a process that helps a person explore and understand this dual paradigm. In actual practice most people are very aware of how their arthritis is affecting their emotional state; level of stress; abilities for working, exercising, parenting, playing, and having sex. But they are less aware of how their functioning in these activities can influence their arthritis. The dual paradigm also extends to the relationship between the person and the environment and community, including quality of air, food, water, noise, and living situation.

Holistic therapy is individually determined. The role of OT in helping the patient to gain an understanding of the holistic approach to health, described above, depends on the individual therapist and how much importance he or she believes people should place on this approach to health and illness. It would require another book to define holistic therapy in sufficient detail to teach it adequately. Thus this chapter focuses on the process of empowerment feasible for every therapist—patient education.

For education to empower it must fill a need; it must be helpful in some concrete way. Understanding the rheumatological, medical, and psychological contingencies described in this chapter can help the therapist make the needs assessment necessary for an effective learning–teaching experience.

THE MYTH OF THE RHEUMATOID PERSONALITY

In 1950, Franz Alexander wrote the first major text on psychosomatic medicine, identifying rheumatoid arthritis (RA) as one of the seven major psychosomatic diseases.[2] His work sparked a surge of research during the late 1940s through the 1960s to prove or to disprove his intriguing claims. At the time clinicians conducting research with RA patients were primarily in large county or university medical centers (before Medicare broke up centralized care). It appeared to many that the patients shared similar personality traits of repressed hostility, passive-aggressive behavior, and depression. This spurred an interest in determining whether personality characteristics could predispose a person to RA or have an etiological connection. (Keep in mind that this was during the pre-cortisone and early cortisone eras and before the advent of most current arthritis medications, except aspirin.)

A number of research articles were published that *appeared* to document a predominant personality pattern in RA patients, as described above.[3-26] These created the concept of an RA personality. But this research was seriously flawed. The most frequently made mistake was the omission of chronicity as a controlled factor and excessive attention to negative personality traits.[27,28] Most of the research involved personality testing on patients who had established severe disease of variable duration. In essence the researchers determined the personality characteristics of people who had had RA for a number of years. These characteristics were later deemed the *result* of chronic RA rather than the *cause*. Since then, studies have shown that these traits are common in people with other chronic diseases and even in those without disease.[1,24,29,30] Furthermore, greater psychosocial variance has been found within a single disease entity than is evident in a comparison of RA with other chronic diseases.[30]

Although subsequent research has ruled out a specific RA personality, this does not mean that the psyche cannot initiate a chain of biochemical events that result in RA—a true psychosomatic origin. In Europe and many other countries, RA is still considered one of the seven major psychosomatic disorders. In the United States, the medical and rheumatology literatures describe and treat RA as a purely physical disorder. The truth, as always, probably lies somewhere in the middle, with some patients having a psychosomatic disease and others having a somatopsychic disease. Keep in mind that the term **psychosomatic** does not mean imaginary or totally psychological. It means that the initiating event was psychological.

In my practice (over 18 years), I would estimate that about one third of my patients with RA can clearly identify a stressful psychological event preceding the onset of the RA. Approximately another third of the patients reveal a long insidious episodic history of joint pain, often starting in high school or grade school. The remaining third have variable modes of onset that do not fall into a particular pattern. I believe that for some patients the initiating event is psychological (i.e., psychosomatic) and that for others it is physical (i.e., somatopsychic) and that, once the disease starts, both the psyche and the body play integral roles in perpetuating the disease and in healing. It best serves the patient to approach the disease from both perspectives—psychosomatic and somatopsychic—because each approach opens different doors to insight and healing.

A discussion on the psychological aspects of the rheumatic diseases is essentially a discussion on the psychological aspects of chronic disease. *The natures of the diseases vary, but the patient response is to the illness and chronic disability.*[31–34] Therefore, the psychological and educational factors relevant to treating patients with rheumatic diseases can be generalized to treatment of patients with other chronic conditions.

The psychological responses necessary to cope with the trauma of arthritis can be compared with those necessary to cope with personal death, as identified by leading theorists and researchers in the field of **thanatology** (the study of death and dying).[35] Encountering a life-threatening disease, such as cancer, or sustaining a limb amputation involves a very obvious and absolute personal loss. Psychologists and other theorists have carried out a great deal of research in order to understand patient response to amputations and terminal disease and to develop approaches for helping patients cope with the trauma of loss.[36,37] The results of this research can also be applied to patients with rheumatic diseases for, although the loss involved with the rheumatic diseases is not as obvious as in the above conditions, its effect on the patient can be equally traumatic. For instance, the loss involved in arthritis can be conceptualized in two ways. First, it is a loss of a joint or body part. Second, it is the loss or death of "a self," of the ability to carry out a personal, family, or societal role (because we consist of many "selves" in many roles). The permanent loss of the ability to fulfill one or more of these roles is an emotional trauma equal to that of losing a limb.

From a practical viewpoint, the emphasis in therapy must be placed on the psychological reaction of the individual to the disability rather than to the etiological or predispositional factors involved.

PSYCHOLOGICAL FACTORS RELATED TO PATIENT EDUCATION AND COOPERATION

The psychological issues relevant to patient instruction and compliance cluster around two processes: the patient's response to the disability and the interaction of, or relationship between, the patient and the health professional.

Patient Response to Disability

Disability carries a distinct meaning for each person, and each person's method of coping is unique. It is important to identify each patient's response, to find out how he or she perceives the disease, to determine what is most important to him or her, and then to relate the method and content of the instruction to the individual's needs.

Although individual response patterns are unique, certain responses occur more frequently and have a stronger influence on patient–professional interaction. These responses are denial, depression, need for control, dependency, and acceptance.[35,36] Denial and depression are the two most common specific responses that have the potential for inhibiting therapy. The need for control and dependency issues are two fundamental concerns that are always present and, therefore, continually need to be considered. Acceptance, as defined later in this section, has a strong positive influence on therapy and allows maximal utilization of health resources to take place. Many other responses—such as those concerning family, cultural, and societal contingencies—influence the patient's response to disability, but a thorough discussion of patient psychology is beyond the scope of this text.

Denial

Denial is an amazing defense mechanism. Very few processes will allow one to wipe out bad events so neatly. If a denial mechanism is in good working order, a person can be told he or she has RA or cancer and it will not affect his or her outlook on life in the least. Denial, like other defense mechanisms, comes into existence when an issue becomes a threat to a person's reality. Therefore, it is a very valuable and necessary process for that person.

However, although denial can be a positive mechanism for the patient, it can at the same time be a negative mechanism for the therapist or physician who believes that the patient needs to understand the disease and appropriate treatment for optimal care.

If a person does not believe that he or she has a serious disease, or a painful wrist, there is no reason to learn the treatment procedures.

This brings up the question of how to determine whether denial is present. This is done simply by talking to the patient, by finding out how the patient perceives the disease and disability, by determining what his or her expectations and attitudes are regarding complying with the instructions, and by establishing the source of discrepancies between the patient's and therapist's perspectives.

It may or may not be possible to reconcile the needs of the patient and the professional concerning denial, but certain measures can help. If the health professional's goal is to do what is best for the patient, it is important to recognize the positive value of denial for the patient. The patient needs the denial or it would not be there. When denial is present, the major concern is to protect the patient from self-harm through actions he or she may take, such as not taking medication or discarding splints. Therefore, it is not necessary to eliminate the denial but to work around it. In fact, it is impossible for the professional to alter the denial; only the patient can do that. Any attempts to eliminate it by "making him or her face reality" probably will be in vain or will only increase the patient's stress.

It is possible to work around the denial by acknowledging the patient's beliefs and designing the treatment regimen to accommodate them. This is somewhat easy to do with the rheumatic diseases because the course is variable and the definite prognosis is not known in the early stages. So, one can honestly give patients the hope of remission while asking them to comply with the current physical problems.

Before dealing with the issue of denial it is extremely important to make sure the patient has accurate information about the disease. It is not enough to describe the disease or to give the patient literature to read. No matter how the patient obtains information, it is absolutely essential to have him or her explain the information to you. For example, I once asked a patient to read a pamphlet about rheumatoid arthritis prepared by the Arthritis Foundation. When she had finished I answered her questions.

About three months later I learned that she had interpreted the passage that read "RA *can* cause disease in the lungs, skin, blood vessels, muscles . . . " to mean "RA *will* cause disease in the lungs, skin, blood vessels, muscles." We cannot protect patients from all misinterpretations, but the only way we can find out what they actually understand is by asking. Had the woman's misinterpretation not been corrected, she might have expected all her organs to become seriously damaged. This is not a specific example of denial, but misconceptions about the severity of the disease may needlessly elicit defense mechanisms such as denial.

A point of crisis often causes a person to interpret information literally or to amplify the meaning, thus making a casual statement into something definite and absolute. This often stems from an acute need for structure and definition at a time of emotional chaos when nothing, not even the individual's body, seems to be stable.

The patient's accurate understanding of both positive and negative aspects of his or her condition is important in helping him or her deal honestly with the condition.

Depression

Psychological depression is probably the most difficult response to identify and to work with, especially in patients with systemic diseases, because the symptoms of depression are identical to those of systemic illness (e.g., fatigue, loss of appetite, malaise, decreased motivation, and diminished sexual drive).[38] The identification of depression becomes further complicated by several issues:

1. There are many medications that cause depression.
2. There are two forms of depression: *reactive, exogenous,* in which the depression is linked with a specific cause; and *endogenous,* in which the severe depression occurs without a discernible cause. The latter category includes depression related to physiological changes.[35]
3. Sadness over loss (grief) appears similar to depression.
4. Symptoms of depression, e.g., fatigue, malaise, and decreased motivation, may be secondary to a sleep disorder. (See Chapter 5 on Fibromyalgia.)

5. Patients with medical problems often attribute the symptoms of mild depression to the physical ailment, thus deferring diagnosis and treatment of the real problem.

The following methods are often helpful in identifying depression.

1. The nature of the fatigue can be a key to distinguishing depression from systemic symptoms. Systemic fatigue is related to activity level and commonly occurs after 4 to 6 hours of activity, whereas fatigue associated with depression is usually constant.
2. Question the patient regarding depressed behavior. When asked, many patients can clearly identify their depression. Patients who initially attribute their depressed behavior to a physical ailment without considering a psychological source often gain insight simply from discussion about possible sources. Depression can result from a variety of causes with the most common being suppression of anger.
3. It is important to distinguish true depression from sadness. When a person encounters loss in any form, it is vital that he or she fully experience the associated grief or sorrow to get beyond it.
4. There are psychological assessments available to help identify depression. These tests are not recommended for routine use in occupational or physical therapy clinics; however, they are helpful in learning what to look for when evaluating for depression. (There are several depression inventories. Their availability changes yearly. A listing of current tests and their reliability and validity scores can be found in Buros, OV (ed): *The Eighth Mental Measurements Yearbook.* Gryphon Press, Highland Park, NJ, 1979.)

The symptoms of depression can pose a real threat to the therapy program. Patients experiencing a sense of hopelessness and futility are not likely to participate in programs designed to make the future brighter. When treatment procedures require rigorous compliance, assessment of depression should be part of the pre-evaluation, and the depression should be addressed before treatment is started. For instance, marked depression has become such an obvious deterrent to rehabilitation of total knee arthroplasties that it is now considered a contraindication at some centers.

It is easy to talk about resolving a depression but significantly harder to do. It is difficult even to discuss methods of working with depression, inasmuch as the method of choice depends upon the patient—why he or she is depressed, the need to be depressed, and how the depression is interfering with the treatment.

Once a person develops strong feelings about something, he or she has difficulty seeing or avoids seeing the opposite viewpoint. This can happen with a health problem. To the patient, the disease is a bad event, and the patient focuses on the negative aspects, which can feed a depressive cycle. The health professional can best help the patient and himself or herself by acknowledging the negative aspects, by acknowledging the person's need to relate those aspects, and by giving the patient positive issues to which to respond. Patients who need to be depressed will stay depressed no matter what is said, but patients in a depressive cycle who are ready to break out of it will pick up on the positive issues mentioned.

Along this line, two specific approaches are often helpful. First, whenever doing an evaluation that focuses on what the patient *cannot do,* such as an assessment of activities of daily living (ADL) or a hand function test, end the procedure on items that the patient can do successfully. This reinforces the patient's awareness of function rather than of dysfunction. Second, have the patient clarify the meaning of his or her negative generalities. When a patient says he "has arthritis all over," asking him to be specific will probably turn up several uninvolved joints. Statements like "I can't cook anymore," may really mean the person can no longer lift heavy pots or open cans. Almost all statements like "I'm no good," "I'm a terrible mother," or "I'm a failure" can become less overwhelming and more realistic and positive by having the patient be more specific.

Need for Control

Basic to life, sanity, and happiness is the need for sensing control over one's body, actions, and environment. Most people who are afflicted with an illness of unknown cause, especially if it strikes suddenly, have a prevailing feeling of incredible helplessness. There is no reason for, or

control of, the situation. "Why me?" becomes a repetitive, forever-unanswered question.

Through the health profession, society has devised an incredible answer to this problem. When people become ill and sense no control over their bodies, they are placed in a hospital, in which they have no control over their environment. Even a healthy person in the hospital for a routine physical examination becomes acutely aware of a lack of control in the hospital environment.

There are many ways for the patient to gain or to restore control. Some people do it by being cooperative and agreeable during clinic interaction, then follow their own wishes when authority figures are not around. This is commonly referred to as a **passive-aggressive** approach. Other people may overtly establish control by refusing to comply and by managing their own treatment.

Everyone needs to sense control over his or her environment. The professional's awareness of how patients maintain a sense of control when they are ill and in a structured environment allows for more effective treatment planning. For example, if the patient's method of gaining control is to resist treatment, then the health professional can reduce the resistance and increase the patient's sense of control by telling the patient the treatment methods available and the alternative to treatment (a consequence of no treatment) and letting the patient choose the option.

Dependency

Another psychological factor that often comes to the forefront when illness strikes is dependency.[36] The conflict between autonomy and dependency is with us from the first year of life. Unresolved conflicts in this area become dominant factors when a person is placed in a position of dependency by becoming disabled or independency by having to take care of someone disabled. (In the second situation the person is no longer able to be dependent.) A person with strong unresolved dependency needs may assume an independent posture in defense of being overpowered by the desire to be taken care of. Examples of behavior patterns that allow symbolic or unconscious satisfaction for dependency but that maintain control of the situation are (1) demanding behavior; for example, constant requests for attention, water, pills, equipment; (2) supercooperative behavior that manipulates others into caring for them without directly requesting care; (3) indecisive behavior, in which there is difficulty making or carrying out decisions. The last is a more overt dependent behavior, especially when it consistently results in people other than the patient making the final decisions.[36,39]

Any of these behaviors can negatively affect a treatment program. When the above behaviors are serving dependency needs, cognizance of that fact can allow the professional to respond to the patient's needs rather than to get caught up in the patient's demands or manipulations, which will only perpetuate a cyclical process. For example, responding to a demanding patient by retaliation and not giving attention to the patient only increases the dependency conflict, whereas increasing the attention often helps reduce the need and demand.

Treatment programs and discharge planning should also take dependency issues into consideration. A patient with strong dependency needs is not likely to follow through on a program that requires independent action or perseverance.

Acceptance

The ideal situation exists when the patient can experience and deal with the emotional trauma of disability and arrive at some point of acceptance.

Acceptance of a disability is a difficult concept to define because it is a process unique for each person. However, in general terms, acceptance can describe an *honest* relationship with the disability—one in which the person acknowledges and experiences the anger, rage, fear, sadness, and helplessness associated with having to live with a miserable disease but at the same time acknowledges those aspects of life not affected by the disease. For example, arthritis of the knees may stop a man from playing basketball with his son but it does not need to interfere with his ability to be a loving husband, father, and competent provider for his family. Nonacceptance may be indicated when the man does not acknowl-

edge the limitations of the arthritis and continues to play ball, possibly causing unnecessary joint damage and greater debility. On the other hand, if he becomes depressed over the inability to play with his son, he will allow the depression to interfere with his role as a husband and provider. In this case, acceptance means anger at the limitations imposed by the arthritis but also recognition of what the true limitations are. Ultimately, the person needs to resolve the anger to develop a healthy working relationship with the illness.

This example is a simplified version of a complex process, and acceptance or nonacceptance is never the sole issue because it is extremely difficult for people to deal openly with issues that threaten their physical existence. However, it *is* possible, and it is a process that can be facilitated by health professionals who are oriented to helping patients deal honestly with all health issues.

Patient-Professional Relationship

The relationship between a patient and the health professional is an extremely sensitive one. The stakes are high: for the former it is an issue of health and of life at a basic survival level; for the latter it is personal satisfaction and good job performance. In spite of these contingencies, it is hoped that, with each encounter, optimal patient care will result and the patient will emerge with a greater sense of well being.

These goals can be achieved only if both parties have a clear understanding of their responsibilities and if the health professional is aware of the effect of his or her behavior on the achievement of these goals.

In general, the optimal treatment situation occurs when the patient takes responsibility for his or her own health care by (a) actively seeking skilled advice, (b) understanding the illness and treatment rationale, and (c) following through with prescribed therapy; and when the health professional takes responsibility by (a) providing competent treatment and (b) providing the appropriate environment and sufficient information for the patient to carry out his or her responsibilities.

The health professional's philsophy and

approach is the keystone to the method of patient care described above. Some of the processes essential to sharing responsibility are:

Education. Many patients believe that a person goes to a hospital or to therapy to be taken care of. They are not aware of the active role they need to play in order to make the system work. In other words, patients need to have their role and responsibility clearly defined.

Modeling the process. The professional's role in the relationship needs to be defined and he or she must carry out the appropriate responsibilities.

Un-mothering. The professional should not assume the patient's responsibilities; once a professional does that, there is no reason for the patient to assume those responsibilities.

In the patient-professional relationship only one person can comply with the treatment instructions, and that is the patient. No one can do it for him or her. The odds on the patient carrying out that responsibility appear to be increased if the patient is assuming responsibility for his or her health care throughout the treatment process.

MEDICAL FACTORS RELATED TO PATIENT EDUCATION AND COOPERATION

Three medical contingencies that can influence learning for people with joint disease are invariably present in the clinic: pain or discomfort, concern about illness (or health), and the effect of medication. The patient with systemic lupus erythematosus may additionally have central nervous system involvement that can interfere with learning. Also, fatigue secondary to a sleep disorder can interfere with learning. This is reviewed in Chapter 5 on Fibromyalgia.

Pain or Discomfort

Pain and the influence it can have on the therapeutic relationship are extremely complex issues. The significance of experiencing pain is unique for each patient and the significance of being with someone in pain is unique for each professional. Pain presents competing stimuli for attention and in general is an inhibitor to learning. However, it does not have to stop the learning process, and when motivation or desire is strong enough a person can learn even when pain is present. The amount of instruction should be adjusted to the amount of patient participation, this being influenced by the severity of pain.

Concern About Health

Concern over one's health status with such reactions as anxiety or fear may not only limit learning in a given session but also prohibit it altogether. This reference to the client's day-to-day concern over health differs from the general psychological response to the disease. It is often more contingent upon sudden changes in his or her health status or upon misinformation obtained from such sources as friends or the news media. Along this line, arthritis creates a double problem. It is a common but extremely misunderstood condition and it is the only chronic disease that carries extensive folklore. Consequently, patients are often inundated with misinformation about their specific type of arthritis, a fact that can be extremely disconcerting. For example, (1) a patient with mild degenerative joint disease of the hands may believe his or her hand will become deformed like those of the patient with rheumatoid arthritis on the other side of the clinic waiting room, (2) a patient with a misconception that the rheumatoid nodule on his or her forearm is cancerous may be scared to mention it to anyone and his or her anxiety may severely interfere with learning, or (3) a patient may have a remission of certain symptoms and believe the disease is cured and therefore believe that he or she does not need to learn a certain necessary procedure.

Many patients are very open about such concerns and seek correct information, but others have been conditioned to listen to the health professional rather than to talk or to disclose their own concerns. However, most patients will respond to encouragement to discuss such issues.

Effect of Medication

The effect of medication on learning ability has both positive and negative features. If the medication relieves pain, it removes a block from learning and thus can facilitate the process. This is often the case with medications taken for a specific or focal problem. However, common rheumatic disease medications can have side effects. Sometimes a side effect such as nausea can be an obvious distraction to learning. More often the side effects are so subtle, such as very slight lightheadedness or vague uneasiness, that the patient might not mention it or may not even be able to define the feeling. In some older patients, aspirin products can impair hearing. These mild effects can also compete with the learning process. Corticosteroid therapy in particular can produce a wide range of emotional side effects. Euphoric responses create such emotional detachment that the patient is not able to attend to instructions. Health professionals need to be well versed on the effects of medication. (See Drug Therapy, Chapter 3, for a review of the side effects.) When patients are on medication that can affect learning or retention, *all instructions should be written out* and should be reviewed at a later date if possible.

PATIENT INSTRUCTION

Methods of instructing patients in the presence of pain, anxiety, or drug side effects are the same for all factors. First, it is important to find out what factors are competing for the patient's attention with the information you want to get across. This can be done only by asking the patient; that is, finding out how he or she feels, if anything about the arthritis is particularly worrisome to the patient, or if he or she is aware of any side effects from medication.

The competing factors must be acknowledged if their influence on the teaching process is to be dealt with. Many professionals believe that if they don't talk about the patient's pain the patient will ignore it and pay attention to the instruction. However, it is impossible to ignore pain or other conflicting stimuli. It is just a matter of overt or covert attention to it.

Conversely, this raises the issue of what to do with the patient who wants to talk incessantly about his or her pain or concerns. When this occurs it is usually the patient's talking that becomes the hindrance to teaching rather than the pain itself. Therefore, it is essential to acknowledge the specific hindrance and to deal with it before learning can take place. For example, if it appears that the patient is more interested in talking than in learning or is not able to take in instruction, I take a very direct approach—"Mrs. Smith, is there anything in particular that you would like to know about the arthritis (exercise, drugs, and so forth) that is not clear, that I could help you with?" This will give you an inside track on where the patient is at and it puts the patient in control. Often in these situations the patient's response is so far removed from what I believe he or she should be learning, that it becomes immediately clear why he or she cannot attend to the topic or process of the moment.

This chapter has focused on the patient's psychological reaction to disability, his or her responsibility for health care, and the influence pain and medications can have on the learning process. This focus was chosen because these issues are often overlooked in the teaching session and are neglected in the literature on education for the arthritis patient, and because these factors need to be considered preliminary to initiating patient instruction. The structure of the actual teaching process has been mentioned only briefly but is equally important for a successful educational–instructional program.

Components for an Effective Instructional Program

First: The patient has to be willing and psychologically ready to learn the material.

Second: The therapist needs to be clear about what he or she wants the patient to learn; there must be specific educational goals.

These may be informal and formulated as one teaches. But before teaching the patient anything, the therapist should determine the teaching objective.

Third: The material must be presented clearly.

Fourth: There must be an assessment of the learning. This can be very informal, such as having the patient put on an orthosis independently or reciting the most important elements learned from a teaching session.

A therapist can never know whether a patient understood the instructed material the way it was intended unless he or she hears from the patient what was learned.

The following material illustrates how to put these four principles into operation.

Guidelines for Patient Instruction

The following guidelines identify the key factors that provide structure for a successful learning–teaching experience with patients who have arthritis.

A. Preliminary considerations
 1. Does the patient *need* education about arthritis or medical care? Does the patient have incorrect information or misconceptions about these issues? Before any other factor is considered, *the patient's educational needs must be evaluated.*
 2. Is the patient ready or interested in participating in an educational session?
 3. Is the patient's medical condition controlled sufficiently to allow effective instruction? If the patient is feeling ill or is in severe pain, instruction should be delayed if possible.
 4. Is the patient's psychological response to the disability conducive to learning more about the disease and treatment? Or is the patient so depressed or angry about the arthritis that he or she is not ready to start taking positive actions to help the arthritis?
 5. Does the patient understand his or her responsibility for health care and his or her role in medical treatment of the condition?
 6. Will the patient's medication interfere with learning? (See Chapter 3.)

 7. What are the patient's goals and interests in learning about the disease and medical and health care?
 8. Determine the patient's track record with regard to arthritis education.
    a. Has the patient ever participated in an arthritis education program before? Was it helpful? What helped and what did not? Was the patient able to incorporate the suggestions made? Can the patient identify factors that facilitated or hindered compliance with instructions? (This may be the most valuable information you will receive for structuring the teaching format.)
    b. Has the patient actively sought information about arthritis or read any books on the topic? If the patient is an avid reader and has not sought any information on arthritis, why not? What does reading or learning about the disease mean to the patient?

B. The learning–teaching session
 1. Explain your educational concerns to the patient: the material you think would be helpful for the patient to learn and why it is important. (Your views may alter the patient's personal goals.)
 2. Establish *both* the learning and teaching goals with the patient. Sometimes it is helpful to make a verbal contract with the patient to establish clear expectations and responsibilities. For example, the therapist might say, "I will teach you methods for reducing the stress and pain in your fingers, if you will practice the techniques for two days." The contract may be of any format desired. This can be a very effective method for making roles and responsibilities explicit rather than implicit and therefore subject to confusion.
 3. After the goals are established, the duration and number of educational sessions need to be planned with the patient.
 4. The teaching objective for each session should be realistic for the learning capabilities of the patient.
 5. The teaching session should be con-

ducted in a distraction-free location.

6. Family members should be included when appropriate.

7. Whenever possible, use teaching examples and materials that are relevant to the patient's personal and home situation, to maximize carry-over of the information. For example, if the therapist is teaching a patient with early joint involvement, examples or slides showing patients with severe deformities may be more distractive than illustrative to the patient.

8. If specific techniques are being taught, provide opportunity, space, and equipment for the patient to practice.

9. Before teaching any techniques, find out how the patient performs the activity. Often the patient's own method is correct or acceptable. Positive reinforcement of the patient's own method validates his or her intelligence and ingenuity. It also encourages correct process and eliminates the need to teach that particular step.

10. Whenever possible use printed handouts to reinforce the material being taught. If a commercial booklet on the topic does not express the full philosophy of your facility, adapt it. Cross out sections that are not relevant to the patient, circle or star the most important section, or add a supplementary page or a favorite diagram. Make the booklet into a dynamic teaching aid. Also, explaining the changes to the patient reinforces the content.

11. All major or key instructions should be provided in writing. This is particularly important if you are teaching a lot of new material in a short period of time.

12. Throughout the teaching process, it is critical to evaluate if the patient has learned the material correctly. This is usually done by having the patient demonstrate the technique or explain the process to the therapist. Positive reinforcement is a valuable tool for helping the patient learn new skills. The therapist should provide support and use positive reinforcement at every opportunity.

If the patient has not learned the material correctly, it is a signal that the teaching process needs to be modified and repeated. During this process it is important to keep in mind an old adage: "If the student didn't learn, then the teacher didn't teach."

Documentation of Patient Education

One last word about patient education. In many hospitals and outpatient clinics, therapists spend a great deal of time teaching patients about arthritis and medical or rehabilitative treatment. Often the teaching is done informally, during an interview or while making orthoses. The therapist provides this information because he or she has determined (by some method) that the patient lacks information and the therapist believes that the patient would be helped by knowing the information. Paradoxically, the same therapist who believes in the value of patient education and in his or her ability to provide it generally does not mention either the assessment or the process in the patient's chart. Consequently, therapists often do a considerable amount of patient education, but no one else on the medical team is aware of the therapist's skills or interest in these areas. Therapists can promote team communication and appreciation for the value of patient education simply by documenting the patient's knowledge about arthritis or his or her information needs in the initial evaluation. This does not have to be an elaborate process. A couple of succinct sentences can suffice; for example, the patient believes his arthritis (OA) is due to too much calcium and has avoided dairy products for this reason. He is not aware of the side effects of his medication. (There is a strong possibility that a few comments like this in the medical chart will increase the staff's awareness of the need for patient education.) If it is apparent that the patient needs information then patient education, even if it is informal, should be included in the treatment goals and plan. Documentation of the education and learning can also be included in the progress or discharge notes.

In many instances, such as the example above, the therapist's educational assessment may reveal that the patient lacks information in an area other than the thera-

pist's area of expertise. In these cases, it is certainly appropriate to document that education will be coordinated with a nurse, dietitian, or other health professional.

REFERENCES

1. Brody, H, and Sobel, DS: A systems view of health and disease. Holistic Health Review 3(3):163–178, 1980.
2. Alexander, F: Psychosomatic Medicine. Norton, New York, 1950.
3. Boynton, BL, Leavitt, LA, Schnur, RR, Schnur, HL, and Russell, MA: Personality evaluation in rehabilitation of rheumatoid spondylitis. Arch Phys Med Rehab 34:489, 1953.
4. Cleveland, SE, and Fisher, S: Behavior and unconscious fantasies of patients with rheumatoid arthritis. Psychosom Med 16:327, 1954.
5. Cobb, S: Contained hostility in rheumatoid arthritis. Arthritis Rheum 2:419, 1959.
6. Cobb, S, Bauer, W, and Whiting, I: Environmental factors in rheumatoid arthritis. JAMA 113:668, 1939.
7. Cobb, S, Miller, M, and Wieland, M: On the relationship between divorce and rheumatoid arthritis. Arthritis Rheum 2:414, 1959.
8. Fisher, S, and Cleveland, SE: Comparison of psychological characteristics and physiological reactivity in ulcer and rheumatoid arthritis groups. Psychosom Med 22:283, 1960.
9. Hellgren, L: Rheumatoid arthritis in both marital partners. Acta Rheum Scand 15:135, 1969.
10. Hellgren, L: Marital status in rheumatoid arthritis. Acta Rheum Scand 15:271, 1969.
11. King, SH: Psychosocial factors associated with rheumatoid arthritis. J Chronic Dis 2:287, 1955.
12. King, SH, and Cobb, S: Psychosocial factors in the epidemiology of rheumatoid arthritis. J Chronic Dis 7:466, 1958.
13. King, SH, and Cobb, S: Psychosocial studies of rheumatoid arthritis: Parental factors compared in cases and controls. Arthritis Rheum 2:322, 1959.
14. Kirchman, MM: The personality of the arthritic patient. Am J Occup Ther 19(3):160, 1965.
15. Lewis-Faning, E: Report on an enquiry into the aetiological factors associated with rheumatoid arthritis. Ann Rheum Dis (Suppl) 9, 1950.
16. Lugwig, AO: Rheumatoid arthritis: Psychiatric aspects. Medical Insight. Insight Publishing, December 1970.
17. Moos, RH, and Solomon, GF: Personality correlates of the rapidity of progression of rheumatoid arthritis. Ann Rheum Dis 23:2, 1964.
18. Mueller, AD, and Lefkovits, AM: Personality structure and dynamics of patients with rheumatoid arthritis. J Clin Psychol 12:143, 1956.
19. Mueller, AD, Lefkovits, AM, Bryant, JE, and Marshall, ML: Some psychosocial factors in patients with rheumatoid arthritis. Arthritis Rheum 4:275, 1961.
20. Nalven, FB, and O'Brien, JF: Personality patterns of rheumatoid arthritis patients. Arthritis Rheum 7:18, 1964.
21. Polley, HF, Swenson, WM, and Steinhilber, RM: Personality characteristics of patients with rheumatoid arthritis. Psychosomatics 11:45, 1970.
22. Rimon, R: A psychosomatic approach to rheumatoid arthritis. Acta Rheum Scand (Suppl) 13, 1969.
23. Robinson, H, Kirk, RF, and Frye, RL: A psychological study of rheumatoid arthritis and selected controls. J Chronic Dis 23:791, 1971.
24. Robinson, H, et al: Psychological study of patients with rheumatoid arthritis and other painful diseases. J Psychosom Res 16:53, 1972.
25. Ward, D: Rheumatoid arthritis and personality: A controlled study. Br Med J 2:297, 1971.
26. Wolff, BB, and Farr, RS: Personality characteristics in rheumatoid arthritis. Arthritis Rheum 7:354, 1964.
27. Wolff, BB: Current psychological concepts. Bull Rheum Dis 22:656, 1971.
28. Spergel, P, et al: The RA personality—a psychodiagnostic myth. Psychosomatics 19(2):79, 1978.
29. Kinnealey, M: The relationship between self concept and hand deformity in RA (thesis abstract). Am J Occup Ther 24:294, 1970.
30. Bourestom, NC, and Howard, MT: Personality characteristics of three disability groups. Arch Phys Med Rehab 46:626, 1965.
31. Shan, LL: The world of the patient in severe pain of long duration. J Chronic Dis 17:119, 1964.
32. Simon, J: Emotional aspects of physical disability. Am J Occup Ther 25(8):408, 1971.
33. Shontz, FC: Physical disability and personality. In Neff, WS (ed): Rehabilitation Psychology. American Psychological Association Publication, 1970.
34. Shontz, FC: Physical disability and personality: Theory and recent research. Psychological Aspects of Disability 17:51, 1970.
35. Kübler-Ross, E: On Death and Dying. Macmillan, New York, 1969.
36. Psychological Aspects of Disability and Rehabilitation. The Menninger Foundation Seminar, Topeka, Kansas. Division of Vocational Rehabilitation, February 1962.
37. Friedmann, LV: The Psychological Rehabilitation of the Amputee. Charles C Thomas, Springfield, IL, 1978.
38. Zaphiropoulus, G, and Barry, HC: Depression in rheumatoid disease. Ann Rheum Dis 33(2):132, 1974.
39. Wright, B: Physical Disability: A Psychological Approach. Harper & Bros, New York, 1960.

ADDITIONAL SOURCES

Psychological Aspects of Rheumatoid Arthritis

Cobb, S, Schull, WJ, Harburg, E, Kasl, SV, et al: The intrafamilial transmission of rheumatoid arthritis, I-VIII. J Chronic Dis 22:193, 1969.

Edwards, MH, and Calabro, JJ: Patient's attitudes and knowledge concerning arthritis. Arthritis Rheum 7:425, 1964.

Ehrlich, GE: Arthritis management: Treating rheumatoid arthritis with behavioral and clinical strategy. Practical Psychology for Physicians, Harcourt, Brace, Jovanovich, July 1975.

Geist, H: The Psychological Aspects of RA. Charles C Thomas, Springfield, IL, 1966.

Hoffman, AL: Psychological factors associated with R.A.: Review of the literature. Nurs Res 23(3):218, May–June 1974.

Ignatavicius, DD: Meeting the psychosocial needs of patients with rheumatoid arthritis (continuing education credit). Orthop Health Saf 56(5):60, 63–64, 1987.

Katz, S, Vignos, PJ, Moskowitz, RW, Thompson, HM, and Svec, KH: Comprehensive outpatient care in rheumatoid arthritis. JAMA 206:1249, 1968.

Medsger, AR, and Rohenson, H: A comparative study of divorce in rheumatoid arthritis and other rheumatic diseases. J Chronic Dis 25:269, 1972.

Meyerowitz, S: Psychosocial factors in the etiology of somatic disease. Ann Intern Med 72:753, 1970.

Meyerowitz, S: The continuing investigation of psychosocial variables in rheumatoid arthritis. In Hill, AGS (ed): Modern Trends in Rheumatology, ed 2. Butterworths, London, 1971.

Moldofsky, H, and Chester, WJ: Pain and mood patterns in patients with rheumatoid arthritis: A prospective study. Psychosom Med 32:309, 1970.

Moldofsky, H, and Rothman, AI: Personality, disease parameters, and medication in rheumatoid arthritis. Arthritis Rheum 13:338, 1970.

Moos, RH: Personality factors associated with rheumatoid arthritis: A review. J Chronic Dis 17:41, 1964.

Moos, RH, and Solomon, GF: Minnesota Multiphasic Personality Inventory response patterns in patients with rheumatoid arthritis. J Psychosom Res 8:17, 1964.

Moos, RH, and Solomon, GF: Personality correlates of the rapidity of progression of rheumatoid arthritis. Ann Rheum Dis 23:145, 1964.

Moos, RH, and Solomon, GF: Psychologic comparisons between women with rheumatoid arthritis and their nonarthritic sisters. L Personality test and interview rating data. Psychosom Med 27:135, 1964.

Moos, RH, and Solomon, GF: Psychologic comparisons between women with rheumatoid arthritis and their nonarthritic sisters. II. Content analysis of interviews. Psychosom Med 27:150, 1965.

Moos, RH, et al: Psychological orientations in the treatment of R.A. Am J Occup Ther 19(3):153, 1965.

Padilla, GV: Conditions under which an arthritic patient is held responsible and receives negative sanctions for her illness. Dissertation, University of California, Los Angeles, 1971.

Pincus, T, Callahan, LF, Bradley, LA, Vaughn, WK, and Wolfe, F: Elevated MMPI scores for hypochondrias, depression, and hysteria in patients with rheumatoid arthritis reflect disease rather than psychological status. Arthritis Rheum 29(12):1456–1466, 1986.

Pow, JM: The role of psychological influences in rheumatoid arthritis. J Psychosom Res 31(2):223–229, 1987.

Prick, JJG, and Van de Loo, KJM: The Psychosomatic Approach to Primary Chronic Rheumatoid Arthritis. FA Davis, Philadelphia, 1964.

Rekola, JK: Rheumatoid arthritis and the family. Scand J Rheum (Suppl 3) 2, 1973, 117 pages. (Psychiatric study comparing families with RA, schizophrenia and neurosis.)

Rimon, R: Depression in R.A. Ann Clin Res 6(3):171, June 1974.

Robb, JH, and Rose, BS: Rheumatoid arthritis and maternal deprivation: A case study in the use of a social survey. Br J Med Psychol 38:147, 1965.

Scotch, NA, and Geiger, JH: The epidemiology of rheumatoid arthritis: A review with special attention to social factors. J Chronic Dis 15:1037, 1962.

Semple, JE: Rheumatoid Arthritis—Conflict and challenge. NZ J Physiother (Wellington) 10(3):24–26, 1982.

Sizemore, JD, and Duncan, DF: Psychosocial epidemiology of rheumatoid arthritis in a rural population. Psychol Rep 29 (Pt 2):866, 1986.

Skevington, SM: Psychological aspects of pain in rheumatoid arthritis: A review. Soc Sci Med 23(6):567–575, 1986 (review).

Skevington, SM, Blackwell, F, and Britton, FF: Self-esteem and perception of attractiveness: An investigation of early rheumatoid arthritis. Br J Med Psychol 60(Pt 1):45–52, 1987.

Solomon, GF, and Moos, RH: The relationship of personality to the presence of rheumatoid factors in symptomatic relatives of patients with rheumatoid arthritis. Psychosom Med 27:351, 1955.

Southworth, JA: Muscular tension as a response to psychological stress in rheumatoid arthritis and peptic ulcer. Genet Psychol Monogr 57:337, 1958.

Strauss, GD, Spiegel, JS, Daniels, M, Spiegel, T, et al: Group therapies for rheumatoid arthritis. A controlled study of two approaches. Arthritis Rheum 29(10):1203–1209, 1986.

Vargo, JW: Some psychological effects of physical disability. Am J Occup Ther 32(1):31, 1978.

Vignos, PJ, Thompson, HM, Fink, SL, Moskowitz, RW, Svec, KH, and Katz, S: The effect of psychosocial factors on rehabilitation in chronic rheumatoid arthritis. Paper read at the 5th Annual Meeting of the Allied Health Professions Section of The Arthritis Foundation, Detroit, June 20, 1970.

Vollhardt, BR, Ackerman, SH, and Schindledecker, RD: Verbal expression of affect in rheumatoid arthritis patients. A blind, controlled test for alexithymia. Acta Psychiatr Scand 74(1):73–79, 1986.

Wallace, DJ: The role of stress and trauma in rheumatoid arthritis and systemic lupus erythematosus. Semin Arthritis Rheum 16(3):153–157, 1987 (review).

Williams, GH: Lay beliefs about the causes of rheumatoid arthritis: Their implications for rehabilitation. Int Rehab Med 8(2):65–68, 1986.

Wolff, BB: Rheumatoid arthritis—Assessment. In Nichols, JR, and Bradley, WH (eds): Proceedings of a Symposium on the Motivation of the Physically Disabled. National Fund for Research into Crippling Diseases, London, 1968, pp 16–20.

Wolff, BB: Experimental pain parameters and pain perception as predictive indices for rehabilitation of the disabled chronic arthritic patient. Final Report, SRS Grant #RD-1733-P, 1970.

Psychological Aspects of Systemic Lupus Erythematosus

Cares, RM, and Weinberg, F: The influence of cortisone on psychosis associated with lupus erythematosus. Psychiatr Q 32:94, 1958.
Clark, EC, and Bailey, AA: Neurological and psychiatric signs associated with systemic lupus erythematosus. JAMA 160:455, 1956.
Guze, SB: The occurrence of psychiatric illness in systemic lupus erythematosus. Am J Psychiatry 123:1562, 1967.
Heine, BE: Psychiatric aspects of SLE. Acta Psychiatr Scand 45:307, 1969.
Johnson, RT, and Richardson, EP: The neurological manifestations of systemic lupus erythematosus. J Lab Clin Med 74:369, 1969.
Kreindler, S, and Cancro, R: An ego psychological approach to psychiatric manifestations in systemic lupus erythematosus. Dis Nerv Sys, February 1970, p 102.
McClary, AR, Meyer, E, and Weitzman, DJ: Observations on role of mechanism of depression in some patients with disseminated lupus erythematosus. Psychosom Med 17:311, 1955.
Stern, M, and Robbins, ES: Psychoses in systemic lupus erythematosus. Arch Gen Psychiatry 3:205, 1960.

General Resources

Anderson, KO, Bradley, LA, McDaniel, LK, Young, LK, et al: The assessment of pain in rheumatoid arthritis. Validity of a behavioral observation method. Arthritis Rheum 30(1):36–43, 1987.
Balaban, DJ, Sagi, PC, Goldfarb, NI, and Nettler, S: Weights for scoring the quality of well-being instrument among rheumatoid arthritics. A comparison to general population weights. Med Care 24(11):973–980, 1986.
Carraccio, CL, McCormick, MC, and Weller, SC: Chronic disease: Effect on health cognition and health locus of control. J Pediatr 110(6):982–987, 1987.
Weinberger, M, Hiner, SL, and Tierney, WM: In support of hassles as a measure of stress in predicting health outcomes. J Behav Med 10(1):19–31, 1987.

Other Rheumatic Diseases

DeForge, BF, and Sobal, J: Psychological evaluation of well-being in the multidisciplinary assessment of osteoarthritis. Clin Ther 9 (Suppl B):43–52, 1986.
Goldenberg, DL: Psychologic studies in fibrositis. Am J Med 81(3a):67–70, 1986.
Johnson, RK: Psychological evaluation of patients with industrial hand injuries. Hand Clin 2(3):567–575, 1986.
Krick, JP, Sobal, J, and DeForge, BR: Psychosocial aspects of the multidisciplinary assessment of osteoarthritis. Clin Ther 9 (Suppl B):43–52, 1986.

Patient Compliance

Berkowitz, NH, et al: Patient follow-through in outpatient department. Nurs Res 12:16, 1963.
Carpenter, J, and Davis, L: Medical recommendations—Followed or ignored? Factors influencing compliance in arthritis. Arch Phys Med 57(5):241, 1976.
Coomes, EN: Physician's assessment of functional overlay. Ann Rheum Dis 29:562, 1970.
Davis, MS: Physiologic, psychological, and demographic factors in patient compliance with doctors' orders. Med Care 6:115, 1968.
Davis, MS: Variations in patients' compliance with doctors' advice: Empirical analysis of patterns of communication. Am J Public Health 58:274, 1968.
Davis, MS, and Eichhorn, RL: Compliance with medical regimens: Panel study. J Health Hum Behav 4:240, 1963.
Diamond, MD, et al: The unmotivated patient. Arch Phys Med 49:281, 1968.
Feinberg, J, and Brant, KD: Use of resting splints by patients with rheumatoid arthritis. Am J Occup Ther 35(3):173, 1981.
Francis, V, Korsch, BM, and Morris, MJ: Gaps in doctor-patient communications: Patients' response to medical advice. N Engl J Med 280:535, 1969.
Gersten, HR, Gray, RM, and Ward, JR: Patient noncompliance within the context of seeking medical care for arthritis. J Chronic Dis 26:689, 1973.
Gordis, L, Markowitz, M, and Lilienfeld, A: Why patients don't follow medical advice: A study of children on long-term antistreptococcal prophylaxis. J Pediatr 75:957, 1969.
Korsch, BM, Gozzi, EK, and Francis, V: Gaps in doctor-patient communication. I. Doctor-patient interaction and patient satisfaction. Pediatrics 42:855, 1968.
Lowe, ML: Effectiveness of teaching as measured by compliance with medical recommendations. Nurs Res 19:59, 1970.
Marston, M-V: Compliance with medical regimens: A review of the literature. Nurs Res 19:312, 1970.
Mayo, NE: Patient compliance: Practical implications for physical therapists. A review of the literature. Phys Ther 58(9):1083, 1978.
Moon, MH, et al: Compliancy in splint wearing behavior of patients with rheumatoid arthritis. NZ Med J 83(564):360, 1976.
Oakes, TW, et al: Family expectations and arthritis patient compliance to a hand resting splint regimen. J Chronic Dis 22:757, 1970.

Patient Education

An Interdisciplinary Educational Program for Patients with Rheumatic Diseases: A Guide for Professional Staff. Columbia Hospital, Rheumatic Disease Program, 2025 East Newport, Milwaukee, WI 53211.
Arthritis Information Clearinghouse. Provides listings of available print and nonprint educational ma-

terials through bibliographies, fact sheets, and newsletters. Arthritis Information Clearinghouse, PO Box 34427, Bethesda, MD 20034.

Arthritis Teaching Slide Collection for the Arthritis Health Professional. Contains 198 slides covering comprehensive management of arthritis. Includes a 216-page instructional guide. This is an excellent patient education resource. Available from the Arthritis Foundation, 3400 Peachtree Road, NE, Atlanta, GA 30326.

Educational Materials Exhibit. Arthritis Health Professions Association Annual Meeting. Each year this exhibit includes all current professional and patient education materials. The catalog for this exhibit is an excellent resource. It is available from the Arthritis Foundation.

Freedman, CR: Teaching Patients. Courseware, Inc., Department HT-4, 10075 Carroll Canyon Road, San Diego, CA 92131.

Kaye, RL, and Hammond AH: Understanding rheumatoid arthritis—Evaluation of a patient education program. JAMA 50:57, 1976.

Lawrence, SV: Hospital develops educational program for arthritis patients. Forum on Medicine, July 1978, p 34.

Locke, EA: Motivational effects of knowledge of results: Knowledge of goal setting. J Appl Psychol 31:325, 1967.

Norberg, B, and King, L: Third-party payment for patient education. Am J Nurs 46:1269, 1976.

Patient Education in Arthritis—"How to" packet. Arthritis Foundation, 3400 Peachtree Road, NE, Atlanta, GA 30326.

Rand, PH: Evaluation of patient education programs. Phys Ther 58(7), 1978.

Vignos, P, Parket, W, and Thompson, H: Evaluation of a clinic education program for patients with rheumatoid arthritis. J Rheum 3(2):155, 1976.

Wallace, R, Heiss, ML, and Bautch, JC: Staff Manual for Teaching Patients about Rheumatoid Arthritis. American Hospital Association, 840 North Lake Shore Drive, Chicago, IL 60611. (This also contains the "How to" packet listed above and an excellent bibliography.)

Williams, G.H, Wood, PH: Common-sense beliefs about illness: A mediating role for the doctor. Lancet 2(8521–22):1435–1437, 1986.

Wright, V: What the patient means: A study from rheumatology. Physiotherapy 64(5):146, 1978.

Chapter 3

Drug Therapy

SALICYLATES (ASPIRIN AND ASPIRIN-CONTAINING
  COMPOUNDS)
NONACETYLATED SALICYLATES (NONASPIRIN
  SALICYLATES)
NONSTEROIDAL ANTI-INFLAMMATORY DRUGS (NSAIDs)
INTRASYNOVIAL CORTICOSTEROID INJECTIONS
DISEASE-MODIFYING DRUGS (DMDs)
    Gold Salts
    Antimalarial Therapy
    Sulfasalazine
    Penicillamine
IMMUNOREGULATORY DRUGS
    Methotrexate
    Azathioprine (Imuran)
CORTICOSTEROIDS
ANALGESICS
DRUGS USED TO TREAT GOUT

Drug therapy for rheumatoid arthritis (RA) is constantly changing and, in fact, is going through a considerable evolution from a standard sequential selection of 5 to 7 drugs in the 1960s to a current armamentarium of 20 or more effective medications.

Over the last 10 years the development of **nonsteroidal anti-inflammatory drugs** (NSAIDs) has created a new classification of antirheumatic medications and greatly extended the flexibility of medical management.

There have been over 100 variations of these NSAIDs developed internationally. As each drug is developed, it is compared with aspirin and/or placebo. This extensive comparison process, particularly in the last 5 years, has generated extensive data on drug therapy and has resulted in a greater appreciation of individual patient response to medication and dosage regimens, as well as a greater appreciation of the benefits and limitations of aspirin.

Drug therapy, like painting a picture or rearing a child, is a creative process. There are basic rules that are essential to each activity, but no single method is recommended over all other methods. The variables in drug management are always changing. Patients and their needs and concerns change; more information about the use of medications becomes available; and physicians change in response to their patient care experience. It is congruent with this total picture that drug therapy for rheumatic diseases varies widely across the country among medical schools and among rheumatologists. Each physician develops his or her own philosophy and systematic approach to medical management of rheumatic diseases. Therapists and other arthritis health professionals need to understand the medical protocols used by the rheumatologists, internists, and family practitioners at their facility.

Understanding medical management is

critical to effective rehabilitative treatment planning, particularly since medications can significantly alter objective measurements, such as grip strength, hand function, range of motion, muscle strength, dressing time, and so forth. The **fast-acting anti-inflammatory and analgesic drugs,** such as aspirin, indomethacin, phenylbutazone, propionic acids, steroids, and propoxyphene hydrochloride (Darvon) can *influence objective assessments* in as short a period of time as a half hour. Slow-acting medications, such as gold, antimalarial drugs, and penicillamine, which take 3 to 4 months to effect change, can influence longitudinal assessments. Therefore, prior to each assessment, it is important to note the type, amount, and time of the last medication dose. This should be checked even with patients who are on a constant medicine regimen, inasmuch as they may take additional analgesic drugs on bad days. Additional medication can result in significant measurement changes. *Thus, quantitative assessments may reflect only the benefits of medication and not the results of rehabilitative treatment.* The converse situation may also occur. If a patient comes to the clinic complaining of increased discomfort, his or her medication pattern should be investigated. He or she may have delayed or missed the morning medication dosage.

Another issue to consider is that joint exacerbations of RA may be chronic and last for months, or they may be responsive to fast-acting medications in a couple of days. Equipment such as assistive devices or splints and instruction in adaptive methods may not be necessary if the flare is responsive to medications.

Therapists can also play an important role in facilitating patient compliance by reinforcing the rationale for anti-inflammatory medications and adherence to the prescribed regimen. Even when physicians do a thorough job of patient education, patients often have questions after they leave the physician's office. Patients frequently raise these questions in therapy, providing an opportunity for the therapist to correct misunderstandings or to reaffirm accurate information. *However, this aspect of patient education can be done only if therapists are familiar with the referring physician's medication protocols.* Excellent articles are available on patient drug education, methods of increasing compliance, and drug usage in the elderly. (See Additional Sources at the end of this chapter.)

Therapists can also facilitate medical care by being alert for serious medication side effects in patients and by advising patients to report the symptoms to their physicians. For example, if an outpatient is noticeably pale and complaining of tiredness, it is appropriate to recommend that the patient see his or her physician because these symptoms may be related to severe anemia. Table 3–1 identifies the trade and generic names for the common medications used for rheumatic diseases.

A word about terminology for therapists unfamiliar with the "war" vocabulary that is often invoked in the "battle against arthritis." Medications are often referred to as part of a "drug armamentarium." Drugs of choice may become "first-line" drugs, denoting the first line of soldiers in battle; second-choice drugs are "second line," and so forth. Occasionally corticosteroids, or "big gun" drugs, are reserved for last choice. In the future we may want to explore the psychotherapeutic implications of participating in battle for women or men patients who are not inclined to join the armed forces.

The rationale for drug use for specific diseases is described at the end of each chapter in Part II, Major Rheumatic Diseases, and in Chapter 14, Juvenile Rheumatoid Arthritis. This chapter discusses the specific drug properties, side effects, and implications for arthritis health professionals. This chapter is not referenced, as all objective data can be found in the major reviews of drug therapy listed in Additional Sources at the end of the chapter.

SALICYLATES (ASPIRIN AND ASPIRIN-CONTAINING COMPOUNDS)

Salicylates are the oldest and most widely used of the antirheumatic drugs and are still the first drugs of choice in the treatment of rheumatoid arthritis and most other inflammatory arthritides. These drugs are popular because they are effective

Table 3–1 Common Medications Used with Rheumatic
Diseases

Generic Name	Trade Name
acetaminophen	Datril, Tylenol
allopurinol	Zyloprim, Lopurin
aspirin (previously acetylsalicylic acid [ASA])	See Table 3–2
auranofin	Ridaura
azathioprine	Imuran
betamethasone	Celestone (Celestone Phosphate and Celestone Soluspan)
chlorambucil	Leukeran
chloroquine	Aralen, Avloclor
choline magnesium trisalicylate	Trilisate
choline salicylate	Arthropan
colchicine	(no trade name)
cyclophosphamide	Cytoxan
dexamethasone	Decadron
diflunisal	Dolobid
fenoprofen calcium	Nalfon
gold sodium thioglucose	Solganal
gold sodium thiomalate	Myochrysine
hydrocortisone	Cortef, Solu-Cortef
hydroxychloroquine	Plaquenil
ibuprofen	Motrin, Rufen, Advil, Medipren, Nuprin
indomethacin	Indocin
levamisole	Ketrax
magnesium salicylate	Magan, Mobidin
meclofenamic acid	Meclomen
methotrexate	Methotrexate, Mexate
methylprednisolone	Medrol, Depo-Medrol
naproxen	Naprosyn
oxyphenbutazone	Oxalid, Tandearil
paramethasone acetate	Haldrone
penicillamine	Cuprimine, Depen
phenylbutazone	Butazolidin, Butazolidin Alka, Azolid
piroxicam	Feldene
prednisone	Deltasone, Meticorten, Delta-Cortef
probenecid	Benemid
propoxyphene	Darvon
quinacrine hydrochloride	Atabrine
salicylsalicylic acid	Disalcid
sulindac	Clinoril
sulfasalazine	Azulfidine
sulfinpyrazone	Anturane
tolmetin sodium	Tolectin
triamcinolone	Aristocort, Kenacort

and inexpensive and have a tolerable incidence of side effects. Aspirin* (acetylsalicylic acid, or ASA) is the most commonly used derivative of salicylic acid (Table 3–2). Other salicylate compounds are also effective and used extensively in the treatment of rheumatic disorders (see Table 3–3).

Salicylates offer an advantage over other antirheumatic drugs in that their level in the blood can be measured by a simple laboratory test. Measurement of **salicylate levels** is valuable for determining proper

*Aspirin, previously a trade name, is now considered the generic term replacing acetylsalicylic acid.

Table 3–2 Common Forms of Aspirin*

There are multiple brands of aspirin in various forms (time released, chewable, suppositories)

Aspirin (with enteric coating to prevent absorption of the aspirin until it reaches the small intestine)
  Cosprin
  Easprin
  Ecotrin (regular and safety coated)

Aspirin with antacids
  Bufferin
  Ascriptin

Aspirin combinations
  APC (with codeine)
  Anacin (with caffeine): regular or maximum strength
  Equagesic (with meprobamate, a relaxant): may be habit forming
  Excedrin (with acetaminophen and caffeine): regular or extra strength
  Midol (with an antispasmodic)
  Vanquish (with acetaminophen, caffeine, and buffering agents)

*These are prescribed in a dosage equivalent to aspirin. Common aspirin contains 5 grains per tablet, equal to 300 mg or 0.3 g. Average anti-inflammatory doses are 12–24 (5-grain) ASA tablets per day or 3.6–7.2 g per day.

blood absorption of the drug. A therapeutic anti-inflammatory level is between 15 and 30 mg per deciliter (dl). Many patients develop side effects that require discontinuation of the drug before a therapeutic blood level is achieved.

When aspirin is used in large doses (12 to 20 tablets per day), it is effective as an anti-inflammatory agent. Used in low doses (fewer than 9 tablets per day), it works primarily as an **analgesic** (pain reliever). The usual dose for children is 80 to 100 mg per kg in 4 divided doses per day.

Toxicity from high dosage of aspirin in adults is indicated by **tinnitus** (persistent ringing or buzzing sound in the ears). Tinnitus is *not* used as a guideline for monitoring aspirin in children. The recommended adult dosage is the amount just lower than that which causes tinnitus. For example, if a dosage of 16 aspirin a day produces tinnitus, the patient is advised to reduce the dosage one tablet per day until the tinnitus stops. In most adults tinnitus corresponds to a serum salicylate level of 20 to 30 mg per dl. In all adult patients, therapeutic anti-inflammatory levels of salicylates (approximately 25 mg per dl) cause a totally reversible 20-decibel hearing loss at

Table 3–3 Salicylates and Nonsteroidal Anti-inflammatory Medications

Purpose: All these medications, to some degree, serve the same purpose or function. They all have anti-inflammatory, analgesic, antipyretic, and anticoagulant properties.

Toxic side effects: Since all these medications inhibit prostaglandin production, they share similar side effects. Some of the side effects have a higher incidence with certain medications, but all of the following can occur with each drug: (1) gastrointestinal side effects, such as indigestion, heartburn, nausea, abdominal pain, diarrhea, ulcers, constipation; (2) fluid retention; (3) anemia; (4) decreased clotting ability; (5) lightheadedness, nasal stuffiness; (6) allergic skin rash; and (7) possible mild stimulant or depressant effects. Related to pregnancy: All drugs that inhibit prostaglandin synthesis may prolong gestation and labor. Salicylates create an additional risk of ante- and postpartum hemorrhage and pulmonary hypertension in the neonate. Indomethacin is contraindicated during pregnancy, but all of these drugs should be avoided during pregnancy.

Precautions: To reduce the side effects on the gastrointestinal system, all of these medications should be taken with food or milk. Antacids can be used with all *except* enteric-coated aspirin. Other precautions include the following: (1) Patients on anticoagulant therapy (Coumadin) who need these medications must be under careful medical supervision because these medications can increase Coumadin blood levels to a dangerous level. (2) Patients with asthma or a history of asthma need to be careful because prostaglandin inhibition can elicit an asthma attack. (3) Patients with hypertension need to be observant because excessive fluid retention can increase hypertension. (4) Patients who drink alcohol need to be aware that both alcohol and NSAIDs increase gastric irritability; in some individuals the combination can increase the risk of gastric irritation or ulcers. (5) Patients with gout need to be aware that low doses of salicylates can increase uric acid levels.

Contraindications: These drugs should not be taken by people with a history of gastric ulcer or bleeding tendencies.

Table 3–3. Salicylates and Nonsteroidal Anti-inflammatory Medications
(continued)

Trade and Generic Names	Dosage	Additional Toxic Side Effects and Special Precautions
SALICYLATES		
Aspirin (acetylsalicylic acid, ASA) Enteric-coated ASA Ecotrin, Easprin Buffered ASA Bufferin, Ascriptin, and others Zero-order release ASA Zorprin	Adult: Start with 8–12 (5-grain ASA) tablets per day, then monitor blood levels/toxicity. Children: determined by weight (80–100 mg/kg)	Central nervous system: tinnitus, deafness (reversible). Acute toxic reaction to high salicylate levels can include vomiting, psychosis, hyperventilation, alkalosis, and metabolic acidosis.
Nonacetylated Salicylates (nonaspirin salicylates) Arthropan (choline salicylate) Trilisate (choline magnesium trisalicylate) Disalcid (salicylsalicylic acid) Magan (magnesium salicylate)		
Dolobid (diflunisal)	1000 mg in 2 divided doses	
PROPIONIC ACIDS		
Motrin, Rufen, Mediprin, Advil, Nuprin (ibuprofen) 200, 300, 400, 600, 800 mg	1200–3200 mg daily in 3–4 divided doses	
Naprosyn (naproxen) 250, 375, 500 mg	500–1000 mg daily in 2–3 divided doses	
Nalfon (fenoprofen) 300, 600 mg	900–2400 mg daily in 3–4 divided doses	
Orudis (ketoproten)	225 mg in 3 divided doses	
Benoxaprofen (Oraflex) has been removed from the market by the FDA because of severe side effects.		
Flurbiprofen, fenbufen, and carprofen have not yet been released by the FDA.		
INDOLE DERIVATIVES		
Indocin or generic (indomethacin) 25, 50, or 75 mg sustained release or suppository	50–200 mg daily in 1–4 divided doses	Central nervous system: headache, dizziness, detached feelings, drowsiness, and hallucinations. May cause birth defects. May interfere with antihypertensive effects of beta-blockers.
Clinoril (sulindac) 150-, 200-mg tablets (both yellow hexagonal tablets)	300–400 mg daily in 2 divided doses	
Tolectin (tolmetin) 200-mg white, round tablet 400-mg red capsule	600–1600 mg daily in 3–4 divided doses	

Table 3–3. Salicylates and Nonsteroidal Anti-inflammatory Medications
(*continued*)

Trade and Generic Names	Dosage	Additional Toxic Side Effects and Special Precautions
FENAMATES		
Meclomen (meclofenamic acid) 50-mg (two-tone gold) capsule 100-mg (gold and white) capsule	200–400 mg daily in 3–4 divided doses	Main complications are diarrhea and abdominal cramps.
OXICAMS		
Feldene (piroxicam) 10- or 20-mg capsules Zomepirac (Zomax) has been removed from the market by the FDA because of severe side effects.	10–20 mg daily in 1–2 doses	
PARAZOLONES		
Butazolidin Alka (phenylbutazone) 100-mg (red, round) tablets	100–400 mg daily in 2–3 divided doses	Serious side effects such as aplastic anemia, agranulocytosis, and thrombocytopenia are rare. Should not be used with sulfa drugs and their derivatives, and some coagulants. Not recommended for the elderly.
Tandearil (oxyphenbutazone) 100-mg tan, round tablets	100–400 mg daily in 2–3 divided doses	Should not be used by patients with liver or renal disease.

all frequencies. This hearing loss may be unacceptable to individuals with pre-existing hearing impairment. Occasionally deafness occurs when aspirin reaches a toxic level. Pre-existing hearing patterns return when the aspirin dosage is reduced. All older adult patients should be cautioned to observe for changes in hearing ability when they take aspirin.

Gastrointestinal symptoms such as nausea and heartburn are the most common side effects of aspirin. Because patients often have to be on aspirin for long periods of time, it is important that they take measures to prevent these side effects. They should take the aspirin with milk or with meals and never on an empty stomach. Technically, aspirin is absorbed more efficiently on an empty stomach, but for daily use ingestion without food creates too high a risk for gastric side effects. For some patients buffered aspirin reduces these symptoms. Enteric-coated aspirin is another useful alternative for some patients, because it is not dissolved until the tablet reaches the

small intestine. Disalcid also does not dissolve in the stomach and may be better tolerated than regular aspirin. Zorprin is compounded in such a way that steady amounts of aspirin are released independently of the amount of drug remaining in the intestine. This is referred to as **zero-order kinetics.** More serious complications of aspirin include gastrointestinal bleeding and allergic reactions such as asthma and hay fever. Aspirin should not be used by patients with documented peptic ulcer or with bleeding tendencies. Aspirin is also associated with an increased risk of antepartum and postpartum hemorrhaging in pregnant women, and it may induce pulmonary hypertension in the neonate.

NONACETYLATED SALICYLATES (NONASPIRIN SALICYLATES)

These salicylate derivatives have gained increasing popularity because, compared with aspirin, they may be better tolerated and have fewer side effects, they are often more readily absorbed, and they deliver almost twice as much salicylate per dose than aspirin, making the medication easier to take. Their main disadvantage is that they cost more than aspirin. The drugs in this category are magnesium salicylate (Magan, Mobidin), choline salicylate (Arthropan—a liquid), choline magnesium trisalicylate (Trilisate), and salicylsalicylic acid (Disalcid). Diflunisal (Dolobid) is another agent often classified as an NSAID, but it actually is a salicylate derivative (see Table 3–2).

Most physicians prescribe aspirin first. If the patient has problems with absorption or side effects, the physician may try another salicylate preparation as an alternative. Some of the newer agents offer all the benefits of aspirin with either fewer symptomatic side effects (nonacetyl salicylates) or better compliance because of twice-a-day administration (Zorprin, Dolobid).

NONSTEROIDAL ANTI-INFLAMMATORY DRUGS (NSAIDs)

Like salicylates, these medications (see Table 3–3) reduce but usually do not completely stop the signs and symptoms of joint inflammation. They are fast-acting medications in that they can influence functioning within an hour, although the maximal therapeutic effect may take 5 to 10 days. They are effective only while therapeutic blood levels are maintained. Although chemically diverse, all the NSAIDs (and salicylates) share the property of inhibiting the production of prostaglandins. This property not only accounts for some of their anti-inflammatory action but also explains why these drugs produce similar side effects such as gastric distress, ulcer formation, fluid retention, bleeding tendencies, and the rare occurrence of asthma and renal failure. Only two of these drugs are approved by the Food and Drug Administration (FDA) for use with children: naproxen and tolmetin. Other NSAIDs are used with children on an experimental basis in pediatric arthritis centers (please refer to Chapter 14).

The more expensive NSAIDs are selected over salicylates when patients cannot tolerate, or do not respond to, salicylates or when the individual prefers the convenience of taking one to four tablets per day rather than 12 to 15 aspirin tablets per day.

Many patients who do not respond to aspirin or one of the NSAIDs may respond to another NSAID. There is no way to predict which will be the most efficacious drug for an individual except by trial use. The third or alternative drug is usually selected from a different chemical class. For example, if one of the propionic acid derivatives is not effective, it is not likely that another will be; therefore the next trial drug will be from outside that group, such as an indole derivative.

Only one NSAID drug should be used at a time and should be used in maximum doses before it is stopped because of a lack of efficacy. Generally, aspirin should not be used with a NSAID because both drugs compete for serum protein binding sites. One may displace the other, lowering blood levels of the other NSAID. In addition, gastric side effects may increase. Despite this, some patients find such a combination synergistic in relieving their symptoms. All these drugs can be used with a corticosteroid or any of the disease-modifying drugs. Many new agents will probably be approved in the next few years. Flurbiprofen, fenbufen, and voltaren are three that are used extensively in other parts of the world. (Fenbufen is not available in the United States; voltaren has recently been approved for use in the United States.)

During lactation, all NSAIDs can be transferred to the infant through the mother's milk. In an excellent review of rheumatic drugs, Needs and Brooks recommend that the best NSAID for a nursing mother is one (1) with a short half-life; (2) found in minimal quantities in mother's milk; and (3) with inactive metabolites also found in small quantities. They believe that ibuprofen, flurbiprofen, and declofenac meet these criteria best. In order to reduce the quantity of the drug in the infant, they recommend that the drug be taken by the mother at the time of breast-feeding, with the next feeding occurring after a time period equivalent to one half-life of the drug. (See Additional Sources, Drug Therapy Related to Child-Bearing at the end of this chapter.)

INTRASYNOVIAL CORTICOSTEROID INJECTIONS

Intrasynovial injections of corticosteroids have different purposes, goals, and consequences than daily oral administration or intramuscular injections of steroids. The indications, use, and side effects are the same for adults and children. Corticosteroids injected into a joint, bursa, or tendon sheath provide *localized* suppression of inflammation in a specific area. Negative consequences are related to the effect of the drug on surrounding joint and tendon structures. The classic steroid side effects such as cushingoid features, osteoporosis, and so forth do not occur with local intrasynovial injections unless they are given more frequently than monthly. Injections can have a slight systemic effect at the time of the injection, but it is not significant enough to produce negative systemic side effects.

Local injections do not cure or stop the inflammation, but they can control it in some patients. Response to local injections is variable. Some patients get relief of pain and swelling for 6 weeks or longer; for others relief may last only a few days. If the benefit is transient, lasting less than a week, repeated injection is usually not helpful and not advisable. In small joints such as the proximal interphalangeal (PIP) joint, a single trial is often sufficient to determine effectiveness of this approach. Larger joints, such as the shoulder and hip, may be responsive to a third injection even if the first two have failed.

Intrasynovial corticosteroid injections are particularly valuable in the following situations.

1. Severe inflammation of one or a few peripheral joints, especially if the joint inflammation is preventing function or restricting motion to the point that a deformity is likely to occur if the inflammation is not resolved.

2. Severe flexor tenosynovitis of the wrist or digits and extensor tenosynovitis of the wrist.

3. Acute shoulder or trochanteric bursitis or tendinitis. (Injections are helpful in this condition but not in chronic adhesive capsulitis.)

Injections are not given in a joint if there is a possibility of infection or fracture near or around the joint, because corticosteroids reduce healing potential. It is also impractical to use injections when multiple joints are inflamed; in these instances, systemic medications need to be used.

Complications include

1. Infections, which are infrequent. They may occur despite rigid sterile techniques and are generally due to resistant staphylococcus.

2. Occasionally injections result in a postinjection flare lasting up to 24 hours. This is considered an aseptic process resulting from synovitis induced by corticosteroid crystals. (Ice compresses are recommended until the delayed effect of the corticosteroid reduces the inflammation.)

3. One of the more serious complications is instability in a weight-bearing joint following repeated injections. In the hip this has been seen along with aseptic necrosis of the femoral head.

4. Tendon rupture can occur if the injection is given into the tendon rather than into the tendon sheath, but this is rare. Athletes have been known to rupture tendons following strenuous exercise of tendons or joints that have been repeatedly injected (for instance, weekly).

5. In children, asymptomatic calcium deposits may occur at the injection site.

DISEASE-MODIFYING DRUGS (DMDs)

When synovitis persists despite the use of NSAIDs and conservative measures, it becomes necessary to use stronger medications. Gold salts, antimalarial drugs, methotrexate, and penicillamine are slow-acting medications that can modify RA and related diseases and in some patients can actually reduce the symptoms to the point that the patient appears to be in remission. In the past it was believed that these drugs actually induced a remission and thus were referred to as *remission-inducing drugs,* but recent studies have documented the progression of joint erosions in some patients despite apparent lack of symptoms.

Aspirin and NSAIDs are considered of equal potency and are grouped as first-line drugs. Gold and Plaquenil are referred to as second-line drugs, and penicillamine and methotrexate are third-line drugs. Rheumatologists generally do not advance to a higher-level drug unless all viable options on a given level have been employed.

Gold salts are the most widely accepted of these drugs. Most physicians will try gold first. If it is unsuccessful, they will then try an antimalarial drug (Plaquenil) or penicillamine. Gold is the preferred second-line drug for juvenile rheumatoid arthritis (JRA). Some physicians highly experienced with antimalarials will start with these drugs in selected patients and then try gold as the second option. Generally, methotrexate is reserved for those patients in whom one or more of the DMDs have proven ineffective.

Gold Salts

The value of gold for RA was a serendipitous discovery in the 1920s during an experimental trial using gold for tuberculosis. It was found that joint disease improved in tuberculous patients who also suffered from RA. (Gold is no longer considered beneficial for tuberculosis.)

Although intramuscular gold has been used to treat arthritis since about 1930, the reasons for its effectiveness are still unknown. Nevertheless, gold provides beneficial anti-inflammatory results in a majority of patients (adults and children) who can tolerate the drug. There is a definite price to pay for these benefits, inasmuch as patients must be seen weekly for 20 weeks for gold injections. Each injection is preceded with blood and urinalyses to detect signs of toxicity. This can pose a problem for patients who are employed or who want to return to work, inasmuch as the clinic visits may necessitate taking off a half day from work.

Side effects of gold toxicity include severe skin rashes and stomatitis (mucous membrane ulcerations in the mouth). These may be controlled by stopping or lowering the dosage. More serious complications that may lead to death include bone marrow depression (thrombocytopenia or agranulocytosis) and kidney damage. Early side effects to observe and to report to the person giving injections include

1. Itching (pruritus) anywhere or a mild rash that itches. Itching is often a precursor to severe dermatitis.
2. Metallic taste in the mouth. This may precede stomatitis and is considered a warning sign of mucosal reaction.
3. Mouth ulcers, tongue or gum inflammation, or sore throat, which are all signs of stomatitis (the second most common side effect).

Early signs of hematological and renal damage are detected by complete blood counts with platelet count and urinalysis.

Because of the seriousness of the side effects, gold therapy is reserved only for patients with RA or JRA who are dependable and have a persistent synovitis that is not responsive to more conservative medication or rehabilitation therapy. It is contraindicated for patients with systemic lupus erythematosus (SLE) and previous severe toxicity to gold and for those severely debilitated. It is also contraindicated during pregnancy and nursing. Gold has a long half-life and may take 4 to 5 months to be fully excreted.

In adults, the dosage is 50 mg weekly for 20 weeks, then once every 2 to 4 weeks. In children, the dosage is 1 mg per kg weekly for 5 to 12 months, then every 2 to 3 weeks. If the child has a cessation of symptoms for 6 months, the gold may be stopped. A positive therapeutic response is often not noticeable until 12 to 16 weeks after therapy is started. Gold should not be given concomitantly with penicillamine but may be used with salicylates, NSAIDs, or corticosteroids. Its safety with methotrexate has not been established.

An alternative to injectable gold is **auranofin** (Ridaura), which is a capsule form of gold taken orally. The usual dose is a 3-mg capsule twice a day. It can be taken with or without food, but taking it with food or milk can reduce the incidence of gastrointestinal side effects. The same side effects can be seen as with injectable gold, with the rather common addition of diarrhea or other gastrointestinal symptoms, such as nausea, cramping, or lack of appetite. The same precautions must be taken with auranofin in terms of laboratory monitoring and the reporting of side effects. The contraindications are the same as those for injectable gold. The exact role of oral gold in the treatment of RA is still to be determined. Many physicians feel that it may not be as effective as intramuscular gold in inducing a therapeutic response, although there seem to be somewhat fewer incidental side effects.

Antimalarial Therapy

Hydroxychloroquine (Plaquenil) is the drug of choice among the antimalarials for the treatment of rheumatic diseases because of its effectiveness and low toxicity compared with other antimalarials. This drug appears to be particularly effective in SLE patients with sun sensitivity and skin rashes. It is also used successfully in both RA and JRA and the spondyloarthropathies.

The use of Plaquenil has increased over the past several years as clinical experience demonstrates that the risk of visual loss or blindness is minimal with current low-dose administration. A variety of **ocular reactions** are possible and need to be observed through periodic ophthalmological examinations (including slit-lamp assessment). Patients should have an eye examination before starting the drug and approximately every 6 months thereafter. The drug is discontinued if visual changes occur. The visual symptoms to be alert for are impaired reading ability, poor distance vision, night blindness, blurred vision, halos around lights, and scotomas (spots in the visual field without vision). Inasmuch as the eyes can become sensitive to the sun, it is recommended that patients wear sunglasses outdoors. Fortunately, visual symptoms at recommended doses are very rare.

Other side effects include a wide range of neurological conditions, including migraine-like headaches, tinnitus, vestibular problems, dermatological conditions, and gastrointestinal disorders. Essentially any unusual symptom in these categories could be related to the drug.

A factor that often influences the selection of this drug over gold salts is the method of administration. Hydroxychloroquine is in tablet form and does not require weekly clinic visits as does gold therapy.

Quinacrine hydrochloride (Atabrine) given at a dose of 100 mg per day is an alternative nonchloroquine-derivative antimalarial that may be used instead of hydrochloroquine for the dermatological manifestations of SLE. The major side effect is yellowing of the skin, secondary to deposition of the yellow drug in the skin.

Sulfasalazine

This drug is a compound that is part sulfa and part salicylate. It has been used since 1980 as a treatment for ulcerative colitis. Over the last few years it has been used as a second-line medication for patients who have RA.

The most common side effects of sulfasalazine are anorexia, nausea, vomiting, and gastric distress. These symptoms can occur with both the regular and the enteric-coated forms. Although rare, almost every *severe* hematological, dermatological, gastrointestinal, renal, and neurological hypersensitivity reaction has been reported. For this reason, patients need to be monitored with frequent complete blood counts and urinalysis. The incidence of adverse reaction is reduced with a dosage of less than 4 g per day for adults. (This drug is not approved for children with JRA.)

Penicillamine

This medication is generally used as the third DMD alternative following gold or Plaquenil or the fourth following methotrexate for the treatment of adult RA. It has been used with children in the past, but recent studies at Children's Hospital of Los Angeles have found the efficacy of penicillamine to be equal to placebo, and they no longer use the drug for JRA.

The toxicities and side effects that may be produced by penicillamine are many and diverse and have limited its clinical use. These side effects can be severe and include

1. Hematological changes, including acute bone marrow depression with neutropenia, thrombocytopenia, and aplastic anemia.

2. Renal changes, including nephropathy and nephrotic syndrome.

3. Dermatological changes. A wide range

of skin rashes can occur and appear similar to the rashes seen with gold therapy.

4. Mucous membrane lesions can occur (both oral and genital) and are dose related.

5. Secondary immune complex diseases can result from penicillamine, including systemic lupus erythematosus (SLE), myasthenia gravis, polymyositis, Goodpasture's syndrome, pemphigus, and Sjögren's syndrome.

6. Hypogeusia (blunting or loss of taste perception) is another common side effect. This may persist for up to 3 months following onset. It gradually clears, even with the continuation of therapy.

7. Delayed wound healing, which may prolong postoperative recovery and therapy.

Dosage is 250 mg per day, *taken on an empty stomach.* This amount is taken for 12 weeks. If there is no response, it is increased by 250 mg. Maximum dosage is 1 mg per day. A therapeutic response takes 2 to 4 months. It is contraindicated during pregnancy because generalized connective-tissue defects have been reported, and it should be discontinued 3 to 4 months before conception to allow full excretion. It is also not given to people with previous renal disease.

IMMUNOREGULATORY DRUGS

Many drugs that affect the regulation of the immune system are effective in reducing the inflammation of RA. Some are very toxic and consequently rarely used (e.g., cyclophosphamide [Cytoxan]). Two have a definite role in the management of RA: methotrexate and azathioprine (Imuran).

Methotrexate

Methotrexate (MTX) was introduced in 1948 as a treatment for childhood leukemia. Later it was used extensively for treatment-resistant psoriasis. It wasn't until the early 1980s that it was determined that low-dose MTX could be used safely for the treatment of RA.

In high doses (75 to 250 mg per week), such as those used for cancer, MTX is considered a potent suppressor for cellular and humoral immunity; it is a folic acid analog that interferes with folic acid metabolism necessary for deoxyribonucleic acid (DNA) synthesis and cell division. It essentially kills rapidly proliferating cells. In low doses (7.5 to 15 mg per week) used for RA, MTX appears to act as an anti-inflammatory medication. The specific mechanism of action of MTX in this dosage is not known at this time, but it may turn out to be different from the above description for high dosage.

In low doses it has proven to be a well-tolerated medication, when given by either oral or intramuscular means in treating RA, psoriatic arthritis, Reiter's syndrome, polymyositis, and JRA. In RA, doses from 5 to 15 mg *given only once a week* are used. A therapeutic effect is usually seen in 6 to 8 weeks.

Methotrexate can be used with an NSAID or corticosteroids, but it is not usually used with salicylates. (Salicylates can reduce excretion of MTX.) It should not be taken with diuretics or antibiotics because they can increase the risk of toxicity. The combination of an NSAID plus a diuretic and MTX creates an exceptionally high risk for toxicity. Immediate toxic effects are dose related and reversible when the medication is stopped or reduced. Symptoms of toxicity include stomatitis (the most common), which includes a burning erythema in the mouth as well as ulcers; abdominal pain; diarrhea; intestinal bleeding; and bone marrow suppression (leukopenia, anemia, thrombocytopenia). Pneumonitis can also occur characterized by dyspnea, nonproductive cough, fever, rales, and hypoxemia. (Previous lung disease may be a risk factor for this side effect.)

Careful clinical laboratory monitoring is mandatory when using methotrexate. It is absolutely contraindicated during pregnancy because it can induce abortion or cause malformations—such as hydrocephalus, cleft palate, and hare lip—if it is given during the first trimester. It is recommended that neither partner use the drug for 4 months before conception. Liver damage (fibrosis/cirrhosis) has been seen in the past when the drug was used daily for the treatment of psoriasis, but its incidence when a weekly dosage schedule is used appears minimal at present. High alcohol intake appears to be a risk factor for liver damage. Long-term studies are in progress to determine this risk in its use for RA.

Azathioprine (Imuran)

Azathioprine (Imuran) is an immuno-suppressive drug approved by the FDA for adults with refractory RA. It is given orally in a dose of 2 to 3 mg per kg body weight daily with meals. It can be given with salicylates, NSAIDs, and corticosteroids but not gold, Plaquenil, or penicillamine. Mild side effects can include gastrointestinal distress and stomatitis (mouth ulcers). Severe side effects include bone marrow suppression and liver dysfunction, requiring careful monitoring. The drug has been shown to be effective in controlling inflammatory manifestations of RA and SLE. The major drawback to its wider use is the uncertainty of the incidence of lymphoreticular malignancies when used for RA. Intercerebral lymphomas show a definite increased incidence in kidney transplant patients who receive azathioprine to prevent transplant rejection. It is contraindicated during pregnancy.

CORTICOSTEROIDS

Corticosteroid preparations are the most powerful anti-inflammatory agents known. Their use may be lifesaving in polymyositis and in certain manifestations of SLE; however, their rational use on a long-term basis for other inflammatory joint diseases is restricted to patients who would be severely disabled without them.

Cautious use of these drugs is essential, since long-term use produces serious and undesirable side effects. These include cushingoid features, such as moon facies and buffalo humps, secondary to deposition of subcutaneous fat, obesity, purpura, and skin striae; severe osteoporosis that can lead to compression fractures of the spine or other pathological fractures; avascular necrosis of the femoral or humeral head; cataracts; peptic ulcers and nausea; and a myopathy similar to polymyositis. In addition, corticosteroids can cause hypertension, exacerbate diabetes, lower the body's resistance to infection, and decrease the ability to heal. These drugs can also affect the central nervous system by diminishing the psychological awareness of pain or by enhancing a sense of well-being. They can also produce aberrant psychological states, such as euphoria or severe psychosis. Probably the most depressing and significant consequences for the patient are the side effects that alter physical appearance.

The occupational or physical therapist and nurse should keep several conditions or consequences in mind:

1. If there is severe osteoporosis, transfers and passive range of motion should be done cautiously.

2. Effects of corticosteroids on the central nervous system can significantly affect the patient's ability to learn and comply with instruction. All instructions must be written out.

3. For patients on long-term steroid therapy, the signs of myopathy (i.e., drooping shoulders and difficulty stepping up steps and arising from a chair, not resulting from joint problems) should be observed for and reported to the patient's physician.

Corticosteroids are used in the lowest dose for the shortest period of time needed to achieve the desired clinical effect. Prednisone in various combinations of 1- to 5-mg tablets currently is the most commonly used oral preparation. As a rough guide, less than 10 mg is considered a low dose, 10 to 30 mg a moderate dose, and 30 to 100 mg a high dose. Other corticosteroid drugs used include triamcinolone, dexamethasone, and methylprednisolone.

There are many ways in which a patient can reduce the side effects of corticosteroids.

1. Once they get a satisfactory response, patients should know how to cut back slowly on their dosage in order to be on the lowest dose possible. If they cut back too fast, this can cause an exacerbation of symptoms. The key to reducing dosage is to do it gradually. For example, a person on 15 mg per day can reduce the dosage to 15 mg and 14 mg on alternate days for a week. If that is successful (no flare-ups) the dosage can be reduced to 14 mg daily for a week, followed by reduction to 14 mg and 13 mg on alternate days, and so on. This may sound slow but it is better to reduce gradually and successfully than to reduce rapidly and have an exacerbation. Patients should have clear guidelines for dose reduc-

tion from their physicians. Any sudden reduction or withdrawal from this drug can cause marked fatigue, nausea, vomiting, exacerbation of arthritis, and a drop in blood pressure.

2. Fluid retention and weight gain can be partially controlled by eating a low-sodium diet.

3. Patients need to guard against infections (i.e., exposure to people or children with colds or influenza) since corticosteroids reduce resistance to infection.

4. Stomach irritation can be reduced by taking the medication with a meal or with low-fat milk.

5. Participation in a gentle fitness exercise program (not just range of motion), if possible, can help reduce the effects of osteoporosis, fluid retention, weight gain, and general debilitation.

6. It is recommended that people wear or carry a "medical alert" identification of some form.

ANALGESICS

In this text and in clinical rheumatology, the term **analgesics** refers to those medications primarily used for pain relief that do not have anti-inflammatory properties. Technically, aspirin and all the drugs listed in Table 3–2 are considered analgesics, but in rheumatology these drugs are used primarily for their anti-inflammatory properties.

The most common mild analgesic is acetaminophen (e.g., Tylenol, Anacin-3, Datril, Nebs, and Percogesic). It can be effective in relieving myalgias and pain that do not involve inflammation. It does not have an anti-inflammatory effect on the muscles or joints. Acetaminophen can also be used by people who cannot take aspirin or NSAIDs, such as those (1) allergic or sensitive to salicylates; (2) on anticoagulant therapy; (3) with a history of bleeding ulcers, gastritis, or hiatal hernia; or (4) with hemophilia.

All of the stronger analgesics have the potential for psychological and physical addiction. These drugs should only be used on an occasional basis, if at all, by people with chronic pain. Drugs in this category include Darvon, Darvocet, codeine, Talwin, Vicodin, Dilaudid, Percocet, Percodan, Fiorinal, Demerol, and morphine.

Many patients with severe rheumatic diseases will take a stronger analgesic on particularly bad days. These drugs are very fast acting (20 to 30 minutes) and can significantly alter objective assessments, such as grip strength, range of motion, walking time, and so forth. Patients often do not mention this to therapists. But the use of these drugs on one therapy day and not on another can skew therapy reassessments and the therapist's subjective assessment of a patient's progress in therapy. Thus before all assessments, it is helpful to find out what anti-inflammatory *and* analgesic medications the patient has taken.

Topical analgesics are nonprescription creams, gels, and lotions that are applied topically to painful muscles and joints to relieve soreness and pain. They primarily work as a counterirritant and mild local anesthetic. Common commercial brands include Absorbine Arthritic, Aspercreme, Myoflex Creme, Teragesic, Ben-Gay, Heet, Icy Hot, and Mentholatum rubs. Aspercreme contains 10 percent trolamine salicylate rather than aspirin and cannot be used instead of aspirin as a treatment for arthritis. Some salicylate absorption occurs with this drug but it is minimal. The value of these agents is subjective. The recommendation and use of these products are generally left up to the patient.

DRUGS USED TO TREAT GOUT

The rationale for and use of these drugs are discussed in Chapter 13. Side effects vary for each drug. Colchicine may cause nausea, vomiting, loss of appetite, diarrhea, weakness, skin rash, fever, and sore throat. Clinically, probenecid has almost no side effects except possibly minor skin rashes, although any of the previously described reactions can occur. Allopurinol, however, can result in skin rashes and, rarely, a severe form of hepatitis.

ADDITIONAL SOURCES

Drug Therapy for Rheumatic Diseases

Bellamy, N, and Buchanan, WW: Interpreting clinical trials of antirheumatic drug therapy. Bull Rheum Dis 36(2):1–10, 1986.

Doyle, DV, and Lanham, JG: Routine drug treatment of osteoarthritis. Clin Rheum Dis 10(2):277–291, 1984 (review) .

Flower, RJ, Moncada, S, and Vane, JR: Drug therapy of inflammation. In Gilman, AG, Goodman, LS, and Gilman, A (eds): The Pharmacological Basis of Therapeutics. Macmillan, New York, 1980, pp 682–728.

Hart, CB, Rhymer, AR, and Miola, SR: Indocin SR (indomethacin MSD) in the treatment of moderate to severe rheumatoid arthritis. Semin Arthritis Rheum 12(2 Suppl 1):147–151, 1982.

Hollister, JR: Immunosuppressant therapy of juvenile rheumatoid arthritis. Arthritis Rheum 20(2 Suppl):544–547, 1977.

Kelly, WN, Ruddy, S, Harris, ED, and Sledge, CB: Textbook of Rheumatology, ed, 2. WB Saunders, Philadelphia, 1987. (This text includes separate chapters on each group of drugs.)

Langley, GB, Sheppeard, H, and Wigley, RD: Placebo therapy in rheumatoid arthritis. Clin Exp Rheumatol 1(1):17–21, 1983.

Lisberg, RB, Higham, C, and Jayson, MI: Problems for rheumatic patients in opening dispensed drug containers. Br J Rheumatol 22(2):95–98, 1983.

Lombardino, JG: Mechanism of action of drugs for treating inflammation and arthritis. Eur J Rheumatol Inflamm 6(1):24–35, 1983 (review) .

Maksymowych, W, and Russell, AS: Antimalarials in rheumatology: Efficacy and safety. Semin Arthritis Rheum 16(3):206–221, 1987.

Mason, DI, and Florence, AT: Medication problems of rheumatic patients assessed by domicilary visits by pharmacists. J Clin Hosp Pharm 7(4):261–268, 1982.

Miller, DR, Letendre, PW, DeJong, DJ, and Fiechtner, JJ: Methotrexate in rheumatoid arthritis: An update. Pharmacotherapy 6(4):170–178, 1986.

Moller, PW: Common errors in the treatment of rheumatoid arthritis. Drugs 21(4):297–301, 1981.

Neuberger, GB: The role of the nurse with arthritis patients on drug therapy. Nurs Clin North Am 19(4):593–604, 1984.

Pullar, T., and Capell, HA: A rheumatological dilemma: Is it possible to modify the course of rheumatoid arthritis? Can we answer the question? Ann Rheum Dis 44(2):134–140, 1985 (review).

Simon, LS, and Mills, JA: Nonsteroidal antiinflammatory drugs. Part I. N Engl J Med 302:1179–1185, 1980.

Simon, LS, and Mills, JA: Nonsteroidal antiinflammatory drugs. Part II. N Engl J Med 302:1237–1243, 1980.

Trice, JM, and Pinals, RS: Dimethyl sulfoxide: A review of its use in the rheumatic disorders. Semin Arthritis Rheum 15(1):45–60, 1985.

Aspirin and Nonsteroidal Anti-inflammatory Drugs

Dromgoole, SH, Furst, DC, and Paulus, HE: Rational approaches to the use of salicylates in the treatment of rheumatoid arthritis. Semin Arthritis Rheum 11:257–283, 1981.

Ward, JR: Update on ibuprofen for rheumatoid arthritis. Am J Med 77(1A):3–9, 1984 (review).

Disease-Modifying Drugs

Iannuzzi, L, Dawson, N, Zein, N, and Kushner, I: Does drug therapy slow radiographic deterioration in rheumatoid arthritis? N Engl J Med 309(17):1023–1028, 1983.

Leden, I: Antimalarial drugs—350 years. Scand J Rheumatol 10(4):307–312, 1981.

Lipsky, PE: Remittive therapy in rheumatoid arthritis: Clinical uses and mechanisms of action. Agents Actions (Suppl) 14:181–204, 1984 (review).

Maksymowych, W, and Russell, AS: Antimalarials in rheumatology: Efficacy and safety. Semin Arthritis Rheum 16(3):206–211, 1987.

Muirden, KD: The use of chloroquine and D-penicillamine in the treatment of rheumatoid arthritis. Med J Aust 144(1):32–34, 36–37, 1986 (review).

Pullar, T, and Capell, HA: Variables affecting efficacy and toxicity of sulphasalazine in rheumatoid arthritis. A review. Drugs 32 (Suppl 1):54–57, 1986 (review).

Stein, HB, Patterson, AC, Offer, RC, et al: Adverse effects of d-penicillamine in rheumatoid arthritis. Ann Intern Med 92:24–29, 1980.

Disease-Modifying Drugs—Gold

Davis, P: Auranofin. Clin Rheum Dis 10(2):369–383, 1984 (review).

Evers, AE, and Sundstrom, WR: Second course gold therapy in the treatment of rheumatoid arthritis. Arthritis Rheum 26:1275–1278, 1983.

Fam, AG, Gordon, DA, Sarkozi, J, et al: Neurologic complications associated with gold therapy for rheumatoid arthritis. J Rheumatol 11:700–706, 1984.

Furst, DE: Mechanism of action, pharmacology, clinical efficacy and side effects of auranofin. An orally administered organic gold compound for the treatment of rheumatoid arthritis. Pharmacotherapy 3:284–298, 1983.

Husby, G: Gold in rheumatoid arthritis therapy today. Dosage. Scand J Rheumatol (Suppl) 51:122–124, 1983 (review).

Kean, WF, Forestier, F, Kassam, Y, Buchanan, WW, and Rooney, PJ: The history of gold therapy in rheumatoid disease. Semin Arthritis Rheum 14(3):180–186, 1985 (review).

Schlumpf, U, Meyer, M, Ulrich, J, et al: Neurologic complications induced by gold treatment. Arthritis Rheum 26:825–831, 1983.

Souliere, CY: Home administration of gold therapy for rheumatoid arthritis. Home Health Nurse 3(4):28–32, 1985.

Immunoregulatory Drugs

Bookbinder, SA, Espinoza, LR, Fenske, NA, Germain, BF, and Vasey, FB: Methotrexate: Its use in the rheumatic diseases. Clin Exp Rheumatol 2(2):185–193, 1984 (review).

Clements, PJ, and Davis, J: Cytotoxic drugs: Their clinical application to the rheumatic diseases. Semin Arthritis Rheum 15(4):231–254, 1986 (review).

Furst, DE: Clinical pharmacology of very low dose methotrexate for use in rheumatoid arthritis. J Rheumatol 12 (Suppl 12):11–14, 1985 (review).

Groff, GD, Shenberger, KN, Wilke, WS, et al: Low dose oral methotrexate in rheumatoid arthritis: An uncontrolled trial and review of the literature. Semin Arthritis Rheum 12:333–347, 1983.

Healey, LA: The current status of methotrexate use in rheumatic diseases. Bull Rheumatic Dis 36(4):1–10, 1986.

Hollister, JR: Immunosuppressant therapy of juvenile rheumatoid arthritis. Arthritis Rheum 20 (2 Suppl):544–547, 1977.

Huskisson, EC: Axathioprine. Clin Rheum Dis 10:325–332, 1984.

Kremer, JM, and Lee, JK: The safety and efficacy of the use of methotrexate in the long-term therapy of rheumatoid arthritis. Arthritis Rheum 29:822–831, 1986.

Letendre, PW, DeJong, DJ, and Miller, DR: The use of methotrexate in rheumatoid arthritis. Drug Intell Clin Pharm 19(5):349–358, 1985.

Miller, DR, Letendre, PW, DeJong, DJ, and Fiechtner, JJ: Methotrexate in rheumatoid arthritis: An update. Pharmacotherapy 6(4):170–178, 1986 (review).

Truckenbrodt, H, and Hafner, R: Methotrexate therapy in juvenile rheumatoid arthritis: A retrospective study. Arthritis Rheum 29:801–807, 1986.

Weinblatt, ME: Toxicity of low dose methotrexate in rheumatoid arthritis. J Rheumatol 12 (Suppl 12):35–39, 1985 (review).

Corticosteroids

Gray, RG, Tenenbaum, J, and Gottlieb, NL: Local corticosteroid injection treatment in rheumatic disorders. Semin Arthritis Rheum 12:231–254, 1981.

Lockie, LM, Gomez, E, and Smith, DM: Low dose adrenocorticosteroids in the management of elderly patients with rheumatoid arthritis: Selected examples and summary of efficacy in the long-term treatment of 97 patients. Semin Arthritis Rheum 12:373–382, 1983.

McDonough, AL: Effects of corticosteroids on articular cartilage: A review of the literature. Phys Ther 62(6):835–839, 1982.

Nahata, MC: Corticosteroids and NSAIDs in rheumatoid arthritis (continuing education credit). J Pract Nurs 36(1):17–23, 1986.

Drug Therapy Related to Child-Bearing

Blau, SP: Metabolism of gold during lactation. Arthritis Rheum 16:777–778, 1973.

Needs, CJ, and Brooks, PM: Antirheumatic medication in pregnancy. Br J Rheumatol 24(3):282–290, 1985 (review).

Needs, CJ, and Brooks, PM: Antirheumatic medication during lactation. Br Rheumatol 23(3):291–297, 1985 (review).

Ostensen, M, and Husby, G: Antirheumatic drug treatment during pregnancy and lactation. Scand J Rheumatol 14(1):1–7, 1985.

Ostensen, M, Aune, B, and Husby, G: Effect of pregnancy and hormonal changes on the activity of rheumatoid arthritis. Scand J Rheumatol 12:69–72, 1983.

Rao, JM: Drugs and breast feeding: Avoiding complications. Curr Ther 25:55–58, 1984.

Drug Therapy for the Elderly

Brooks, PM, Kean, WF, Kassam, Y, and Buchanan, WW: Problems of antiarthritic therapy in the elderly. J Am Geriatr Soc 32(3):229–234, 1984 (review).

Pfeiffer, RF: Drugs for pain in the elderly. Geriatrics 37(2):67–69, 73, 76, 1982.

Todd, B: Drugs and the elderly: For arthritis—plain aspirin or an aspirin alternative? Geriatr Nurs (New York) 3(3):191–194, 1982.

PART II

MAJOR RHEUMATIC DISEASES

This section reviews the signs and symptoms of the most common rheumatic diseases. The presentation of the diseases in this section has been ordered roughly on the basis of their incidence in the adult population. The high frequency of rheumatoid arthritis in occupational therapy clinics frequently makes this disease appear to be far more common than it is in the total scheme of rheumatic disorders.

This section can be used as a resource for the clinician new to treating these diseases. That is, the chapters provide a succinct overview correlating disease treatment to clinical manifestations. For example, if you have never treated a person with systemic lupus erythematosus and you receive a referral that reads "Jane Smith, Dx: SLE. Evaluate and treat," Chapter 9, which deals with this topic, was written for you.

I highly recommend that all therapists read Chapter 4 on osteoarthritis and Chapter 5 on fibromyalgia to become familiar with detecting and treating these two conditions. Osteoarthritis occurs in people with other rheumatic diseases, such as rheumatoid arthritis, with the same incidence that it occurs in the general population. Frequently many of the problems one encounters in an older person with a primary diagnosis of rheumatoid arthritis, ankylosing spondylitis, or polymyalgia rheumatica are due to osteoarthritis. Typically the osteoarthritis is not listed as a secondary diagnosis because it is often asymptomatic. Fibromyalgia is also a common condition, and people with a chronic illness are at high risk for developing it. In fact, it is not uncommon for a person with rheumatoid arthritis to have joint involvement that is well controlled or in remission and have fibromyalgia as the predominant problem. In addition, the symptoms of fibromyalgia can easily be mistaken for carpal tunnel syndrome, radiculitis, or tendinitis. It is critical that therapists be able to differentiate the symptoms of osteoarthritis and fibromyalgia from other primary diagnoses.

The chapters on osteoarthritis and rheumatoid arthritis are relevant solely to adults. The other chapters originally written for treatment of adults have been edited and revised to include relevance to children.

Chapter 4

Osteoarthritis (Degenerative Joint Disease)

Osteoarthritis (OA) refers to disorders of the joints characterized by deterioration of the articular cartilage and secondary new bone formation. Onset is noninflammatory but secondary inflammation is common. Typically the disease is slowly progressive, but OA can have remissions and cartilage regeneration.[1]

ETIOLOGICAL FACTORS AND AGE AND SEX AFFECTED

OA is viewed as a disease of the cartilage that can be initiated by genetic, metabolic, systemic, and traumatic factors. It is likely that no single one of these processes can be the cause of OA. Like other rheumatic diseases, it results from a combination of factors.[2]

OA is *no longer* considered a part of aging or simply a "wear-and-tear" process. Some researchers believe that OA is due to a physiological imbalance between the stress applied to a joint and the ability of the physiological shock absorbers, soft tissue, cartilage, and bone to deal successfully with the stress of loading.[2,3] This theory is supported in large part by the fact that OA tends to start as a focal process in the joint at the point of habitual loading, surrounded by healthy cartilage. This also explains how diametrically opposed forces such as excessive weight-bearing and immobilization can trigger OA.[2]

Osteoarthritis is classified as primary, secondary, or spinal.

Primary Osteoarthritis

Three major subsets have been identified so far in this category.[2,4,5]

1. OA confined to the distal interphalangeal (DIP) and proximal interphalangeal (PIP) joints (with the Heberden's and Bouchard's nodes): This is the most common form of OA. It may be asymptomatic or produce deformity, stiffness, and occasional pain. It is generally not very disabling.[5,6]

2. Generalized primary OA: This is considered hereditary and occurs in women more than in men. It affects the hands in the classic distribution: DIP, PIP, and carpometacarpal (CMC) joints, and occasion-

---

Table 4–1 Classification of Osteoarthrosis

Primary
  A. Idiopathic
  B. Primary Generalized Osteoarthrosis
  C. Erosive Osteoarthrosis

Secondary
  A. Congenital or Developmental Defects
      Hip dysplasias
      Shallow acetabulum
      Morquio's syndrome
      Legg-Calvé-Perthes disease
      Slipped capital femoral epiphysis
      Femoral neck abnormalities
      Primary protrusio acetabuli
      Multiple epiphyseal dysplasia
      Osteochondritides
  B. Traumatic
      Acute
      Chronic
      Charcot's arthropathy
  C. Inflammatory
      Rheumatoid arthritis
      Psoriatic arthritis
      Reiter's disease
      Septic arthritis (bacterial and tuberculous)
      Recurrent gout or pseudogout
      Chronic inflammatory bowel disease and arthritis
  D. Endocrine Diseases and Their Influence
      Acromegaly
      Diabetes
      Sex hormone abnormalities
      Iatrogenic hypercortisonism
      Hypothyroidism with myxedema
  E. Metabolic
      Gout
      Hemochromatosis
      Ochronosis
      Chondrocalcinosis
      Paget's disease

From Bland, JH, and Stulberg, SD: Osteoarthritis: Pathology and clinical patterns. In Kelly, WN, Harris, ED, Ruddy, S, and Sledge, CB (eds): Textbook of Rheumatology. WB Saunders, Philadelphia, 1985, with permission.

ally the scaphotrapezoid joint; the knees; and the great toe (first metatarsophalangeal [MTP] joint). The course may be asymptomatic for years until there is an acute episode of inflammation or severe cartilage loss and mechanical pain.

3. Erosive OA: This appears as a form of severe inflammatory OA of the DIP and PIP joints. It differs from the subset listed as 1, above, in that there is a proliferative synovitis, severe cartilage destruction, bony erosions, ankylosis, and marked deformity. Rheumatoid factor is negative, and sedimentation rate is often normal. Some clinicians believe that this is distinct from both OA and rheumatoid arthritis (RA). Others believe that it represents a variant of seronegative RA superimposed over pre-existing OA.[7,8]

Secondary Osteoarthritis

If the etiological factors of cartilage destruction are known, the term **secondary OA** is applicable. OA can occur in adolescents and adults secondary to congenital defects, trauma, inflammation, endocrine and metabolic diseases, and occupational use (see Table 4–1). There is no typical distribution because the involvement of joints depends on the underlying causative factors. However, weight-bearing joints are the most frequently involved.[2]

Osteoarthritis of the Spine

OA of the spine occurs in two distinct articular systems: the posterior diarthrodial (apophyseal) joints and the intervertebral discs (spondylosis).[2,5]

OA of the apophyseal facet joints is often referred to as **spinal OA** and is similar to OA of other diarthrodial joints. It is characterized by cartilage degeneration (joint space narrowing), cyst formation, sclerosis, and osteophyte formation. Osteophytosis can narrow the neural foramina and the vertebral artery foramina in the cervical spine.[2,4]

Involvement of the intervertebral fibrocartilage discs is more properly referred to as **spondylosis,** or discogenic disease of the spine. This typically results in narrowing of the disc, decreased resilience, and flexibility of the disc, reducing its shock-absorbing properties and osteophytosis around the body of the vertebrae.[2] When the intervertebral discs degenerate, osteophytes are formed from the involved vertebrae, probably as an ineffective effort at repair of the damaged discs. This leads to the typical radiological appearance of disc space narrowing in the presence of osteophytes.

The most common sites of involvement are the areas of the spine that receive the most stress from movement, that is, the fifth to eighth cervical and the fourth lumbar to the first sacral vertebrae. Some degree of spondylosis of the spine occurs in everyone over the age of 40 years.[2]

DIAGNOSIS

The diagnosis of primary OA is made clinically by the presence of bony enlargement around the involved joints and the classical distribution of the involvement. Secondary OA and OA of the spine are diagnosed on the basis of radiographic evidence of characteristic cartilage loss and osteophyte formation.

COURSE AND PROGNOSIS

Symptoms do not necessarily correlate with the degree of radiological involvement of the joints. For example, a person can have severe radiographic changes in the joint and have no pain or discomfort. Likewise, another person can have only minor changes in radiographic readings but be disabled by pain. In general, prognosis for functional use is excellent for the upper extremity and back, fair for the knees, and poor for the hips.[9] Some people have a totally asymptomatic course throughout their lives. Others are asymptomatic at the start, then develop an acute bout of inflammation (often related to excessive joint stress), and go on to an episodic symptomatic course. Exercise, weight loss, diet, medications, improved posture, and altering functional use patterns can influence disease course.[1]

OA was once thought to be an unrelenting, progressive disease. There is now evidence that in some people with secondary OA, the disease can go into remission and that the cartilage can actually remodel and regenerate cartilage, which is a combination of hyaline and fibrocartilage, during periods of remission.[1,2]

SYMPTOMATOLOGY AND IMPLICATIONS FOR OCCUPATIONAL THERAPY

General Symptoms of all Forms of Osteoarthritis

Symptoms are common to all forms of OA and may occur in any combination or be concurrent. They include (1) joint pain with secondary muscle spasm and muscle inhibition; (2) aching during cold weather (considered a response to the change in barometric pressure); (3) stiffness after prolonged (15 to 30 minutes) static positioning (this is usually not as pronounced as in rheumatoid arthritis); (4) crepitation upon motion; (5) limited joint motion and joint deformity caused by osteophyte formation (bony enlargement); (6) muscle weakness and atrophy as a result of disuse; and (7) joint effusions, which are usually minimal, but can be severe.[2]

Therapy

Treatment goals are to assess functional ability in order to eliminate aggravating factors; to reduce stiffness, pain, and inflammation; to maintain range of motion (ROM); to maintain or increase muscle strength; to reduce joint stress; and to increase functional independence.[4,9,10] Treatment methods are the same as for noninflammatory joint disease and are outlined in Chapter 1. The discussion in Chapter 1 was written to be used as a companion piece to this chapter.

Primary Osteoarthritis

Typically the finger DIP and PIP joints and the thumb CMC joint are involved. Less frequently the scaphotrapezoid is also involved. Treatment of joints other than the thumb and fingers is discussed in this chapter under Secondary Osteoarthritis and Osteoarthritis of the Spine.

Fingers

The DIP joints are most commonly affected; the PIP joints are affected to a lesser degree. Deforming bony protuberances, osteophytes, on the margins and dorsal surfaces of the DIP joints **(Heberden's nodes)** and PIP joints **(Bouchard's nodes)** are characteristic, and therefore diagnostic, of primary OA.

In primary OA the process of **cartilage degeneration** and **osteophytosis** may cause mild stiffness or decreased ROM but is generally painless. In the hand, pain is primarily associated with inflammation even if there are no other signs, such as swelling, redness, or warmth. Mechanical pain due to impingement or stretch of the capsule or presence on subchondral bone can occur during specific movements or at the end of range. Persistent pain or aching is associated with inflammation. The inflammation associated with primary OA is generally milder than that seen with RA and is less responsive to thermal modalities. However, acute episodes with swelling and warmth may respond to cold applications. In the PIP and DIP joints, mild or even moderate inflammation is generally not responsive to orthotic immobilization, but occasionally severe acute inflammation will respond to this method of treatment.

In OA of the hands without inflammation, ROM essentially becomes limited for one reason only; that is, osteophytes blocking mobility. Loss of flexion is due to volar osteophytes. Loss of extension is due to dorsal osteophytes. Lateral deviation deformity can result from unilateral cartilage degeneration or osteophyte formation. In the presence of noninflammatory primary OA (excluding erosive OA) alone, people do not develop joint contractures due to swelling, soft tissue limitations, or tendon involvement. People generally use their full available ROM during hand function except as limited by bony block. ROM lag is not associated with this condition. For this reason, exercises for *maintaining or increasing ROM* are simply not needed or are of no value because they cannot change or alter available motion. Limbering exercises, such as squeezing a Nerf ball in warm water in the morning, can be quite helpful as a flexibility exercise for decreasing stiffness.

When significant inflammation is present, the patient may not use the joint through full ROM, or swelling or pain may prevent full ROM, resulting in contracture of the collateral ligaments or capsule. Patients should be taught early that if they lose mobility during a flare-up, they should see a therapist to regain it when the inflammation subsides.

When the DIP joints have chronic pain or develop severe flexion or angulation deformity, arthrodesis in about 5-degree flexion can provide an effective functional and cosmetic solution. For severe pain or deformity of one or two PIP joints, an implant arthroplasty is a possible solution. If a person does physically hard work, arthrodesis of the index finger PIP joint in 20- to 40-degree flexion may be the preferred operation with implant arthroplasty of the remaining PIP joints. (See Chapter 29.)

The MCP joints and extensor mechanisms seldom are involved; therefore, it is not associated with ulnar drift. However, it is possible to have a swan-neck deformity result from imbalance created by a mallet deformity secondary to OA of the DIP joint.

Therapy

For Pain and Inflammation

1. For acute inflammation of an isolated DIP joint, a thermoplastic cylinder orthotic is a feasible solution. For some it works well; for others it does nothing.

2. When one or two PIP joints are involved, a cylinder orthotic may help if the imposed limitation to function is tolerable. For some patients, cutting a digit sleeve off a thermoelastic glove (Futuro brand), hemming the ends, and wearing it over the PIP joint as a sleeve can be useful in two ways. First, it provides warmth, which increases circulation and helps decrease inflammation, pain, and stiffness. Second, it provides a reminder to "go easy" when using the digit, which decreases joint stress. Again, this does not work for everyone.

3. In OA of the digit, heat is generally more effective than cold for decreasing discomfort even when overt inflammation is present. If heat is not helpful, cold (e.g., an ice water soak for 2 to 3 minutes) should be tried.

4. Joint protection consists of "going easy" on the joint and avoiding forceful use. This is often accomplished by adapting handles. (See Chapters 24 and 25.)

For Stiffness

1. Digit stiffness is usually greatest in the morning. Squeezing a soft sponge or Nerf ball in or under warm water in the bathroom sink is a helpful flexibility exercise.

2. If excessive stiffness limits functional ability, I recommend a trial of using Futuro thermoelastic gloves at night. (I find them more effective than Isotoner gloves, although for some patients any type of stretch gloves will work.)[11-13] *Note:* Since OA is usually a bilateral condition there is an opportunity for the patient to apply the above treatments to one hand and use the other as control. This way the patient can tell if the treatment actually works. Treatment for OA is only of value if it gets results. Therapists need to be very clear in their instruction about the rationale and goals for each treatment.

For Limited Flexion

When limited flexion reduces functional ability, the only solution is to build up handles so the person can apply power within his or her available range. (See Chapter 25, Assistive Devices.)

Thumbs

The first CMC joint is the most common site of involvement and may be the first or only symptomatic joint. In a review of 200 thumbs with OA *selected for surgery*, Swanson and de Groot-Swanson found significant involvement of all four trapezium joints: trapezium–first metacarpal (CMC) joint, 100 percent; trapezium–second metacarpal joint, 86 percent; trapezio-scaphoid, 48 percent; and trapeziotrapezoid, 35 percent.[14] **Pan-trapezial arthritis** refers to involvement of all four joints.

The thumb is responsible for 45 percent of hand function.[15] Consequently the highly versatile and mobile CMC joint is subject to considerable occupational stress over a lifetime. Early signs and symptoms include tenderness, aching, throbbing, and crepitation. There can also be swelling, redness, and warmth. Stiffness is generally not a common complaint related to the CMC joint, possibly because the CMC joint has a limited arc of motion. The disease can progress to instability, decreased retroversion, decreased retroversion or extension, decreased strength, and subluxation or adduction contracture. The joint tends to sublux in a radial–proximal direction producing a characteristic "**squaring**" of the joint.[14] An adduction contracture of the CMC joint can result in a secondary hyperextension or lateral deviation deformity of the thumb MCP joint. Symptoms of CMC joint arthritis are aggravated by repetitive pinch, grasp, or wringing prehension activities and nonprehension application of force with the heel of the hand or thenar area.

If chronic pain persists despite orthotics, medications, and other conservative measures, or if deformity limits function, surgery may be indicated. There are several surgical options for OA of the CMC joint, including resection arthroplasty either of the trapeziometacarpal joint with or without a condylar implant, or of the entire trapezium with a trapezium implant.[14] This is a rapidly advancing area of surgery. Surgical techniques are improving continually so patients are often advised to wait for the surgery if at all possible. (See Chapter 29.)

Pain associated with inflammation can radiate distally down the thumb or proximally up the forearm. These symptoms can be easily confused with those of **de-Quervain's tenosynovitis** of the first dorsal compartment. Therapists should be certain that the problem is in the CMC joint before fabricating orthotics. The orthotics used for these two conditions are completely different. (See Chapter 23.) The "**grind test**" is a specific test for localizing pain or crepitus to the CMC joint. The adapted **Finklestein test** is specific for localizing pain in the first dorsal tendon compartment. (See Chapter 19.)

Apprehension of pain during functional activities can result in muscular guarding that extends up the entire extremity into the neck. About one-third of the patients referred to our center for CMC orthoses have neck tension or aching secondary to muscular guarding of the limb to protect the thumb.

Therapy
For Pain and Inflammation
1. A CMC–MCP joint immobilization thermoplastic orthosis that provides a C-bar (to maintain the web space) but allows full interphalangeal (IP) joint and wrist mobility is preferred.[11] (See Chapter 23 for wearing instructions.)

2. If there is swelling and warmth, ice packs are usually effective. Inflammation of the CMC joint differs from that of the PIP and DIP joints in that repetitive trauma seems to be a frequent initiating event. Also, the CMC joint area is not as sensitive to cold as the fingertips are and therefore tolerates it better.

3. Provide instruction in relaxation techniques for the entire extremity. Patients need to be taught to relax and let the orthosis do the work.

4. Assess the daily activities that aggravate the joint and provide instruction in adaptive methods or assistive devices that can reduce stress to the joint.

   a. In addition to pinch activities, applying pressure with the heel of the hand, such as squeezing oranges or stapling, can cause direct trauma to the joint.

   b. The aggravating factor may not be the activity itself but the force and tension with which it is carried out. Some people hold a pen lightly, some very tightly, but they all write. People, especially women with CMC joint arthritis, may need to learn how to accomplish activities with a lighter touch.

Secondary Osteoarthritis

The weight-bearing joints (spine, knees, hips, and ankles) are the most common sites of involvement, but any joint can be involved secondary to trauma, stress, or infection.[2,16]

Knees

The knees are the most common site of secondary OA. In the early stages, pain may be present only when bearing weight or climbing stairs. Again, the course may be asymptomatic or have episodic bouts of acute inflammation with mild to severe effusions. Chronic inflammation increases the risk of ligamentous instability, which allows greater forces to occur in the joint during ambulation.[2] Associated spasm of the knee flexors and inhibition of the extensors interfere with ambulation and encourage knee flexion contractures.

OA primarily affects the medial compartment so progressive loss of cartilage and ligamentous laxity typically result in a varus (bow-legged) deformity. Valgus deformity is less common but can occur, whereas valgus deformity and lateral compartment involvement are more the rule in RA.[16,17] When severe deformity develops or inflammation persists despite adequate medical management, surgical options include osteotomy and parital or total joint replacement. (See Chapter 34, Knee Surgery.)

In a young or middle-aged person with early signs of OA in the knee, it is critical that posture alignment, gait, and foot alignment be analyzed as contributing to pressure forces in the knee. Often physical therapy or foot orthotics can correct faulty alignment and prevent stress on the joint. (See Chapter 24.)

Some people walk hard, others walk lightly, but they all get to their destination. Altering the forces on the knees may require changing the way a person walks rather than limiting his or her walking. Discrepancy of leg lengths can also be an aggravating factors for OA of the knee. If this is suspected, appropriate referral should be made to correct length difference with shoe lifts.

Therapy

The incorporation of **work-simplification** methods to minimize ambulation and motion and the use of elevated chairs and joint protection principles to minimize stress and pain are priority treatment objectives.[4,18]

Patient education is a crucial issue. Many people have misconceptions about what to do for their arthritis. The classic example of this is the patient with OA of the knees who continues, by choice, to live in an upstairs apartment because he believes that climbing the stairs three of four times a day will keep his legs strong. In fact, this will wear down the cartilage. There are non-weight-bearing ways, such as isometric exercise, to keep leg muscles strong.[11] If obesity is an aggravating factor, it is important to reinforce diet planning. If the patient lacks nutritional knowledge, refer him or her to a dietitian or community weight-control program when possible.

The use of a cane is a valuable aid for reducing stress to a knee. The cane should be used in the hand *opposite* the involved knee. Patients who have difficulty ambulating should be counseled on how to adapt their home to reduce architectural barriers and reduce safety hazards.[18,19] (See the section on home assessment in Chapter 22.)

Patients with knee involvement are seen in physical therapy for modalities to decrease inflammation (e.g., ice, phonophoresis), gait training, and muscle strengthening. Joint protection, positioning, and exercise are the same for OA as for other types of arthritis and are reviewed in the specific chapters for these topics in Part V.

Hips

Hip involvement is common, and severe involvement affects women almost twice as often as men.[20] Hip involvement is more frequently unilateral than bilateral. Eighty percent of the cases are considered secondary to congenital defects in the hip (i.e., hip dysplasia).[2] Abnormal alignment alters the shape of growing cartilage, producing incongruent surfaces that ultimately wear unevenly. The most typical situation is for mild **dysplasia** to go undetected until OA sets in in the fourth, fifth, or sixth decade. Children in whom severe dysplasia was not detected until age 2 or 3 years may develop severe OA during the teens or early twenties. Slipped capital femoral epiphysis can occur in children ages 10 to 15 years, resulting in secondary OA in the fifth or sixth decade.[2,20] **Legg-Calvé-Perthes disease**, or avascular necrosis of the proximal capital femoral epiphysis, is another condition in childhood that can result in OA in adulthood. (This disease primarily affects boys 4 to 8 years of age.[2])

The initial symptoms of OA of the hip may be limited ROM or stiffness. Pain typically occurs in the groin or inguinal area but can refer to the lateral buttock or proximal thigh or distal thigh–knee region. Pain over the trochanteric area, especially upon rising or stair climbing, usually indicates trochanteric bursitis. Early in the disease course the hip may be pain free in flexion but painful during extension or rotation. Internal rotation is the first motion lost, followed by loss of extension, abduction, and flexion. With disease progression, there is a concentric loss of motion. Loss of motion is due to osteophytosis limiting range rather than to soft tissue or muscular contractures, which occur secondary to the joint limitation.

Hip *flexion* contractures will alter the person's ability to stand straight or require the person to keep his knees bent to compensate for hip angle, thereby promoting knee flexion contractures.[9,16] Hip *extension* contractures are a greater functional limitation than flexion contractures. A person who can flex his or her hip to only 60 degrees (from neutral) will not be able to sit straight in a regular chair. Hip flexion less than 90 degrees can also cause excessive pressure against the spine when the person attempts to sit in a straight-back chair. (This can be a source of complaints of lower back pain in patients with OA of the hip.) Also, lack of hip flexion can cause the patient to drop into a chair rather than to sit down, causing additional stress to the spine and hip. Hip *adduction* contractures (limited abduction) are also of frequent consequence. For women, adduction contractures can seriously interfere with feminine hygiene and positioning during sexual intercourse.[21,22]

Discrepancy in leg length can influence hip involvement. Referral for evaluation and possible shoe lift correction are indicated if there is a discrepancy.[16] Progression of severe disease results in cartilage loss and reduces the actual leg length. The femur may sublux upward and lateral into the acetabulum, referred to as **protrusio acetabuli.** Loss of leg length reduces the efficiency of the hip extensor–abductor muscles. This, combined with decreased motion, results in rapid atrophy of these muscles as well as the quadriceps muscles (from lack of use). These limitations result in either an antalgic gait with the trunk lurching to the affected side or a Trendelenburg gait with pelvis dropping on the opposite side during the stance phase.[4]

For the older patient age 65 years plus with severe OA, especially sedentary people, the total hip arthroplasty has made an enormous difference in their functional ability. For the patient younger than 65 years of age, especially active men with monoarticular disease, the surgery of choice has been an osteotomy. If only the painful joint was replaced, the men tended to become too active (e.g., they resumed playing tennis) and the cemented replace-

ments began to loosen and fail. The advent of the new cementless total hip replacements provides new options, especially for the younger, more vigorous patient. (See Chapter 33.)

Therapy

Work-simplification and joint-protection methods to minimize ambulation, standing, and stress are priority treatment objectives.[10]

Lying prone daily is an important adjunct to maintenance of ROM of the hip, ideally for two 30-minute periods per day.[4] However, if there is also back involvement, see Chapters 24 and 28 for back-protection methods in joint-protection and positioning methods before advising the patient to lie prone. Use of a cane also can greatly reduce the amount of stress to an affected joint.[4,23]

Hip involvement often limits ability for transfer, lower extremity dressing, and perineal care. (See Chapter 25, Assistive Devices, for solutions to common problems.) When hip involvement interferes with sexual activities, the patient should be referred to a staff member knowledgeable in sexual counseling to discuss alternative positioning methods that minimize stress.[24–27] Elderly patients should not be left out of this process.[26]

Lack of hip flexion necessitates specially designed chairs or seats (including toilet seats) that will allow the patient to sit upright with less than a 90-degree flexion. (See Chapter 25, Assistive Devices, for solutions to common problems.)

If there is a decrease in ambulation status and the patient needs to use a crutch, walker, or wheelchair, it is important that the patient receive training in how to do daily activities with the required ambulation aids. Also, patients with thumb adduction contractures secondary to OA may require an adapted (narrowed or padded) crutch or cane handle to prevent thumb pain or allow a secure grip.

Ankles

Involvement of the ankle is fairly rare, and the role of occupational therapy is minimal. Polyethylene molded supports (UC-BL support), short leg braces, and ambulation aids may be prescribed. Ambulation should be minimized. Counseling on work-simplification methods to reduce ambulation may be indicated.

Shoulders

OA of the shoulder occurs in only about 5 percent of all patients with painful shoulder conditions. The majority of shoulder problems (85 percent) are the result of periarticular involvement (e.g., tendinitis, bursitis, rotator cuff tears, and adhesive capsulitis).[28]

Therapy

Occupational therapy for shoulder conditions consists of a combination of joint-protection methods designed to eliminate unnecessary shoulder motion or stress and activities planned to maintain strength of shoulder muscles and increase ROM in joints. Relaxation training using biofeedback is extremely helpful for reducing muscular tension and pain.

Codman exercises are recommended when a painful shoulder condition severely limits shoulder motion.[28] In these exercises the patient bends from the waist, allowing gravity to assist shoulder flexion to 90 degrees.[29] It is important that effective ROM be done in the acute stages to avoid shortening of the inferior aspect of the capsule and **frozen shoulder syndrome**. If a patient has **subacromion bursitis**, *exercises such as wall walking and finger ladder climbing are contraindicated since active flexion or abduction against gravity only causes greater impingement of the subacromion bursa.*[28] Also during acute flares of bursitis, ice compresses are more effective than heat for reducing swelling and pain.[30]

Treatment should not be narrowly focused on the shoulder joint but should take into consideration the entire body, as the shoulder is the intersection of the musculature of the spine, trunk, and upper extremity. This is often best done in physical therapy using whole-body, hands-on techniques.

Elbows and Wrists

Actual OA of these joints is rare. Elbow pain frequently is due to inflammation at the point of origin of the extensor muscles (lateral epicondylitis, tennis elbow) or flexor muscles (medial epicondylitis, golfer's elbow) rather than a result of OA.

Therapy

Evaluation of self-care or occupational tasks that aggravate affected muscles is an essential part of therapy. Treatment includes (1) instruction in joint (tendon) protection and work simplification; (2) training in performing the activity without stress to the involved muscles; and (3) if there is pain over the muscle origins upon resistance to wrist extension or flexion, application of a rigid wrist orthosis may be effective in resting the flexor and extensor muscles and to promote healing. (It must totally limit both flexion and extension.) *It is important that patients be taught to relax into the orthosis and let it do the work.* (4) If the source of aggravating stress is a twisting wrist motion, a leather or canvas wrist gauntlet orthotic may be sufficient by preventing circumduction but allowing flexion and extension.

Osteoarthritis of the Spine (Spondylosis)

The process of OA is the same throughout the spine. The entire spine is an integral unit. The concept of treating the neck or back as separate entities is fallacious because they cannot be separated and must be treated as a unit.

OA of the spine involves both the hyaline cartilage of the apophyseal joints (spinal OA) and the fibrocartilage of the discs (spondylosis)—two distinct articular systems. Degeneration of the disc results in diminished resilience and capacity to respond to physical stress and diminution in height (disc space narrowing). This reduces the distance between the vertebrae, diminishing the flexibility of the spine. Osteophytosis around the body of the vertebrae further limits flexibility of the spine with bony block. This degeneration of the discs is often referred to as **spondylosis.**[2,5]

OA in the apophyseal joints of the spine is similar to that of the peripheral diarthrodial joints, with cartilage degeneration, cyst formation, fibrosis, and osteophytosis. Involvement of these joints is often referred to as **spinal OA.** The osteophytes may narrow the neural foramina and compress the nerve roots as they exit from the spinal cord (radiculopathy), producing pain and sensory changes or loss. Motor impairment is less common but can occur as a result of OA. In the cervical spine, osteophytes may also encroach upon the foramina through which the vetebral artery travels.[1,2,5]

Involvement of both articular systems is most common in the lower cervical spine and the lower lumbar spine. In women, OA of the mid-thoracic area around T10 at the level of the brassiere line seems to be a common phenomenon that is seldom discussed in the literature.

Symptoms of OA in the spine include stiffness, especially after sleeping or prolonged static positioning; decreased range of motion; pain, especially acute, indicating inflammation in the absence of nerve compression; and muscle tightness and spasm.[2]

Most people with OA have postural or alignment problems that contribute to stress to the involved area. Physical therapy for assessment, strengthening, postural improvement, and reduction of muscle spasm and pain and muscular imbalance is a critical part of therapy for OA of the spine.[31]

Therapy

Assessment

1. Occupational use that aggravates the involved area.[32,33] See Chapter 22 for evaluation of activities of daily living and vocational assessment.
2. Posture during reading, writing, driving, watching television, work, and recreation.[32–34]
3. Muscular tension or emotional stress during an activity that may contribute to pain and muscle spasm. This may be done with or without electromyographic (EMG) biofeedback instrumentation.[34]
4. Sensorimotor evaluation if neurologic signs are present.
5. Sleep posture and type of pillow and mattress used. (See Chapters 24 and 28 on joint protection and positioning.)

Treatment

1. Instruction on how to incorporate postural recommendations into daily activities.

2. Instruction in joint protection and energy conservation. (See section on Back and Neck Protection Methods in Chapter 24.)
3. Fabrication of semirigid Plastazote neck collars if commercial collars are not effective.
4. Assessment and instruction in how to adapt daily activities to accommodate cervical collars.
5. Instruction in adapted methods and assistive equipment to encourage correct posture or compensate for loss of ROM. (See Chapter 25, Assistive Devices.)
6. Fabrication of lumbar supports with thermoplastic inserts. Instruction in adaptive corset or brace dressing techniques.
7. Instruction in relaxation techniques.
8. Coordination of Occupational Therapy and Physical Therapy.

The sleep position and type of pillow that a patient uses at night can have a strong influence on neck pain and stiffness. Patients with cervical arthritis should not sleep on their stomachs, since this position requires prolonged positioning at the extreme of range. If a patient complains of greater neck pain at night or upon awakening than during the day it may be due to the type of pillow he or she is using. When a person uses a regular pillow the shoulders and occipital area of the head are supported. This positioning causes a flattening of the normal lordotic curve of the cervical spine and places stress on the cervical joints and ligaments. A pillow that supports the neck in a normal lordotic curve and provides support to the cervical muscles can be very effective in reducing muscle spasm and associated pain and stiffness.[32]

The Jackson Cervipillo was designed for this purpose.[32] A survey of patient response to using the pillow revealed that the majority of patients found the pillow reduced symptoms. Of the 50 patients surveyed, 31 returned the questionnaires. Of those who responded, 30 stated that the pillow was beneficial and 13 of these 30 rated their pain as severe with a regular pillow and minimal to absent with the Cervipillo.[36]

Not all patients need a special pillow. Some patients may be attaining sufficient support with a soft feather pillow that they can shape around the neck. Also the Cervipillo is not effective for all patients. Compliance appears to be the highest when the concept of cervical support is explained to the patient and the patient determines to try the pillow on an experimental basis.[36]

DRUG THERAPY

Aspirin or acetaminophen in analgesic doses (650 mg every 4 to 6 hours) is often sufficient for symptomatic relief of stiffness, aching, and mild pain. If pain persists or there are frank signs of inflammation, nonsteroidal anti-inflammatory drugs (NSAIDs) or intra-articular corticosteroid injections may be beneficial. All of the NSAIDs have been shown effective for treating the symptoms of OA. Aspirin in anti-inflammatory doses may be used but hearing loss (**ototoxicity**) may occur with even low doses in the elderly. Indomethacin is often particularly effective in relieving pain related to OA of the hips, shoulders, and knees, but it has a greater number of side effects than the other NSAIDs. (See Chapter 3 for precautions and side effects of specific drugs.) Disease-modifying drugs, immunosuppressive drugs, and systemic corticosteroids are *contraindicated* in the treatment of OA.

REFERENCES

1. Bland, JH, and Cooper, SM: Osteoarthritis: A review of the cell biology involved and evidence for reversibility. Semin Arthritis Rheum 14(2):106–133, 1984.
2. Bland, JH, and Stulberg, SD: Osteoarthritis: Pathology and clinical patterns. In Kelley, WM, et al (eds): Textbook of Rheumatology, ed 2. WB Saunders, Philadelphia, 1985.
3. Radin, EL, et al: Mechanical aspects of osteoarthrosis. Bull Rheum Dis 26(7):862–865, 1975.
4. Robinson, WD: Management of degenerative joint disease. In Kelley, WM, et al (eds): Textbook of Rheumatology, ed 2. WB Saunders, Philadelphia, 1985.
5. Moskowitz, RW, Howell, D, Goldberg, UM, and Mankin, AH: Osteoarthritis: Diagnosis and Management. WB Saunders, Philadelphia, 1984.
6. Labi, M, and Gresham, GE: Hand function in osteoarthritis. Arch Phys Med Rehab 63:438–440, 1982.
7. Ehrlich, GE: Inflammatory osteoarthritis— The clinical syndrome. J Chronic Dis 25:317, 1972.
8. Peter, JB, Pearson, DM, and Marmur, C: Erosive osteoarthritis of the hands. Arthritis Rheum 9:365a, 1966.
9. Stevens, J: Osteoarthritis of the hip: A review with special considerations of the problem of bilateral malum coxae senilis. Clin Orthop 71:152, 1970.
10. Wickersham, B: Physical therapy management of the patient with DJD. Arthritis Foundation Newsletter, Vol 13, No 1, Spring, 1979.
11. Ehrlich, G, and DiPierro, AM: Stretch gloves: Nocturnal use to ameliorate morning stiffness in arthritic hands. Arch Phys Med Rehab 52:479, 1971.
12. Culic, DD, et al: Efficacy of compression gloves in rheumatoid arthritis. Am J Phys Med 58(6):278–284, December 1979.
13. Melvin, JL: Rheumatic Disease—Occupational Therapy and Rehabilitation. FA Davis, Philadelphia, 1977.
14. Swanson, AB, and de Groot-Swanson, G: Osteoarthritis in the hand. Clin Rheum Dis 11(2):393–420, 1985.
15. Swanson, AB, Goran-Hagert, C, and Swanson, G: Evaluation of impairment of hand function. In Hunter, JM, Schneider, LH, Macken, EJ, and Bell, JA (eds): Rehabilitation of the Hand. CV Mosby, St Louis, 1978.
16. Polley, HF, and Hunder, GG: Rheumatologic interviewing and physical examination of the joints. WB Saunders, Philadelphia, 1978. (Sections on evaluation of the shoulder, hand, and knee.)
17. Eyanson, S, and Brandt, KD: Osteoarthritis. Primary Care 11(2):259–269, 1984.
18. Haviland, N, and Jette, AM: Joint protection for osteoarthritis. Audiovisual program from the University of Michigan Media Library, G1302, Towsley Center, University of Michigan Medical Center, Ann Arbor, MI 48109. (Program includes booklet.)
19. Tillman, F, and Haviland, N: 602 Elm Street: Overcoming barriers to independence. Audiovisual program from the University of Michigan Media Library, G1302, Towsley Center, University of Michigan Medical Center, Ann Arbor, MI 48109. (Program includes booklet.)
20. Jerring, K: Osteoarthritis of the hip: Epidemiology and clinical role. Acta Orthop Scand 51(3):523–530, 1980.
21. Currey, HLF: Osteoarthritis of the hip joint and sexual activity. Ann Rheum Dis 29:488, 1970.
22. Todd, RC, Lightowler, CD, and Harris, J: Low fraction arthroplasty of the hip joint and sexual activity. Acta Orthop Scand 44(6):690, 1973.
23. Petty, B, and Harrison, S: Compliance with medical instruction. Audiovisual program from the University of Michigan Media Library, G1302, Towsley Center, University of Michigan Medical Center, Ann Arbor, MI 48109. (Program includes booklet and examples of using a cane and taking medications.)
24. Conine, TA, and Evans, JH: Sexual reactivation of chronically ill and disabled adults. J Allied Health 11(4):261–270, 1982.

25. Hamilton, A: Sexual problems in arthritis and allied conditions. Int Rehab Med 3(1):38–42, 1981.
26. Hobson, KG: The effects of aging on sexuality. Health Soc Work 9(1):25–35, 1984.
27. Richards, JS: Sex and arthritis. Sexual Disability 3:97–104, 1980.
28. Bland, JH, Merrit, JA, and Boushey, DR: The painful shoulder. Semin Arthritis Rheum 7(1):21, 1977.
29. Cailliet, R: Shoulder Pain. FA Davis, Philadelphia, 1964.
30. Rocks, JA: Intrinsic shoulder pain syndrome: Rationale for heating and cooling in treatment. Phys Ther 59(2):153, 1979.
31. Jackson, O (ed): Physical Therapy of the Geriatric Patient. Churchill Livingstone, New York, 1983.
32. Jackson, R: The Cervical Syndrome, ed. 4. Charles C Thomas, Springfield, IL, 1978.
33. Flower, A, Naxon, E, Jones, RE, and Mooney, V: An OT program for chronic back pain. Am J Occup Ther 35(4):243–248, 1981.
34. Cailliet, R: Neck and Arm Pain. FA Davis, Philadelphia, 1964.
35. Abildness, AH: Biofeedback strategies. Rockville, MD, American Occupational Therapy Association, 1982.
36. Melvin, JL: Cervical support pillow to reduce neck pain: Follow up survey of patient response. Paper presented at the AOTA Physical Disabilities Specialty Section Meeting, San Antonio, 1981.

ADDITIONAL SOURCES

Adler, S: Self care in the management of the degenerative knee joint. Physiotherapy (London) 71(2):58–60, 1985.
Affleck, A, Bianchi, E, Cleckely, M, Donaldson, K, McCormack, G, and Polon, J: Stress management as a component of occupational therapy in acute care settings. Occupational Therapy in Health Care 1(3), 1984.
Altman, RD: Review of ibuprofen for osteoarthritis. Am J Med 77(1A):10–18, 1984.
Bland, JH: Cervical spondylosis. In Roth, SH, et al: Rheumatic Therapeutics. New York, McGraw-Hill, 1985.
Bland, JH: The reversibility of osteoarthritis: A review. Am J Med 74(6A):16–26, 1983.
Bohannon, RW, and Gajdosik, RL: Spinal nerve root compression—some clinical implications. A review of the literature. Phys Ther 67(3):376–382, 1987 (review).
Bohlman, HH: Neck pain. In Nickel, VL (ed): Orthopedic Rehabilitation. Churchill Livingstone, New York, 1982, pp 467–480.
Capra, P, Mayer, TG, and Batchel, R: Adding psychological scales to your back pain assessment. J Musculosk Med 2(7):41–52, 1985.
Chamberlain, MA: Socio-economic effects and therapy in osteoarthrosis. Br J Rheum (London) 23(3):185, 1984.
Chamberlain, MA, Care, G, and Harfield, B: Physiotherapy in osteoarthrosis of the knees. A controlled trial of hospital versus home exercises. Int Rehab Med 4(2):101–106, 1982.

Cogen, L, Anderson, LG, and Phelps, P: Medical management of the painful shoulder. Bull Rheum Dis 32(6):54–58, 1982.
Cooke, TD: Pathogenetic mechanisms in polyarticular osteoarthritis. Clin Rheum Dis 11(2):203–238, 1985.
DeForge, BR, and Sobal, J: Psychological evaluation of well-being in the multidisciplinary assessment of osteoarthritis. Clin Ther 9 (Suppl B):43–52, 1986.
Dequeker, J: The relationship between osteoporosis and osteoarthritis. Clin Rheum Dis 11(2):271–296, 1985.
Downing, DS, and Weinstein, A: Ultrasound therapy of subacromial bursitis. A double blind trial. Phys Ther 66(2):194–199, 1986.
Gross, M: Psychosocial aspects of osteoarthritis: Helping patients cope. Health Soc Work 6(3):40–46, 1981.
Grosshandler, SL, Stratas, NE, Toomey, TC, and Gray, WF: Chronic neck and shoulder pain. Focusing on myofascial origins. Postgrad Med 77(3):149–151, 154–158, 1985.
Hess, EV, and Herman, JH: Cartilage metabolism and anti-inflammatory drugs in osteoarthritis. Am J Med 81(5B):36–43, 1986 (review).
Huskisson, EC, Doyle, DV, and Lanham, JG: Drug treatment of osteoarthritis. Clin Rheum Dis 11(2):421–431, 1985.
Jubb, RW: Therapeutic progress: Review XXV. Osteoarthritis—are we making progress? J Clin Pharmacol Ther 12(2):81–90, 1987 (review).
Keefe, FJ, Caldwell, DS, Queen, K, Gil, KM, et al: Osteoarthritic knee pain: A behavioral analysis. Pain 28(3):309–321, 1987.
Keefe, FJ, Caldwell, DS, Queen, KT, Gil, KM, et al: Pain coping strategies in osteoarthritis patients. J Consult Clin Psychol 55(2):208–212, 1987.
Krick, JP, Sobal, J, and DeForge, BR: Psychosocial aspects of the multidisciplinary assessment of osteoarthritis. Clin Ther 9 (Suppl B): 43–52, 1986.
LaBorde, JM, Dando, WA, and Powers, MJ: Influence of weather on osteoarthritics. Soc Sci Med 23 (6):549–554, 1986.
Lewis, RJ: Degenerative arthritis. In Nickel, VL (ed): Orthopedic Rehabilitation. Churchill Livingstone, New York, 1982, pp 515–524.
Loy, TT: Treatment of cervical spondylosis: Electro-acupuncture versus physiotherapy. Med J Aust (Sydney) 2(1):32–34, 1983.
Moldofsky, H, Lue, FA, and Saskin, P: Sleep and morning pain in primary osteoarthritis. J Rheumatol 14(1):124–128, 1987.
Moratz, V, Muncie, HL Jr, and Miranda-Walsh, H: Occupational management in the multidisciplinary assessment and management of osteoarthritis. Clin Ther 9 (Suppl B):24–29, 1986.
Muncie, HL Jr: Medical aspects of the multidisciplinary assessment and management of osteoarthritis. Clin Ther 9 (Suppl B):4–13, 1986.
Nitz, AJ: Physical therapy management of the shoulder. Phys Ther 66(12):1912–1919, 1986.
Peyron, JG: Osteoarthritis. The epidemiologic viewpoint. Clin Orthop (213):13–19, 1986 (review).
Peyron, JG: Review of the main epidemiologic-etiologic evidence that implies mechanical forces as factors in osteoarthritis. Eng Med 15(2):77–79, 1986.

Pipino, F, Patella, V, Bancale, R, and Moretti, B: The present day value of simple displacement osteotomy in surgical treatment of osteoarthritis of the hip. Orthopedics 9(10):1369–1378, 1986.

Pybus, PK: The control of pain and stiffness in the osteoarthritic hand (letter). S Afr Med J 59(15):514, 1981.

Quinet, RJ: Osteoarthritis: Increasing mobility and reducing disability. Geriatrics 41(2):36–50, 1986.

Randolph, JW: The Role of occupational therapy in back school. OT in Health Care 1(3), 1984.

Rydevik, B, Brown, MD, and Lundborg, G: Pathoanatomy and pathophysiology of nerve root compression. Spine 9(1):7–15, 1984.

Schank, JA, Herdman, SJ, and Bloyer, RG: Physical therapy in the multidisciplinary assessment and management of osteoarthritis. Clin Ther 9 (Suppl B):14–23, 1986.

Chapter 5

Fibromyalgia

Fibromyalgia is a syndrome of soft tissue rheumatism characterized by diffuse musculoskeletal aching, pain, and stiffness, accompanied by a nonrestorative sleep pattern, chronic fatigue, and increased tenderness at specific "tender points." Associated conditions include peripheral paresthesias, irritable bowel syndrome, headaches, and arthralgia (see Table 5–1).

ETIOLOGICAL AND EPIDEMIOLOGICAL FACTORS

Fibromyalgia is currently considered one of the most common forms of musculoskeletal pain. The incidence of fibromyalgia in outpatient rheumatology clinics has been assessed at 15 to 20 percent.[1,2] The prevalence in the community is not known. However, as physicians and the public become more familiar with this condition as a specific syndrome, undoubtedly its prevalence in rheumatology and general practice will increase. Some estimate that this syndrome is the second most common rheumatological condition after osteoarthritis. The highest incidence is in people between 40 and 60 years of age, although it can occur at any age including childhood.[2,3] Currently, it is estimated that fewer than 15 percent of all patients are men, creating approximately a 5:1 female-to-male ratio.[1,2]

Fibromyalgia can occur alone without associated disease or trauma; in these cases it is referred to as **primary fibromyalgia.**[4] It can also occur in conjunction with a wide variety of rheumatic, infectious, myopathic, endocrine, malignant, or depressive disorders (e.g., rheumatoid arthritis and hypothyroidism).[5,6] Fibromyalgia can occur in a person with any systemic disease that has fatigue as a prominent component (e.g., influenza).[5] (The associative relationship is not known and may be stress, sleep

Table 5-1 Misnomers of Fibromyalgia

The following terms have been used to describe the syndrome currently described as fibromyalgia:

Fasciitis
Fibromyositis
Fibrositis
Myalgia
Myofascial pain syndrome*
Myofascial trigger point syndrome*
Myofascitis
Myositis
Muscular rheumatism
Nonrestorative sleep syndrome
Psychogenic rheumatism
Pain amplification syndrome
Strain or sprain
Tension rheumatism

*Distinct disorders frequently confused with fibromyalgia.

disturbance, or an unknown factor.) This is referred to by some authors as **secondary fibromyalgia,** indicating that the underlying disease has a causal relationship to the fibromyalgia.[4] However, *there is no evidence that it is truly secondary,* and it may, in fact, be simply a concomitant condition.[1,6] The onset of symptoms may be triggered by seemingly unrelated events, such as acute emotional stress, physical trauma, severe influenza, or sleep-deprivation problems (e.g., restless leg syndrome).

The research studies of causal factors for this condition are relatively few and are not conclusive at this time. Although studies have demonstrated associations with sleep disturbance,[7] depression,[8] and autoimmune phenomenon,[9] none have adequately explained the etiology or pathogenesis of fibromyalgia. Clinicians have hypothesized that the syndrome is a result of referred pain from deep structures (pain amplification),[5] or a pain–spasm cycle,[4] repetitive stress to the muscle,[4] or reactivation of a latent virus.

Clinically fibromyalgia appears to be a musculoskeletal system response to stress, much as an ulcer is a gastrointestinal system response to stress, although for some patients there seems to be a predominant viral component. The relationship to viral symptoms is not well understood and is the subject of current research. Conditions such as hypertension, fibromyalgia, and ulcers have powerful psychological (stress-related) and physical components that need attention for long-lasting resolution.

DIAGNOSIS

The diagnosis of fibromyalgia is made by the presence of characteristic clinical symptoms and objective **tender points,** 14 of which have been identified by Smythe and Moldofsky.[10] These sites are sensitive or tender in normal individuals. However, patients with fibromyalgia are more sensitive

Table 5-2 Diagnostic Criteria for Fibromyalgia Developed by Yunus and Associates[4]

Obligatory criteria
  Presence of generalized aches and pains or prominent stiffness, involving three or more
    anatomical sites, for three or more months
  Absence of secondary causes, such as trauma or other diseases
Major criterion
  Presence of at least five consistent tender points
Minor criteria
  Change of symptoms with physical activity
  Change of symptoms with warm weather, exacerbation by cold
  Change of symptoms with anxiety or stress
  Poor sleep
  General fatigue
  Anxiety
  Chronic headache
  Irritable bowel syndrome
  Subjective swelling
  Nonradicular or nondermatomal numbness

(tender) than normal individuals in these specific spots. As noted below, not all 14 sites must be painful to qualify for the diagnosis of fibromyalgia.[10]

Because the symptoms of fibromyalgia can be associated with many systemic conditions, diagnosis is based, in part, on a process of exclusion. Laboratory tests are used to rule out the diseases most frequently associated with fatigue, muscle aching, and stiffness (i.e., rheumatoid arthritis [RA], polymyalgia rheumatica, hypothyroidism, polymyositis, and systemic lupus erythematosus [SLE]).

Yunus and colleagues compared the clinical symptoms of people with fibromyalgia to matched normal controls, resulting in the diagnostic criteria for fibromyalgia listed in Table 5–2.[4] (A multicenter study is currently underway to validate the diagnostic criteria for fibromyalgia.)

Rice[11] proposes simpler "working criteria" for diagnosing fibromyalgia: (1) musculoskeletal pain or tenderness in characteristic locations unexplained by associated structural or systemic disease; (2) duration of symptoms of longer than 3 months; and (3) associated sleep disturbance and/or chronic fatigue.

COURSE AND PROGNOSIS

The extent of fibromyalgia varies greatly. Some people have fibromyalgia localized in a specific region of the body (e.g., the back or neck and shoulders) and appear to have a "**localized**" condition. Others have migrating symptoms or have fibromyalgia diffusely located throughout the back and upper and lower extremities, and appear to have a "**generalized**" condition.

Long-term longitudinal studies that clearly outline the natural course of this condition have not been done. It is common to find patients who can tell you that their symptoms have been consistent for 10 to 20 years. Others report a more episodic course with exacerbations but no complete remissions. Most patients can reduce or control their symptoms to a very low level and continue to live very active lives.[12,13] It is likely that many people have had episodes of fibromyalgia and then become asymptomatic, never seeking medical care

or simply stopping medical care, so we have no data on remission rates.

It appears at this time that the greatest determinant to overall outcome is the patient's attitude and approach to the illness. A diligent approach to seeking physicians, therapists, and helpful health programs and an openness for exploring and resolving physical and psychological factors that contribute to stress generally lead to a good prognosis. The ability to resolve or reduce psychological or internal stress factors that keep muscles tight depends on how severe the stress factors are. Many patients have abusive life situations, and some have lifelong depression or anxiety. Stressors of this type are not resolved quickly.

At this writing the most beneficial nonmedication treatments are processes that have a direct impact on improving the patient's systemic health, such as aerobic and nonaerobic exercise,[14–16] meditation,[17] nutrition,[18] deep relaxation techniques,[19] and psychotherapy—all of which involve active participation and motivation. Patients overtly depressed or in denial of the problem, which is common,[8,20] may have more difficulty participating in these types of programs and, therefore, have a less favorable outcome. The most successful treatment approaches we have seen combine physical fitness, stress-reduction programs, and psychological counseling (individual or group).

SYMPTOMATOLOGY AND IMPLICATIONS FOR OCCUPATIONAL THERAPY

The symptoms are divided for purposes of discussion but they are all interwoven clinically and must be approached as a whole. Therapy is addressed after all symptomatology is reviewed.

Pain, Aching, and Stiffness

The pain or discomfort of fibromyalgia presents in a wide variety of patterns. Most (but not all) patients have aching and stiffness in the back of the neck and upper back,[4,7] and one or more of the following **patterns of pain** or "aching": (1) radiating to the mid to upper arm or to the forearm; radiating distal to the mid or lower back; (2) in the hands radiating up the forearm; (3) in the quadriceps (often distal portion); (4) in the feet radiating up to the mid leg; (5) around the ribs with or without aching in the sternocostal and costovertebral joints; and (6) in the sacral area radiating to the buttocks, lateral borders of the hip, and thigh. (These are the most typical patterns but other patterns are possible.) The symptoms tend to be bilateral and symmetric (but can have unilateral prominence) and proximal rather than distal. Some patients complain of "pain and aching," whereas others describe the sensation as "aching and stiffness." Typically the pain is constant, although the severity and sites of pain may shift over time.[5] The **pain** in fibromyalgia appears as a *referred pain of deep origin* that does not correspond to dermatomal distribution.[13]

The sensation of pain is influenced by many factors:

1. When physical trauma initiates pain, the symptoms of trauma and fibromyalgia may be confused.

2. Pain in the neck can elicit muscular guarding throughout the extremities and trunk. The amount of guarding varies; excessive guarding can contribute to pain in the associated muscles.

3. Psychological denial can alter what patients perceive. It is not uncommon for a patient, when asked about pain in a specific area (e.g., the thighs), to answer with a negative response, and then two weeks later report pain in the thighs ever since the therapist asked about it. Patients who are having difficulty coping with predominant symptoms may deny new symptoms because they cannot handle additional problems.

4. Deconditioned muscles are more susceptible to strain. A functional activity, such as shopping, may stress weak muscles, increasing discomfort.

5. Medications can mask certain symptoms at the time of interview.

6. Fear can result in denial or amplification of symptoms. If patients handle crisis situations in stride, they may minimize symptoms. If patients don't handle a crisis well and feel overwhelmed by it, they may exaggerate symptoms.

Patients usually report that the symptoms are aggravated by stress; fatigue; unaccustomed exertion; irritants, such as traffic, crowds, loud noise, or emotional conflicts; and cold damp weather or changing weather conditions.[4,7,8,13] Consequently, symptoms are often reduced by warmth, particularly hot baths and Jacuzzi tubs (if not indulged to the point of severe fatigue), massage, vacations, and light exercise.[5,13]

The **stiffness** associated with fibromyalgia is typically worse in the morning[5] and resolves with morning activity to the level that remains for the rest of the day. Stiffness coincides with the aching or discomfort and responds to heat and other interventions in the same manner. In a study of 50 patients with fibromyalgia, Yunus found that eight patients had no stiffness, four had stiffness only in the evening after work, and two had stiffness all the time. The median amount of stiffness was 40 minutes.[4]

In clinical practice, pain and tenderness at the site of tendon insertions are common and are frequently misdiagnosed as tendonitis, bicipital supraspinatus tendonitis, epicondylitis, or trochanteric bursitis. Pain at these locations is more likely the result of referred pain from active trigger points in the muscle rather than from true inflammation. This becomes quite evident when the symptoms do not respond to localized rest or anti-inflammatory medications. The aching in the upper arms typically appears as referred pain and often is most tender around the insertion of the deltoid, a common site for referred pain.[5] In the wrists, tenderness over the insertion of the extensor carpi ulnaris and extensor carpi radialis longus and brevis muscles in association with referred pain is common and can be bilateral and unilateral. Treatment must be directed toward inactivating the trigger points. This is not responsive to intervention used for traumatic tendonitis. Orthotic immobilization of the wrist will rest the wrist muscle, which tends to diminish pain, but discomfort persists. (Despite this fact, many patients prefer to wear orthoses for whatever amount of relief they offer.)

The muscles in the neck, shoulders, and upper back (i.e., trapezius, posterior cervical, and rhomboids) are vulnerable to three forms of muscular stress: emotional tension (including depression), fatigue/strain, and postural stress. There is a unique neurophysiological relationship between the postural (trunk) muscles and the psyche that does not appear to exist in the peripheral muscles. The slumped, round-shouldered posture reflective of depression is a result of posterior trunk inhibition and anterior trunk stimulation. Conversely, the chest-high, shoulder-protracted stance of someone who is exuberant reflects posterior stimulation and anterior inhibition.[21] Our language reflects this process as we "shoulder burdens" and "embrace triumph." It is much easier to determine a person's psychological state by looking at their posture than by looking at the position of their arms or legs. One cannot lose sight of this neurophysiological relationship when working with tension, pain, or spasm in this region. It is likely that the years of stress on these muscles contribute to a muscular stress syndrome like fibromyalgia.

Studies of muscle pathology on tender muscles have demonstrated definite, but not specific, tissue abnormalities. Biopsy studies of involved muscles demonstrate minor histopathological abnormalities but no evidence of inflammation. Electron microscope studies have shown Type II fiber atrophy. Muscle energy metabolism was studied by chemical analysis of biopsy specimens, which were shown to have excessive lactic acid accumulation in the tender muscles of patients with fibromyalgia after exercise as compared to control muscles and control patients.[20] However, the physical therapist at my center reports that when massaging these patients, the muscles with fibromyalgia feel very "hard" to the touch just under the surface (different from muscle spasm) and that this hardness diminishes as the fibromyalgia decreases. Some patients with fibromyalgia prefer a deep pressure massage: it is as if they need the deep pressure to get through the density, or hardness, of the muscle. But response to massage is highly variable. Some patients cannot tolerate massage and find that even light massage makes them more sore the next day. A small minority find deep pressure massage painful but helpful the next day. We encourage patients to try it but to pursue it only if it helps demonstrably.

Middle and lower back involvement may be due directly to fibromyalgia or be referred from the upper back. It may also reflect postural strain secondary to guarding or compensating for neck and shoulder pain.

Aching of the "thighs" (common) and lower leg (infrequent) is not specifically addressed in the medical literature but is loosely grouped with all distal symptoms as "referred pain of deep origin."[5,13] Patients may report that their legs fatigue easily, "feel weak," or "feel like lead when they climb stairs or walk long distances," but generally the lower extremity symptoms are tolerable and do not cause dysfunction compared to the neck, shoulder, and upper extremity pain.

Tender Points, Trigger Points, and Nodules

In the presence of fibromyalgia or other muscular stress, certain localized musculoskeletal areas can become exceptionally tender.[11] These are referred to as **tender points**.[10,11,13,22,23] In fact, a tender point is defined as one that is *excessively* tender with direct pressure. Some of these points may actually become "trigger points," and some may not. The exact relationship between these phenomena is not known.[22,23] A trigger point is defined as an area of localized tenderness that, spontaneously or when palpated, produces referred pain at a distant site.[22–24] Travell defines trigger points as follows.

> Myofascial trigger points are hyperirritable loci in muscle or fascia and are usually activated by acute or chronic overload of the muscle. They are identified by objective and subjective findings. Objective signs include a palpably firm, tense band in the muscle, production of a local twitch response, restricted stretch range-of-motion, weakness without atrophy, and no neurologic deficit. Subjectively, the patient reports stiffness and easy fatigability, spontaneous pain in a distribution predictable for that trigger point and exquisite deep tenderness specifically at the tender point; *sustained pressure on tender point induces referred pain in the predicted pattern.*[25,26] They are classified as active or latent.[26]

The physical medicine literature championed by Travell and Simons includes fibromyalgia under "myofascial trigger point syndromes."[24-29] They do not address it as a separate condition. They advocate management of myofascial pain through direct treatment of the trigger points with hyperstimulation analgesia.[26] This is produced by stimulating the trigger point with a dry needle, saline injection acupuncture, intense cold (Fluori-Methane spray and stretch), intense heat, or chemical irritation to the skin.[26] Most rheumatologists would agree with the above description except that many do not see a consistent relationship between trigger points and referred pain and may see tender points as a symptom, not a cause, of fibromyalgia.[23] It is common practice in rheumatology to use hyperstimulation analgesia if there are a few (1 to 3) problematic tender points. It is an impractical technique if there are many symptomatic points. In physical therapy, the most common form of hyperstimulation analgesia used is the application of Fluori-Methane spray to the trigger point while the muscle is under stretch. This procedure is described in detail by Travell and Simons.[26]

Simons and Travell do not address the systemic features frequently associated with fibromyalgia, such as chronic fatigue, malaise, mild influenza-like symptoms, irritable bowel syndrome, Raynaud's phenomenon, paresthesias, headaches, and positive test for antinuclear antibodies.[26,30] So it appears that myofascial pain syndrome is a localized disturbance that can be clearly defined by specific patterns of referred pain related to identifiable trigger points. Fibromyalgia is a generalized condition that is usually bilateral with a systemic component. Active trigger points may be a treatable source of pain in fibromyalgia but they are not the cause of the syndrome.

Many patients form fibrositic nodules (bandlike or nodular thickenings in the muscles). The nodules are firm, often tender, and most commonly found in the periscapular and sacral areas.[4,5] Fibrositic nodules must be distinguished from fibrofatty nodules, which are firm mobile nodules that develop in the sacral and posterior iliac crest area unrelated to fibromyalgia. Patients frequently point to them as evidence that they have a real physical disease. But the role and nature of these noninflammatory thickenings is not known.[13] They are considered separate from tender points yet may have the same role.[13] They are often absent in patients with chronic rheumatic complaints, and, conversely, similar nodules can be found in symptom-free people (50 percent of one control group[4]).[10]

Neurological Symptoms

Neurological symptoms of tingling, subjective numbness, or paresthesias in the hands and feet radiating proximally are common in fibromyalgia (84 percent of 161 patients in one review).[31,32] People also frequently report "swelling" in the hands but without objective changes. This is described as subjective swelling and may be a type of paresthesia. Neurological symptoms are usually bilateral, involving either the upper extremities alone or both upper and lower extremities. It is not uncommon for these symptoms to be part of the initial presentation of the condition. Many of these patients are suspected of having carpal tunnel syndrome even though objective signs (i.e., dry skin, positive Phalen's and percussion [Tinel] tests, and diminished sensation) are lacking. These patients are often unnecessarily subjected to invasive nerve conduction studies or even surgery before being correctly diagnosed with fibromyalgia.[32] These symptoms wax and wane over time but do not progress into a more serious problem. If the paresthesias are due to fibromyalgia, wrist orthoses are *not* indicated.

Stress, Fatigue, and Sleep Disturbance

Fatigue may be the most disruptive factor in life-style.[4,5,11] Patients may not have the energy to go places with their family or friends, especially for evening activities. Several factors may contribute to fatigue: (1) lack of deep restorative sleep, (2) chronic pain, (3) emotional stress, and (4) depression (overt, masked, or cyclic). Compounding the issue of fatigue is a sense of subjective weakness, secondary to the presence of pain, and deconditioning, associated with diminished physical activity or exercise.

Portrait of a Night

Sleep is a state of mind and body—regular, recurrent, easily reversible, ultimately irresistible. Sleepers look quiet and seem unresponsive to the world around them, but sleep is not a passive state. It is a dynamic process, made up of two types of rest: active and quiet. Active sleep is characterized by movements of the eyeballs beneath closed lids and more intense activity in the brain than during quiet sleep; it is referred to as Rapid Eye Movement or REM sleep. Quiet sleep consists of four distinct stages, all categorized as non-REM or NREM sleep.

Each night you literally turn yourself down for sleep. As you rest, your body begins to slow down, and muscular tension decreases. The brain produces steady, small waves at a rate of nine to twelve cycles per second. In Stage 1 NREM sleep, your brain waves become smaller and much more pinched, irregular and variable. Mundane thoughts drift through your mind, and pulse and respiration become more even. If awakened from this twilight zone, you may deny having slept. As you enter Stage 2, your brain waves become larger, characterized by occasional sudden bursts of activity. Your eyes become unresponsive to stimuli; if your eyelids were lifted, you would not see. Your bodily functions slow still more, and your eyes may roll slowly back and forth. In Stage 3, your brain waves are about five times the size of those in Stage 1 and much slower (about one cycle per second). In Stage 4, the most profound state of unconsciousness, very large brain waves appear in a slow jagged pattern.

The full journey to the depths of tranquility usually takes more than an hour. Then you begin your ascent, not to consciousness but to active or REM sleep. The muscles of your middle ear begin to vibrate. Your brain waves resemble the patterns of waking more than of deep sleep; they are pinched and irregular. The muscles of your face, limbs, and trunk are slack, but there may be quick bursts of activity in the central nervous system that cause twitches, particularly in the toes and fingers. Your pulse and breathing quicken, and your brain temperature and blood flow increase. Your eyes dart back and forth. Males have erections, whether they are seven months or seven decades old. When sleepers have been awakened from REM sleep in laboratories, 80 percent have reported vivid dreams.

The initial REM period of the night is short, usually only 10 minutes. The 90 to 100-minute REM-NREM cycle is repeated four to five times, with deep NREM Stages 3 and 4 growing shorter and REM periods growing longer during the night. Dreams may occur all through the night, but those recalled from NREM periods tend to be mundane and simple, while REM dreams are usually more dynamic and complex. In an 8-hour night, you will spend 2 hours in REM sleep; in the course of a lifetime, 5 or 6 years are spent in REM sleep and three times that amount in NREM sleep.

As you shift from stage to stage of sleep, your body goes through assorted changes—physical, chemical, hormonal, muscular. Various levels of brain chemicals, including the so-called "sleep juice" serotonin, rise and fall. Body temperature drops to its lowest levels; you breathe less oxygen and burn up fewer calories. In REM, these processes are orchestrated from the brain stem, a region of the brain no larger than your little finger. Your brain, unlike all others in the world, organizes your sleep in a pattern that reflects your sex, age, and health. Your sleep style may be totally different from your bed partner's, but it will be remarkably consistent night after night.

Dianne Hales
The Complete Book of Sleep
Addison-Wesley, 1980

One of the most prominent features of fibromyalgia is a sleep disturbance.[5,7] This typically takes the form of "going to sleep easily, but waking up in the early morning (from 3 to 5 AM) unable to go back to sleep or go back to deep sleep." Technically, this is described as a nonrapid eye movement (non-REM) or deep (restorative) sleep disturbance.[5,7] Even if patients sleep through the night, if they don't sleep deeply (stage

4), they will wake up exhausted, feeling as if "hit by a truck." (This pattern is also indicative of diminished restorative sleep.) Starting the day tired increases irritability and sensitivity, and reduces tolerance for stress and pain, creating a vicious cycle.

When individuals wake up in the morning, they may or may not feel tense or anxious. However, they tend to ruminate over daily events that appear stress provoking (e.g., financial difficulties, discontent at work, and marital or family problems). My psychotherapeutic experience with these individuals shows that the "stresses" that can be acknowledged and verbalized in the early morning are generally not the stress stimuli for the fibrositis or sleep disturbance, which is often denied or subconscious. It is profound denial of the problem that makes it so difficult for the patient to see the connection between the actual stressor and the stress response (the sleep disturbance). Consequently, behavioral cognitive stress-management techniques that focus on verbalized early morning ruminations are not successful in ameliorating the symptoms. Being able to connect with and resolve the deeper emotional conflicts is clearly the most effective and profound treatment for this disorder, but this takes time and the patient's willingness to walk through the subconscious "door of fear" that creates the denial (see the section on denial in Chapter 2).

To complicate matters, patients unable to get help for their symptoms because physicians have told them "It's all in your head" often need to prove that *it isn't* to all concerned (spouse, employer, children, physician, and so on). These patients often become focused on the physical and resist exploring the psychological issues and thus further limit their options for resolution.

Any process that improves sleep can go a long way in improving the patient's energy and endurance. Such interventions include

1. **Medications:** Low-dose tricyclic antidepressants, such as Elavil, or muscle relaxants, such as Flexeril or cyclobenzaprine, have proven effective for improving deep sleep.[4,5,13,33]

2. **Stress management and stress reduction:** Strategies may be developed for reducing known stresses or altering one's response to stress.

3. **Deep relaxation:** Practicing deep muscular relaxation right before sleep, such as systematically focusing on and relaxing (letting go) of each muscle group will clearly demonstrate how much tension someone is holding in his or her muscles even in a most relaxed state or comfortable position. Individuals who sleep with their muscles tense generally awake feeling tired.[34] It is a common misconception that a person is relaxed when he or she sleeps. The existence of bruxism (teeth grinding), night screams, somnambulism, and fist-clenching testifies to the body's ability for muscular tension during sleep.

4. **Nutrition:** Our food intake can affect sleeping in several ways. First, a high-energy, healthy diet (i.e., one low in fats, sugar, and chemicals, and high in complex carbohydrates, such as vegetables, grains, and fruits) can increase energy, allowing a person to participate in more physical activities, which reduce stress and improve sleeping.[18] A person who is feeling energetic is more likely to exercise during the day. Second, specific foods and substances can encourage or interfere with sleep. For example, highly acidic foods, such as tomatoes, citrus fruits, or wine, consumed late at night can disrupt sleep.[34] Alcohol, especially wine, can induce sleep but may wake up the person in the middle of the night. Alcohol consumption or lack of sufficient water intake can also lead to dehydration, fatigue, headaches, and disturbed sleep. Drugs such as caffeine and nicotine are known stimulants that remain in the system for a long period. For example, a cup of coffee drunk at 3:00 in the afternoon can keep a person sensitive to caffeine awake in the evening. Chocolate desserts may contribute sufficient caffeine to affect some people. Some patients also report that sugar acts as a stimulant at night. On the other hand, supplements such as calcium–magnesium (400 to 600 mg) taken 45 minutes before retiring can encourage muscle relaxation and deeper sleep.

5. **Exercise:** Patients with fibromyalgia who participate in a safe, moderate exercise program (e.g., walking, swimming, or soft aerobics) report that it is one of the most beneficial approaches they have tried for reducing symptoms. Exercise helps decrease anxiety and improves endurance and the ability to relax and sleep.[34–36] Exercise that

increases the heart rate significantly (aerobics) is beneficial, in part because it improves nutrition and circulation to the deep dense tissues (e.g., tendons, joints, ligaments). It improves the functioning and health of every cell in the body. The side effects of exercise, such as increased self-esteem, better posture, and increased energy, are the effects people with chronic pain need most (see Therapy, below).

Gastrointestinal Symptoms

Irritable bowel syndrome (IBS) is a common symptom associated with fibromyalgia. Published reports estimate that IBS may be present in 30 percent of patients with primary fibromyalgia.[4,13] It is present in about 80 percent of the patients I treat. IBS is characterized by periodically altered bowel habits (diarrhea or constipation) associated with excessive gas and lower abdominal cramping or distention, usually relieved by bowel movements. There are no abnormalities on colonoscopy examination to suggest organic disease.[4] The symptoms of IBS are often related to emotional stress and correlated with anxiety.[1]

Fats, dairy products (e.g., ice cream), and spicy foods are frequent irritants. Most cases of IBS can be controlled by a high-fiber, low-fat diet and bulk fiber supplements. Treatment is the same whether the problem is diarrhea or constipation. For patients with chronic anxiety the unpredictability of IBS attacks frequently causes them to curtail their social or community activities.

Headaches

Yunus found in his study that 22 of 50 patients reported **migraine or tension headaches.**[4] Most migrainous attacks occurred during the patients' younger years. Non-migrainous headaches (25 percent) were described as dull, pressure-like ache over the occipital area, spread diffusely in the skull or frontal area around one or both eyes. These headaches are associated with trigger points in the suboccipital muscle insertion areas, other muscles in the scalp, and deep cervical ligaments.[4] This type of

head pain is frequently associated with **numbness, paresthesias,** or **localized swelling** in the face. If severe or chronic it can be quite dysfunctional, making it impossible for the person to think, work, read, or do daily activities.

Depression and Anxiety

The role of depression and psychological disturbance in fibromyalgia is controversial and undefined at present because controlled studies have produced conflicting results. Some studies implicate depression, hypochondriasis, and obsessive-compulsive and anxiety disorders as causal factors; other studies refute this.[37] I have a psychotherapy practice with about 70 percent fibromyalgia patients. From this clinical perspective, it is clear that many patients have definable psychiatric disorders, such as those listed above, that precede the fibromyalgia and contribute to muscle tension and sleep disorders. Others, probably the majority, would not qualify for any specific psychiatric diagnosis but have considerable tension and stressful life situations that contribute to muscle tension and sleep disorders. And others, especially those with mild episodic involvement, have exacerbations of symptoms that directly correspond to stressful life events. This does not mean that fibromyalgia is a purely psychosomatic disorder, as it has been referred to in the past; but it does indicate that there is a psychobiological conponent that can have a profound effect on the body in general and muscle health in particular.[37]

Another consideration that further complicates the process of sorting out physical from psychological factors is the fact that the symptoms associated with depression, such as altered mood, sleep disturbance, anergy (lack of energy), appetite changes, decreased libido, irritability, myalgias, withdrawal of interest, weakening of relationships, and increased somatic preoccupation, can occur secondary to a chronic sleep disorder (chronic fatigue) or the emotional sequela of chronic pain.[38-39] Ultimately you can have: **pain, depression,** and **fatigue** (sleep disorder) each supporting the other two, creating three vicious cycles.

In my experience, factors contributing to

psychological stress and anxiety must be addressed if people are going to have success in correcting a sleep disorder and reducing muscle tension. The patients at my center who make the most progress are those who are committed to a holistic or mind-body approach to health, who work through the psychological factors contributing to depression, anxiety, or stress and their associated physiological changes.

Anxiety also plays a key role in perpetuating this syndrome for *some* patients. Yunus[4] found in a review of 50 patients that 70 percent "admitted to being unduly anxious" and 68 percent reported that symptoms were made worse by anxiety and mental stress. Patients with identifiable anxiety should seek the services of a psychotherapist. There are several specific anti-anxiety medications available. Drug therapy for anxiety should be monitored by a psychiatrist or psychopharmacologist, as some of the drugs can be addictive. Medical treatment of underlying anxiety can often make it possible for patients to participate successfully in physical fitness and rehabilitative programs.

Therapy

Occupational therapy and physical therapy both play a role in helping to improve the health or integrity of the muscles. However, in my experience, a holistic approach, which addresses the internal psychological conflicts that create stress as well as the physical factors, is most successful for achieving resolution of symptoms. Patients at our center who seek *only* a physical approach make some improvement—they feel better and the quality of their life may improve—but the symptoms do not totally resolve. It is often these patients who have the most serious denial about the psychological stress issues in their lives.

Therapists can play a vital role in educating the patient about the relationship between stress, lack of restorative sleep, and muscle pain and the importance of addressing both the psychological and physical aspects of "muscle health." For their patients, therapists can identify community or staff resources for psychotherapy, group therapy, sleep counseling (including mattress and pillow recommendations), and safe fitness programs.

Occupational therapy intervention includes (1) analysis of stress factors (i.e., emotional factors such as tension, anger, or fear), physical factors (lifting, repetitive, or static activities), and postural factors that aggravate the involved muscles; (2) conscious deep muscle relaxation, stress-management techniques, meditation, biofeedback, and deep breathing exercises (or referral for this component); and (3) analysis of posture and strain during vocational activities, activities of daily living (ADL), and leisure activities, and sleeping. Educate patients about these adaptive methods or recommend equipment to reduce the strain to the neck and shoulder region. (The approach to therapy is the same as for joint protection for osteoarthritis of the neck; see Chapter 4.)

Physical therapy intervention includes (1) massage, which can be helpful as part of a total relaxation program but seems to have little benefit as a sole treatment; (2) trigger point therapy; (3) relaxation training, biofeedback, or deep breathing; (4) exercises to correct postural deficits; and (5) guidance on a fitness program.

Exercise

The value of exercise for fibromyalgia is fourfold. (1) By improving the strength of the affected muscles, you can make them more resistant to the effects of stage 4 sleep deprivation.[7] (2) Strengthening the entire body can improve posture and efficiency in carrying out functional activities, reducing strain on the muscles. (3) Exercise can help release emotional stress and reduce depression.[36] (4) Exercise can increase relaxation and improve sleep.[34] *All of these outcomes can be achieved with nonaerobic exercises.* Exercise that improves cardiovascular efficiency (usually aerobic, but nonaerobic exercise can serve this function for very weak people) improves health at cellular and systemic levels as well as achieving the above goals.[15]

An aerobic exercise program is ideal for most people, but for the majority of patients with fibromyalgia an aerobic program (even a low-impact one) is too vigorous in the beginning of treatment but should be gradually added to the program whenever possible.

Exercise for People Who Do Not Exercise

In the beginning, the goal is to get the patient into an exercise program that he or she can (1) accomplish without exacerbating his or her symptoms, (2) enjoy, and (3) achieve the four desirable outcomes listed above. Enjoying one's exercise program is important for participation over a long duration. (Misery in exercise will only increase depression.) The following factors can influence the achievement of this goal and must be considered when prescribing exercises:

1. **Fear.** Prior to diagnosis, patients are very fearful of pain, and almost all report that exercise makes it worse. Following counseling and education about fibromyalgia and the therapeutic value of exercise, these same patients can usually successfully participate in a gentle exercise program. If a patient's fear about exercise causing pain or reinjury is not addressed, the patient will not be able to participate in exercise successfully. (In some patients, this fear may actually become a phobia.)

2. **Compulsivity or perfectionism.** Patients with an all-or-none approach to exercise, or life, need skilled supervision during exercise. Often these patients "overdo" when they first start working out and then have a setback, creating fear of, instead of confidence in, exercise.

3. **Anxiety.** Patients who are generally anxious or anxious in groups or group activities (evidence of performance anxiety) may participate in activities or exercises with excessive tension in muscles. Therefore, a blanket recommendation to "use an exercise cycle or join a soft-aerobics class" could prove to be a failure and might increase an anxious patient's distrust in the above processes.

4. **Excessive muscular tension and stiffness.** Some patients need individual physical therapy to relax and mobilize musculature that has been bound by immobility and tension for years before successful participation in even a gentle exercise program is possible.

It is best to start out with a gentle exercise class, two to three times per week, that moves the entire musculature in integrated spiral or functional patterns with an emphasis on active rather than resistive toning. The class should be led by an exercise instructor who understands fibromyalgia and does not push patients beyond their limits. The patients need to be taught how to assess the effect of exercise on their bodies and to be in control of progressing their programs.

We have conducted classes of this nature at our center for four years. These classes, developed by a physical therapist and movement therapist, have been very well received by patients, and most have achieved the above-described outcomes. After patients are able to participate successfully in this type of program, we encourage them to move on to exercise that provides greater cardiovascular conditioning, perhaps an exercise class, swimming, or fast walking. Many choose to stay in the class but add swimming or walking to their regimen.

Exercise for People Who Exercise but Without Results

Some people, often exercise enthusiasts, are already participating in their own exercise program at the time of diagnosis. The exercise typically is swimming, running, or aerobics classes. For these patients, it is important to determine "how" they are exercising. Is their manner of exercising (i.e., tension, vigor, and style) increasing stress on the muscles? If they are exercising appropriately, they need to focus their therapeutic energy in the area of psychotherapy, stress management, and relaxation work.

DRUG THERAPY

In fibromyalgia the most valuable function of medications is to improve the quality of sleep. Because there is generally no inflammation, aspirin and other NSAIDs do not have a dramatic effect and work only as mild analgesics. However, NSAIDs are often effective for patients with severe muscle spasm or concomitant osteoarthritis.

Sleep Enhancers

Tricyclic antidepressants such as amitriptyline (Elavil) and imipramine (Tofranil) are the most common and successful medications used to improve sleep. They may work in fibromyalgia by reducing alpha-wave intrusion and contribute to a more normal late-morning sleep pattern.[40] These agents block re-uptake of norepinephrine and serotonin. It is theorized that they also raise endorphin stimulation levels, contributing to their therapeutic effect.[41] Used in low doses before going to sleep, these medications *do not* have a mood-altering effect. They must be taken in high doses (amitriptyline at 100 to 250 mg per day) to have an antidepressant effect. If amitriptyline is used simply as a sleep enhancer, a patient would start with a dosage of 10 mg, adding 10 mg per week up to a maximum of 30 to 50 mg, until the desired effect is achieved. The most common side effects are morning drowsiness or lethargy, nightmares, and mouth dryness,[41] but most side effects can be avoided if a patient starts with a low dose. Morning or next-day drowsiness can often be avoided by taking the medication earlier in the evening. The goal of this therapeutic approach is to have the patient sleep through the night and wake up feeling rested. Often the medications help patients sleep through the night, which is an improvement, but they still wake up feeling tired, which indicates that they are not getting sufficient restorative sleep.

Another medication that is effective with fibromyalgia is cyclobenzaprine (Flexeril). Classified as a muscle relaxant, it differs from other muscle relaxants because it is a tricyclic derivative. Cyclobenzaprine functions very much like low-dose amitriptyline and similarly does not have an antidepressant effect. This drug is reported to act primarily at the brain stem level with the net effect of reduced tonic autonomic motor activity.[41] As with all tricyclics, morning lethargy may be a problem; again, this can be reduced if the dosage is taken earlier in the evening. Dry mouth is another common side effect.

Controlled trials have shown that as little as 10 to 20 mg of this drug can be effective in improving global response and reducing muscle spasm, pain, tenderness, sleep disturbance, and morning fatigue. Essentially all parameters improved except morning stiffness.[41,42]

REFERENCES

1. Wolfe, F, and Cathey, M: Prevalence of primary and secondary fibrositis. J Rheumatol 10(6):965–968, 1983.
2. Wolfe, F: The clinical syndrome of fibrositis. Am J Med 81(Suppl 3A):7–14, 1986.
3. Yunus, M, and Masi, AT: Juvenile primary fibromyalgia syndromes: A clinical study of thirty-three patients and matched normal controls. Arthritis Rheum 28:138–145, 1985.
4. Yunus, M, Masi, AT, Calabro, JJ, Miller, KA, and Feigenbaum, SL: Primary fibromyalgia (fibrositis): Clinical study of 50 patients with matched normal controls. Semin Arthritis Rheum 11(1):151–171, 1981.
5. Smythe, HH: Fibrositis and other diffuse musculoskeletal syndromes. In Kelly, WN, Harris, ED, Ruddy, S, and Sledge, CB (eds): Textbook of Rheumatology. WB Saunders, Philadelphia, 1985.
6. Goldenberg, DL: Fibromyalgia syndrome. An emerging but controversial condition. JAMA 257(20):2782–2787, 1987 (review).
7. Moldofsky, H, Searisfrick, P, Englund, R, et al: Musculoskeletal symptoms and non REM sleep disturbance in patients with fibrositic syndrome and healthy subjects. Psychosom Med 37:341–351, 1975.
8. Hudson, JI, Hudson, MS, Plener, LF, Goldenberg, DL, and Pope, HG: Fibromyalgia and major effective disorders: A controlled phenomenology and family history study. Am J Psychiatry 142(4):441–446, 1985.
9. Dinerman, H, Goldenberg, DL, and Felson, DT: A prospective evaluation of 118 patients with the fibromyalgia syndrome. J Rheumatol 13:368–373, 1986.
10. Smythe, H, and Moldofsky, H: Two contributions to understanding of the "fibrositis" syndrome. Bull Rheum Dis 28(1):928–931, 1977.
11. Rice, JR: Fibrositis syndrome. Med Clin North Am 70(2):455–568, 1986.
12. Felson, DT, and Goldenberg, DL: The natural history of fibromyalgia. Arthritis Rheum 29:522–526, 1986.
13. Bennett, RM: Fibrositis: Misnomer for a common rheumatic disorder (medical progress). West J Med 134(5):405–413, 1981.
14. Vaccaro, P, et al: The effects of aerobic dance conditioning on the body composition and maximal oxygen uptake of college women. J Sports Med Phys Fitness 21(3):291–294, 1981.
15. Rodgers-Gould, G: Soft aerobics. Am Health, 56–63, November 1985.

16. McCain, GA: Role of physical fitness training in the fibrositis/fibromyalgia syndrome. Am J Med 81(3a):73–77, 1986.
17. Kanellakos, DP, and Lucas, JP: The Psychobiology of Transcendental Meditation. WA Benjamin, Hunter, NY, 1974.
18. Bland, J: Your health under seige—Using your diet to fight back.
19. Achterberg, J, McGraw, P, and Lawlis, GF: Rheumatoid arthritis: A study of relaxation and temperature biofeedback training as adjunctive therapy. Biofeedback Self Regul 6(2):207–223, 1981.
20. Bengtsson, A, Henriksson, KG, and Larsson, J: Reduced high-energy phosphate levels in the painful muscles of patients with fibromyalgia. Arthritis Rheum 24:817–821, 1986.
21. Lowen, A: Depression and the body: The biological basis of faith and reality. Coward, McCann, and Geohegan, New York, 1973.
22. Campbell, SM, Clark, S, Tindell, EA, Forehand, ME, and Bennett, RM: Clinical characteristics of fibrositis. I. A blinded controlled study of symptoms and tender points. Arthritis Rheum 26(7):817–824, 1983.
23. Wolfe, F: Tender points, trigger points and the fibrositis syndrome. Clin Rheum Dis 2:36–38, 1984.
24. Travell, J: Identification of myofascial trigger point syndromes: A case of atypical facial neuralgia. Arch Phys Med Rehab vol 62, 1981.
25. Melzack, R: Myofascial trigger points: Relation to acupuncture and mechanisms of pain. Arch Phys Med Rehab 62:114–117, 1981.
26. Travell, JG, and Simons, DG: Myofascial Pain and Dysfunction: The Trigger Point Manual. Williams & Wilkins, Baltimore, 1983.
27. Simons, DG: Muscle pain syndromes. Part I. Am J Phys Med 54(6):289–311: Part II. Am J Phys Med 55(1):15–42, 1976.
28. Simons, DG: Myofascial trigger points: A need for understanding. Arch Phys Med Rehab 62:97–99, 1981.
29. Rubin, D: Myofascial trigger point syndromes: An approach to management. Arch Phys Med Rehab 62(3):107–110, 1981.
30. Simons, DG: Fibrositis/fibromyalgia: A form of myofascial trigger points? Am J Med 81(Suppl 3A):93–98, 1986.
31. Simms, R, Goldenberg, D, and Felson, D: Neuropathic symptoms in fibromyalgia. Arthritis Rheum 30:s, (abstract), 1987.
32. Goldenberg, D: Fibromyalgia syndrome. JAMA 257(20):2782–2787, 1987.
33. Goldenberg, D, Felson, D, and Dinerman, H: A randomized controlled trial of amitryptilene (AM) and naproxen (N) in the treatment of patients with fibromyalgia. Arthritis Rheum 29:1371–1377, 1986.
34. Hales, D: The complete book of sleep—How your nights affect your days. Addison-Wesley, Reading, MA, 1981.
35. Griffin, SJ, and Trinder, J: Physical fitness, exercise and human sleep. Psychophysiology 15:447–450, 1978.
36. McCann, IL, and Holmes, DS: Influence of aerobic exercise on depression. J Pers Soc Psych 46(5):1142–1147, 1984.
37. Goldenberg, DL: Psychologic studies in fibrositis. Am J Med 81(Suppl 3A):67–70, 1986.
38. Blumer, D, and Heilbrunn, M: Chronic pain as a variant of depressive disease—The pain-prone disorder. J Nerv Ment Dis 170(7):381–394, 1982.
39. Lopez-Ibor, JJ: Masked depression. Br J Psychiatry 120:245–258, 1972.
40. Hauri, P: The Sleep Disorders. The Upjohn Company, Kalamazoo, MI, 1977, p 51.
41. Gatter, RA: Pharmacotherapeutics in fibrositis. Am J Med 81(Suppl 3A):63–66, 1986.
42. Bennett, RM, Gatter, RA, Campbell, SM, et al: A double-blind study of cyclobenzoprine versus placebo in patients with fibrositis. Arthritis Rheum 27 (S76), 1984.

ADDITIONAL SOURCES

Bennett, RM: Current issues concerning management of the fibrositis/fibromyalgia syndrome. Am J Med 81(3a):15–18, 1986.

Danneskold-Samsoe, B, et al: Regional muscle tension and pain ("fibrositis"): Effect of massage on myoglobin in plasma. Scand J Rehab Med (Stockholm) 15(1):17–20, 1982.

Hadler NM: A critical reappraisal of the fibrositis concept. Am J Med 81(3a):26–30, 1986.

Hench, PK, and Mitler, MM: Fibromyalgia. 1. Review of a common rheumatologic syndrome. Postgrad Med 80(7):47–56, 1986 (review).

Hench, PK, and Mitler, MM: Fibromyalgia. 2. Management guidelines and research findings. Postgrad Med 80(7):57–64, 1986 (review).

Moldofsky, H: Sleep and musculoskeletal pain. Am J Med 81(3a):85–89, 1986.

Smeltzer, KJ: Fibromyalgia: The frustration of diagnosis and management. Orthop Nurs 6(3):28–31, 1987.

Smeltzer, KJ: The fibrositis/fibromyalgia syndrome: Current issues and perspectives. Symposium proceedings. Am J Med 81(Suppl 3A):1–115, 1986. (Includes review articles by all the leading researchers in the field.)

Chapter 6

Rheumatoid Arthritis

Rheumatoid arthritis (RA) is a chronic inflammatory disease of the synovium with a course characterized by exacerbations and remissions. It is a systemic disease and in some people may involve the lungs, blood vessels, heart, or eyes.

ETIOLOGICAL FACTORS AND AGE AND SEX AFFECTED

Although no etiological agent has been identified, much has been learned about the inflammatory process involved in RA. The disease seems to be perpetuated by a continued, unknown immune reaction in synovial tissue that leads to inflammation; hypertrophy of the synovium; weakening of the capsule, tendons, and ligaments; and eventual destruction of cartilage and bone. Since the etiology is unknown, drug treatment is aimed at modifying the immunological reaction and inflammatory process in the synovial membrane.[1]

Three of four cases of RA occur in women although severe seropositive erosive disease affects men and women almost

> Studies of the pathogenesis of rheumatoid arthritis continue to focus on one recurring fact: there are an enormous number of different types of cells and pathways of communication among cells that are activated in this disease. Despite this confluence of stimuli, rheumatoid arthritis occasionally goes into remission spontaneously or in response to treatment. The inference from this is an optimistic one: that apparently minor interventions affecting a few crucial mediators of inflammation or restoring a few inhibitory pathways in and around the joints may be sufficient to restore a balance leading to remission.
>
> Edward Harris
> Pathogenesis of Rheumatoid Arthritis
> Am J Med 80, Suppl 4B 4/28/86

equally. It can occur in any race and at any age, but the greatest incidence is during the third and fourth decades.

DIAGNOSIS

The first indication of RA usually is a polyarthritis affecting the small joints of the hands and feet in a symmetric fashion although occasionally it starts with systemic manifestations. Large joints and the cervical spine can also be involved, but the thoracic and lumbar spine is usually spared. The diagnosis may be confirmed by the presence of subcutaneous rheumatoid nodules, by radiological demonstration of cartilage destruction or bony erosions, and by the presence of an antibody in the serum called **rheumatoid factor (RF).**[2]

The American Rheumatism Association (ARA) has revised the diagnostic criteria for RA. The terms *classical, definite, probable,* and *possible,* previously used to distinguish RA, have been eliminated. The new criteria can be used in two formats. The "tree" format is considered slightly more accurate in clinical use (see Table 6–1). The traditional format is given in Appendix 1 for reference. Both can be used by clinicians and researchers.[3]

COURSE AND PROGNOSIS

The majority of people (60 to 70 percent) have a slow insidious onset over a period of weeks to months. Some people (15 to 20 percent) have an intermediate onset, developing symptoms within days or weeks, while others (8 to 15 percent) have acute severe onset, often "waking up with swollen joints." It is not uncommon for all symptoms of RA to take 6 months to 2 years to emerge fully, making an accurate diagnosis possible.[2]

The **course of the disease** roughly falls into 3 patterns:[2]

1. Intermittent: Approximately 20 to 30 percent of all patients have a variable course of remissions and flare-ups. Disease may progress with each exacerbation. For patients in this category, *it is extremely im-*

Table 6–1 The 1987 Classification Tree Criteria and Definitions for Rheumatoid Arthritis (RA)*,[3]

Criterion	Definition
1. Arthritis of three or more joint areas	At least three joint areas simultaneously have had soft tissue swelling or fluid (not bony overgrowth alone) observed by a physician. The 14 possible joint areas are right or left PIP, MCP, wrist, elbow, knee, ankle, and MTP joints.
2. Arthritis of hand joints Wrist MCP MCP or wrist MCP and wrist	Soft tissue swelling or fluid (not bony overgrowth alone) of the specified area observed by a physician. Where two areas are specified, involvement must have been simultaneous.
3. Symmetric swelling (arthritis)	Simultaneous involvement of the same joint areas (as defined in 1) on both sides of the body. Bilateral involvement of PIPs, MCPs, or MTPs is acceptable without absolute symmetry.
4. Serum RF	Demonstration of abnormal amounts of serum RF by any method for which the result has been positive in <5% of normal control subjects.
5. Radiographic changes of RA	Radiographic changes typical of RA on posteroanterior hand and wrist radiographs, which must include erosions or unequivocal bony decalcification localized in or most marked adjacent to the involved joints (osteoarthritis changes alone do not qualify).

*To make the diagnosis of RA using this tree the patient must have two of these five criteria and have a clinical diagnosis of RA by his or her physicians. Criteria 1, 2, and 3 must have been present for at least 6 weeks.

portant to emphasize the need to regain range of motion (ROM) and function after each exacerbation.

2. Long clinical remissions: A person may have one or a few bouts of inflammation and then go into a prolonged remission for 10 to 30 years, or there may be years of remission between episodes. The exact number of people in this category is not known because they often discontinue medical care with the remission.

3. Progressive unremitting course: Progress may be slow or rapid. This group can be divided into those who respond to disease-modifying drugs and those who do not. Although patients who develop a severe, rapid destructive course with class IV functional ability comprise only 3 percent of all people diagnosed with RA, they represent a much higher percentage of patients in rehabilitation programs.

The long-term prognosis cannot be predicted in the beginning, although an acute onset is considered to have a more favorable outcome. The presence of rheumatoid nodules and extra-articular features is associated with a more severe course. (See Appendix 2 for classification of progression of RA).[2]

Joint involvement is usually bilateral (symmetric). That is, the joints involved may be symmetric but the residual deformities may be asymmetric (e.g., a person can have boutonnière deformities on the left hand and swan-neck deformities on the right). Peripheral joints are involved more frequently than proximal ones.

The patient's **functional ability** can vary considerably between exacerbations and remissions. He or she may be independent during remissions and maximally assisted during flare-ups. The ARA Functional Classification roughly delineates function by the following parameters:

Class I: Complete functional capacity with ability to carry on all usual duties without handicaps.

Class II: Functional capacity adequate to

Pathogenesis of Joint Disease in Rheumatoid Arthritis

The initiating factors in rheumatoid arthritis remain undefined, but our understanding of the cellular interactions leading to joint inflammation and tissue destruction have increased significantly in the past few years. The mononuclear cells of the macrophage type interact with the T lymphocytes. This interaction, in consort with B cells, causes local production of antibody. Antigen–antibody complexes form within the joint and are subsequently phagocytized by polymorphonuclear leukocytes and the synovial lining cells. In the course of their ingestion, a variety of biologically active inflammatory mediators are released, which give rise to the redness, swelling, and pain characteristic of rheumatoid synovitis. Simultaneously, the macrophages and T cells are communicating through soluble mediators with the unusual dendritic cells of the synovial lining. These, by their ability to produce and release compounds with destructive potential, cause bone and cartilage erosion that result in the characteristic rheumatoid disability and deformity. Viewed in this context, drug therapy has the potential for modifying these reactions at a variety of points. Indeed, it seems that the polypharmacy characteristically employed by rheumatologists on an empiric basis has a good theoretical foundation. Disease-modifying agents, such as gold, penicillamine, and antimalarials, most likely influence macrophages and T cells; nonsteroidal anti-inflammatory drugs block the generation of arachidonate metabolites; corticosteroids, even in small doses, can interfere with opsonization, chemotaxis, and the release of prostaglandins and collagenases from cultured synovial cells. Cytotoxic drugs, such as cyclophosphamide, have a direct effect on the production of antibodies by B cells. In the future, one can anticipate that agents will be developed that more specifically pinpoint discrete steps in this reaction sequence.

Nathan J. Zvaifler, M.D.
Pathogenesis of the Joint Disease of RA
Am J Med 12/30/83

conduct normal activities despite handicap or discomfort or limited mobility of one or more joints.

Class III: Functional capacity adequate to perform only a few or none of the duties of the patient's usual occupation or of self-care.

Class IV: Largely or wholly incapacitated with patient bedridden or confined to a wheelchair, permitting little or no self-care.

SYMPTOMATOLOGY AND IMPLICATIONS FOR OCCUPATIONAL THERAPY

The symptoms of RA fall into three categories:

1. Articular and periarticular symptoms, including those of inflammatory joint disease and associated soft tissue involvement.

2. Systemic manifestations such as fever, malaise, fatigue, anorexia, and generalized stiffness (morning stiffness).

3. Symptoms associated with involvement of organs, including lung, vascular, and cardiac complications.[4]

Articular and Periarticular Involvement

The joint deformities that develop with this disease can also occur in other chronic inflammatory arthritic diseases. For example, a person with systemic lupus erythematosus or psoriatic arthritis who develops a chronic inflammatory arthritis of the metacarpophalangeal (MCP) joints can develop the same deformities typically seen in RA. Since the common hand deformities are not unique to RA, they are discussed and referenced in detail in Chapter 19. The following is a brief cursory review of the common physical and functional consequences of chronic inflammatory disease of the extremity joints and cervical spine associated with RA. (Basic treatment for joint involvement is described in Chapter 1.) The section on surgical rehabilitation (Chapters 29 to 35) also contains a referenced review of the specific pathodynamics for each joint.

In this section, the joints are discussed in the order of frequency of occurrence and pattern of involvement in RA (i.e., hands, wrists, feet, ankles, knees, hips, elbows, and shoulders).

Hands and Wrists

Metacarpophalangeal (MCP) Joints. Synovitis weakens and distends the joint capsule and associated ligaments. It is theorized that, in addition, the stretch of the capsule leads to a protective reflex spasm of the interosseous and lumbrical muscles. Intrinsic muscle tightness can lead to a flexion contracture **(intrinsic plus) deformity** of the MCP joint as well as contribute to a **swan-neck finger deformity.** (See section on swan-neck deformity in Chapter 19.) Damage to the fibrous flexor sheath (pulley) that supports the flexor tendons allows the tendons to migrate volar and ulnarward to the joint. This alters the mechanical advantage of the flexor tendons, allowing them to pull the proximal phalanx into **ulnar and volar subluxation** during power pinch and grasp activities. These factors, combined with radial deviation of the wrist, stretching of the radial collateral ligaments, the normal ulnar slope of the metacarpal heads, the power advantage of the ulnar interossei over the radial interossei, and dislocation of the long extensors into the ulnar valleys, make MCP ulnar drift a common sequela in adult RA. (See Fig. 19–22 in Chapter 19.) Hand involvement is very different for children; see Chapter 14, Juvenile Rheumatoid Arthritis (JRA).

Wrist Joint. Typically in the adult RA wrist, the synovitis weakens the supporting ligaments. Ligamentous laxity may allow the carpus to slip down the volar slope of the distal radius resulting in **ulnar–volar subluxation of the carpus.** The carpus may rotate during this process, producing radial deviation of the wrist, or it may not rotate, producing **ulnar deviation** of the wrist. In some cases **ulnar translocation** occurs. (See Chapter 19 for referenced detailed discussion of finger and wrist deformities.) Subluxation of the wrist may be further enhanced by **volar displacement of the extensor carpi ulnaris tendon.** Once displaced this tendon loses its effectiveness as an extensor and creates an additional flexor and deviation force on the carpus.

Extensor Tendon Sheath. Tenosynovitis weakens the extensor tendons by direct infiltration and indirectly through pressure, compromising the neurovascular supply of the tendons. Constant movement over the roughened carpal bones can lead to **rupture of the long finger extensor tendons.** *Unlike joint synovitis, tenosynovitis may be painless and without warmth during the active phase.*[5]

Flexor Tendon Sheath. Tenosynovitis can occur at three levels: the wrist, palm, and volar aspects of the fingers and thumb. In the wrist or **carpal tunnel** it can result in entrapment of the median nerve, impairing sensation to the thumb, index, middle, and ring fingers, as well as the ability to abduct the thumb. Wrist tenosynovitis can also impede flexor tendon excursion, creating either a **flexion or extension lag,** typically affecting all four digits. If left untreated, this can result in permanent contractures of the digital joints. Wrist flexor tenosynovitis can also directly invade the tendons, making them vulnerable to rupture. **Digital tenosynovitis** is common and can result in (1) impaired tendon excursion that initially limits distal interphalangeal (DIP) flexion but, if severe, *can limit motion in all of the joints;* (2) thickening or stenosing of the flexor sheath; (3) proliferative tenosynovium that can impair tendon function; and (4) granulomatous plaques that can build up on the tendon. These plaques, as well as tendon nodules, can catch on the fibrous bands of the sheath (**annular ligaments— "pulleys"**), creating a **"trigger finger."** (See Chapter 19, Hand Pathodynamics and Assessment.)

The various combinations of hand deformities are practically boundless. Each hand is unique and the effect of the deformity on hand function depends on how the person uses his or her hands in daily activities. Similar to not judging a book by its cover, one cannot determine hand function by looking at the appearance of the hand. Actual functional assessment through demonstration is essential for determining hand function.

Therapy

Occupational therapy for hand involvement consists of five areas:

1. Evaluation of hand pathology and function, including the quality of use— tense, relaxed, or strong.
2. Fabrication and use of orthotics to reduce pain and inflammation, maintain joint integrity, and improve function.
3. Instruction in joint-protection techniques, adaptive methods, and use of assistive equipment to maintain joint integrity, reduce pain, and improve function.
4. Patient instruction in the use of heat or cold to control inflammation, enhance mobility, and facilitate exercise.
5. Instruction in activities or exercises to maintain or improve hand function, joint mobility, and muscular strength.

Specific therapy procedures can be found in Chapter 19, Hand Pathodynamics and Assessment; Chapter 23, Orthotic Treatment for Arthritis of the Hand; Chapter 24, Joint-Protection and Energy-Conservation Instruction; Chapter 25, Assistive Devices; Chapter 26, Functional Activities; Chapter 27, Exercise Treatment; and Chapter 28, Positioning and Lying Prone.

Feet and Ankles

Initial RA involvement typically includes the metatarsophalangeal (MTP) joints. MTP joint involvement is painful and is frequently described by the patient as "feels like walking on marbles." It interferes with the push-off phase of ambulation, thereby shifting the effect of weight bearing on other joints. **Synovitis in the MTP joints** weakens the joint capsules and supporting ligaments, which makes them extremely vulnerable to the stress of weight bearing. The result of MTP synovitis is flattening of the anterior arch (**splayed forefoot**), **plantar subluxation of the metatarsal heads** with **plantar callosities, spasm** of the intrinsic and extrinsic muscles, and secondary **cock-up or hammer toe deformities.** The subconscious attempt to avoid weight bearing on painful toes often elicits hyperactivity of the long toe extensor, contributing to cock-up toe deformities as well as **hindfoot varus** or **valgus.** (Try walking across the room pretending you have painful MTP joints. Note extensor muscle activity, whether you walk on the inside or outside of your feet, and how it limits active knee and hip ROM.)

The synovium lines the ankle (tibiotalofibular) and subtalar joints, the sheaths of the tendons that cross the ankle, and the Achilles bursa. Although it is possible for all of these structures to become inflamed, many (possible the majority) patients with RA have involvement of only the MTP and subtalar (hindfoot) joints and possibly the tendons but never develop true ankle joint disease, which limits flexion and extension. Subtalar involvement increases the natural tendency of the talus to glide forward, downward, and medially. Subsequent pressure on the calcaneus and spring ligament results in **hindfoot pronation** (valgus) and **flattening of the longitudinal arch.** This diminishes inversion and eversion mobility necessary for adjustment to uneven ground. Ambulation with the ankle in this position necessitates medial pressure against the large toe and contributes to a hallux valgus deformity of the first MTP joint and alters weight-bearing forces on the knee. (See Chapter 35 for further discussion on foot pathodynamics.) Foot and ankle pain diminishes the desire to walk and stand and necessitates walking slowly; thus the time spent performing daily activities is lengthened. This must be kept in mind during the activities of daily living (ADL) assessment and when recommending active ADL measures.

The true ankle joint is involved less frequently than the subtalar, but when it is involved, it severely limits ankle flexion and extension.

JRA foot involvement is different from that in adult RA. (See Chapter 14.)

Therapy

Occupational therapy programs for foot involvement vary considerably. They may consist of (1) evaluation to determine the degree of foot involvement and how the pain affects the person's daily activities; (2) patient education regarding appropriate exercise and rest for the foot and ankle during synovitis, proper positioning in bed, and appropriate shoe support; and (3) fitting of Plastazote shoe liners. In some clinics, particularly in Canada, the therapist's role extends to constructing and fitting shoe adaptations. (See Chapter 24, Joint-Protection and Energy-Conservation Instruction, for a discussion of foot orthotics and recommended shoe requirements.)

The foot should be treated as thoroughly and aggressively as the hand. What follows is my personal approach for management of early RA foot involvement.

For Early MTP Synovitis

1. Referral to a podiatrist for a custom Plastazote orthosis with MTP pad, which can be used in various shoes to reduce weight bearing on the MTP joints.

2. Counseling regarding proper shoe requirements (see Chapter 24).

3. Recommend using orthoses and good-quality athletic walking shoes as much as possible, especially for any distance walking.

4. Daily active and passive ROM exercises to the toes and foot to prevent contractures secondary to muscle spasm and altered gait. (Ideally this is done during a tub bath or when drying the feet after a shower.)

For Subtalar Synovitis

1. Use of a custom plastic orthosis with a heel cup and MTP bar to reduce inversion and eversion instead of a basic orthosis.

2. For hindfoot valgus, a corrective wedge can be included in the orthosis.

For Tenosynovitis

1. If it is an isolated problem, use cold compresses two times per day.

2. If it is associated with acute synovitis of other joints, contrast baths or simply a cold bath may be helpful.

Patients with severe **hindfoot deformity** or **ankle instability** are usually candidates for surgery (see Chapter 35) or a polypropylene foot–ankle orthosis (see Chapter 25). The increasing interest in running sports and sports medicine has generated many new designs and concepts for management of ankle–foot orthotics and supports. It is likely that some of these new products will have applicability in orthotic management for arthritis.

The occupational therapist needs to be aware of the skills of other team members, such as the physical therapist, podiatrist, orthopedist, and orthotist, and of community shoe resources, so he or she can make appropriate recommendations for referral.

Specific therapy procedures can be found in Chapter 24, Joint-Protection and Energy-Conservation Instruction, and Chapter 28, Positioning and Lying Prone.

Knees

The knee joint contains the largest amount of synovium in any one joint. Consequently synovitis can produce marked hypertrophy and effusions that distend and stretch the joint capsule and the supporting cruciate and collateral ligaments. Pain and stretch of the joint capsule result in reflex spasm of the hamstring muscles and inhibition of the knee extensors. Patients frequently respond by keeping their knees flexed (usually with pillows under the knee or sleeping side-lying) to relieve the joint tension.

Knee flexion contractures, secondary hamstring tightness, and postural adaptation are severe functional problems that disrupt the stability of the joint for weight bearing and ambulation (See Chapter 34, Knee Surgery, for a discussion of knee pathodynamics and use of ambulation aids.)

Therapy

The goal of occupational therapy for knee involvement is to educate the patient in joint protection, proper positioning, and assistive equipment. The latter includes raised chairs and commercial resting splints, which are used to minimize stress and pain and thereby reduce inflammation and increase functional ability. Specific therapy procedures can be found in Chapter 24, Joint-Protection and Energy-Conservation Instruction; Chapter 25, Assistive Devices; and Chapter 28, Positioning and Lying Prone.

Physical therapy for reduction of inflammation and contractures, quadriceps strengthening, and gait training is critical.

Hips

Inflamed synovium confined in a tight fibrous hip capsule produces pain and muscle spasm of the flexor and adductor muscles of the hip. The most comfortable position for someone with hip synovitis is hip flexion and external rotation. Consequently, **fibrous contractures in flexion and external rotation are common** if restriction of motion is prolonged. Pain as a result of hip involvement is commonly felt anteriorly in the groin; occasionally the pain is referred to the medial side of the knee. Severe disease can produce extensive destruction of both the acetabulum and femoral head, a condition that can result in the acetabulum being pushed into the pelvic cavity by the femur (**protrusio acetabuli**).

Pain is the main cause of functional limitation, and it impedes all weight-bearing activities. **Protective muscular spasm** promotes hip flexion contractures in the early stages. This necessitates knee flexion and lumbar lordosis in order to permit a vertical position, and thus producing additional stress to these areas and contributing to knee flexion contractures.

When involvement becomes more intense, limitation of hip flexion and abduction may interfere with sitting comfortably in chairs, walking up steps, positioning during sexual intercourse, and with self-care capabilities, such as those involved with reaching the feet.

Therapy

Occupational therapy for hip involvement is primarily of an educational nature. For example, the patient is instructed in joint-protection techniques and the use of assistive devices; he or she is taught to lie prone to maintain hip extension and shown how to use proper positioning at night. Exercises to improve hip abductor and extensor strength and joint mobility are prescribed in physical therapy.

Elevated chairs and toilet seats can significantly reduce stress to the hip joint and back as well as increase the patient's comfort when there is severe involvement, such as extension contractures. (See the section on hips in Chapter 4, Osteoarthritis, for additional information on severe limitations, and Chapter 33, Hip Surgery, for a discussion on hip pathodynamics.) Assistive aids for dressing and hygiene of the lower extremity may also be indicated.

Specific therapy procedures can be found in Chapter 24, Joint-Protection and Energy-Conservation Instruction; Chapter 25, Assistive Devices; and Chapter 28, Positioning and Lying Prone.

Elbows

The synovial lining is common to both the elbow (humeroradioulnar) and the proximal radioulnar joint. Painful synovitis prompts the patient to keep the arm in flexion and pronation with consequent contractures as the main functional limitation.

Flexion contractures up to 30 degrees usually do not interfere with functional ability; however, when the loss of extension is greater, function is affected. A loss of 30 to 60 degrees of extension interferes with ability for reach such as that needed for pulling on socks, and a loss of 45 to 90 degrees of extension restricts push-off leverage for chair transfers and interferes with mobility required in dressing. Loss of greater than 90 degrees of extension is rare but, when it occurs, it seriously restricts reach and ability for dressing, perineal care, and transfer, and it necessitates trunk flexion for performance of desk work or feeding.

Extension contractures (diminished elbow flexion) are less frequent; they can severely limit one's ability for feeding, grooming, and hygiene. For example, a person who can only flex his or her elbow to 90 degrees generally will not be able to eat even with regular utensils (unless he or she has a long flexible neck).

When loss of forearm rotation is inevitable, the optimal position for ankylosis depends upon shoulder and wrist function; however, 20 degrees of pronation allows easier substitution of shoulder rotation for forearm motion.

Another problem seen in some patients with RFT RA is the presence of **subcutaneous rheumatoid nodules** over the dorsum of the olecranon or shaft of the ulna. (These nodules can also occur over other bony prominences, e.g., ischial tuberosity, occipital bone, and so forth.) They are usually painless but can become painful when irritated by pressure. The nodules are important diagnostically as they indicate a more complex immunological dysfunction.

Therapy

The obvious treatment of choice is prevention. After permanent contractures develop, the only nonsurgical means to improve function is instruction in adaptive methods and use of assistive equipment.

Night splinting of the elbow to provide local rest and proper positioning or to apply sustained passive pressure to reduce developing contractures is a valid approach for some clients.[5] When nodules are aggravated by pressure, pain can be reduced by alleviating the irritating source or redistributing the pressure with a doughnut pad or an elbow protector pad encased in a knit sleeve that slips onto the elbow. Several brands are available from medical supply distributors (see Chapter 28, Positioning and Lying Prone). Some nodules that occur at pressure sites will diminish or disappear once the pressure is alleviated. Lambswool cuffs *should not be used* because they encourage elbow flexion contractures (elbow flexion is needed to keep them in place).

Specific therapy procedures can be found in Chapter 25, Assistive Devices; Chapter 28, Positioning and Lying Prone; and for methods of documenting nodule status, Chapter 19, Hand Pathodynamics and Assessment.

Shoulders

The shoulder is a complex structure that depends upon the coordinated movement of four joints (glenohumeral, acromioclavicular, sternoclavicular, and thoracoscapular) and the smooth gliding of tendons, principally the biceps and supraspinatus tendons, which cross over the glenohumeral joints.

Synovitis affects the glenohumeral joint, thereby causing cartilage loss, damage to the capsule, and severe limitation of motion and function. However, fibromyalgia, tendinitis, bursitis, and capsular fibrosis are far more frequent sources of shoulder pain even in patients with RA.

Patients who complain of aching in the trapezius area radiating into the upper arm or distal to the fingers should have a medical work-up for fibromyalgia. Patients with RA are so used to having pain that both they and their physicians often attribute all musculoskeletal symptoms to RA. The emotional stress and pain of RA frequently interfere with deep sleep, making fibromyalgia a likely consequence (see Chapter 5).

When there is true RA involvement of the shoulder, it is frequently severe and limits functional ability for hair care and dressing. Several factors contribute to this situation. Prime among these are the facts that shoulder joint involvement usually occurs late in the disease process, and that patients, who are concerned with limitations caused by early hand, knee, and foot involvement, frequently neglect shoulder exercises or problems, or both. They are not aware of shoulder limitations until significant mobility restrictions occur. Since only about 90 degrees of shoulder flexion and abduction and 30 degrees of external rotation are necessary for most functional activities, a person can lose up to 50 percent of shoulder mobility before it interferes with his or her ADL.

Therapy

Three factors limit functional use of the shoulder: pain, decreased muscle strength and endurance, and decreased ROM. Any program to improve function must address these issues. Pain and poor endurance usually interfere with function long before decreased ROM is a problem. Functional activities (crafts) are often an effective adjunct to improvement of shoulder strength and endurance, since they can be designed to tax muscle power within a pain-free range.

Remedial exercises usually do not help when there is actual bony destruction. Compensatory measures, such as using assistive equipment and instruction in adaptive methods, are the only nonsurgical means for improving function. Assistive equipment, such as dressing sticks, reachers, and extended combs, brushes, and tableware, is helpful. When prescribing this equipment, however, it is important to assess the entire upper extremity since many extended-handle devices can cause damaging stress to the hands.

Specific therapy procedures can be found in Chapter 24, Joint-Protection and Energy-Conservation Instruction; Chapter 25, Assistive Devices; Chapter 26, Functional Activities; and Chapter 27, Exercise Treatment.

Cervical Spine

Cervical **pain** and **stiffness** are common symptoms in early RA, and radiographic changes are almost universal in advanced cases of RA. The posterior neck muscles, especially the trapezius, are prone to tightness secondary to postural strain and emotional stress in "healthy" individuals. The addition of emotional factors, such as depression, fear, and physical factors, such as pain, deconditioning, altered gait, and functional biomechanics typically associated with RA, take a toll on the cervical region. Consequently **localized myofascial pain syndrome** or **generalized fibromyalgia** are common sequela. Also, **disc degeneration** or **cervical spondylosis** occurs with the same incidence in people with RA as it does in the general population. Chronic synovitis attacks the capsules, ligamentous supports, and joint surfaces of the apophyseal and lateral interbody joints (joints of Luschka). The first to fourth cervical vertebral joints are the most common sites of inflammation, but the entire cervical spine can be involved. Initially there is pain and muscle spasm that limit mobility. Progressive involvement leads to subluxation of the joints, particularly the atlantoaxial joint (first to second cervical). **Subluxation of the low cervical spine** is more likely to produce symptoms of cord root compression than subluxation of the first to fourth cervical vertebrae because the ratio of the spinal cord to the diameter of the spinal canal is less in the upper portion; that is, the cord takes up about half the spinal canal in the first to fourth cervical area but nearly fills the canal along the fourth to eighth cervical vertebrae.

Patients with **atlantoaxial subluxation** present with pain and tenderness in the upper cervical spine and radiation of pain to the suboccipital area, aggravated by full neck flexion or extension. They may have sharp paresthesias or **Lhermitte's sign,** electricity-like pain radiating into the extremities with neck flexion.[6] *These symptoms should be immediately reported to the patient's physician* because they indicate a high risk for cord damage. Patients may also have a feeling of weakness and instability.[6] Occasionally, the patients are able to feel the bones sublux, stating it feels like their head will "slip off."[6] Compression of either of the vertebral arteries may cause visual disturbance (diplopia, blurring), loss of equilibrium, tinnitus, dizziness, or light-headedness.[7,8] Neurological symptoms do not have to be present.[9] If they are present, they can be multiple and varied, including occipital neuralgia, upper motor neuron symptoms, altered reflexes, or quadriparesis. Subjective sensation may be altered, producing feelings of paresthesia, numbness, heat, and cold. (These symptoms need to be distinguished from fibromyalgia and anxiety.) Bulbar disturbance can be sudden and fatal, or it may present with abnormal swallowing or phonation.[7]

Once frank symptoms of cord compression are evident the only measure that will help is cervical fusion. Cervical collars and intermittent halter traction are not sufficient to reduce subluxation.

Therapy

In the early stages treatment is directed to muscular spasm and tightness and improving posture and muscular tone. Physical therapy includes massage, relaxation techniques, postural exercises, deep breathing, myofascial release, and exercises or movements to maintain or improve ROM. For acute muscular spasm, modalities such as ultrasound, neuroprobe, or electric stimulation may be used. Occupational therapy measures include assessment of postural use and strain at home (including sleeping postures), work, and leisure, and counseling in body mechanics and joint-protection techniques to reduce pain and cervical stress, as well as the dynamic forces that contribute to subluxation. For instruction in using relaxation techniques at work or during daily activities keep in mind that the neck is a focal point for emotional stress. Any treatment, such as energy conservation or stress management counseling, that can reduce fatigue or help prevent overexhaustion contributes to reduction of cervical spinal pain and spasm. Cervical pillows can also be effective in reducing muscle spasm and stiffness. (See the section on the cervical spine in Chapter 4, Osteoarthritis; Chapter 28, Positioning and Lying Prone; Chapter 22, Evaluation of Activities of Daily Living, at Home, Work, and Leisure; Chapter 24, Joint-Protection and Energy-Conservation Instruction; and Chapter 25, Assistive Devices.)

Soft neck collars can serve patients in several ways. First, for people with early involvement who do not need a collar for treatment, the collar can be a very helpful device for training patients in ideal cervical alignment during functional activities. For example, a secretary trying to learn how to reduce neck strain while typing will learn very quickly how to position copy material if she wears a collar during typing (not as treatment but as a training technique). Second, for some patients a collar may help relieve muscle spasm because it keeps the neck warm and encourages straighter alignment. Third, collars should be worn by all patients with radiographic evidence of subluxation during high-risk situations, such as driving.

Cervical pillows can also be very effective in reducing muscle spasm and stiffness. My preference is to start with the Jackson cervical pillow (Cervipillo), since it is the least expensive and has a high success rate.

Custom Plastazote collars provide greater restriction of flexion but do not completely immobilize the neck. The Somi brace is a widely used commercial four-post brace and is the most restrictive type of brace. Maximal (nearly complete) immobilization is achieved only with a halo apparatus, with a plaster vest, or by pelvic fixation.[10,11] Fortunately cervical fusions make the halo nearly unnecessary for people with RA. See also Chapters 5, Fibromyalgia, and the section on cervical osteoarthritis in Chapter 4.

Systemic Manifestations

The symptoms of **fatigue, malaise, subjective weakness, anorexia, and decreased motivation** accompany all systemic illnesses to some degree. In addition to these, generalized stiffness is part of RA. The severity of systemic symptoms is roughly correlated with the degree of inflammatory activity in the joints and tends to increase with energy expenditure. Consequently, fatigue and associated manifestations often become apparent after about 4 to 6 hours of activity.

Many of the symptoms of systemic disease are identical to those of psychological depression and distinguishing these two phenomena can be difficult. A helpful feature is that systemic fatigue is usually related to the person's energy expenditure, whereas fatigue associated with depression is more constant.

Therapy

For fatigue resulting from systemic involvement, instruction in work simplification and energy conservation can improve the patient's endurance for functional activities. Assess the individual's rest patterns and reinforce the need for 10 to 12 hours of rest per day to allow the body's restorative processes to help combat disease. Another compounding factor is that pain and stiffness at night often cause the patient to lose sleep, which further enhances fatigue and muscular pain (fibromyalgia).

When the disease is under control or in a chronic-active phase, patient participation in a community program of body conditioning or exercise two to three times a week can be effective for improving endurance, muscle tone, balance, posture, and self-esteem. However, patients often need guidelines for determining which exercises to do and how to monitor the effects of exercise on their arthritis.

When fatigue associated with depression interferes with the person's ADL, refer the patient to a person (physician, psychologist, psychotherapist, counselor, or social worker) or agency (community counseling service) that can arrange for ongoing counseling to help him or her work through the depression.

Specific therapy procedures can be found in Chapter 2, Psychological Considerations in Patient Education and Treatment; Chapter 24, Joint-Protection and Energy-Conservation Instruction; and Chapter 22, Evaluation of Activities of Daily Living at Home, Work, and Leisure. Also see Chapter 5, Fibromyalgia.

Associated Organ Involvement

A small percentage of people with RA develop various degrees of pulmonary and cardiac involvement.[4] There are no specific occupational therapy measures for these conditions except to be aware that they can exist. If cardiac or pulmonary involvement may influence the therapy program, it should be verified with the physician before starting a treatment program. This usually does not create a problem since patients with significant cardiac or lung involvement normally would not be on a stressful therapy regimen.

There can also be a rare but severe vasculitis associated with RA. (See Chapter 12 for more information.)

DRUG THERAPY

Anti-inflammatory medications are the mainstay of drug treatment for RA. **Aspirin** and aspirin-type medications work as analgesics when given in small doses; they are effective as anti-inflammatory agents when given in large doses. The dosage is adjusted to maintain a blood salicylate level just below toxicity, which is evidenced by tinnitus (ringing or sound in the ears). Any of the other **nonsteroidal anti-inflammatory drugs** (NSAIDs) may be used in place of a salicylate. These drugs have been shown to be as effective as acetylsalicylic acid (ASA) in controlling the inflammation of RA. For many individuals, NSAIDs have less gastrointestinal side effects, and they have the advantage of easier administration, requiring 1 to 4 tablets per day.

When synovitis is nonresponsive to aspirin and other nonsteroidal anti-inflammatory medications, the second line of attack (or defense, depending on one's perspective) is to use **disease-modifying drugs** (DMDs). These medications have the potential for serious side effects, but they also have the potential for controlling the long-term effects of the disease and in some cases effecting a near remission. Medications in this category include **injectable gold salts, oral gold, antimalarial drugs** (Plaquenil), **penicillamine, low-dose methotrexate,** and **azathioprine** (Imuran). Gold therapy is the most widely used and is generally tried first; Plaquenil is often the second choice (but may be the first choice); and until recently, penicillamine was the typical third choice; now low-dose methotrexate is often used in those patients unresponsive or intolerant to gold. Methotrexate and azathioprine are used in patients unresponsive or intolerant to the others.

Gold salts given by injection can be an effective form of therapy for some patients, particularly in the acute or subacute stages of their disease. Injections are given weekly for 20 weeks, and if there is a good response, they are continued at 2- to 4-week intervals. Auranofin (oral gold) now provides an alternative to injection therapy.

Antimalarial medication is in tablet form and does not require weekly clinic visits as does gold therapy. The current practice of using lower doses has significantly reduced the risks of permanent visual loss; however, patients must be responsible for obtaining appropriate ophthalmological evaluations every 6 months.

Low-dose methotrexate is given in a weekly dosage either orally or parentally. It has proven to be a very effective anti-arthritic medication. In low dosage it does not have the side effects associated with the dosage used to treat cancer. Occasionally, however, life-threatening side effects such as bone marrow suppression or acute allergic pulmonary involvement can occur even at low doses.

Corticosteroids such as prednisone are effective anti-inflammatory agents. Their undesirable side effects usually preclude their long-term use in RA, except in small doses in conjunction with other medications.

Experimental drugs such as **cyclophosphamide** (Cytoxan) and **chlorambucil** are used occasionally and can benefit selected patients. However, these drugs may have an immunosuppressive action as well as an anti-inflammatory effect. Their undesirable side effects frequently preclude their use.

The procedure of removing large quantities of plasma, or **plasmaphoresis,** has been claimed to be effective in reducing inflammation in RA. This treatment must be considered purely experimental until well-controlled studies have been performed.

REFERENCES

1. Harris, ED: Pathogenesis of rheumatoid arthritis. In Kelley, WM, et al (eds): Textbook of Rheumatology, ed 2. Philadelphia, WB Saunders, 1985.
2. Harris, ED: Rheumatoid arthritis: The clinical spectrum. In Kelley, WM, et al (eds): Textbook of Rheumatology, ed 2. WB Saunders, Philadelphia, 1985.
3. Arnett, FC, Edworthy, SM, Bloch, DA, et al: The American Rheumatism Association 1987 revised criteria for the classification of rheumatoid arthritis. Arthritis Rheum 31(3):315–324, 1988.
4. Decker, JL, and Plotz, PH: Extra-articular rheumatoid disease. In McCarty, DJ (ed): Arthritis and Allied Conditions. Lea & Febiger, Philadelphia, 1979.
5. Melvin, J: Rheumatic Disease—Occupational Therapy and Rehabilitation, ed 2. FA Davis, Philadelphia, 1982.
6. Thomas, WH: Surgical management of the rheumatoid cervical spine. Orthop Clin North Am 6(3):793, 1975.
7. Jackson, R: The Cervical Syndrome. Charles C Thomas, Springfield, IL, 1977.
8. Lipson, SJ: Rheumatoid arthritis of the cervical spine. Clin Orthop Rel Res 182:143–149, 1984.
9. Fielding, JW, and Bjorkengren, AG: Surgery for arthritis of the cervical spine. In Kelly, WM, et al (eds): Textbook of Rheumatology, ed 2. WB Saunders, Philadelphia, 1985.
10. Johnson, RM, et al: Cervical orthoses: A study comparing their effectiveness in restricting cervical motion in normal subjects. J Bone Joint Surg 59A:3, 1977.
11. Hart, DL, Johnson, RM, Simmons, EF, and Owen, J: Review of cervical orthoses. Phys Ther 58(7), July 1978.

ADDITIONAL SOURCES

Bland, JH: Rheumatoid arthritis of the cervical spine. J Rheumatol 3:319–341, 1974.
Boulware, DW, Weissman, DN, and Doll, NJ: Pulmonary manifestations of the rheumatic diseases. Clin Rev Allergy 3(2):249–267, 1985.
Bulmash, JM: Rheumatoid arthritis and pregnancy. Obstet Syn Annu 8:223, 1979.
Calabro, JL: Rheumatoid arthritis. Clinical Symposia, CIBA, Vol 23, No 1, 1971.
Carty, EA, Conine, TA, and Wood-Johnson, F: Rheumatoid arthritis and pregnancy: Helping women to meet their needs. Midwives Chron 99(1186):254–257, 1986.
Cavender, D, Haskard, D, Yu, CL, Iguchi, T, Miossec, P, et al: Pathways to chronic inflammation in rheumatoid synovitis. Fed Proc 46(1):113–117, 1987 (review).
Ehrlich, GE: Social, economic, psychologic, and sexual outcomes in rheumatoid arthritis. Am J Med 75(6A):27–34, 1983.
Fox, RI, Lotz, M, Rhodes, G, and Vaughan, JH: Epstein-Barr virus in rheumatoid arthritis. Clin Rheum Dis 11(3):665–688, 1985.
Harris, CJ: Rheumatoid arthritis and the pregnant woman. Am J Nurs 85(4):414–417, 1985.
Jorizzo, JL, and Daniels, JC: Dermatologic conditions reported in patients with rheumatoid arthritis. J Am Acad Dermatol 8(4):439–457, 1983.
Kovarsky, J: Otorhinolaryngologic complications of rheumatic diseases. Semin Arthritis Rheum 14(2):141–150, 1984.
Kowanko, IC, Knapp, MS, Pownall, R, and Swannell, AJ: Domiciliary self-measurement in the rheu-

matoid arthritis and the demonstration of circadian rhythmicity. Ann Rheum Dis 41(5):453–455, 1982.

Levine, JD, Collier, DH, Basbaum, AI, Moskowitz, MA, and Helms, CA: Hypothesis: The nervous system may contribute to the pathophysiology of rheumatoid arthritis. J Rheumatol 12(3):406–411, 1985.

Makisara, GL, et al: Prognosis of functional capacity and work capacity in RA. Clin Rheum 1(2):117–125, 1982.

McCookey, B, Fraser, GM, and Bligh, AS: Transparent skin and osteoporosis. Annu Rheum Dis 24:219–223, 1965.

McDuffie, FC: Morbidity impact of rheumatoid arthritis on society. Am J Med 78(1A):1–5, 1985.

Nitz, AJ: Physical therapy management of the shoulder. Phys Ther 66(12):1912–1919, 1986.

Polly, HF, and Hunder, GG: Rheumatologic Interviewing and Physical Examination of the Joints. WB Saunders, Philadelphia, 1988.

Roschmann, RA, and Rothenberg, RJ: Pulmonary fibrosis in rheumatoid arthritis: A review of clinical features and therapy. Semin Arthritis Rheum 16(3):174–185, 1987 (review).

Santavirta, S, Kankaanpaa, U, Sandelin, J, Laasonen, E, et al: Evaluation of patients with rheumatoid cervical spine. Scand J Rheumatol 16(1):9–16, 1987 (review).

Scott, DL, and Farr, M: Assessing the progression of joint damage in rheumatoid arthritis. Drugs 32(Suppl 1):63–70, 1986 (review).

Skevington, SM, Blackwell, F, and Britton, NF: Self-esteem and perception of attractiveness: An investigation of early rheumatoid arthritis. Br J Med Psychol 60(Pt 1):45–52, 1987.

Steinbach, L, Hellmann, D, Petri, M, Gillespy, T, et al: Magnetic resonance imaging: A review of rheumatologic applications. Semin Arthritis Rheum 16(2):79–91, 1986 (review).

Wallace, DJ: The role of stress and trauma in rheumatoid arthritis and systemic lupus erythematosus. Semin Arthritis Rheum 16(3):153–157, 1987 (review).

Audiovisual

Caruso, L, and Mathiowetz, V: Rheumatoid Arthritis: Occupational Therapy Evaluation and Treatment Planning. Midwest Arthritis Treatment Center, Columbia Hospital, Milwaukee, 1984.

Chapter 7

Psoriatic Arthritis

Psoriatic arthritis (PA) is a distinct systemic disease in which psoriasis is associated with inflammatory arthritis and a negative serological test for rheumatoid factor (RF). The arthritis can range from mild to severely erosive and can affect single or multiple peripheral joints as well as the spine. The disease is characterized by exacerbations and remissions.[1]

Psoriasis is a chronic, occasionally acute, dermatitis, consisting of discrete pink or dull-red lesions surrounded by a characteristic silvery scaling.[2]

ETIOLOGICAL FACTORS

The specific cause of psoriasis or of PA is not known. The high incidence of psoriasis within families clearly indicates a genetic component to the pathogenesis of the disease.[3] The antigen HLA-B27 is seen in one subtype of PA in which spondylitis is present but not in the nonspondylitic subtypes.[4]

AGE AND SEX AFFECTED

Psoriasis occurs in about 1 percent of the population, with a peak incidence in the third decade of life. About 7 percent of adults with psoriasis develop some form of PA. The adult male-to-female incidence is nearly 1:1.[4] Both psoriasis and PA are generally not seen under the age of 6 years and are uncommon in older children.

DIAGNOSIS

In the majority of adult patients (75 percent), the psoriasis precedes the arthritis; in 10 percent, it has an onset synchronous with that of the arthritis. In adults, the diagnosis is based on the presence of an inflammatory polyarthritis in the presence of psoriasis along with a negative serological test for RF. Certain characteristic features, such as arthritis confined to the distal interphalangeal (DIP) joints, "sausage swelling" of fingers or toes, asymmetric distribution of the arthritis in the hands and feet, absence of subcutaneous nodules, specific peripheral or axial radiographs, and a history or PA in first-degree family members, are supportive of the diagnosis.[1,3,5,6] In children, RF seronegativity is not a distinguishing feature so diagnosis is based on the characteristic clinical features.[7]

In 15 percent of cases, in which the arthritis occurs first, PA can only be suspected if there is a combination of *classic signs,* such as *severe erosive DIP involvement* and *seronegative test for RF, or asymmetric sausage swelling, negative RF, and a family history of psoriasis.*[5,8]

The incidence of psoriasis in patients with seropositive arthritis is similar to the incidence of psoriasis in the general population, about 1 percent. Therefore, it is possible to have a coincidental occurrence of psoriasis and RA.[9]

Initially considered a variant of RA, PA is now recognized as a distinct disease that shares features with other forms of arthritis that occur with diseases of the skin, urethra, bowel, or spine. These diseases are called **spondyloarthropathies** and include Reiter's syndrome, ulcerative colitis, regional enteritis, and ankylosing spondylitis, in addition to PA. Besides asymmetric inflammatory arthritis, these diseases share the following features: (1) negative test for RF; (2) absence of subcutaneous (rheumatoid) nodules; (3) ocular inflammation; (4) sacroiliitis and/or spondylitis; and (5) evidence of HLA-B27 antigen.[3,5]

COURSE AND PROGNOSIS

Joint inflammation in PA occurs in a wide spectrum of presentations, ranging from mild, insidious monoarticular involvement to a rapidly destructive arthritis mutilans.[3] In general, there is no correlation between the severity of the skin disease and the extent of joint involvement. Exacerbations of joint and skin disease *may* or *may not* coincide.[3]

The course and prognosis depend on which type of involvement is present. In general, the outcome for functional independence is better for PA than for RA. The following five clinical patterns of adult joint involvement have been identified by Moll and Wright.[1]

Group 1. Predominant involvement of the DIP joints of the hands. This pattern is described as the classic pattern because it was the first type of arthritis clearly related to psoriasis, even though it represents only 5 to 10 percent of patients with PA.[5,10] These patients may have asymmetric involvement of other joints. The arthritis can range from minimal to severely erosive with osteolysis of the terminal tuft. DIP joint involvement is almost always associated with psoriatic nail changes.[5]

Group 2. Arthritis mutilans (osteolysis of the bones in the involved joints). Typically, this process occurs in the phalanges (hands and feet), metacarpals, metatarsals, and occasionally, the distal ulna. When it occurs in the digits, the ends of the bones resorb and shorten. The overlying redundant skin creates a telescoping appearance to the fingers **("opera glass hand").** This condition may happen to one or all of the digits.[8,11] When it occurs in several fingers, it may severely limit functional dexterity. This pattern occurs in a minority of cases, approximately 5 percent of all PA patients.[10] These patients also have a high incidence of spinal involvement and are prone to bony ankylosis in joints not affected with mutilans.[5,9,10]

Group 3. Symmetric peripheral polyarthritis similar to the distribution seen in RA. Any synovial joints can be affected, including the temporomandibular joint. As in RA, all degrees of involvement can be seen in this group. Some patients with acute inflammation can rapidly progress to ankylosis.[5,11]

Group 4. Asymmetric, oligoarticular arthritis (affecting a single or few joints) of the fingers or toes.[8] This distribution accounts for 70 percent of all cases of PA.[3,5,10]

Group 5. Ankylosing spondylitis associated with psoriasis. This may occur in a pattern similar to idiopathic ankylosing spondylitis or may be in association with severe peripheral joint disease.[5] (See Chapter 8.)

This classification describes five typical patterns; it is possible for patients (adults and children) to have mixed patterns of joint involvement.

SYMPTOMATOLOGY AND IMPLICATIONS FOR OCCUPATIONAL THERAPY

Articular Involvement

Hand Involvement

Patients in Groups 3, 4, or 5 often present with diffuse swelling of one or more entire digits, typically referred to as **sausage swelling** to distinguish it from **fusiform swelling,** which denotes swelling confined to the joint capsule.

This diffuse swelling is attributed to a combination of interphalangeal (IP) or IP and metacarpophalangeal (MCP) joint synovitis and flexor tendon sheath effusion.[5,9] The swelling is firm or hard when palpated, and it appears to be throughout the entire digit, not isolated to the volar aspect as flexor tenosynovitis is in RA. Radiographs often reveal periosteitis along the shaft of the bone, when there is sausage swelling, but this may be a reflection of generalized tenosynovitis rather than a causal factor.[11]

In addition to the sausage digits, hand involvement in *PA differs from that seen in RA* in the following features:

1. There may be severe involvement of the DIP joints. Mallet finger deformities are common.[3,5]
2. PIP and MCP joint involvement is random or asymmetric.[5]
3. There is a higher incidence of bony ankylosis, particularly in the digits, as well as in the wrist (bony ankylosis in RA tends to occur in the wrists).[5,12]
4. It is rare to have extensor tenosynovitis and extensor tendon ruptures in PA.[5,12]
5. Ulnar drift is less common and occurs in patients with chronic MCP synovitis.[6]
6. PIP flexion contractures are common, but swan neck and boutonnière can also occur.[12]
7. Marked synovial hypertrophy is less common.[12]
8. The most common deformities are contractures due to periarticular swelling and generalized capsular fibrosis.

Other Joint Involvement

Joint inflammation in all joints except the hands, toes, and spine is similar to that seen with RA. (See Chapter 3 and Part VI for consequences of chronic synovitis in specific joints.) The toes often have a destructive arthritis of the IP joints similar to that in the fingers and can also have the sausage digital swelling. Rarely, the feet may be involved before the hands.[5]

Spinal involvement may encompass the entire spine, identical to ankylosing spondylitis.[5,10] (See Chapter 8 for symptomatology and treatment.) More commonly, the spinal involvement may be asymmetric and even skip vertebrae as the involvement ascends the spine.

Therapy

Occupational therapy is the same for PA as it is for RA or ankylosing spondylitis (if the spine is involved), except in the following areas.

1. Some patients with severe arthritis are prone to developing rapid contractures. These patients need to have their range of motion (ROM) carefully monitored. Proper bed positioning, especially for neck, wrists, knees, and ankles, is critical. Hand and ankle splints may be the only effective means of preventing nonfunctional contractures. (See Chapter 23, Orthotic Treatment for Arthritis of the Hand, and Chapter 28, Positioning and Lying Prone.)

Wearing orthoses is often difficult in the presence of severe psoriasis. A cotton (not nylon) stockinet worn over the extremity in addition to foam orthotic lining often increases comfort. Plastic orthoses should not be applied directly to skin with psoriatic lesions. All orthoses and linens should be washable.

2. The diffuse digital swelling seen in PA is one of the most perplexing hand problems to treat. From personal experience, none of the conventional means of reducing this edema has been effective in diminishing swelling. Methods tried have included string wrapping, Coban* wrapping,

---

*Coban is a soft stretch tape manufactured by the 3M Corporation. It adheres to itself and is reusable. The one-inch width is convenient for gentle, sustained tension to digit joints. It is available through 3M distributors.

and use of Futuro thermoelastic gloves. Neither heat (paraffin) nor ice compresses have reduced digit circumference or increased ROM. On a couple of occasions, heat has increased edema and decreased ROM. Joint-protection techniques can be helpful in reducing joint stress and inflammation.

When only one or a few MCP or proximal interphalangeal (PIP) joints are involved, wrapping the joint into flexion with Coban has proven an effective means of applying gentle sustained pressure and *maintaining* flexion range. (Sustained pressure achieves greater ROM by pushing or compressing the edema, not by stretching the capsule. See Chapter 27.)

Some patients are able to accomplish gentle sustained ROM manually. Teaching patients how to measure fingertip to crease provides them with an easy method for determining that they have achieved their goal of maintaining or improving motion.

Skin and Nail Changes

Except for the fact that DIP joint synovitis is always associated with nail changes, other forms of PA are not associated with any particular pattern of skin involvement. Within any of the PA groups, the psoriasis can range from a minuscule flake in an unnoticeable area, such as the scalp or umbilicus, to generalized exfoliative lesions covering the entire body.[1]

The **psoriatic lesions** consist of sharply demarcated erythematous papules or plaques covered with overlapping shiny or slightly opalescent scales. Itching is usually absent or mild but occasionally can be considerable. The lesions heal *without* scarring.[2]

Psoriasis characteristically involves the scalp (including postauricular regions), the extensor surface of the elbows and knees, the back and buttocks, the nails, eyebrows, axillas, umbilicus, and anogenital region.[2]

The most common nail lesions seen in psoriasis are multiple pits, as if one stuck the nail with a pin, and **onycholysis,** which is the discoloration and loosening of the nail beginning at the free border. These lesions, however, are not unique to this disease and can be associated with fungal and bacterial infection, trauma, and other conditions.[2,3,12,13]

Therapy

Effective therapy of localized psoriasis for most patients is the use of topical coaltar preparations, topical corticosteroid preparations (with or without occlusive dressing), and ultraviolet light or sunlight exposure. Systemic treatment with methotrexate may be considered in patients unresponsive to local therapy. Systemic corticosteroids are contraindicated not only because they are ineffective but because the disease may worsen when the dose is tapered.[4]

Ocular Involvement

Ocular inflammation has been identified with all of the seronegative spondyloarthritides. Iritis is the most significant involvement and is identical to that seen in ankylosing spondylitis.[4,14]

DRUG THERAPY

As in the therapy of RA, nonsteroidal anti-inflammatory medications (NSAIDs) are the initial drugs of choice in controlling the symptoms of PA. Aspirin or any of the other nonsteroidal anti-inflammatory medications may be used. These medications will control the inflammatory symptoms in most patients.[4] When only one or two joints are inflamed, intra-articular injections of corticosteroids may control the process without the need for systemic medication.

Gold salts have been reported to be effective in patients unresponsive to the NSAIDs even though some physicians feel that gold injections may aggravate the skin disease. Penicillamine has not received adequate trial, and the antimalarial drugs are probably contraindicated. Weekly administration of methotrexate in doses of 5 to 20 mg may be effective in controlling more severe skin and joint disease.

REFERENCES

1. Moll, JMH, and Wright, V: Psoriatic arthritis. Semin Arthritis Rheum 3:55, 1973.
2. Sauer, GC: Manual of Skin Diseases, ed 4. JB Lippincott, Philadelphia, 1980. (Excellent dermatological resource for therapists.)
3. Bennett, RM: Psoriatic arthritis. In McCarty, DJ (ed): Arthritis and Allied Conditions, ed 9. Lea & Febiger, Philadelphia, 1979, pp 642–655.
4. Wright, V: Psoriatic arthritis. In Kelley, WM, et al (eds): Textbook of Rheumatology. WB Saunders, Philadelphia, 1981.
5. Wright, V, and Moll, JMH: Seronegative Polyarthritis. Elsevier North-Holland, Amsterdam, 1976.
6. Kammer, GM, Soter, NA, et al: Psoriatic arthritis: A clinical, immunological and HLA study of 100 patients. Semin Arthritis Rheum 9(2), 1979.
7. Singsen, BH: Psoriatic arthritis in childhood. Arthritis Rheum 20:408, 1977.
8. Redisch, W, Messina, EJ, Hughes, G, and McEwen, C: Capillaroscopic observations in the rheumatic diseases. Ann Rheum Dis 29:244, 1970.
9. Baker, H, Golding, N, and Thompson, M: Psoriasis and arthritis. Ann Intern Med 58:909, 1963.
10. Roberts, MET, Wright, V, Hill, AGS, et al: Psoriatic arthritis: Followup study. Ann Rheum Dis 35:206, 1976.
11. Forrester, DM, Brown, JC, and Nesson, JW: The Radiology of Joint Disease. WB Saunders, Philadelphia, 1978.
12. Belsky, MR, Feldon, PG, Millender, LH, Nalebuff, EA, and Phillips, CA: Hand involvement in psoriatic arthritis. J Hand Surg 7:203, 1982.
13. Zaias, N: Psoriasis of the nail: A clinico-pathological study. Arch Derm 99:567, 1969.
14. Lambert, JR, and Wrist, V: Eye inflammation in psoriatic arthritis. Ann Rheum Dis 35:354, 1976.

ADDITIONAL SOURCES

Fassenbender, HG: Pathology of Rheumatic Diseases. Springer-Verlag, New York, 1975, p 245. (Includes a section on pathology of sausage swelling in the digits.)
Laurent, MR: Psoriatic arthritis. Clin Rheum Dis 11(1):61–85, 1985.
Reid, DM, Kennedy, NS, Nicoll, JJ, Smith, MA, Tothill, P, and Nuki, G: Total and peripheral bone mass in patients with psoriatic arthritis and rheumatoid arthritis. Clin Rheum 5(3):372–378, 1986.

Chapter 8

Ankylosing Spondylitis

Ankylosing spondylitis (AS) is a chronic systemic disease in which the primary sites of inflammation are the ligamentous, capsular, and tendinous insertions into bone—the **enthesis.** AS has a predilection for the sacroiliac, spinal apophyseal, and axial joints. Other symptoms may include asymmetric or peripheral arthritis, or ocular, cardiac, or pulmonary involvement.[1]

ETIOLOGICAL FACTORS

There is a definite genetic predisposition to AS and other spondyloarthropathies. A genetically determined histocompatibility antigen, HLA-B27, has been found in greater than 90 percent of people with AS. It is estimated that 10 to 20 percent of in-dividuals with the HLA-B27 antigen will develop one of the spondyloarthrop-athies.[1,2]

AGE AND SEX AFFECTED

The classical form of this disease, with severe spinal involvement, primarily affects men (9 of 10 cases). Over the past 10 years investigations have revealed a milder form of this disease that primarily affects women.[3] The HLA-B27 antigen is found more frequently in white people; therefore, all of the spondyloarthropathies are more common in the white race.[3]

Primary AS usually develops in the second or third decade of life, but juvenile spondyloarthropathy can occur in children.

(See the discussion on pauciarticular onset, subset II, in Chapter 14.)

DIAGNOSIS

Diagnosis is based on history or presence of sacroiliac or lumbar back pain, morning stiffness, and characteristic radiological changes in the sacroiliac or spinal joints. A positive test for the HLA-B27 antigen may help confirm the diagnosis, but it is not essential and is frequently negative.[1]

The disease is considered **primary** if no other rheumatological disorder is present and **secondary** if the sacroiliitis is due to another spondyloarthropathy, such as Reiter's syndrome or psoriatic arthritis.[3]

COURSE AND PROGNOSIS

The course varies widely. Some people have one or two bouts of sacroiliitis in high school or college, then the pain stops. They attribute the problem to a sports- or activity-related strain and never have the problem diagnosed. Years later the characteristic sacroiliac joint changes become a serendipitous discovery on a radiograph. Others, especially men, can develop steadily progressive classical spinal involvement that ascends from the sacroiliac joint to the lumbar, thoracic, and cervical spine. Typically people with active AS experience some peripheral arthritis or enthesopathy. This may be mild and episodic or chronic. They may also develop extra-articular involvement of the eyes, lungs, and heart. The disease process may stop at any stage, with residual pain-free deformity or limitations. People with severe spinal involvement have an excellent prognosis in terms of work, with about 75 percent continuing with full employment.[1-3]

Women can have a severe course as described above. But it is now recognized that the majority of women with this disease have more cervical and peripheral involvement and less dramatic spinal changes (including sacroiliac joint changes). They also tend to have a more slowly progressive, milder course and less extra-articular features.[1]

SYMPTOMATOLOGY AND IMPLICATIONS FOR OCCUPATIONAL THERAPY

Back and Neck

Pain often is a result of both the inflammatory process and paravertebral muscle spasm secondary to inflammation. Usually the pain is episodic and may be more severe at night. Stiffness in the morning and after inactivity commonly accompanies the pain and is usually confined to the involved joints or enthesis.[1] It usually lasts longer than with mechanical spinal problems. The joint pain may not be well localized by the patient, who may describe it as centered in the lower back or buttocks with minimal radiation.

When there is spinal involvement, typical deformities include a reversed lordotic curve and kyphosis that is compensated for by neck flexion. The vertebrae eventually become joined by bony bridges, forming the characteristic **bamboo spine image** on roentgenography.[2] Involvement of the thoracic spine leads to markedly limited chest expansion, a common sequela of this disease.[4]

Therapy

In women with milder cervical involvement, treatment is the same as for osteoarthritis of the neck and fibromyalgia. (See Chapters 4 and 5, which deal with these conditions, and Chapter 24 for joint protection techniques.)

For people with spinal involvement, proper positioning during activities, leisure, and sleep is crucial in preventing back deformities. Posture habits during activities such as watching television, reading, and desk work need careful evaluation. Assistive equipment may be necessary to ensure proper posture. A reasonably functional life can be anticipated if proper posture is maintained.[4]

Proper neck positioning at night is a critical factor and can literally prevent neck deformity in patients with cervical AS.[4] *Ideally the positioning method should support the cervical muscles* (to allow relaxation and reduce muscle spasm) *and maintain the normal lordotic curve to the neck without causing cervical flexion* (i.e., the occipital skull should be touching or close to the mattress).[5] Sleeping without a pillow flattens the lordotic curve.[5] It may be possible to find a cervical pillow that meets the above requirements, but most are too thick or maintain the neck in flexion. The best solution at this time is to adapt a pillow like the Jackson Cervipillo[5] (Trueze Corp.) by removing some of the filler to create the correct thickness. (It may be necessary to return the filler later when the pillow becomes compressed by use.)

The patient should have a firm mattress that does not sag but that has a soft top layer of foam to reduce pressure on bony prominences. Hospital beds should be kept flat at night and have only the back raised during the day. Do not use the semi-Fowler position (with the head raised and knee gatch partially raised). Ideally the patient should sleep supine rather than side-lying with legs bent.[4] (See Chapter 28, Positioning and Lying Prone.)

Trunk-stretching exercises for posture in the erect and supine positions with emphasis on extension and hamstring stretching are part of the physical therapy program as well as deep breathing exercises to maintain chest expansion.

Once patients are over the acute phase, they should be encouraged to participate in an ongoing community sports or exercise group. Almost any sport or game is acceptable as long as it does not aggravate involved joints or tendons. Swimming is universally recommended because it exercises all the muscles in a non-weight-bearing situation and it improves respiration and chest excursion. The only sports not recommended are springboard diving (because of the risk of neck injury) and distance bicycling (because of the static flexion posture required).

In Great Britain and in Europe, the therapeutic approach to AS is far more vigorous than in the United States. At the Royal National Hospital for Rheumatic Disease in Bath, patients take an intensive 3-week group physiotherapy program. In Austria, there are spas that offer a 6-week intensive exercise and sports program for people with AS. These programs have demonstrated the value of active exercise.[6] One study (n

= 21) reported that patients in a 2-week, inpatient program of bedrest and postural and mobilizing exercises made significant improvements in function, early morning stiffness, spinal pain, lumbar extension, lateral spinal flexion, finger to floor distance, and ear (tragers) to wall distance. Improvement was greater in the spine than in the neck. Gains were maintained at the 2-month follow-up assessment.[7]

Activities of Daily Living

Bed mobility often is limited and can be facilitated by grab bars, cloth ladders, or blanket cradles. Electric blankets or matress covers help reduce stiffness.

Daily activities such as transferring, dressing, hygiene, toileting, driving, and vocational skills need special consideration. The need for training in adaptive methods for performing these activities varies with each person.

Sitting and standing postures during work activities need evaluation. If a person cannot maintain an erect posture during a specific task, a soft neck collar or back support may be valuable solely as a postural reminder during the activity.

For clients with fused backs, special consideration is needed with regard to safety precautions against falling. This is especially true during bending activities (dressing, gardening, or bathing), when a shift in the center of gravity can cause a loss of balance. These patients in particular are vulnerable to neck fractures.[4] Safety while driving is another factor that needs consideration, since cervical ankylosis reduces the visual driving field. Elongated clip-on rearview mirrors are readily available in auto supply stores and allow people to see side blind spots without turning around. Wright and Moll describe an ingenious right angle mirror that attaches to the hood of the car, which allows the driver to see cars approaching from both left and right directions, while facing straight ahead.[4]

Patients with fused backs also find it helpful to have a comfortable chair at home with a swivel base. This allows them to face people easily during conversations and to expand their visual field. Executive office chairs (with casters removed) work well for this purpose and often can be purchased at a reasonable cost at used office furniture stores.

Joint Stiffness

Stiffness is often prominent after rest, sitting, or prolonged static positioning. Usually clients are more comfortable if they can change positions frequently and avoid sustained postures. Exercise, repetitive movement, and heat application (hot showers and heating pads) help relieve stiffness and pain secondary to muscle spasm. Some patients have reported that wearing warm undershirts helps increase back comfort. Those with neck pain may find that wearing a turtleneck collar (a dickie) under a blouse or shirt helps at work, especially if there are air conditioning drafts.

Hips

About 30 percent of all AS patients develop clinically significant arthritis of the hips. The consequences of hip disease in AS are often identical to the problems seen in both rheumatoid arthritis and degenerative joint disease.[4] Many of these patients develop hip-flexion and/or hip-extension contractures and may develop compensatory knee-flexion contractures. To stand vertically, they compensate for the hip flexion by flexing the knees, and thus cause knee contractures.[1] Adduction contractures can also develop and interfere with perineal care and ability for sexual intercourse for women.[4] (Also see the sections on hip involvement in Chapter 3 and Chapter 10.)

Therapy

In addition to proper positioning at rest, as mentioned previously in this chapter, instruction in lying prone to stretch the hip flexors is important. Begin with lying prone to tolerance and progress to at least 60 minutes per day. Therapeutic exercise or physical therapy may improve mobility.

Hip involvement often limits ability for transferring and lower extremity dressing. If extension contractures are present, the patient will have difficulty sitting straight in a normal chair. (See Chapter 25, Assistive Devices.)

Treatment for joint inflammation is the same as for inflammatory joint disease in

Chapter 1 and for rheumatoid arthritis. Specific therapy procedures can be found in Chapter 24, Joint-Protection and Energy-Conservation Instruction, and Chapter 28, Positioning and Lying Prone. Patients with severe hip limitations may be candidates for hip surgery. (See Chapter 33).

Shoulders

The development of a bicipital or supraspinatus tendinitis occurs quite frequently. Inflammation of the sternoclavicular and acromioclavicular joints or glenohumeral joints is seen in some patients.[4]

Treatment for joint disease of the shoulders is the same as for rheumatoid arthritis (see Chapter 6).

Peripheral Arthritis

Not all patients with AS develop arthritis in the peripheral or distal joints. When it occurs, it usually affects the knees, elbows, ankles, and wrist joints, often asymmetrically. Outside of the hips, the knees are the most frequently affected. Small joint peripheral arthritis tends to be transitory and seldom causes residual deformity. Occasionally the wrists or an isolated finger joint develops severe disease.

Treatment is the same as for rheumatoid arthritis except that for the hands or wrists instruction in joint protection techniques needs to be carefully individualized because people with AS generally do not develop ulnar drift or swan-neck deformities.

Other Manifestations

Ocular Involvement

Iritis and **conjunctivitis** occur in approximately 25 percent of patients with AS. Symptoms of iritis may involve acute, painful red eyes with blurring of vision, or may be insidious and progressive, thus leading to visual impairment before it is recognized. Iritis may also continue to be present long after the AS has become inactive.[4]

There are no occupational therapy measures for this symptom; however, the therapist needs to be alert for signs of eye involvement and to have the patient report any symptoms to the physician.

Cardiovascular Involvement

Heart disease occurs more frequently in people with more severe spondylitis. If affects 3 to 10 percent of patients but may not become symptomatic until 25 to 30 years after onset.[1] Aortic valve disease, cardiomegaly, and conduction defects are the most common findings.[1] Since patients with heart involvement tend to be more seriously limited, they are generally not involved in vigorous activity. A patient who has new cardiovascular symptoms should report them to his or her physician. Any home or exercise program should take symptomatic cardiac involvement into account.

Pulmonary Involvement

Patients with severe spondylitis may develop upper lobe pulmonary fibrosis as an uncommon, late manifestation, typically in the fifth decade of life. It presents in a manner very similar to tuberculosis, with cough, dyspnea, and sputum. It is progressive and can be fatal.

Associated Conditions: The Spondyloarthropathies

At one time AS was believed to be a variant of rheumatoid arthritis. AS is now identified as a separate disease and is a member of a group of diseases called **seronegative spondyloarthritides.**[8,9] Other diseases in this classification include psoriatic arthritis, Reiter's syndrome, enteropathic spondylitis (arthritis associated with regional enteritis or ulcerative colitis), and the arthritides of Whipple's disease and Behçet's syndrome. The four major diseases in this classification—AS, psoriatic arthritis, Reiter's syndrome, and enteropathic spondylitis—share the following characteristics: (1) small joint involvement tends to be asymmetric; (2) there is frequent arthritis of the sacroiliac joints and spine similar to AS; (3) iritis may be associated with any of these diseases; (4) HLA-B27 antigen is present in a high percentage of these patients; and (5) the overall prognosis in terms of disability is better than in rheumatoid arthritis.[3,4,8,9]

DRUG THERAPY

Indomethacin (Indocin) or any of the NSAIDs are recommended drugs of choice to relieve the inflammatory manifestations of AS. Aspirin, given in anti-inflammatory doses (8 or more per day) can be given but is generally not very effective. Phenylbutazone is considered if all other drugs are ineffective.

See Chapter 3 for precautions and side effects of specific drugs.

REFERENCES

1. Calin, A: Ankylosing spondylitis. In Kelley, WM, et al (eds): Textbook of Rheumatology, ed 2. WB Saunders, Philadelphia, 1985.
2. Bluestone, R: Ankylosing spondylitis. In McCarty, DJ (ed): Arthritis and Allied Conditions. Lea & Febiger, Philadelphia, 1978.
3. Calin, A (ed): Spondyloarthropathies. Grune & Stratton, Orlando, FL, 1984.
4. Wright, V, and Moll, HMH: Seronegative Polyarthritis. Elsevier North-Holland, Amsterdam, 1976.
5. Jackson, R: The Cervical Syndrome, ed. 4. Charles C Thomas, Springfield, IL, 1978.
6. O'Driscoll, SL, Jayson, MI, and Baddeley, H: Neck movements in ankylosing spondylitis and their response to physiotherapy. Ann Rheum Dis 37(1):64, 1978.
7. Wordsworth, BP, Pearcy, MJ, and Mowat, AG: In-patient regime for the treatment of ankylosing spondylitis: An appraisal of improvement in spinal mobility and the effects of corticotrophin. Br J Rheumatol 23(1):39–43, 1984.
8. Hart, FD: The ankylosing spondylopathies. Clin Orthop 74:7, 1971.
9. Haslock, I, and Wright, V: The arthritis associated with intestinal disease. Bull Rheum Dis 24:750, 1974.

ADDITIONAL SOURCES

Alaranta, H, Karppi, SL, and Voipio-Pulkki, LM: Performance capacity of trunk muscles in ankylosing spondylitis. Clin Rheumatol 2(3):251–257, 1983.

Booth, J, and Weatherley, C: Ankylosing spondylitis. Nurs Times 82(4):28–31, 1986.

Bulstrode, SJ, Barefoort, J, Harrison, RA, and Clarke, AK: The role of passive stretching in the treatment of ankylosing spondylitis. Br J Rheumatol 26(1):40–42, 1987.

Calabro, JJ, Eyvazzadeh, C, and Weber, CA: Contemporary management of ankylosing spondylitis. Compr Ther 12(9):11–18, 1986.

Chamberlain, MA: Socioeconomic effects of ankylosing spondylitis in females: A comparison of 25 female with 25 male subjects. Int Rehabil Med 5(3):149–153, 1983.

Chamberlain, MA: Socioeconomic effects of ankylosing spondylitis. Int Rehabil Med 3(2):94–99, 1981.

Engst-Hastreiter, U: [Psychological adjustment to disease in patients with ankylosing spondylitis.] Z Rheumatol 43(6):299–302, 1984.

Koh, TC: Tai Chi and ankylosing spondylitis—A personal experience. Am J Chin Med 10(1–4):59–61, 1982.

Ledo, KM: Ankylosing spondylitis. Orthop Nurs 2(6):39–40, 1983.

Moll, JMH: Ankylosing Spondylitis. Churchill Livingstone, Edinburgh, 1980.

Richter, MB: Management of the seronegative spondyloarthropathies. Clin Rheum Dis 11(1):147–169, 1985.

Rogers, F: Helping patients to live with ankylosing spondylitis. Practitioner 227(1381):1187–1189, 1983.

Shah, BC, and Khan, MA: Review of ankylosing spondylitis. Compr Ther 13(3):52–59, 1987.

Swezey, RL (ed): Straight Talk on Ankylosing Spondylitis. Ankylosing Spondylitis Association, Sherman Oaks, CA, 1985.

Urbanek, T, Sitajova, H, and Hudakova, G: Problems of rheumatoid arthritis and ankylosing spondylitis patients in their labor and life environments. Czech Med 7(2):78–89, 1984.

Wenneberg, B, Kopp, S, and Hollender, L: The temporomandibular joint in ankylosing spondylitis. Correlations between subjective, clinical, and radiographic features in the stomatognathic system and effects of treatment. Acta Odontol Scand 42(3):165–173, 1984.

Wordsworth, BP, and Mowat, AG: A review of 100 patients with ankylosing spondylitis with particular reference to socioeconomic effects. Br J Rheumatol 25(2):175–180, 1986.

Chapter 9

Systemic Lupus Erythematosus

Systemic lupus erythematosus (SLE) is a systemic inflammatory disease character-ized by small vessel vasculitis with a di-verse clinical picture. Manifestations of the disease depend on the organ systems in-volved and may include any or all of the following: fever, an erythematous rash, polyarthritis, pneumonitis, polyserositis (especially pleurisy and pericarditis), myo-sitis, anemia, thrombocytopenia, and renal, neurological, psychological, and cardiac ab-normalities. (SLE is different from discoid lupus. See the Glossary.)

ETIOLOGICAL FACTORS

Many of the clinical manifestations can be explained by the deposition of antigen-antibody complexes in the walls of small blood vessels. There is also a hereditary predisposition. Although a viral agent may be linked etiologically, none has been iden-tified to date.[1]

AGE AND SEX AFFECTED

Nine of every ten patients are women, primarily in the age range of young adult and adolescence, but the disease can occur at any age, including in the elderly. There is a higher incidence of SLE in black women when compared with the incidence in white women. It is now considered a relatively common disease, since it occurs more frequently than cystic fibrosis, muscular dystrophy, multiple sclerosis, or leukemia.[2]

DIAGNOSIS

Diagnosis is made clinically by the presence of multiorgan system involvement not explained by other diseases. A facial rash and glomerulonephritis are the most frequent diagnostic features. Confirmatory tests include the presence of antinuclear antibodies (ANA) in the serum or characteristic histological changes in a kidney or skin biopsy. The diagnosis should always be made on clinical grounds because ANA may be present in many people for reasons other than SLE.

COURSE AND PROGNOSIS

The course and prognosis are highly variable and depend on the organs affected, age of the patient, severity of disease, and responsiveness to treatment. Earlier diagnosis and improved treatment have reduced associated morbidity dramatically over the last 20 years. The disease can be life threatening if there is renal, neurological, or myocardial involvement. Mortality tends to be highest in the first year following diagnosis, with 80 percent surviving 5 years or longer. The long-term outlook is often good if the disease is limited to the joints or skin.[2,3]

SYMPTOMATOLOGY AND IMPLICATIONS FOR OCCUPATIONAL THERAPY

Patients with an associated arthritis, myositis, neuropathy, or functional psychosis are frequently referred for rehabilitation. Unfortunately, patients with only general systemic manifestations are often not referred because physicians are not aware of occupational therapy measures for these symptoms. Patients limited by fatigue can often benefit from instruction in energy conservation methods and stress management techniques as well as general body conditioning. Biofeedback has proven to be a valuable adjunct in the management of Raynaud's phenomenon.[4-7]

A word of caution is needed regarding patient instruction for those taking high-dose corticosteroids. This medication can produce a wide range of side effects, including **euphoria** and a false sense of well-being. This does not occur in all patients, but when it is present, even in mild form, patient instruction is extremely difficult. When a patient is euphoric, he or she cannot perceive the seriousness of the condition or the need for instruction. Many of these patients are in the process of having their medications stabilized. If possible, patient education should be delayed until the medication is reduced. *Also, all patient education for patients on high-dose corticosteroids should be reinforced with written instructions.*

Polyarthritis

Polyarthritis occurs in 90 percent of SLE patients. The arthritis associated with SLE has the same distribution as rheumatoid arthritis; that is, it is symmetric and affects the small peripheral joints more frequently than the larger joints. Unlike rheumatoid arthritis, *the arthritis associated with SLE typically does not erode the cartilage but primarily affects the capsule and supporting structures.*[8] Deformities are not as common as in RA, but they do occur and can include all of the typical rheumatoid-type deformities (e.g., ulnar drift, swan neck, or boutonnière). The deformities in SLE are primarily due to capsular and ligamentous involvement, rather than erosive cartilage and bone changes. Therefore, joint instability and subluxation are common sequelae, and contractures and ankylosis are unusual.

Complications of corticosteroid therapy that can be misinterpreted as arthritis include (1) ischemic (aseptic) necrosis of the bone mast, frequently in the hip and less frequently in the shoulder or knees, which presents with pain and decreased range of motion and function of the affected joint;[9] and (2) accelerated osteoporosis resulting in compression fractures, especially in middle-age or older women, which can present as acute back or rib pain. Therapists should be alert for these symptoms and have the patient report them to his or her physician.

Therapy

Treatment for the acute, subacute, and chronic stages is the same as outlined for inflammatory joint disease in Chapter 1. See also Chapter 6, Rheumatoid Arthritis, for information on the functional and physical consequences of arthritis in the peripheral joints.

Systemic Manifestations

Symptoms include fever, malaise, fatigue, weight loss, anorexia, and weakness. **Fatigue** can become very disruptive to the patient's life-style and family and social relationships. Patients may feel too tired to play with their children, maintain a job, have sexual relations, or participate in social events. As with all systemic diseases, these systemic manifestations need to be distinguished, if possible, from the symptoms of depression. See the section on systemic manifestations in Chapter 6, Rheumatoid Arthritis, and the section on depression in Chapter 2, Psychological Considerations in Patient Education and Treatment.

The level of fatigue is also affected by sleeping and rest patterns. Some patients taking high doses of corticosteroid may have a great deal of difficulty sleeping at night, resulting in greater fatigue during the day.[1]

Women with SLE are also at high risk for developing **fibromyalgia**, which is associated with symptoms of fatigue, subjective sense of muscle weakness, muscular aching and pain, headaches, paresthesias in the hands (occasionally the face), and sleep disorder. Frequently the symptoms of fibromyalgia are misinterpreted as SLE symptoms. This confusion is compounded by the fact that about 25 percent of patients with fibromyalgia may test positive for ANA. Therapists working with patients with SLE should also be aware of the diagnostic, evaluative, and treatment approaches for fibromyalgia. We have seen several women who developed a malar rash, sun sensitivity, Raynaud's phenomenon, borderline positive ANA, arthralgias, and fibromyalgia. Further symptoms of lupus never developed and the fibromyalgia became the primary problem.

Therapy

It is critical that patients with SLE get sufficient rest. Some patients perform best when they have 10 hours of sleep per night; others may need 8 or 9 hours with a nap during the day.

Exercise should be in moderation and not to the point of exhaustion. Yoga and general body toning and stretching exercises can improve endurance and help a patient stay in shape without excessive stress. All exercise programs should be built up gradually and reduced if they appear to cause an increase in systemic manifestations.

Since this is a systemic disease, it is important to consider the patient's daily hospital or home routine when planning a treatment program. Instruction in energy conservation and work simplifications as well as specific training in conscious relaxation can be of benefit in improving the patient's functional endurance. Specific therapy procedures can be found in Chapter 24, Joint Protection and Energy Conservation Instruction.

Muscle Involvement

The most common muscle involvement is an **inflammatory myositis.** It presents similarly to polymyositis with initial proximal muscle weakness but is usually milder than idiopathic polymyositis. Patients can also develop a noninflammatory myopathy secondary to steroid or antimalarial therapy.[1]

Therapy

Because myositis or myopathy is a relatively common development, a therapist should be alert to the signs of proximal muscle weakness in all patients with SLE or on steroid or cloroquine therapy. Typical signs include difficulty in rising from a chair without assistance (not resulting from joint involvement); tiredness or difficulty in stabilizing the neck; waddling gait; drooping of and/or tiredness in the shoulders; difficulty stepping up onto a step or curb; and dysphagia. If these signs are observed in a patient, a group muscle test should be done to determine any actual proximal weakness and the findings should be reported to the physician. Occupational therapy for this type of myositis is the same as for polymyositis (see Chapter 11, Polymyositis and Dermatomyositis).

Skin Involvement

An erythematous rash, which is often symmetric, occurs over the face, neck, extremities, hands, and elbows. It may form a characteristic butterfly shape when it is over the nose and cheeks. The rash may be episodic or chronic and with or without scarring. In some cases it appears to be a healthy-looking blush. Frequently, exposure to sunlight or ultraviolet light can cause the rash or systemic manifestations to flare up.[1,3]

Therapy

The patient who is sun-sensitive should be advised to report sensitivity to his or her physician, avoid sun exposure when possible, wear protective clothing, and use a *sun block* lotion containing para-aminobenzoic acid (PABA) over exposed areas. (It is helpful to give the patient some brand names so that he or she does not buy a suntan lotion by mistake.) A pharmacist can advise which commercial sun blocks have the greatest amount of PABA. A PABA sun-protection factor of 15 or more is recommended.

Neuropsychological Involvement

Psychological reactions may include anxiety, depression, hyperirritability, confusion, hallucinations, phobias, paranoias, and autistic behavior. Psychotic episodes during exacerbations may be secondary to lupus cerebritis, corticosteroid treatment (drug-induced), or psychological need (functional). Neurological findings may include headaches, organic brain syndrome, seizures, acute cranial nerve dysfunction, cerebrovascular accident, subarachnoid hemorrhage, transverse myelitis, myelopathy, movement disorders, motor and sensory neuropathies, and delirium. Peripheral motor and sensory loss is usually responsive to corticosteroid therapy.[10-13]

Therapy

It is important to report observed neurological or personality changes to the referring physician. Patients with psychiatric disorders need a psychiatric occupational therapy program while they are in the hospital. Other secondary neurological syndromes are treated the same way a primary condition would be.

Crafts employed as a therapeutic modality can be effective during psychotic periods to enhance the patient's reality testing and as evaluation tools to assess the patient's psychological status, problem-solving ability, or judgment.

Other Manifestations

Other manifestations of SLE may include the following:

1. Pleurisy and pneumonitis. (Occurs in 50 percent of patients.)
2. Raynaud's phenomenon. (Raynaud's phenomenon associated with SLE differs from that seen with systemic sclerosis in that it often resolves if the SLE goes into prolonged remission. Instruct the patient in appropriate precautions; see Chapter 10.)
3. Pericarditis or myocarditis. (It is important to determine the patient's cardiac status and observe work tolerance carefully.)
4. Nephritis accounts for 50 percent of all fatalities.
5. Ulcerations of the mouth, pharynx, or vagina. (These ulcers are usually painful; mouth ulcers may make talking uncomfortable for the patient.)
6. Alopecia. (Usually there is eventual regrowth. If the alopecia is severe, purchase of a wig is warranted.)
7. Transverse cord myelopathy is rare but has been reported in 28 cases. It can result in quadriplegia or paraplegia.[14]

Other conditions that occur in association with SLE are Sjögren's syndrome and avascular necrosis (osteonecrosis), usually of the femoral head.

Pregnancy and SLE

SLE primarily affects women during the childbearing years. The concerns about pregnancy—how it will affect the mother, the child, and the lupus—are common ones. Pregnancy may cause an exacerbation of the lupus, most frequently in the last trimester and in the early postpartum period. The effect of an exacerbation varies from patient to patient depending on how extensive the lupus is and which organs are involved. For example, a patient with kidney involvement could be placed at high risk for renal failure. Women with SLE also have a higher incidence of miscarriages, premature births, and stillbirths compared to women in the general population. Despite these risks, patients with mild disease can have a safe and successful pregnancy. For women who are planning to have children it is recommended that conception be planned when the disease is mild or in remission. For many women the disease can be kept under control with corticosteroids during the pregnancy. So far, there is no evidence that corticosteroid therapy affects the fetus.

Another major concern is whether SLE can be genetically transmitted. The answer to this question is uncertain. It appears that people who develop SLE have a genetic predisposition to it. Occasionally SLE will run in families, or various rheumatic diseases will run in a family. It is also possible for people to have a genetic predisposition to a disease but never develop the disease, as demonstrated in studies of identical twins. To date, no specific genetic defect has been detected.[15,16] A condition called **neonatal SLE** occurs rarely in infants born to mothers who have one type of ANA, called **anti-RO (SS-A).** These infants have congenital heart block and annular-type skin rashes. The condition seems to be secondary to transplacental passage of the antibody.

The first few months after the birth of a baby are difficult both physically and emotionally for healthy parents. The risk of a lupus flare at this time makes adjustment even more difficult. Patients may need counseling to plan realistically for the child care and psychological support needed during the postpartum period.

Practicing conscious relaxation or meditation twice a day for 15 minutes can be very supportive in controlling systemic symptoms, reducing stress, and improving functional endurance. Developing a daily discipline of this type reinforces one's self-esteem and sense of control, and the fact that it is okay, indeed necessary, to take care of one's self as well as the baby, husband, other children, house, relatives, and pets.

DRUG THERAPY

Medications used in SLE depend on the organ systems involved with the disease.

Skin disease may be controlled with local steroid creams or with oral administration of antimalarial drugs such as hydroxychloroquine sulfate (Plaquenil Sulfate) or quinacrine (Atabrine).

The inflammatory manifestations such as arthritis and pleurisy often can be controlled with anti-inflammatory drugs such as aspirin in high doses or with one of the nonsteroidal anti-inflammatory drugs. This may be combined with an antimalarial drug or with prednisone if manifestations are not controlled.

For life-threatening conditions, such as with central nervous system, cardiac, or hematological involvement, corticosteroids such as prednisone are used in high dosages.

In certain types of renal disease, steroids may be combined with an immunosuppressive drug such as azathioprine (Imuran) or cyclophosphamide (Cytoxan).

Some physicians administer corticosteroids in alternate-day doses, for example, 20 mg every other day, or alternating a high and a low dose. This is done to encourage the patient's adrenal glands to produce natural steroids on alternate days and to reduce side effects. Patients on this type of program often vary in their functional ability, depending on the day and dose. An activities of daily living (ADL) evaluation needs to take this dual functional pattern into account.

See Chapter 3 for precautions and side effects of specific drugs.

REFERENCES

1. Rothfield, N: Clinical features of systemic lupus erythematosus. In Kelley, WM, et al (eds): Textbook of Rheumatology. WB Saunders, Philadelphia, 1981.
2. Dubois, EL: Lupus Erythematosus: A Review of the Current Status of Discoid and Systemic Lupus Erythematosus and Their Variants, ed 2. University of Southern California Press, Los Angeles, 1974.
3. Fries, JF, and Hollman, HR: Systemic Lupus Erythematosus: A Clinical Analysis. WB Saunders, Philadelphia, 1975.
4. Taub, E, and Strobel, CF: Biofeedback in the treatment of vasoconstrictive syndromes. Biofeedback Self Regul 3(4):363, 1978.
5. Sunderman, RH, and Delk, JL: Treatment of Raynaud's disease with temperature biofeedback. South Med J 71(3):340, 1978.
6. Sedlacek, K: Biofeedback for Raynaud's disease. Psychosom Med 20(8):535, 1979.
7. Green, E, and Green, A: General and specific applications of thermal biofeedback. In Basmajian, JV (ed): Biofeedback—Principles and Practice for Clinicians. Williams & Wilkins, Baltimore, 1979.
8. Labowitz, R, and Schumacher, HR: Articular manifestation of systemic lupus erythematosus. Ann Rheum Dis 33:204, 1974.
9. Zizic, TM, Hungerford, DS, and Stevens, MD: Ischemic bone necrosis in systemic lupus erythematosus. Medicine 59:134–148, 1980.
10. Gibson, T, and Myers, AR: Nervous system involvement in systemic lupus erythematosus. Ann Rheum Dis 35:398, 1976.
11. Small, P, et al: CNS involvement in SLE. Arthritis Rheum 20:869, 1977.
12. Baker, M: Psychopathology in systemic lupus erythematosus. Part I. Psychiatric observations. Semin Arthritis Rheum 3(2):95, 1973.
13. Adelman, DC, Saltiel, E, and Klinenberg, JR: The neuropsychiatric manifestations of systemic lupus erythematosus: An overview. Semin Arthritis Rheum 115(3):185–199, 1986.
14. Thakarar, P, and Greenspun, B: Transverse myelopathy in systemic lupus erythematosus. Arch Phys Med Rehab 60:323, 1979.
15. Medsger, TA, and Chetlin, SM: Lupus and Pregnancy. Pennsylvania Lupus Foundation, 1978.
16. White, JF: Teaching patients to manage systemic lupus erythematosus. Nursing '78 8:27, 1978.

ADDITIONAL SOURCES

Ansari, A, Larson, PH, and Bates, HD: Cardiovascular manifestations of systemic lupus erythematosus: Current perspective. Prog Cardiovasc Dis 27(6):421–434, 1985.
Arnett, FC, Reveille, JD, Wilson, RW, Provost, TT, and Bias, WB: Systemic lupus erythematosus: Current state of the genetic hypothesis. Semin Arthritis Rheum 14(1):24–35, 1984.
Ballou, SP: Systemic lupus erythematosus. Controversies in management. Postgrad Med 81(8):157–159, 163–164, 1987 (review).
Brasington, RD, and Furst, DE: Pulmonary disease in systemic lupus erythematosus. Clin Exp Rheumatol 3(3):269–276, 1985.
Doherty, NE, and Siegel, RJ: Cardiovascular manifestations of systemic lupus erythematosus. Am Heart J 110(6):1257–1265, 1985.
Dray, GL, Millender, LH, Nalebuff, EA, and Phillips, C: The surgical treatment of hand deformities in SLE. J Hand Surg 6(3):339, 1981.
Gossat, DM, and Walls, RS: Systemic lupus erythematosus in later life. Med J Aust 1(7):297–299, 1982.
Joyce, KM, Austin, HA 3rd, and Balow, JE: The patient with lupus nephritis: A nursing perspective. Heart Lung 14(1):75–79, 1985.
Lewis, KS: Systemic lupus erythematosus: The great masquerader. Nurse Pract 9(8):13–22, 1984.
Schidt, M: Oral manifestations of lupus erythematosus. Int J Oral Surg 13(2):101–147, 1984.
Segal, AM, Calabrese, LH, Ahmad, M, Tubbs, RR, and White, CS: The pulmonary manifestations of systemic lupus erythematosus. Semin Arthritis Rheum 14(3):202–224, 1985.
Sutton, JD, Navarro, A, and Stevens, MB: Systemic lupus erythematosus XI: Nonpharmacological management. Md State Med J 33(6):469–472, 1984.

Pregnancy

Burkett, G: Lupus nephropathy and pregnancy. Clin Obstet Gynecol 28(2):310–323, 1985.
Hayslett, JP, and Reece, EA: Systemic lupus erythematosus in pregnancy. Clin Perinatol 12(3):539–550, 1985.
Lockshin, MD: Lupus pregnancy. Clin Rheum Dis 11(3):611–632, 1985.

Neuropsychiatric Symptoms

Allen, TX, and Glicksman, MS: Psychologic involvement in systemic lupus erythematosus: A psychometric approach. Clin Rheum Prac 4(2):64, 1986.
Bluestein, HG, Pischel, KD, and Woods, VL Jr: Immunopathogenesis of the neuropsychiatric manifestations of systemic lupus erythematosus. Springer Semin Immunopathol 9(2–3):237–249, 1986 (review).
Central nervous system involvement in systemic lupus erythematosus [clinical conference]. Johns Hopkins Med J 149(4):140–142, 1981.
Hall, RC, Stickney, SK, and Gardner, ER: Psychiatric symptoms in patients with systemic lupus erythematosus. Psychosomatics 22(1):15–19, 1981.
Harris, EN, and Hughes, GR: Cerebral disease in systemic lupus erythematosus. Springer Semin Immunopathol 8(3):251–266, 1985.
Kinash, RG: Physiologic responses of patients with systemic lupus and implications for rehabilitation. Rehab Nurs 9(5):32–34, 1984.

Kulesha, D, Moldofsky, H, Urowitz, M, and Zeman, R: Brain scan lateralization and psychiatric symptoms in systemic lupus erythematosus. Biol Psychiatry 16(4):407–412, 1981.

Lahita, RG: The influence of sex hormones on the disease systemic lupus erythematosus. Springer Semin Immunopathol 9(2–3):305–314, 1986 (review).

Lee, BA: Living with lupus. J Pract Nurs 36(5):37–39, 1986.

Liange, MH, Rogers, M, Larson, M, Eaton, HM, Murawski, BJ, Taylor, JE, Swafford, J, and Schur, PH: The psychosocial impact of systemic lupus erythematosus and rheumatoid arthritis. Arthritis Rheum 27(1):13–19, 1984.

Nashel, DJ, and Ulmer, CC: Systemic lupus erythematosus: Important considerations in the adolescent. J Adoles Health Care 2(4):273–278, 1982.

Schur, PH (ed): The Clinical Management of Systemic Lupus Erythematosus. Grune & Stratton, New York, 1983. (Provides guidelines for physicians.)

Silber, TJ, Chatoor, I, and White, PH: Psychiatric manifestations of systemic lupus erythematosus in children and adolescents. A review. Clin Pediatr 23(6):331–335, 1984.

Patient Education

The following resources can be ordered from the Lupus Foundation of America, Inc., 1717 Massachusetts Avenue, NW, Suite 203, Washington, DC 20036:

Aladjem, H: Lupus—Hope through understanding. 1982.

Aladjem, H: Understanding Lupus. 1985. $8.00

Carr, R: Lupus Erythematosus: A Handbook for Physicians, Patients, and Their Families. 1986. $2.75.

Jameson, EJ, and Bloom, SL: A Legal Manual for Lupus Patients. 1982. $8.00.

The following publications must be ordered directly from the publisher:

Bell, LR: The Red Butterfly: Lupus Patients Can Survive. 1984. Order from Branden Press, 21 Station Street, Brookline, MA 02147. $4.95 plus postage.

Blau, S, and Schultz, D: Lupus: The Body Against Itself. 1985. Order from Doubleday and Co., Direct Mail Order Division, 501 Franklin Avenue, Garden City, NJ 11530, $12.95.

Lewis, K: Successful Living with Chronic Illness. 1985. Order from LFA, Atlanta Chapter, 2814 New Spring Road, Room 304A, Atlanta, GA 30339. $8.00.

Lupus and You: A Guide for Patients. 1986. Order from Park Nicollet Medical Foundation, Communications Department, 5000 West 39th Street, Minneapolis, MN 55416. Also available are *Lupus and You* slides and sound tape. $45.00.

Nass, T: Lupus Erythematosus: Handbook for Nurses. 1985. Order from Lupus Society of Wisconsin, Inc., PO Box 16621, Milwaukee, WI 53216. $5 plus postage.

Phillips, RH: Coping with Lupus. 1984. Order from Avery Publishing Group, Inc., 350 Thorens Avenue, Garden City Park, NY 11040. $7.95 plus postage.

Additional Sources for Children with Lupus

Butterflies and Sunshine, from the Pediatric Arthritis Center of Hawaii. 1984. Order from Wilma B. Schiner, Director, Training and Education, 1319 Punahou Street, Honolulu, HI 96826.

Walsh, D: Lucy Lupus Wolf: A Story Book about Lupus for Children Who Have Lupus. Order from Doris Walsh, LFA Central New York Chapter, 419 West Onondaga Street, Syracuse, NY 13202. $4.00 plus postage.

Chapter 10

Systemic Sclerosis (Scleroderma)

Systemic sclerosis (SS), or scleroderma, is a generalized disorder of the small blood vessels and connective tissues, characterized by fibrotic, ischemic, and degenerative changes in the skin and internal organs. Its systemic nature is evidenced by frequent involvement of the alimentary tract, synovium, lungs, heart, and kidneys. SS frequently is associated with calcinosis, Raynaud's phenomenon, esophageal dysfunction, sclerodactyly, and telangiectasis (the CREST syndrome).

ETIOLOGICAL FACTORS

The specific cause of excess deposition of fibrous tissue is not known. There are two current theories on pathogenesis: vascular and immunological.[1] Some believe the primary event is vascular damage resulting from endothelial cell injury.[2] This is supported by the early Raynaud's phenomenon, capillary and renal vascular changes, and a serum factor toxic to endothelial cells.[1,2] The immune theory holds that the initial event is T- and B-cell immunity to previously unrecognized tissue antigens.[3] The activated lymphocytes produce lymphokines, which stimulate fibroblast migration and proliferation, and collagen production (fibrosis). Products from the activated lymphocytes and macrophages cause endothelial cell injury and the microvascular changes of scleroderma.[1]

AGE AND SEX AFFECTED

SS usually occurs during the third to fifth decades and three of four patients are women. Onset is rare in children and uncommon in the elderly.[4]

DIAGNOSIS

Diagnosis is made by the presence of characteristic tightening of the skin. In the early stages this may involve only the fingers but often it progresses proximally to a more generalized involvement. The presence of Raynaud's phenomenon and abnormalities of esophageal mobility are other diagnostic features.[4]

The current classification of SS is[5]

1. With symmetric, diffuse involvement of the skin (scleroderma)—affecting trunk, face, and proximal as well as distal portions of the extremities, and a tendency toward the relatively early appearance of disease of the esophagus, intestine, heart, lung, and kidney—classical disease.

2. With relatively limited involvement of the skin—often confined to the fingers and face. Prominence of calcinosis, Raynaud's phenomenon, esophageal dysfunction, sclerodactyly, telangiectasis, and prolonged delay in appearance of distinctive internal manifestations (including severe pulmonary arterial hypertension and biliary cirrhosis)—the CREST syndrome.

3. "Overlap" syndromes, including sclerodermatomyositis and mixed connective tissue disease. These patients share features with other closely related disorders such as systemic lupus erythematosus (SLE) polymyositis or rheumatoid arthritis (RA).

Table 10-1 Classification of Scleroderma

1. **Generalized scleroderma (systemic sclerosis)**
   a. Diffuse scleroderma (acute and chronic)
   b. CREST syndrome (calcinosis, Raynaud's phenomenon, esophageal hypomotility, sclerodactyly, telangiectasia)
   c. Overlap or mixed connective tissue syndromes
      (1) Sclerolupus
      (2) Sclerodermatomyositis
      (3) Scleromyxedema
      (4) Primary biliary cirrhosis
      (5) Sjögren's syndrome
2. **Localized scleroderma**
   a. Morphea
   b. Linear
3. **Scleroderma-like syndromes** (diseases with skin changes resembling scleroderma)
   a. Occupational
      (1) Associated with vinyl chloride
      (2) Associated with vibration ("jackhammer disease")
      (3) Associated with silicosis
   b. Fasciitis with eosinophilia
   c. Scleredema of Buschke (often postinfectious)
   d. Metabolic
      (1) Porphyria
      (2) Amyloid
   e. Immunological
      (1) Graft-versus-host reaction
   f. Juvenile onset diabetes mellitus (results in digital sclerosis and joint contractures)
4. **Scleroderma-associated syndromes**
   a. Inherited
      (1) Werner's syndrome
      (2) Phenylketonuria
      (3) Brandywine triracial isolate
   b. Tumor-associated
      (1) Carcinoid syndrome
      (2) Bronchoalveolar carcinoma

Fibrosis of skin (scleroderma) is one symptom of SS. It is also a symptom of several other conditions and syndromes (Table 10–1). When patients with these syndromes develop hand, upper extremity, or facial involvement they are often referred to occupational therapy to improve functional ability.

COURSE AND PROGNOSIS

Onset is gradual and the course is highly variable. The disease is not always fatal, and many clients have a normal life expectancy. Death is usually secondary to visceral involvement.

In some patients the symptoms are confined to the hand for years (sclerodactyly). In others, the skin sclerosis may progress to total body involvement within the first year. Involvement is usually symmetric and occurs in the hands first.

SYMPTOMATOLOGY AND IMPLICATIONS FOR OCCUPATIONAL THERAPY

Characteristic Skin and Joint Involvement

Early changes show edema that is gradually replaced by fibrosis, giving the skin a tight, hard, smooth appearance. Hyperpigmentation or hypopigmentation may occur in spots or in blotches. The changes are often symmetric and progress proximally to include the arms, neck, face, trunk, and lower extremities.[4]

Patients usually are referred to therapy when they begin to lose range of motion (ROM), particularly in the hands. Limitation of ROM is secondary to a combination of decreased skin mobility, edema, fibrosis, arthritis, and thickening of the subcutaneous tissues, muscles, tendons, synoviums, and joint capsules. The patient usually perceives any of these changes as stiffness. For evaluation purposes, this must be distinguished from any morning stiffness, because the morning stiffness tends to wear off. Leathery creaking is often audible where tendons pass over joints and is secondary to fibrinous deposits on the surfaces of the tendon sheaths and overlying fascia.[4]

When the patient is beginning to lose function due to joint limitations it is easy for the patient, physician, and therapist to become focused solely on physical joint treatment. But for complex chronic conditions such as SS with no predictable cure, the most effective treatment is holistic in nature. That is, it takes a broad integrative approach, addressing all spheres of a person's life that can influence his or her health, such as exercise, nutrition, attitude, interpersonal relationships, response to stress, productive work, social role, leisure, and enjoyment. Table 10–2 outlines a comprehensive holistic team approach to care of the person with SS.[6]

Therapy

Because of the nature of the disease, the primary goal in treatment is to *maintain maximal ROM* since it is very difficult to increase ROM. In some cases it is possible to increase joint range, but treatment in this area is highly experimental. The possibility of increasing ROM is more favorable when the disease is in the early stages

---

Table 10–2 Comprehensive Team Care for the Patient with Systemic Sclerosis

1. Counseling to help the patient explore and work through the psychological, familial, social, and vocational ramifications of an uncommon disease with visible deformities.
2. Education about symptoms and treatment options (and treatments to avoid).
3. Specific medications and modalities (e.g., biofeedback, relaxation techniques) to control symptoms, relieve pain, and improve function.
4. Effective exercise program to maintain joint mobility, facial mobility, and chest excursion.
5. Counseling about nutrition and dental care.
6. Instruction in adaptive methods and assistive devices to compensate for functional loss.

and edema is a major cause of range loss. *The ideal situation is to have the patient referred to therapy before he or she loses ROM.* This allows the therapist to determine the patient's normal measurements and use them as the baseline or objective for treatment.

Many physicians do not refer patients to therapy because they believe it is impossible to prevent joint contractures caused by SS. There is partial truth to this concept. Sometimes the sclerosis is so severe that contractures develop despite diligent daily exercises. However, far more frequently contractures develop as a result of disuse, inappropriate ROM or lack of ROM exercise, and improper positioning. *Contractures that develop from these processes are preventable.*

Any method for increasing ROM is applicable. The most effective means for diminishing established contractures is gentle passive, slow stretch applied through exercise or dynamic orthotics. (*Precaution:* if range limitation is secondary to active synovitis, excessive or forceful stretching may increase inflammation and fibrosis. Additional information can be found in Chapter 27, Exercise Treatment, and Chapter 28, Positioning and Lying Prone.)

Mild heat applications such as warm-water soaks, wrapping the part, or use of a heating pad, and the use of massage can increase circulation and thus help reduce edema and stiffness and increase mobility prior to exercise. Most heat modalities, including paraffin baths, can be used safely in the early stages, if the patient can tolerate them. All heat modalities must be used with caution because the blood supply to the skin is compromised. Specific precautions for the hands are discussed below under therapy for hands. A cylindrical facial vibrator is excellent for reducing stiffness, particularly for patients with painful fingers who find massage difficult.

ROM and function can be improved for clients with established range limitations when part of the contracture is recent and when function is limited by multiple joint involvement. To clarify the first point, when a patient presents with a 40-degree flexion contracture of the metacarpophalangeal (MCP) joint, it is usually not known how longstanding the entire contracture is. The patient might have lost the last 10 de-

grees in the previous week. The time factor is significant because recent losses can often be regained. In the second point, being able to gain 5 degrees of range in a single joint is not significant but, if function is limited by multiple joints, a 5- to 10-degree increase over several joints can be significant. For example, for the patient unable to perform palmar pinch and lacking one inch between finger and thumb pads, a few degrees gained at each finger and thumb joint can make a significant difference. The more joints involved in limiting function, the greater the chances of improving functional ability; for example, if a patient is unable to reach his toes for foot dressing, a gain of 10 degrees each in the knees, hips, back, and elbows can make the difference between dependence and independence in this task.

Hands

The characteristic early hand deformities that occur in systemic sclerosis are

1. Loss of flexion of the MCP joints and loss of extension of the proximal interphalangeal (PIP) joints. This is probably due to early fibrosis of the delicate dorsal expansion in a shortened position.
2. Loss of thumb abduction, opposition, and flexion.
3. Loss of wrist motion in all planes.

As involvement progresses, motion is usually lost in all joints in all planes. In order to preserve hand function, the primary objectives of hand therapy in the early stages are to maintain MCP joint flexion and thumb abduction and to prevent wrist flexion contractures.

Patients with SS generally do not develop ulnar drift or swan-neck deformities unless they have a chronic inflammatory arthritis of the MCP joints prior to sclerotic changes.

Typical skin and vascular changes include painful small ulcerations over the fingertips and dorsum of the proximal interphalangeal (PIP) joints and Raynaud's phenomenon.[7]

The painful ulcerations over the fingertips are caused by ischemia and tight skin. These can severely limit hand function, especially for fine tasks such as writing, buttoning, sewing, and using zippers, and they impair strong grasp. The ulcers may heal after sufficient atrophy has occurred and the blood flow becomes adequate for the remaining tissue.[4] Calcium deposits may occur in or under the skin, creating a painful pressure area with skin breakdown over the deposit.[4] Later in the disease, bony resorption of the distal phalanges can result in shortening of the fingers.

Handwriting is often a difficult task for patients with painful ulcers. Rubber slip-on pencil holders are often helpful in reducing the pressure required for writing. They are available from stationery stores.

Raynaud's phenomenon is an episodic vasospasm of the digital arteries causing cyanosis or blanching during the spasm and erythema of the skin following the spasm. It is most often precipitated by cold but may be induced by emotional stress. It occurs in 90 percent of all patients with SS.[4]

Therapy

The objective of therapy is not to prevent all contractures, because some limitations are inevitable, but to prevent unnecessary contractures due to inadequate daily ROM, poor positioning, and disuse. It is important that the patient is also aware of these realistic objectives so that he or she does not have false expectations or false guilt if limitations develop. (Patients often assume guilt for hand limitations, when in fact the limitations may have developed despite the patient's efforts.)

Range of Motion. The type of ROM program used with other patients is not sufficient for scleroderma patients. For example, if a patient has a maximum of 80 degrees of MCP flexion, that patient needs to achieve 80 degrees every day to maintain mobility. Typically, two things happen to patients when they do passive exercises: (1) they may achieve 75 degrees one day, 72 degrees the next, and so forth, not realizing that they are not achieving the same amount; or (2) they may waste a lot of energy or time trying to achieve more than 80 degrees, not realizing that they are at their maximum. Since patients with scleroderma have so many exercises to do, the therapist must encourage them to work on the exercises that will bring the most results.

Patients seem to maintain mobility more effectively when they have a precise ROM program with objective goals to aim for and to measure their progress by. The challenge to the therapist is to help the patient develop a system of applying sustained gentle passive stretch to all affected joints. This is often difficult for patients with sensitive painful fingertip ulcers who are unable to apply pressure with their fingers. Arthritis can also be a limiting factor. Swollen painful joints should be ranged gently, and anti-inflammatory medications should be taken prior to exercising. The ROM program and instruction can be simplified if the patient has already developed an effective method for exercising certain joints; or the therapist can tell the patient the objective of the exercise program and let him or her determine the exercise. The patient who develops his or her own exercise is more likely to remember it and follow through. This also means less learning and less teaching.

Evaluation. Goniometric measurement should be taken of all joints in all planes of motion, and a tracing of the hand should be made to document digit abduction and thumb web space. Ideally, measurements should be taken before and following a heat and exercise program. Measurements taken before exercise will tell you how much mobility the patient maintains easily; and measurements taken after exercise determine exercise objectives. If a patient has not been exercising, this type of initial evaluation (especially if it follows the physician's evaluation) may make the patient's hands somewhat sore and stiff the next day. It is helpful to forewarn the patient about this.

Exercise Programs for Specific Joints and Muscles

1. MCP Joints. MCP flexion is the most important motion to maintain. If a patient is capable of doing only one exercise, this is the one recommended. Some patients can effectively maintain motion by passive manual pressure applied to the dorsum of the proximal phalanges using the heel of the other hand. Others may need the help of a dynamic flexion-assistance device, a wrist strap with leather finger cuffs that slip over the proximal phalanges. The tension on the rubber bands should allow gentle pressure for at least a half hour. If the patient can tolerate only 10 minutes, the bands are too tight. For most patients this type of device is most comfortable if the wrist cuff is placed around a simple volar wrist orthosis. One cuff and splint can often be used alternately on each hand. Such a device allows a patient to apply sustained pressure while watching TV or doing other activities. Not all patients can tolerate this type of device. All splints have to be carefully monitored for their effect on edema, decreased circulation, and skin vulnerability. One method for allowing the patients to determine if they are achieving maximal flexion is to have them use a template, with the desired degree angle cut out of it. These can easily be made of cardboard or wood. For example, take a 3-inch circle of cardboard and cut a 90-degree wedge out of it. If the patient can fit the wedge over the flexed joint, he or she knows that the goal has been achieved. The amount cut out of the template should correspond with the patient's ROM goals. Many patients need only one or two templates.

2. Finger–Thumb Abduction. Patients can monitor their abduction and thumb web space by having a copy of their hand tracings at home. They should do active and passive abduction and adduction of each MCP joint, until they achieve their span goal each day. If the fingers are tight, passive stretch can be achieved by wedging a tissue or piece of cloth between each finger for 5 minutes each or longer. If a patient is starting to loose thumb web space, the only effective method for maintaining it is to use a thumb carpometacarpal-metacarpal (CMC-MC) stabilization orthosis with a C-bar. The one described in Chapter 23 has worked well with several patients. Wearing it at night is usually sufficient. Patients in an acute episode should also wear it during prolonged bedrest and inactivity.

3. Finger Hyperextension. In the early stages, finger hyperextension is an important motion to maintain, since it is often the first to be lost. With hands together in a prayer position, patients can measure their hyperextension span against a ruler or a marking on an index card.

4. Finger Intrinsic Muscles. Exercising the interossei and lumbricals is valuable for mobilizing dorsal expansion; for example, resistance applied to PIP extension with the MCP joints flexed; spreading a rubber band apart with the middle phalanges and thumb; active PIP joint flexion with the MCP joints extended; resistance to abduc-

tion; or trapping an index card between the fingers to provide resistance to the adductors. It appears that fibrosis of the dorsal expansion creates the characteristic scleroderma hand deformity of MCP extension and PIP flexion.

General Guidelines. When possible, exercises should be done daily to maintain motion in all joints and in all planes. This includes flexion and extension of all the finger and thumb joints; finger and thumb abduction and adduction; thumb circumduction, wrist flexion, extension, deviation, and circumduction; and forearm supination and pronation. It is not feasible to list every possible ROM method that can be used with scleroderma patients. Each program needs to be developed with creativity and sensitivity to the patient's ability to carry out a program. Some patients can only manage three or four exercises despite the twenty or more that could be recommended. It is better that they perform three or four exercises effectively than none at all.

Other Considerations. When patients have fixed deformities that limit function, the only recourse is to adapt equipment to accommodate the deformity. Typically this includes built-up handles and cuffs. An example of this is a universal cuff (adjustable plastic slip-on handcuff that holds utensils).

There is also increased vulnerability of the skin to infection and irritation. Avoid any abrasive activities, materials, or substances that irritate the skin. Patients should be careful about traumatizing the skin over the dorsum of the finger joints. In some patients the use of thin cotton laboratory gloves helps protect sensitive skin during housework or routine activities.

If the patient has skin ulcers, it is important to assess hand function, in particular for fine tasks such as writing and buttoning.

Raynaud's Phenomenon. Vasospasm of the digital arteries can result in blanching, erythema, or cyanosis of the fingers and hand. The arteries may spasm in various patterns, causing either a uniform color change or the presence of blanching, erythema, and cyanosis at one time. The spasm may last from a few seconds to 20 minutes or longer. It can be painless or there may be associated aching, numbness, burning, or sharp pain.

Arterial spasm in clients with this form

of vasomotor instability can occur spontaneously or be triggered by (1) exposure to cold; (2) conscious emotional change, such as excitement, nervousness, anger, or subconscious fears; and (3) trauma.

Patients should observe the following precautions:

1. Avoid tobacco (nicotine) and other vasoconstrictors such as amphetamines and ergotamine.[8]
2. Avoid cold:
    a. Wear mittens in cold weather and gloves in the market when touching items from refrigerated sections.
    b. Use oven mitts or potholders when handling frozen foods or ice.
3. Avoid positions that cause venous stasis in the fingers (e.g., allowing the hand to hang motionless to the side for long periods or to hang over the edge of the bed at night).
4. Wear warm clothing on the trunk to help maintain peripheral vasodilatation.[4]
5. Eat modest meals. Eating a large meal reduces peripheral circulation.[4]

Most clients are aware of events that bring on an attack, especially if the event is associated with pain. However, the client may not relate emotional changes or the use of tobacco or various medications with an attack. Nicotine is a major vasoconstrictor. Patients having difficulty giving up smoking may find it helpful to join a community organization devoted to assisting smokers to quit.

These precautions also are important for the therapist to observe in the clinic, especially during activities of daily living (ADL) training in the kitchen or during hand treatment when there is a tendency to work with one hand and let the other hand hang at the side.

For selected patients biofeedback may be a valuable intervention for helping to manage Raynaud's phenomenon.[9-12] Thermal biofeedback provides the most effective method for teaching patients how to raise their peripheral temperature. After biofeedback training, people are able to raise their temperature at will when they experience vasospasm. The relaxation training required for this process is also valuable for the management of stress and developing a greater sense of control over the disease.

Several resources are available for the therapist interested in learning biofeedback training.[13-17]

Face

Facial mobility may be lost early in the disease. The skin becomes taut and the lips may atrophy and recede. The face takes on a characteristic mask-like appearance.[2] Facial involvement is one of the most devastating aspects of the disease. It robs the patient of personality and individuality in an unparalleled manner. Facial changes can also create a communication problem in that one cannot always rely on facial expressions as a cue to the patient's emotions or understanding of instruction.

One of the major consequences of facial involvement is the limitation of temporomandibular joint excursion secondary to sclerosis of the skin, subcutaneous tissues, and musculature. Limited excursion restricts oral hygiene, dental care, and ability to chew solid foods and reduces verbal articulation.

Therapy

If lack of facial expression is causing a communication problem, discuss it with the patient. He or she usually is aware of facial changes, but the loss of nonverbal communication may be unsuspected. It is also helpful to have the patient bring in a photograph taken before the onset of systemic sclerosis. A photograph may facilitate discussion about the psychological effects of the facial changes and help the therapist to appreciate the individuality of the patient as well as changes the patient has experienced.

Where there is decreased jaw mobility, teach the patient how to measure the mouth aperture (distance between upper and lower teeth) in front of a mirror with a ruler at least once a day in order to monitor the excursion. This method provides visual feedback so stretching exercises can be increased if ROM is being lost. It is important to assess the patient's oral hygiene habits and to educate the patient in the importance of maintaining dental health. If the patient does not know appropriate hygiene measures (e.g., how to brush thoroughly or use dental floss), refer the patient to a dental hygienist for a thorough cleaning and instruction.

If the patient has marked limitation, determine what assistive equipment would facilitate better hygiene, e.g., electric toothbrushes, water jet pics, and dental floss applicators (devices that loop the floss around the tooth).

Maintaining Facial Mobility Through Exercise. When planning therapy for facial involvement it is important to keep in mind that in SS, fibrosis and atrophy take place in all the soft facial structures including the skin, subcutaneous fat, and muscles. The use of exercises to maintain facial mobility is experimental in that clinic studies to prove efficiency have not been performed. In fact, their efficacy may never be proven because of the variability of the disease. However, considering the consequences of tight facial structures (i.e., limited mouth aperture appearance), along with the lack of any other form of treatment, a logical treatment approach can be followed.

Each of the exercises described here is designed to move a specific muscle or group of muscles in order to mobilize the fluid in the tissue and stretch the facial structures. It is literally a ROM program for the facial muscles, skin, and subcutaneous tissue.

Patients who use this program daily report one or more of the following outcomes: (1) an increase in the number of different exercises performed over time; (2) an increase in the ability to perform the exercises; and (3) a subjective sense of increased flexibility and suppleness following the exercises.

Treatment Approach. A client should not be instructed in these exercises unless there is definite evidence of sclerosis (skin changes or hardness) in the facial, neck, shoulder, or chest areas. If there is sclerosis in the chest or shoulder area, the disease is likely to spread to the neck and facial area. However, if there is sclerosis only in the hands or arms, there is no way of predicting the disease course. In some clients the disease may affect only the hands, but these patients should be monitored for disease progression.

All the facial and neck muscles should be exercised no matter what the stage of involvement. Obviously many of the muscles will not move in the moderate or severe stages of sclerosis, let alone respond to exercise; therefore, the program needs to be individually tailored for each client. A client with severe involvement may be able to do only a couple of the prescribed exercises. The lip and mouth exercises are the most important since a limited mouth opening interferes with eating and oral hygiene.

Instructions to the Client
1. Do exercises in front of a mirror.
2. Massage (firm touch) the entire face using small circular motions with the fingertips, a warm washcloth, or a vibrator. Then massage each specific area again just before exercising that part.
3. The number of repetitions necessary to get maximal mobility depends upon the individual. One approach is to do the exercise fast two or three times as a warm-up and then do five repetitions holding each stretch position to the count of five. Sustained stretch is more effective for increasing mobility than are rapid motions.

Exercises. The following directions are designed to isolate, contract, and stretch the major facial muscles.

1. Raise the eyebrows as high as possible. Return to the normal position.
2. Bring the eyebrows down and together as hard as possible as if frowning. Then raise the eyebrows as high and wide as possible.
3. Wrinkle the bridge of the nose by raising the upper lip and then frowning (as if smelling something bad).
4. Close the eyes very tight. Then release the squeeze slowly and raise the eyebrows as high as possible before opening the eyes.
5. Flare the nostrils. Then narrow the nostrils down, pushing the upper lip out.
6. Make an exaggerated tight wink with each eye separately, using the cheek muscles to help close the eye.
7. Cover the teeth with the lips. Then open the mouth as wide as possible without the teeth showing. Close lips and press hard (as if blotting lip gloss).
8. Open the mouth so that the lips are as wide apart as possible.
9. Open the mouth so that the teeth are as far apart as possible.

10. Push the jaw forward to create an underbite (bottom teeth in front of the upper teeth).

11. Make as wide a grin as possible without showing the teeth.

12. Pucker the chin by pushing the lower lip upward.

13. Stick the tongue out as far as possible.

14. Push the lower lip down and outward (as in an exaggerated pout).

15. Keep the mouth closed and puff the cheeks out with air; hold to the count of five and then release the air and suck the cheeks inward.

16. Lean the head back as far as possible and open and close the mouth five times.

Thoracic Area

Chest expansion may decrease secondary to fibrosis of the skin, subcutaneous tissues, and intercostal muscles. In some patients, pulmonary fibrosis may develop, further decreasing vital capacity.[1]

Therapy

The objective of therapy is to maintain normal chest excursion. Treatment includes instructing the patient in deep breathing exercises. Usually this is done in physical therapy. Evaluation of progress or status can be made by measuring the chest circumference during inspiration and expiration at the nipple line or below the breasts.

Mobility is also enhanced by having the patient perform total body/trunk stretching exercises.

Arthritis

Arthralgia and/or **arthritis** occurs in 90 percent of the cases at some time. About one third of the patients have articular symptoms first.[2]

Typically the arthritis is a polyarticular, inflammatory, small joint, symmetric arthritis. The arthritis is nonerosive and usually self-limited. Because of fibrosis, swelling is less obvious. Pain in the joints is indicative of arthritis and is often the only symptom.

Therapy

Treatment for arthritis in SS is the same at outlined for RA *except* that people with SS generally *do not* develop the same hand deformities. For example, they usually do not develop ulnar drift or swan-neck deformities. The other major exception is that cold modalities are contraindicated in the hands. (See Chapters 1 and 6.)

Muscle Involvement

Involvement of the skeletal muscles is insidious and often difficult to detect in the early stages. Pathologic changes in the muscles include atrophy and necrosis of the fibers, fibrosis of the fiber sheaths with increased production of connective tissue, diminished number of capillaries and perivascular infiltrates of lymphocytes and plasma cells, and electromyographic abnormalities.

Muscle weakness may be the result of muscle pathology, secondary to disuse, or caused by the inhibition of muscle strength by joint pain.

Patients with SS can develop proximal muscle weakness similar to polymyositis. Difficulty in stepping up on a curb or raising arms overhead is often the first symptoms of proximal muscle weakness. (See Chapter 11.)

Calcinosis

There are two types of subcutaneous calcification. The more common form occurs as a localized deposit (**calcinosis circumscripta**) around joints or near body prominences that may become painful if constantly irritated by pressure.[1] This is especially true over the elbows and ischial tuberosity. Rarely, there may be a diffuse encasing calcification of the skin and subcutaneous tissues that may contribute to severe joint contractures.

Therapy

T-foam cushions, convoluted cushions, or slip-on foam elbow-protector sleeves may help relieve pressure and discomfort.

Telangiectasis

Chronic dilation of capillaries and small arterial branches produces small reddish spots in the skin, called **telangiectasia.** The condition usually is benign and is an indication of internal vascular changes.[3] No therapy is available; the condition is primarily of cosmetic concern.

Visceral Involvement

Viscera are usually involved in all patients with SS. The severity, however, ranges from being entirely asymptomatic to causing death.[1]

Gastrointestinal Involvement

Involvement of the alimentary tract most frequently results in a slowing or absence of the peristaltic waves throughout the tract. The esophagus is usually involved first. The effects of this hypomotility are more pronounced in the recumbent position. **Hypomotility** results in difficulty swallowing (dysphagia), reflux esophagitis, heartburn, bloating, nausea, vomiting, and regurgitation with the risk of aspiration.[2] More extensive involvement of the bowel may lead to malabsorption with consequent severe weight loss and weakness.[1]

Patients with gastrointestinal symptoms are at high risk of developing nutritional deficiencies directly from the symptoms, from a decreased interest in food, or from difficulty in planning or preparing full meals. Patients often start omitting foods that are difficult to eat without making appropriate substitutions for the nutritional loss.[18]

Therapy

The symptoms of hypomotility, reflux, and dysphagia can be reduced or alleviated by sitting very erect while drinking or eating in order to align the esophagus optimally and to allow gravity to assist motility; by eating smaller, more frequent meals; by chewing food well and concentrating on the chewing and swallowing process; and by sleeping with the head of the bed elevated 8 inches on blocks to allow gravity to assist motility.[2,13]

All patients who have difficulty eating or who cannot eat certain foods should receive counseling from a nutritionist.

Pulmonary Fibrosis

The majority of patients develop pulmonary fibrosis, which can reduce vital capacity. In the early stages, this is often asymptomatic because patients have restricted physical activity. Progressive exertional dyspnea and a cough can occur with increasing severity of fibrosis.

Therapy

Occupational therapy primarily involves instructing the patient in energy-conservation methods. Physical therapy instruction in diaphragmatic breathing may also be helpful. Training in adaptive self-care methods should be correlated to diaphragmatic breathing principles.

Cardiac Fibrosis

The most common forms of cardiac involvement include pericardial effusion, myocardial necrosis with fibrosis, and involvement of the large and small vessels of the coronary arteries. Myocardial infarctions are rare.[2]

The symptoms of cardiac involvement are similar to those of pulmonary involvement (i.e., shortness of breath at rest and dyspnea on exertion). Orthopnea, cardiomegaly, and dependent edema indicate primary cardiac disease.

Therapy

It is important to determine the status of the heart from the physician who is treating the patient, since the overall treatment program should be relevant to this aspect of the patient's condition. Observe work-simplification principles in the clinic.

Renal Involvement

Renal failure is the most common cause of death in SS. Patients with proteinuria, hypertension, azotemia, or hyperreninemia are at high risk for developing renal failure.[2]

Therapy

Patients with renal failure are treated with aggressive antihypertensive therapy and with renal-support measures of dialysis. Nephrectomy and kidney transplantation have been used successfully with selected patients.[2]

Associated Conditions

Associated conditions in SS are **myositis,** which is indistinguishable from polymyositis (see Chapter 11); and **Sjögren's syndrome,** a disease of the lacrimal and parotid glands.

DRUG THERAPY

No single drug or combination of agents has been proven to be valuable. Current drug therapy is symptomatic. Steroids such as prednisone are usually contraindicated except in those patients with inflammatory complications such as polymyositis. Antihypertensive drugs should be used to control hypertension, and calcium channel blocking drugs may be helpful in the control of Raynaud's phenomenon.

See Chapter 3 for precautions and side effects of specific drugs.

REFERENCES

1. Sternberg, EM: Pathogenesis of scleroderma: The interrelationship of the immune and vascular hypotheses. Surv Immunol Res 4(1):69–80, 1985.
2. Leroy, EC: Pathogenesis of scleroderma (systemic sclerosis). J Invest Dermatol 79(Suppl 1):87, 1982.
3. Postlethwaite, AE, and Kang, AH: Pathogenesis of progressive systemic sclerosis. J Lab Clin Med 103:506–510, 1984.
4. LeRoy, EC: Scleroderma (systemic sclerosis). In Kelley, WM, et al (eds): Textbook of Rheumatology. WB Saunders, Philadelphia, 1981.
5. Rodnan, GP, Jablonski S, and Medsger, TA Jr: Classification and nomenclature of progressive systemic sclerosis (scleroderma). Clin Rheum Dis 5:5–13, 1979.
6. Melvin, JL, Brannan, KL, and LeRoy, EC: Comprehensive care for the patient with systemic sclerosis (scleroderma). Clin Rheum Prac 2(3):112, 1984.
7. Entin, MA, and Wilkinson, RD: Scleroderma: A reappraisal. Orthop Clin North Am 4:1031, 1973. (Only specific resource on hand problems.)
8. Winkleman, RK, Kierland, RR, Perry, HO, et al: Management of scleroderma. Mayo Clin Proc 46:128, 1971.
9. Yocum, DE, Hodes, R, Sundstrom, WR, and Cleeland, CS: Use of biofeedback training in treatment of Raynaud's disease and phenomenon. J Rheumatol 12(1):90–93, 1985.
10. Freedman, RR, Ianni, P, and Wenig, P: Behavioral treatment of Raynaud's phenomenon in scleroderma. J Behav Med 7(4):343–353, 1984.
11. Sunderman, RH, and Delk, JL: Treatment of Raynaud's disease with temperature biofeedback. South Med J 71(3):340, 1978.
12. Surwit, RS, Pilon, RN, and Fenton, CH: Behavioral treatment of Raynaud's disease. J Behav Med 1:323, 1978.
13. Abildness, AH: Biofeedback Strategies. AOTA, Rockville, MD, 1982.
14. Rogers, SR, Shuer, J, and Herzig, S: The use of biofeedback techniques in occupational therapy for persons with chronic pain. OT in Health Care 1(3), 1984.
15. Green, E, and Green, A: General and specific applications of thermal biofeedback. In Basmajian, JV (ed): Biofeedback—Principles and Practice for Clinicians. Williams and Wilkins, Baltimore, 1979.
16. Olton, DS, and Noonber, AR: Biofeedback: Clinical Applications in Behavioral Medicine. Prentice-Hall, Englewood Cliffs, NJ, 1980. (Contains a chapter on the treatment of Raynaud's disease.)
17. Biofeedback Society of America. (This organization can provide information about resources and training opportunities in your area. Write to Francis Butler, Executive Secretary, University of Colorado Medical Center, 4200 East 9th Ave., Denver, CO 80220.)
18. Silverman, EH, and Elfant, IL: Dysphagia: An evaluation and treatment program for the adult. Am J Occup Ther 33(6):382, 1979.

ADDITIONAL SOURCES

General

Baron, M, Lee, P, and Keystone, EC: The articular manifestations of PSS. Ann Rheum Dis 41(2):147–152, 1982.
Blom-Bulow, B, Jonson, B, and Bauer, K: Factors limiting exercise performance in PSS. Semin Arthritis Rheum 13(2):174–181, 1983.

Callen, JP: Mixed connective tissue disease: An overview. South Med J 75(11):1380–1384, 1982.

Connolly, SM: Scleroderma: Therapeutic options. Cutis 34(3):274–276, 1984.

Fleischmajer, R, and Perlish, JS: The vascular, inflammatory, and fibrotic components in scleroderma skin. Monogr Pathol 24:40–54, 1983.

Fleischmajer, R, Perlish, JS, and Duncan, M: Scleroderma: A model for fibrosis. Arch Dermatol 119(12):957–962, 1983.

Goplerud, CP: Scleroderma. Clin Obstet Gynecol 26(3):587–591, 1983.

Haustein, UF, and Ziegler, V: Environmentally induced systemic sclerosis-like disorders. Int J Dermatol 24(3):147–151, 1985.

Ingram, VW: Scleroderma—The silent disease. J Nephrol Nurs 3(2):55–59, 1986.

Jayson, MI: The micro-circulation in systemic sclerosis. Clin Exp Rheum 2(1):85–91, 1984.

Jayson, MI: Systemic sclerosis—A microvascular disorder? J R Soc Med 76(8):635–642, 1983.

Lovell, CR, et al: Joint involvement in systemic sclerosis. Scand J Rheum 8(3):154–160, 1979.

Petersen, P, et al: Therapeutic intervention in scleroderma. Clin Rheum Prac 3(3):107–115, 1985.

Rehabilitation Institute of Chicago: Clinical Evaluation of Dysphagia. Rockville, MD, Aspen Publishers, 1985.

Walker, L: Clinical problems: Progressive systemic sclerosis. Nurs Pract 7(3):60–62, 1982.

Behavorial Treatment for Raynaud's Phenomenon

Freedman, RR, et al: Biofeedback treatment of Raynaud's disease and phenomenon. Biofeedback Self Regul 6(3):355–365, 1981.

Surwit, RS, Allen, LM 3rd, Gilgor, RS, and Duvic, M: The combined effect of prazosin and autogenic training on cold reactivity in Raynaud's phenomenon. Biofeedback Self Regul 7(4):537–544, 1982.

Wilson, E, Belar, CD, Panush, RS, and Ettinger, MP: Marked digital skin temperature increase mediated by thermal biofeedback in advanced scleroderma [letter]. J Rheumatol 10(1):167–168, 1983.

Hand Treatment

Askew, LJ, Beckett, VL, An, KN, and Chao, EY: Objective evaluation of hand function in scleroderma patients to assess effectiveness of physical therapy. Br J Rheumatol 22(4):224–232, 1983.

Baron, M, et al: Prostaglandin E1 therapy for digital ulcers in scleroderma. Can Med Assoc J 126(1):42–25, 1982.

Seeger, MW, and Furst, DE: Effects of splinting in the treatment of hand contractures in progressive systemic sclerosis. Am J Occup Ther 41(2):118–121, 1987.

Body Image

Murray, RLE: Principles of nursing interventions for the adult patient with body image changes. Nurse Clin North Am 7:697, 1972.

Trust, D: Disfigurement: Something to face up to. Med Times 109(7):88–92, 1981.

Facial/Oral Treatment

Craig, M: Miss Craig's Face Saving Exercises. Random House, New York, 1970. (Written by a physical therapist but designed for the public, this book is an excellent resource regarding facial musculature. However, it is too detailed to be used by patients with SS for the purposes described in the exercises in this chapter.)

Marmasy, Y, et al: Scleroderma: Oral manifestations. Oral Surg 52(1):32–37, 1981.

Naylor, WP: Oral management of the scleroderma patient. J Am Dent Assoc 105(5):814–817, 1982.

Naylor, WP, Douglass, CW, and Mix, E: The nonsurgical treatment of microstomia in scleroderma: A pilot study. Oral Surg Oral Med Oral Pathol 57(5):508–511, 1984.

Children

Ansell, B, et al: Scleroderma in childhood. Ann Rheum Dis 35(3):189–197, 1976.

Peskett, SA, Ansell, BM, Fizzman, P, and Howard, A: Mixed connective tissue disease in children. Rheum Rehabil 17(4):245–253, 1978.

Singsen, BH: Scleroderma in childhood. Ped Clin North Am 33(5):1119–1139, 1986.

Patient Resources

Scleroderma patient groups are being developed around the country. These groups can be invaluable for helping patients cope with the complex psychological and social ramifications of this disease. For information on the many local groups write to the following organizations:

The United Scleroderma Foundation
PO Box 724
Watsonville, CA 95076
(Publishes newsletter for patients)

The Arthritis Foundation
3400 Peachtree Road, NE
Atlanta, GA 30326

Scleroderma International Foundation
704 Gardner Center Road
New Castle, PA 16101
(Publishes newsletter for patients)

Chapter 11

Polymyositis and Dermatomyositis

Polymyositis (PM) is a diffuse inflammatory disease of striated muscle that leads to muscle destruction and symmetric proximal muscle weakness. When any of a variety of skin rashes accompanies this condition, it is known as **dermatomyositis (DM).** Frequently PM is associated with other rheumatic diseases such as systemic lupus erythematosus, progressive systemic sclerosis, juvenile rheumatoid arthritis, and Sjögren's syndrome.

ETIOLOGICAL FACTORS

The cause is unknown. In some older adults, there is a link with visceral malignancies.[1]

AGE AND SEX AFFECTED

PM and DM can occur at any age and are found in females in a 2-to-1 ratio over males.[1] In adults, PM is more common; in children, DM is more common.

DIAGNOSIS

Diagnosis is based on proximal muscle weakness, serological evidence of muscle destruction (indicated by elevated muscle enzymes), heliotrope (purple) rash of the eyelids (not always present), characteristic muscle biopsy, characteristic electromyogram, and a lack of neurological findings. The breakdown of muscle tissue is indicated by elevated creatine kinase (CK) levels in the blood (normal is 30 to 225).

The following classification is used for diagnosis:

Group 1. Primary idiopathic PM (adults or children).

Group 2. Primary idiopathic DM (adults or children).

Group 3. DM or PM associated with neoplasia.

Group 4. Childhood DM or PM associated with vasculitis. (This is considered the most severe form and is life-threatening if not treated appropriately.)

Group 5. PM or DM associated with collagen and vascular disease (overlap groups).

COURSE AND PROGNOSIS

This varies in all aspects. Initial symptoms may be muscular, dermal, or articular. Remissions or exacerbations may occur spontaneously. Prognosis is more favorable when onset occurs at a younger age and for those who have a slowly progressive course.[2]

The overall course of the disease can be divided into three types: (1) a monocyclic course of relatively short duration without collapse, (2) a relapsing form, and (3) a long-persisting disease that may endure for many years.

SYMPTOMATOLOGY AND IMPLICATIONS FOR OCCUPATIONAL THERAPY

Proximal Muscle Weakness

Muscle weakness may vary from mild involvement with no functional loss to severe muscle destruction with quadriparesis. The muscle weakness is typically proximal although there are reported cases of predominantly distal weakness.

The pelvic girdle, shoulder girdle, and neck flexor muscles are the most obvious groups involved but the abdominal, back and neck extensor, intercostal, and diaphragm muscles are affected also. Weak pelvic girdle muscles cause a characteristic waddling gait. Muscle involvement may become more distal with severity.

Therapy

When the patient is in an *acute exacerbation,* the following protocol is recommended:

1. *Safety precautions against falling should be taken.* Assistive equipment to ensure safe ambulation should be used and instruction in safe transfer methods should be started early in the course of the disease. A wheelchair or rolling walker should be used to protect the hip muscles.

2. Strict bedrest is advised. Weakened muscle groups should not be used beyond tolerance. Only activities that can be done comfortably without muscle fatigue are recommended. A patient should not perform an activity that cannot be stopped immediately if he or she becomes fatigued (e.g., walking down a long hallway or standing in a shower). Heavy resistive tasks should be *avoided;* these include unassisted walking, difficult unassisted transfer, and wheelchair propulsion with the arms. Muscle stress is believed to enhance tissue destruction and thus elevates enzyme levels.

3. Patient education regarding activity and exercise is important. Many patients believe incorrectly that weak muscles should be used as much as possible.

4. Gentle-passive range of motion (ROM), progressed to active-assisted ROM, should be performed daily. Lying prone is also recommended to maintain hip ROM.

5. During bedrest (sitting or lying), neck and back support should keep the spine in straight alignment. A soft neck collar may be necessary to support the neck when the patient is sitting up.

6. *If* involvement progresses distally, night splinting may be indicated for the knees, elbows, or wrists.

7. For patients with severe weakness, mobile arm supports (or deltoid aid) can be used to increase functional independence for feeding, facial hygiene, and writing.

8. Relaxation training can help a patient regain some sense of control, reduce fear and anxiety, and improve systemic health.

As the patient responds to the medication and gains in strength, functional activities can be progressed as tolerated and an active-assistive exercise program initiated. *All exercise should be performed to toler-*

ance and the muscles should not be fatigued. The program should be progressed gently with patient response carefully observed.

The strengthening program can be continued and progressed to a resistive one as long as the patient continues to gain in strength. The patient is essentially in a chronic-active phase if the inflammatory process decreases then plateaus at a low level. At that point the program emphasis changes from strengthening to one of (1) activities of daily living to tolerance, (2) instruction in energy conservation and work simplification to improve functional endurance, (3) instruction in proper positioning at night and at leisure (see Chapter 28, Positioning and Lying Prone), and (4) physical therapy with exercise to maintain ROM and strength.

Dysphagia and Pulmonary Involvement

The most common type of lung involvement is **aspiration pneumonia.** Patients with PM/DM syndromes are highly susceptible as a result of pharyngeal muscle weakness, impairment of the protective cough clearance mechanism, and blunting of protective body movements (i.e., turning and bending in response to vomiting). Pharyngeal dysfunction and dysphagia are due to weakness of the striated muscle of the soft palate, pharynx, and upper esophagus, which places the patient at high risk for regurgitation and possible asphyxiation.[3]

The lung may be involved directly with interstitial lung disease (5 to 10 percent of patients), or it may be involved secondary to a complication of muscle weakness leading to ventilatory insufficiency, or it may be a sequela of treatment (e.g., drug-induced interstitial pneumonitis or opportunistic infection).[3]

Therapists should be alert for the following symptoms of lung involvement: shortness of breath or dyspnea on exertion, coughing, the symptoms of dysphagia, and difficulty swallowing. These symptoms should be reported to the medical and nursing staffs.

Therapy

Because the risk of regurgitation is life-threatening, dysphagia secondary to muscle weakness is considered a medical emergency. Advise the treating physician promptly if the patient reports symptoms of dysphagia. Patients with established dysphagia should be advised to have several small feedings instead of three large meals per day; to *sit erect* while drinking or eating (with back and head supported if necessary) to optimally align the esophagus and maximize gravity assistance; to chew foods carefully; and to avoid dry, hard foods. The head of the bed should be elevated 8 inches at night or during rest to provide gravity assistance to muscles for swallowing.

Muscle Involvement

When **muscle pain** occurs, it is most common about the shoulders, upper back, upper arms, and forearms, but it can occur in any muscle group. It is not usually a predominant symptom. Also, a patient may interpret muscle weakness or tiredness as pain.[2]

Muscle atrophy is common in later stages of the disease. It is secondary to muscle degeneration and other factors such as disuse.[2]

Therapy

Heat applications and massage often help relieve soreness. (For the inpatient this usually is carried out by physical therapy. Transcutaneous electrical nerve stimulation (TENS) may be useful if pain is specific and limiting. The patient at home may need instruction in use of heating pads.)

Strengthening treatment depends upon the phase of the disease. (See Chapter 27, Exercise Treatment, for a discussion on the relationship between muscle strength and atrophy.)

Joint Contractures

Joint contractures may be due to joint and muscle pain, muscle fibrosis, calcinosis, weakness, or postural adaptations. ROM may be limited early in the disease, being secondary to pain or inflammation. Fixed contractures are typical of later stages of the disease or in cases in which medical treatment has been delayed. Children with severe dermatomyositis differ from adults in that they often develop severe joint contractures rapidly in the early stages of the disease.[4-6]

Therapy

ROM and muscle strength should be watched closely. The distal muscle groups can also be involved in severe cases.

During the acute or subacute phase, gentle-passive ROM with slight stretch to the point of discomfort, not pain, is recommended twice a day to affected joints. If a patient develops contractures in the acute phase, serial casting is the most effective method for reducing them and should be instituted as soon as the patient is medically stable and can tolerate the procedure. If done early, serial casting can reduce contractures in a few days. In the chronic-active phase, active or active-assisted exercises are recommended. In the nonactive phase, a standard ROM program to increase ROM is suitable. Lying prone to tolerance is recommended to prevent hip contractures. (See Chapter 27, Exercise Treatment, and Chapter 28, Positioning and Lying Prone.)

Arthritis

An inflammatory type of polyarthritis may occur with either PM or DM. It differs from rheumatoid arthritis in that it is nonerosive, usually not chronic, and typically subsides without residual deformity. If hand deformities do occur, they usually are due to muscle fibrosis and tendon shortening.[1]

Therapy

Treatment is the same as outlined for inflammatory joint disease (see Chapter 1). Additional information on chronic inflammation of specific joints can be found in Chapter 6, Rheumatoid Arthritis.

Skin Rash

Rashes occur in 40 percent of the patients and may occur in various forms. Typically a rash occurs initially as a scaly erythema over the extensor surfaces of the knuckles and elbows. It may also occur over parts of the body exposed to the sun. The eyelids may be a characteristic heliotrope hue with edema in the periorbital area.[2]

Therapy

The rash *may* be sensitive to the sun, with exposure to sun or ultraviolet light causing it to flare up. The patient should wear protective clothing and sun block lotion with a PABA factor of 15 or more when outside if he or she has a sun-sensitive rash.

Associated Conditions

Malignant neoplasms are common in patients over 40 years of age; however, they are not associated with the childhood form of the disease or when myositis occurs in association with another rheumatic disease. Other conditions that may occur with PM are Sjögren's syndrome, Raynaud's phenomenon, and pulmonary fibrosis.

DRUG THERAPY

The principle of drug therapy in PM is to give an agent that will stop the inflammatory destruction of muscle fibers. Prednisone or other corticosteroid preparations are considered the drugs of choice for this condition. Corticosteroids are initially given in large doses (60 to 100 mg/day) and tapered when signs of activity have abated. Methotrexate very effectively suppresses muscle inflammation and can be used in patients not responding to prednisone or in whom the prednisone needs to be reduced because of side effects.

REFERENCES

1. Bohan, A, and Pelter, J: Polymyositis and dermatomyositis. N Engl J Med (Part I) 292(7):344, 1975; (Part II) 292(8):403, 1975. (Contains current medical information; does not include aspects of rehabilitation.)
2. Pearson, CM: Polymyositis and dermatomyositis.

In McCarty, DJ (ed): Arthritis and Allied Conditions, ed 9. Lea & Febiger, Philadelphia, 1978.
3. Dickey, BF, and Myers, AR: Pulmonary disease in polymyositis/dermatomyositis. Semin Arthritis Rheum 14(1):60–76, 1984.
4. Feallock, B: Dermatomyositis; Case study. Am J Occup Ther 19(5):279, 1965. (Describes occupational therapy treatment for an adolescent with severe involvement.)
5. Jacobs, JC Jr: Treatment of dermatomyositis. Proceedings of the Conference on the Rheumatic Diseases of Childhood. Arthritis Rheum 20(2):338, 1977. (Strong advocacy for steroid therapy.)
6. Sullivan, DB, Cassidy, JT, and Petty, RE: Dermatomyositis in the pediatric patient. Arthritis Rheum 20(2):327, 1977.

ADDITIONAL SOURCES

Bradley, JD: Jaccoud's arthropathy in adult dermatomyositis. Clin Exp Rheum 4(3):273–276, 1986.
Bradley, W: Inflammatory disease of muscles. In Kelley, WM, et al: Textbook of Rheumatology. WB Saunders, Philadelphia, 1981, pp 1255–1275.
Callen, JP: Dermatomyositis. Dis 33(5):237–305, 1987.
Edwards, RHT, et al: Muscle breakdown and repair in polymyositis: A case study. Muscle Nerve, 223–238, May/June 1979.
Fessel, WJ: Muscle disease in rheumatology. Semin Arthritis Rheum 3(2):127, 1973.
Hochberg, MC, Feldman, D, and Stevens, MB: Adult onset polymyositis/dermatomyositis: An analysis of clinical and laboratory features and survival in 76 patients with a review of the literature. Semin Arthritis Rheum 15(3):168–178, 1986.
Hunder, GG, and Michet, CJ: Giant cell arteritis and polymyalgia rheumatica. Clin Rheum Dis 11(3):471–483, 1985.
Kagen, LJ: Dermatomyositis and polymyositis: Clinical aspects. Clin Exp Rheumatol 2(3):2717, 1984.
Mastaglia, FL, and Ojeda, VJ: Inflammatory myopathies: Part 2. Ann Neurol 17(4):317–323, 1985.
Pachman, LM: Juvenile dermatomyositis. Pediatr Clin North Am 33(5):1097–1117, 1986.
Physical Therapy Protocols for Polymyositis and Dermatomyositis. University of Michigan Hospitals, 1985.
Resnick, J, et al: Muscular strength as an index or response to therapy in childhood dermatomyositis. Arch Phys Med Rehabil 62:12–19, 1981.
Sundaram, MB, et al: Polymyositis presenting with distal and asymmetrical weakness. Can J Neurol Sci 8:147–149, 1981.
Walton, J: The inflammatory myopathies. J R Soc Med 76(12):998–1010, 1983.

Chapter 12

Polymyalgia Rheumatica and Arteritic Syndromes

POLYMYALGIA RHEUMATICA
ARTERITIC SYNDROMES
    Giant Cell (Temporal) Arteritis
    Polyarteritis Nodosa
    Wegener's Granulomatosis
    Anaphylactoid Purpura (Henoch-Shönlein Purpura)
    Hypersensitivity Angiitis
    Aortic Arch Arteritis

POLYMYALGIA RHEUMATICA

Polymyalgia rheumatica (PMR) is a syndrome of primarily proximal muscle stiffness and pain. It is not considered an arteritis by itself but is often seen in association with giant cell (temporal) arteritis. Therefore, the two syndromes are discussed together in this chapter.

The precise nature of the relationship between PMR and giant cell arteritis is not known. Some researchers hypothesize that PMR may be a manifestation of subclinical giant cell arteritis, although this has not been proven and all patients with giant cell arteritis do not get PMR. Because of this association with a serious arteritis, PMR is an important syndrome to detect early.[1] It is also one that is frequently misdiagnosed as neck or back pain, osteoarthritis, fibromyalgia, or bursitis, or it may be overlooked in patients with one of these concomitant problems. If these patients are in therapy, the occupational or physical therapist may be the first to detect the symptoms of PMR and direct the patients to

seek consultation with their internist or rheumatologist.

PMR is characterized by marked stiffness and pain of the shoulder muscles but *without* objective weakness (although pain may limit performance of these muscles in a manual muscle test). Other symptoms can include low-grade fever, weight loss, arthralgias, myalgias, malaise, fatigue, depression, morning stiffness, persistent aching, mild synovitis in any joint, and pain at night with movement.[1,2] These symptoms can severely limit the person's ability for activities of daily living (ADL). The diagnostic criteria commonly includes (1) symmetric proximal limb girdle myalgias associated with significant stiffness, (2) duration of symptoms longer than 1 month, (3) age of 50 years or more, (4) Westergren erythrocytic sedimentation rate of 40 mm/hour or more, and (5) absence of other disease processes capable of causing the musculoskeletal symptoms, such as systemic lupus erythematosus.[3]

In the majority of patients, the symptoms dramatically resolve with the administration of short-term, low-dose (<20 mg) corticosteroid therapy.[3] About half the patients need long-term, low-dose corticosteroid therapy for 3 years or longer to control symptoms.[3] In the others, the corticosteroids can be slowly tapered and discontinued. For many elderly women, side effects of prolonged corticosteroid use can create additional health problems (e.g., osteoporosis).[1] When patients respond favorably to low-dose corticosteroids, they generally do not need any occupational or physical therapy. Patients with severe or nonresponsive symptoms, or those unable to tolerate the medications, may need counseling in energy conservation, conscious deep muscle relaxation, methods to reduce postural strain, adaptive methods for ADL, and assistive devices. These patients also need careful instruction in a daily range-of-motion (ROM) program and isometric shoulder exercise program to prevent atrophy and adhesive capsulitis.

ARTERITIC SYNDROMES

These conditions involve inflammation, which is usually segmental, of the arteries (arteritis) or both arteries and veins (vasculitis) associated with a severe systemic disease process. They present in two ways: (1) as a primary disorder with or without secondary joint involvement, or (2) concomitant with a rheumatic disease, usually rheumatoid arthritis or systemic lupus erythematosus.[4] It is because of this second factor, the relationship with the rheumatic diseases, that arteritis and vasculitis are included in this section.

Symptoms of arteritis depend upon the severity and duration of inflammation and the size and location of the affected arteries. Each arteritic syndrome tends to involve arteries of a particular size or location in various combinations, resulting in a more or less characteristic symptom complex.[5]

These conditions are less common than the other diseases discussed in Part II and are included primarily for definition. Patients are not likely to be referred to therapy unless there is significant or prolonged arthritis, central nervous system involvement, muscle weakness, neuropathy, or a major peripheral ischemic complication, such as gangrene.

Giant Cell (Temporal) Arteritis

Giant cell (temporal) arteritis is an inflammation of the temporal and cranial arteries. In three of four cases, it affects women in the 50- to 90-year age range. The onset can be abrupt or insidious. Early symptoms can include constitutional symptoms of fatigue, anorexia, or weight loss; headaches with marked boring or lacerating pain, localized to arteries of the scalp or more diffuse scalp tenderness often in association with the headaches; or low-grade fever, which occurs in half the patients. Visual symptoms may include diplopia, ptosis, or transient or permanent partial or complete blindness (due to ischemia of the optic nerve or tracts secondary to arteritis of the ophthalmic or postciliary arteries). There may be intermittent claudication in the muscles of mastication and swallowing and in the extremities. Psychological and neurological symptoms can include confusion, depression, psychosis, hemiparesis, peripheral neuropathy, acute hearing loss, and brain stem strokes. Cardiac involvement, including angina pectoris, congestive heart failure, and myocardial infarction, has been reported but is far less frequent.[1]

Patients may be referred to occupational therapy for any of the psychological or neurological symptoms or for training in adaptive methods for partial visual loss. Patients with severe visual loss or blindness should be referred to a specialized mobility and ADL training center for the blind. Blindness and serious complications can usually be prevented with early detection of symptoms and treatment with corticosteroids.[1]

Polyarteritis Nodosa

Polyarteritis nodosa (periarteritis nodosa) is an inflammatory disease that destroys the walls of medium and small-sized arteries. In some patients the segmental angiitis creates small aneurysms: if subcutaneous, these appear as nodules, forming the basis of the disease's name. It primarily affects males between the ages of 20 and 50 years, with peak incidence in the fifth and sixth decades. The disease commonly affects the heart, intestinal tract, kidneys, and muscle. Central nervous system and lung involvement are unusual. Onset can range from insidious and mild, similar to an influenza syndrome, to acute and extremely severe.[6] Although the cause is unknown, in some patients there is an association with intravenous use of methamphetamine ("speed") and with the presence in the serum of the hepatitis-associated antigen.[7] Prognosis has been dramatically improved with the use of corticosteroids and cyclophosphamide. The 5-year survival rate is now around 80 percent with these medications. If untreated the 5-year survival rate is only 13 percent.[8]

Referrals may be made to occupational therapy for treatment of a mild arthritis, peripheral neuropathy,[9] or fatigue and weakness from chronic systemic involvement, central nervous system involvement, or for protective splinting for digital gangrene. The vasculitis that occurs rarely in rheumatoid arthritis (malignant rheumatoid arthritis) has the same pathological basis and prognosis as polyarteritis nodosa.[5]

Wegener's Granulomatosis

Wegener's granulomatosis is a destructive arteritis of the upper respiratory tract, lungs, and kidneys that, when untreated, progresses to death from renal failure. Associated symptoms may include a rash, arthralgias, muscle involvement, peripheral neuropathy, and nephritis. Treatment with cyclophosphamide has resulted in cures of this otherwise fatal disease.[4,10]

Anaphylactoid Purpura (Henoch-Schönlein Purpura)

Anaphylactoid purpura is a vasculitis that affects small vessels of the skin, gastrointestinal tract, synovium, and kidneys. It is far more common in children than in adults, occurring from infancy to adolescence with a median age at onset of approximately 6 years. It affects males twice as frequently as females.[11] The clinical picture of characteristic purpuric skin lesions over the buttocks and down the backs of the lower extremities combined with arthritis leads to the diagnosis. Angioedema may occur in half the children. The majority of children develop significant joint pain and swelling that most commonly occur in the knees and ankles but can occur in the fingers and elbows. During the acute stage the arthritis can be quite disabling but it typically resolves without residual deformity or sequelae. Other symptoms can include colicky abdominal pain and gastrointestinal bleeding. The disease usually involves series of continuous acute attacks that can last up to 6 weeks[11] and then resolve for the majority of patients; however, some can have persistent chronic symptoms. Death from renal failure is rare but has occurred.[12]

Hypersensitivity Angiitis

Hypersensitivity angiitis is a general term that refers to inflammation of small vessels that results from drug reactions, serum sickness, or other unidentified inciting factors. The skin and synovium are the most frequently involved sites and can result in a mild self-limited synovitis.[1]

Aortic Arch Arteritis

Aortic arch arteritis (Takayasu's or pulseless disease) is an arteritis of the large muscular arteries that arises from the aortic arch. It is a rare disease of young women. Symptoms reflect insufficient circulation to the areas served by the large vessels and can include central nervous system involvement, involvement of the aortic arch, or intermittent claudication if the lower aorta is involved. Systemic features, such as arthralgia, arthritis, fever, and anemia, may also be present.[11]

REFERENCES

1. Hunder, GG, and Hazlemann, BL: Giant cell arthritis and polymyalgia rheumatica. In Kelley, WM, Harris, ED, Ruddy, S, and Sledge, CB (eds): Textbook of Rheumatology, ed 2. WB Saunders, Philadelphia, 1985.
2. Allen, NB, and Studenski, SA: Polymyalgia rheu-

matica and temporal arteritis. Med Clin North Am 70(2):369–384, 1986.

3. Ayoub, WT, Franklin, CM, and Torretti, D: Polymyalgia rheumatica. Duration of therapy and long term outcome. Am J Med 79:309, 1986.

4. Hunder, GG, and Conn, DL: Necrotizing vasculitis. In Kelley, WM, Harris, ED, Ruddy, S, and Sledge, CB (eds): Textbook of Rheumatology, ed 2. WB Saunders, Philadelphia, 1985.

5. Haynes, BF, Allen, NB, and Fauci, AS: Diagnosis and therapeutic approach to the patient with vasculitis. Med Clin North Am 70(2):355–368, 1986.

6. Pitkin, RM: Polyarteritis nodosa (in pregnancy). Clin Obstet Gynecol 26(3):579–586, 1983.

7. Duffy, J, et al: Polyarteritis and hepatitis B$_{12}$. Medicine 52:19, 1976.

8. Leib, ES, Restivo, C, and Paulus, HE: Immunosuppressive and corticosteroid therapy of polyarteritis nodosa. Am J Med 67:941, 1979.

9. Besole, R, Lister, C, and Kleinert, H: Polyarteritis: A cause of nerve palsy in the extremity. J Hand Surg 3(4):320, 1978.

10. Fauci, AS, Hayes BF, Katz P, et al: Wegener's granulomatosis: Prospective clinical and therapeutic experience with 85 patients for 21 years. Ann Intern Med 98:76, 1983.

11. Hanson, V: Systemic lupus erythematosus, dermatomyositis, scleroderma and vasculitides in childhood. In Kelley, WM, Harris, ED, Ruddy, S, and Sledge, CB (eds): Textbook of Rheumatology, ed 2. WB Saunders, Philadelphia, 1985.

12. Allen, DM, Diamond, LK, and Howell, DA: Anaphylactoid purpura in children. Am J Dis Child 99:833, 1960.

ADDITIONAL SOURCES

Cupps, TA, and Fauci, AS: The Vasculitides. WB Saunders, Philadelphia, 1981.

Ghouse, AT, Smith, KM, and Rooney, PJ: Polymyalgia rheumatica and rheumatoid arthritis: A prodromal or overlap syndrome? Eur J Rheumatol Inflamm 7(2):56–62, 1984.

Hart, FD: Polymyalgia rheumatica: Its correct diagnosis and treatment. Drugs 33(3):280–287, 1987.

Hicks, RV, and Melish, ME: Kawasaki syndrome. Pediatr Clin North Am 33(5):1151–1175, 1986.

Leavitt, RY, and Fauci, AS: Therapeutic approach to the vasculitic syndromes. Mt Sinai J Med 53(6):440–448, 1986.

Littler, T: Polymyalgia rheumatica—The health visitor's role in diagnosis and prevention. Health Visit 56(11):418–419, 1983.

Medicus, L: Kawasaki disease: What is this puzzling childhood illness? Heart Lung 16(1):55–60, 1987.

Rogers, C, Parnassus, W, and Noguchi, TT: Suicide in a patient with undiagnosed periarteritis nodosa. Am J Forensic Med Pathol 8(1):51–55, 1987.

Siemssen, SJ: On the occurrence of necrotising lesions in arteritis temporalis: Review of the literature with a note on the potential risk of a biopsy. Br J Plast Surg 40(1):73–82, 1987.

Sigal, LH: The neurologic presentation of vasculitic and rheumatologic syndromes. Medicine 66(3):157–180, 1987.

Chapter 13

Gout

ETIOLOGICAL FACTORS
AGE AND SEX AFFECTED
DIAGNOSIS
COURSE AND PROGNOSIS
SYMPTOMATOLOGY AND IMPLICATIONS FOR
  OCCUPATIONAL THERAPY
  Acute Gouty Arthritis
  Therapy
  Chronic Tophaceous Gout
  Therapy
DRUG THERAPY

Gout is characterized by acute episodes of arthritis associated with the presence of sodium urate crystals in the synovial fluid or deposits of urate crystals (tophi) in or about the joints and other tissues.

ETIOLOGICAL FACTORS

Primary gout is the most common form and is the type that may lead to chronic tophaceous gout. It occurs alone and is not secondary to any other major disease. It results from elevation of serum uric acid levels **(hyperuricemia)** and deposition of urate crystals in the tissues and joints. Hyperuricemia develops because too much uric acid is being produced, too little is being excreted in the urine, or both.[1]

Secondary gout occurs when hyperuricemia is directly due to an underlying disease (e.g., leukemia or chronic renal disease). This form rarely develops tophi because of the decreased life span resulting from the underlying disease.[1]

AGE AND SEX AFFECTED

Primary gout is found primarily in males (9 to 1); it occurs most commonly in the fifth decade but it can present any time after puberty. It rarely occurs in women until after menopause.[2]

DIAGNOSIS

Diagnosis is confirmed by the presence of monosodium urate crystals in the synovial fluid and hyperuricemia. In patients who present with tophi, the presence of crystals in the tophus establishes the diagnosis.[3]

COURSE AND PROGNOSIS

With appropriate medication: Typically the initial acute attack lasts for a few days; further acute attacks and the development of tophi are prevented.

Without medication: Typically there are recurrent episodes of acute inflammatory monoarticular arthritis that subside spontaneously in about two weeks. If the hyperuricemia persists, tophi may develop. These accumulations of urate crystals can erode into the joints, bones, and periarticular structures, causing functional impairment.[2,3]

SYMPTOMATOLOGY AND IMPLICATIONS FOR OCCUPATIONAL THERAPY

Acute Gouty Arthritis

The acute attack of gout is an excruciatingly painful arthritis, usually affecting a single joint. Lower extremity joints are most commonly affected, particularly the first metatarsophalangeal joint **(podagra)**. The onset is rapid with swelling, heat, and erythema in the affected joint.[1]

Historically gout was thought to be caused by the overindulgence of food or alcoholic beverages; however, with the advent of drugs to control the hyperuricemia, severe dietary restrictions are rarely indicated. Patients are advised to eat a regular diet, avoiding only those foods that are particularly high in purines (purines break down into uric acid) such as fish eggs (caviar) and sweetbreads (calf's thymus glands).[3]

Therapy

Occupational therapy is rarely indicated for an acute attack of gout. However, protective or resting splints may be helpful, especially if the site of the attack is the wrist or hand.

Chronic Tophaceous Gout

Five to ten years after the onset of gout, **tophi** (deposits of urate) may develop. These usually appear as subcutaneous lumps, most commonly in the olecranon bursa and along the cartilage of the ear. When they occur around joints, they may lead to cartilage and bone erosion with residual joint deformity or decreased range of motion secondary to mechanical interference.[2]

The most frequent hand limitations are decreased finger flexion and decreased grip. Other problems related to urate deposition are renal stones and nerve entrapment syndromes; the former are common but the latter are rare.

Tophi can often be reduced or eliminated by proper medication but this usually takes a considerable amount of time—months or even years.[3]

Therapy

The main symptom that would indicate referral to occupational therapy would be decreased hand function secondary to tophi. Physical measures are generally not indicated for deformities directly caused by tophi. Occupational therapy is usually identified in terms of adapted equipment and assistive devices.

DRUG THERAPY

Drugs that reduce inflammation are usually prescribed for acute attacks. Colchicine, indomethacin, and phenylbutazone are the drugs classically used for this purpose. It is now known that any of the nonsteroid anti-inflammatory drugs may be used to abort the acute attack. They should be used at the maximal recommended dose until the inflammation subsides. After the acute attack is controlled, therapy is directed at lowering the serum uric acid.[2]

Sulfinpyrazone or probenecid lowers serum uric acid by increasing the renal excretion of uric acid. High fluid intake is urged with these drugs to minimize the risk of uric acid renal stone formation. Allopurinol effectively lowers serum uric acid by blocking an enzyme needed for the production of uric acid.[2] Dosage is adjusted until the serum uric acid is at the desired level. See Chapter 3 for precautions and side effects of specific drugs.

REFERENCES

1. Gutman, AG (ed): Gout: A Clinical Comprehension. Burroughs Wellcome Co., Research Triangle Park, NC, 1971.
2. Kelley, WM: Gout and related disorders of purine metabolism. In Kelley, WM, et al (eds): Textbook of Rheumatology. WB Saunders, Philadelphia, 1981.
3. Wyngaarden, JB, and Holmes, EW: Clinical gout and the pathogenesis of hyperuricemia. In McCarty, DJ (ed): Arthritis and Allied Conditions, ed 9. Lea & Febiger, Philadelphia, 1979.

ADDITIONAL SOURCES

Bomalaski, JS, and Schumacher, R: Podagra is more than gout. Bull Rheum Dis 34:6, 1984.
German, DC, and Holmes, EW: Hyperuricemia and gout. Med Clin North Am 70(2):419–436, 1986.
Landry, JR, and Schilero, J: The medical/surgical management of gout. J Foot Surg 25(2):160–175, 1986.
Murray, JB: Psychosomatic aspects of gout. J Gen Psychol 103(1st half):131–138, 1980.
Varga, J, Giampaolo, C, and Goldenberg, DL: Tophaceous gout of the spine in a patient with no peripheral tophi: Case report and review of the literature. Arthritis Rheum 28(11):1312–1315, 1985.

PART III

ARTHRITIS IN CHILDREN AND ADOLESCENTS

Thus far over 50 diseases with arthritis as a component have been identified as occurring in children. The most common of these diseases, with chronic joint or muscle symptomatology, comprise the childhood rheumatic diseases. In some centers **juvenile arthritis** is the preferred umbrella term for this spectrum of conditions (see Table III–1).

Juvenile rheumatoid arthritis (JRA) is the main focus of this section because it is the most frequently seen diagnosis and because it provides a prototype for treatment of inflammation in the peripheral joints, as well as the hips, shoulders, and cervical spine; it also serves as a prototype for management of psychosocial and developmental factors of arthritis during childhood. In other words, the protocol for treating wrist inflammation in JRA is the protocol used for treating wrist inflammation associated with any other childhood arthritis such as systemic lupus erythematosus, even if the diagnosis is undetermined at the time of treatment. Rehabilitation for children with rheumatic diseases other than JRA is based on (1) joint management similar to JRA, (2) psychosocial and developmental management as identified for JRA, and (3) disease management as outlined for the specific diseases in Part II of this book.

OCCUPATIONAL THERAPY— DEVELOPMENTAL AND BIOMECHANICAL INTEGRATION

The treatment of children with JRA presents a challenge to the occupational therapist in both the biomechanical context of preserving joint function and the developmental context of promoting normal physical, psychosocial, and cognitive growth. To integrate the biomechanical and developmental approaches, the therapist must be cognizant of normal developmental tasks and appreciate the effects of a chronic disease on the child at each stage of the child's development as well as globally in response to disease/development throughout the course of illness. Occupational therapy must constantly change in response to the progressively mature social behavior expected of the child in order to facilitate physical, psychosocial, and cognitive growth. This requires a critical analysis of the child's daily response to therapy.

Throughout assessment, treatment, and goal setting, the following concepts will assist the therapist in formulating a well-balanced program for the child.

1. The child must be an active participant in therapy. When the child is totally involved in therapy, neuromotor and emotional development is self-directed and physical status is improved.

2. Play or meaningful activity is the primary means for improving function. Exercise should be incorporated into a play scheme whenever possible, but play alone should not substitute for exercise.

3. A child needs control at each stage of development. This can include control over one's own actions, personal care, activity choice, environment, or schedule. If control is not permitted through healthy outlets, manifestations may erupt in noncompliance. For example, infants may cry, not eat, or not take medications; toddlers may not allow examinations, not participate in therapy, or frequently demand to go to the bathroom during therapy; and the adolescent may not comply with orthotic protocols, arrive late for therapy, or execute tasks poorly.

4. Recognize a child's strengths. A child needs to recognize his or her unique strengths. These strengths need to be fostered to promote confidence and a positive self-concept.

5. Hospitalization means separation from family. Children ages 2 to 4 are particularly susceptible to separation trauma. A child may temporarily show regressive behavior by clinging and crying until he or she is more comfortable with the people and surroundings. (See the section on effects of hospitalization in Chapter 15.)

6. The family must be included in all aspects of treatment. Their values, education, beliefs regarding disease, and schedules must be considered before a program is prescribed. The need for the child's discipline and the importance of siblings receiving adequate attention while the patient is in the hospital should always be addressed.

7. Therapy takes place throughout the day. Self-care, home routines, school, after-school therapy, and the home program are all aspects of treatment. The impact of all therapies on the child throughout the day must be considered. When the therapy demands are excessive, it is helpful to consider priorities regarding the most critical therapeutic and emotional needs for the child in order to ensure a balance of work, play, and rest.

8. Frequent and accurate reassessment is critical. Changes in disease, developmental needs, and functional level dictate program changes.

9. Mastery of self-care helps form a basis for self-esteem. Good habits or routines of care should be established. Participation in self-care even though the child may not be independent is important for psychosocial development.

10. Coordination of care between the hospital therapy and the community is essential. This includes the school, transportation, school-based therapy, and group programs such as scouts, summer camps, and recreational activities.

Table III–1 Rheumatic Diseases Affecting Children and Adolescents

I. **Inflammatory**
    A. Collagen vascular diseases
        1. Juvenile rheumatoid arthritis
        2. Systemic lupus erythematosus
        3. Systemic sclerosis
        4. Dermatomyositis
        5. Mixed connective tissue disease
    B. Spondyloarthropathies
        1. Juvenile ankylosing spondylitis
        2. Reiter's syndrome
        3. Postdysenteric arthritis
        4. Reactive arthritis
        5. Arthritis associated with inflammatory bowel disease
        6. Psoriatic arthritis
        7. Enthesopathy syndromes

Table III–1 Rheumatic Diseases Affecting Children and Adolescents
(*Continued*)

    C. Soft tissue conditions
       1. Tendinitis
       2. Tenosynovitis
       3. Bursitis
    D. Vasculitides
       1. Schönlein-Henoch purpura
       2. Kawasaki's syndrome (infantile polyarteritis nodosa)
       3. Systemic vasculitis
       4. Polyarteritis nodosa
       5. Wegener's granulomatosis
    E. Infectious arthritis
       1. Toxic synovitis of the hip
       2. Septic arthritis (bacterial, fungal, tubercular)
       3. Osteomyelitis with sympathetic arthritis
       4. Lyme arthritis
       5. Multicentric osteomyelitis
       6. Brodie's abscess (localized, walled-off osteomyelitis)
    F. Reactive arthritis
       1. Poststreptococcal arthritis
       2. Acute rheumatic fever
       3. Sarcoid arthritis (causative agent unknown)
    G. Foreign body arthritis
       1. Palm thorn synovitis
       2. Sea urchin synovitis
II. Noninflammatory
    A. Traumatic arthritis
       1. Battered child trauma
       2. Hypermobility syndrome
    B. Neoplastic disease
       1. Acute lymphatic leukemia
       2. Neuroblastoma
       3. Osteoid osteoma
       4. Other neoplastic conditions
    C. Avascular necrosis syndromes
       1. Osgood-Schlatter's disease
       2. Legg-Perthes' disease
       3. Long-term corticosteroid therapy
       4. Köhler's disease
       5. Other osteochondritis syndromes
    D. Arthromyalgia syndromes
       1. Limb pain of childhood (growing pains)
       2. Fibromyalgia
       3. Reflex sympathetic dystrophy
    E. Other conditions
       1. Chondromalacia patellae
       2. Discitis
       3. Slipped capital femoral epiphysis
       4. Congenital abnormalities
         a. NOMID (neonatal-onset multisystem inflammatory disease)
       5. Hemophilia (arthritis secondary to bleeding in joints)
    F. Psychiatric disorders
       1. Somatization disorder
       2. Malingering
       3. Conversion disorder (hysterical neurosis)

(Compiled by Jeanne Melvin, O.T.R. and Bram Bernstein, M.D.)

Chapter 14

Juvenile Rheumatoid Arthritis

JEANNE L. MELVIN, O.T.R., M.S.Ed., F.A.O.T.A.
MARCY ATWOOD, M.A., O.T.R.

TERMINOLOGY AND CLASSIFICATION

The identification and classification of juvenile rheumatoid arthritis (JRA) and its subtypes has been one of the major advances in rheumatology over the past 15 years. This classification system has been extremely helpful because it allows the clustering of sequelae in order to determine clinical course, risk of complications, and prognosis.

Juvenile rheumatoid arthritis is delineated into three major types *defined by the symptoms present during the first 6 months following onset:* **systemic-onset, polyarticular-onset,** and **pauciarticular-onset.**[1] These have been further divided according to the type of course the disease follows (Table 14–1).

The terminology used to describe the JRA subtypes is very specific based on the above criteria. This can create some confusion for therapists new to this area of practice. For example, children who have high-spiking fevers in the beginning are classified as "systemic-onset." But, in fact, all forms of JRA are systemic diseases in that they all have an element of fatigue, malaise, and so forth when the arthritis is active. In essence, therefore, they all are systemic, but only the group with high-spiking fevers and marked internal organ involvement is given that designation. Another example is that children with pauciarticular-onset may develop additional joint involvement after the initial 6 months and have polyarthritis, but they will retain the "pauciarticular-onset" classification. Another term that needs clarification is **early.** To avoid confusion, in this text the term **young-onset** is used instead of **early** or **early-onset** to refer to onset of disease at a young age. Some authors, most notably British, use the term **early JRA** to indicate a child referred for treatment *early* in the course of the disease, for example, within the first year.

There are other international differences in terminology in pediatric rheumatology.

The classification in this text, which delineates subtypes by the nature of onset, reflects the preference of American rheumatologists. In the United Kingdom (UK) and Europe, the preference is to delineate subtypes based on the presence of the rheumatoid factor (RF). The terms **juvenile chronic polyarthritis (JCPA)** and **juvenile chronic arthritis (JCA)** refer specifically to chronic seronegative arthritis, the most common situation in JRA. This designation, however, crosses all subtypes recognized by the American Rheumatism Association (ARA). Children with a positive test for rheumatoid factor in Europe are considered to have the juvenile form of rheumatoid arthritis and are referred to as having **seropositive JRA.** There are logical arguments for and reasonable criticisms against both the American and UK/European terminologies, so the controversy continues. At this point, it is important to be aware of the differences in labeling when reading the international literature.

A final point about terminology: the term **juvenile rheumatoid arthritis** implies that it is the childhood equivalent of adult **rheumatoid arthritis.** This is not quite true since JRA represents several distinct subtypes. Only one subtype of JRA (polyarticular-onset, rheumatoid factor positive) resembles adult RA clinically and is considered its childhood equivalent.

DIAGNOSIS

In order for the definitive diagnosis of JRA to be made, the child must be under 16 years of age and have at least a 6-week history of true arthritis that cannot be attributed to any known cause (e.g., infection, trauma, or disease such as systemic lupus erythematosus or rheumatic fever). (See Appendix 4 for a list of the conditions that must be ruled out in order to make this diagnosis.) **Arthritis** is defined as **swelling or limitation of motion with heat, pain, or tenderness.** Pain or tenderness alone is not sufficient to make the diagnosis. All joints are counted individually with the exception that the cervical spine joints, the carpal joints, and the tarsal joints in each extremity are counted as one joint each.[1]

The specific subtype is determined by symptomatology and the pattern of joint involvement present during the first 6 months following onset. Laboratory tests are used to help classify subtypes, but there are no specific diagnostic tests for JRA. The course and prognosis vary for each subtype.

By definition there is no known cause of JRA. In some subtypes genetic predisposition has been demonstrated with the presence of specific antigens, such as DRw5.[2]

EPIDEMIOLOGY

JRA is known throughout the world and affects children of all races and ethnic groups. Over the years there has been a wide variance in the epidemiological studies estimating prevalence of JRA. A few years ago as many as 200,000 children were thought to have JRA. But the most recent study indicates a prevalance of 50 per 100,000 children, with an estimate of 30,000 to 60,000 children with JRA in the United States.[3] This excludes children with other rheumatic diseases. JRA is, therefore, considered a relatively uncommon disease. The age and sex affected vary with each subtype.

SYSTEMIC-ONSET JUVENILE RHEUMATOID ARTHRITIS

This form of JRA can strike at any age but most frequently occurs in those under the age of 10 years.[4] It accounts for about 10 to 20 percent of all JRA and affects boys and girls equally.[5,6] Laboratory tests for rheumatoid factor (RF) and antinuclear antibodies (ANA) are negative.[7] There is no known human lymphocyte antigen (HLA) association for genetic susceptibility. *There is also no eye involvement in this group.*[7]

By definition this type of JRA starts with an episode of marked **systemic symptoms,** including: a high fever (103°F or above), often spiking in the afternoon and then returning to normal; a classic evanescent (meaning it appears and disappears quickly) maculopapular rash; hepatosplenomegaly; lymphadenopathy; polyserositis; myalgia; arthralgia; leukocytosis; and anemia. Pleurisy and pericardial effusions are not uncommon and are occasionally se-

Table 14–1. Comparison Summary of Juvenile

	Systemic		Polyarticular	
Type of onset	Spiking fever Rheumatoid rash Hepatosplenomegaly Lymphadenopathy Polyserositis Myalgia, arthralgia Leukocytosis, anemia		Symmetrical arthritis	
Pattern of joint symptoms	Same as pauciarticular JRA (40% of systemic onset patients)	Same as polyarticular JRA (60% of systemic onset patients)	Arthritis involving upper and lower extremities; both small and large joints (wrists, hands, elbows, shoulders, hips, knees, ankles, feet, jaw, and neck); but not lumbodorsal spine	
Rheumatoid factor	Negative	Negative	Negative	Positive
Course of joint disease	Remitting—40%	Remitting with scarring— 35% Severe, unremitting and destructive— 25%	Remitting May "burn out"	Persistent chronic and destructive
Age at onset (median)	5 years	5 years	3 years	12 years
Sex ratio	M = F	M = F	F >> M	F >>> M
Antinuclear antibody	Absent	Absent	+ in 25%	+ in 75%
HLA-associated	?	?	None	DR4
Uveitis	Rare	Rare	Rare	Absent
Comments	Systemic manifestations usually ultimately remit even if arthritis continues		Extra-articular manifestations generally mild	Childhood onset of classical adult RA Subcutaneous rheumatoid nodules common

(From Jacobs, J: Pediatric Rheumatology. Springer-Verlag, New York, 1982, pp. 182–183,

Rheumatoid Arthritis: Types and Subtypes

Pauciarticular		
Asymmetrical arthritis		
Onset in knee only in 50% of cases. Monarticular in 74%	Few joints at onset (average 2); severe periarticular inflammation; periostitis; enthesopathy; SI joints, low back and first MTP joint; primarily lower extremity. Strong familial pattern	Few joints involved; typically knee, hip, ankle; occasionally spotty involvement of other joints as well
Negative	Negative	Negative
Joint destruction rare but some chronic knee damage	Remitting—occasional rapid destruction, especially of hips; calcification of the inflamed entheses (heel spurs) follows lytic lesions in heel entheses	Remitting; mild enthesopathy; no joint destruction, no calcification of the enthesis
2 years	10 years	6 years
F >>>> M	M >> F	F > M
+ in 50%	Occasionally transiently positive at onset	Absent
DR5	B27	None (? many subsets)
+ in 40% Subacute and chronic	8% in childhood 25% in lifetime (Acute, subacute, and chronic)	Rare
Total blindness in 17% in the past was the major disability. Average number of joints at onset = 1.3	May progress to ankylosing spondylitis; may begin with Reiter's syndrome. Average number of joints at onset = 2.5	Not a well-defined group

with permission.)

vere.[7] The systemic manifestations may occur in any combination.

Classically, the fever peaks (spikes) in the midafternoon or early evening, lasts several hours, then returns to normal. Some patients can have a daily double spike, but this is less common. After treatment is initiated, the fever may spike in the morning. Younger children tend to become very irritable, fretful, and anorexic during the febrile state; lack of appetite can result in serious weight loss.[8] These children may appear severely ill. If the joint symptoms are delayed for weeks or months, the diagnosis can be quite difficult.

The symptoms of arthritis, myalgias, and arthralgias, which limit mobility, correspond to the fever and can be mild or absent when the fever remits. This explains why some children who are nonambulatory in the evening may be quite mobile in the morning.[9] Fatigue and poor endurance are problems, as in all forms of systemic arthritis.

The characteristic evanescent, erythematous rash may occur on the face, trunk, and extremities, but it tends to skip the palms and the soles of the feet. It is *generally* neither painful nor purpuric (itchy); however, some children may be bothered by itching.[8] Reproducing the rash by scratching the skin is called the **Koebner phenomenon** or **isomorphic response.** It may also be induced by a hot bath or emotional stress. The rash also correlates to the presence of fever.[10] The systemic manifestations tend to be consistent for several months and then become inconsistent and stop. Overall, the symptoms are not considered life-threatening; however, children with very serious systemic disease have died of infections, hepatic failure, myocarditis, blood disorders, and neoplasms. In Europe, renal failure secondary to amyloidosis is the leading cause of death in JRA.[11]

Polyarticular Course

Approximately 60 percent of children with systemic-onset develop a symmetric **polyarthritis** in five or more joints. In about 35 percent of these cases, the arthritis will remit with some joint damage, and approximately 25 percent will have a progressive unremitting and destructive arthritis.[7,12] These children often have **generalized growth retardation** and altered bone growth of the long bones and mandible owing to the localized effects of the inflammation on the epiphyseal plate. They can develop the characteristic **micrognathia** (smaller or receding jaw) if the mandible is affected.[7] (Growth retardation also can occur in the nonsystemic-polyarticular type, but it is more common in the systemic-onset unremitting polyarticular course.) Once the rash and spiking fevers stop and the arthritis persists, these children appear identical to children with polyarticular-onset JRA.

The arthritis most frequently occurs in the smaller extremity joints (hands, feet, knees, elbows) and cervical spine (most often at C2-3 apophyseal joints) and less frequently in the hips, shoulders, and axial joints. It generally spares the thoracic and lumbar spine, although children may develop a severe lordosis to compensate for hip contractures. In some cases the arthritis may not appear for weeks or months after the onset of fever and systemic manifestations.[4,5,7,8,10]

Pauciarticular Course

Of all the children with classic systemic manifestations at onset, approximately 40 percent will develop arthritis in four or fewer joints **(pauciarticular arthritis);** a few have no significant arthritis at all. For most of these children, the arthritis goes into full remission.[7,12]

POLYARTICULAR-ONSET JUVENILE RHEUMATOID ARTHRITIS

JRA that starts with inflammation of five or more joints (polyarticular) as the predominant symptom—without the high, spiking fever or rash—accounts for approximately 40 percent of all JRA[7] (see Table 14–1).

The pattern of arthritis is the same as that described for systemic-onset JRA, except that it is in multiple joints from the beginning. The pattern or distribution is essentially the same as that for adult RA; that is, it is symmetric and affects the following joints listed in rough order of descending frequency: the hands, wrists, feet, knees, ankles, elbows, cervical spine, temporomandibular joint, shoulders, and hips.[13] It spares the thoracic and lumbar apophyseal joints. The sequela, however, is often quite different from the adult form, and this is discussed later under specific joint involvement.

Children with polyarticular-onset JRA who test positive for RF have a clinical picture different from those who are negative for RF. Polyarticular-onset is, therefore, further divided into two subgroups based on the presence of RF.

Seronegative Course (Juvenile Chronic Arthritis in Europe)

Approximately 25 percent of all children with JRA have this form. Girls are affected more frequently than boys. It can strike at any age, but the peak age of onset is 3 years. By definition, the test for rheumatoid factor is always negative, but the test for ANA is positive about 25 percent of the time. There is no known HLA association.[14]

The majority of these children tend to have a milder arthritis with a greater remission rate and less systemic features than children who are seropositive for RF.[7] But if the arthritis is prolonged or unresponsive to medications, these children can develop severe joint contractures, localized bone growth alteration, and generalized growth retardation. Pericarditis may occur, but it tends to be mild. Uveitis also can occur but is rare. Approximately 10 to 15 percent of these children become so limited that they require assistance in self-care and ambulation and have American Rheumatism Association (ARA) functional classes of III and IV (see Chapter 18).

Seropositive Course (Juvenile Rheumatoid Arthritis in Europe)

This is the form of JRA that is described as the most like adult RA. It predominantly affects girls and most often occurs after the age of 10 years.[15] The test for RF is always positive; but because a transient positive test for RF can be associated with other diseases, the test must be persistently positive over the course of several months to warrant classification in this category.[16] Recently the DR$_4$ antigen has been identified as a genetic marker in this subgroup.

The pattern of joint involvement is the same as that of the seronegative group, but the small joints of the hands and feet are involved more in the beginning. Distal flexor tenosynovitis seems less common.[8] The hand deformities can be similar to those seen with adult RA (see Table 14-2 later in this chapter).

Systemic manifestations of low-grade fever, malaise, and anorexia are more prevalent during exacerbations. Fatigue can be a major functional problem similar to the way it is in adult RA. Other manifestations similar to those of adult RA include subcutaneous nodules (any location), vasculitis, parenchymal lung involvement, and Felty's syndrome. Uveitis is not associated with this group.[7]

About half of these children will have progressive arthritis into adulthood with severe functional limitations in ARA class III or IV.

PAUCIARTICULAR-ONSET JUVENILE RHEUMATOID ARTHRITIS

This classification designates children who develop arthritis in four or fewer joints during the first 6 months from onset. The age of onset and the presence of the HLA-B27 antigen further define two major subsets in this classification.

Subset I: Young-Onset

Of all the children with JRA, about one third are in this category. This subset primarily affects girls under the age of 5 years. It typically starts as a mild, insidious swelling of one or two middle-sized joints (i.e., the knee, elbow, wrist, or ankle). About 74 percent have monarticular onset and 50 percent have onset in the knee.[7] It is common for the children to appear healthy and to have no complaints of pain. In fact, it may be the presence of a limp or contracture that first alerts the parent to the problem.[8] In younger, especially chubby, children ages 2 to 4 years, it is easy for joint swelling or a mild contracture to go unnoticed. It is not clear why these children do not report pain. The most common theory is that children do not perceive pain in the same way as adults do and thus do not report the sensation as "painful." The perception of pain may be influenced by the neurophysiology of the capsule and bone, which is different in the child compared with that in an adult. (See section on pain in juvenile rheumatoid arthritis.)

On clinical examination the joints are swollen, warm, and frequently limited in motion. Laboratory values, including white blood count, hemoglobin, and sedimentation rate, are generally normal. RF is negative, but the test for ANA is positive in half of the patients. The test for the HLA-DRw5 is positive in children who develop uveitis.[2]

In this subgroup a positive ANA test is an ominous sign, because it correlates with propensity to develop chronic **iridocyclitis** (inflammation of the iris and ciliary body of the eye), which can lead to scarring (synechiae) and visual loss or blindness (17 percent of cases) if it goes undetected or untreated.[17,18] This eye disease is asymptomatic in the beginning, so it can easily go undetected. It is diagnosed by finding inflammatory cells in the anterior chamber of the eye with a "slit-lamp examination." The eye inflammation does not correlate with joint involvement and may start even when the arthritis is in remission. Therefore, all children with pauciarticular-onset JRA, especially if they test positive for ANA, must have periodic ophthalmic examinations every 6 to 12 weeks throughout childhood, even if the arthritis is in remission.[10]

Other possible eye sequelae include calcium deposits on the cornea (**band keratopathy**), cataracts, and secondary glaucoma.[10]

Treatment for the uveitis consists of local corticosteroid drops and mydriatics (drugs to dilate the pupil to prevent adhesions). Severe cases may require systemic corticosteroids.[10,17]

It is typical for the arthritis to remit in 1 to 2 years, although a few may develop arthritis in additional joints and a more prolonged course with exacerbations and remissions. This is not considered a "deforming" arthritis, but it can be as persistent and severe. Joint contractures and localized overgrowth of long bones adjacent to the involved joints are common sequelae. When this occurs in the knee, problems include leg-length discrepancy, which may alter gait, encourage a knee-flexion contracture, or create a pelvic tilt and compensatory scoliosis, tibial subluxation, and quadriceps atrophy. Aggressive treatment of contractures to minimize muscle imbalance and biomechanical malalignment is essential and should include heel lifts, nightly leg orthotics, and exercise. Overall, these children have a good functional prognosis.[7]

Subset II: Late-Onset

This subgroup also may be referred to as "juvenile spondyloarthopathy or seronegative arthritis with enthesopathy." It is far less common and accounts for about 15 percent of all children with pauciarticular-onset JRA. It affects primarily boys after the age of 9. Presence of the HLA-B27 antigen is very strong and helpful in making the diagnosis.[7] RF is negative, and the test for ANA is usually negative.[7]

This form of JRA typically starts as an asymmetric pauciarticular arthritis of the lower-extremity joints, with the hip, ankle, and metatarsophalangeal (MTP) joints being the most frequently affected. Occasionally the wrist or a single digit joint can become involved. The arthritis is described as mild and episodic.[13]

A common—and unique—symptom of this subtype is **enthesopathy**: inflammation at an enthesis (i.e., the site of attachment of tendons and ligaments to bone).[7,19] Common sites include those of the Achilles tendon, metatarsal heads, iliac crest, patella, and tibial tuberosity.[19] Inflammation may be severe and out of proportion to the arthritis. The enthesis may calcify, forming a bone spur.[7]

For most patients the main complaints are joint and/or tendon pain, stiffness in afflicted areas, and some fatigue. In some patients systemic manifestations of fever, weight loss, and malaise are more pronounced. Some children report that muscular aching and stiffness precede the onset of arthritis by several months.[8] A few of these children actually develop the characteristic conjunctivitis and keratoderma blennorrhagica (blistering, pustular skin condition) associated with **Reiter's syndrome.**[5,7]

There is frequently a family history related to Reiter's syndrome, psoriasis, inflammatory bowel disease, reactive arthritis, or ankylosing spondylitis.[7] Uveitis is associated with this subtype, but it is acute and symptomatic and typically not destructive. It is treated with local steroid drops and mydriatics.[18]

These children can have an episodic course for years. They *do not* get sacroiliitis or spondylitis in childhood. It is not known how many go on to develop another seronegative spondyloarthropathy in adulthood.[5]

Subset III: Undefined or Mixed

There are children who develop an arthritis in one to four joints who are neither ANA positive or HLA-B27 positive and do not fit neatly into the above subtypes. Some subsequently go on to have other diseases such as psoriatic arthritis or inflammatory bowel disease. Others, after a year, develop additional joint involvement and a polyarticular pattern. So this is not a true subset, but a means of categorizing cases that do not fit in the other subsets.

PAIN IN JUVENILE RHEUMATOID ARTHRITIS

Synovitis without Pain

One of the striking differences in rheumatology between working with children and working with adults is the way children report pain. A child may have a swollen knee and limp into the clinic, but when asked, "Does the knee hurt?" will reply, "No." Certainly some children with active arthritis will tell you it hurts and will have tenderness with palpation, but the relationship of pain to joint inflammation is highly variable in children, giving the impression that they can have joint synovitis without pain. (In adults it is extremely rare to have joint synovitis without pain.) Consequently "pain" plays a different role as a criterion in assessments and treatment planning.

The most commonly proposed explanation of this phenomenon is that children *perceive pain differently.*[20] Several studies have helped shed some light on this issue.

Laaksonen and Laine[21] were the first to study this phenomenon, comparing joint pain between children and adults. Overall, the children had significantly lower scores on pain with palpation and functional use compared with adults; but, interestingly, they showed equivocal scores for pain in actively inflamed joints passively moved in extreme range (the researchers believed that this demonstrated intact joint neural pathways). They concluded that the difference was due to children reacting differently to pain than adults.[21]

Scott, Ansell, and Huskinsson asked 100 children (ages 2 to 17) to rate their pain using a visual analog scale with 1 to 20 points (increments).[22] They found that the children's scores were lower overall than those found with adults, and the scores did not correlate with activity or severity scores. They concluded that pain can be measured in children using an analog scale but that pain is not a particularly useful measurement for evaluating treatment. This is especially the case when the patient rates the pain low to begin with, for this leaves little room for improvement. The researchers comment on the fact that pain threshold, which rises with age, does not seem to be a factor in this phenomenon; and they note that it is a common observation that children seem to sustain considerable trauma with minimal pain. Yet, clearly, some children have pain that correlates with the severity of the inflammation. They found also that parents assessed the child's pain much higher than did the child; and, in some instances, parents encouraged the child to make a higher score than the child had originally intended. (This is common and must be watched for in the clinic.)

Both of these studies focused on the reporting of pain and did not address the physiological, cognitive, or psychological aspects of pain perception in children.

Children with frank inflammation who do not acknowledge pain clearly do not perceive it as pain. But why they do not is another question that has never really been addressed. Perception of pain is influenced by maturation of the joint and peripheral and central nervous systems as well as cognitive skills and psychological mechanisms, such as denial, fear, and shame. In addition, the entire process of pain perception can be altered or masked by anti-inflammatory and analgesic medications, especially corticosteroids. The reporting of perception is *further influenced* by social learning and communication skills, such as ability to label perceptions of pain and stiffness accurately.[20,23]

Beales, Keen, and Lennox Holt[20] addressed the issue of interpretation of pain based on the child's level of comprehension of joint pathology. Children ages 6 to 12 years and 12 to 18 years were interviewed regarding their joint sensation, which was assessed by presenting a list of 11 descriptive terms (e.g., aching or cutting) and delineating the meaning attributed to these sensations. Results indicated that similar sensations were reported in joints of both groups (100 percent of all children reported an "aching" sensation, and 53 percent reported a "sharp" sensation). The older children interpreted this sensation as more unpleasant, perhaps because of their increased understanding of joint pathology. The younger children attributed negative qualities to the joint sensation only as it interfered with their functional abilities. This study suggested that a child's pain threshold was related to the interpretation of sensory input as an indicator of the child's overall condition. "The more children approximate an adult's appreciation of the significance and implications of the sensation experienced, the more the level of arthritic pain perceived approximates that of adults with RA. These perceptions appear to progress along a cognitive developmental sequence."[20]

It is still entirely possible that the neuroreception of pain in children's joints is different from that of adults, but proving this is beyond the scope of this text. As if this were not complex enough, there are two more concepts that need consideration when using pain as a criterion: that tenosynovitis can occur without pain, and that synovitis can occur without swelling.

Tenosynovitis with and without Pain

In both adults and children, tenosynovitis may be either painful or painless. When pain is present it may be used as a guide for monitoring progress, but swelling and tendon function (gliding) must be used as the primary criteria for detecting, evaluating, and monitoring tenosynovitis.

My clinical experience with treatment of painless tenosynovitis in the hand is that orthotic immobilization *does not help* and often makes the problem worse. This appears to be due in part to the elimination of muscle action as a means for reducing swelling. When tenosynovitis is painful, motion appears to be a stressor to the tendon. Immobilization eliminates the stress, reduces pain, and improves healing. The absence of pain requires that we clearly think through the goals of treatment and our criteria for efficacy (see Chapter 19).

Dry Synovitis

Another type of joint involvement that occurs only in JRA is **dry** or **nonproliferative** synovitis. This is arthritis *without swelling or warmth;* the only symptoms may be pain or tenderness and either gradual or rapid loss of motion.[5,7,8,10] Considering the factors that influence the child's perception and reporting of pain, and the analgesic effect of medications, patients may not even report tenderness in these joints—leaving loss of motion as the prime symptom. In advanced cases the joint can be eroded and progress to ankylosis.

Dry synovitis can produce permanent contractures so rapidly that it can be described only as a devastating experience to witness. The contractures often develop because the physicians, therapists, or nurses are not familiar with *dry* synovitis and do not assess it or recognize the need for immediate treatment. It literally catches everyone by surprise.

Because there is no way of predicting which joints can develop dry synovitis, the only way to have preventive treatment planning is to evaluate each joint for tenderness and limited motion (even those without swelling or pain).

If a child begins to lose motion in a joint when there is no pain, swelling, or tenderness, dry synovitis should be assumed. The recommended treatment is the use of orthoses and devices for positioning and active and passive range-of-motion (ROM) exercises following heat application. (Heat generally works better because dry synovitis is primarily a problem of stiffness rather than of swelling.)

All joints should be monitored carefully in children during all phases of hospitalization, especially early during the admission and when the child is very sick. When a child is very sick, the systemic manifestations often take the attending physician's attention; frequently occupational and physical therapists are not called in until the patient "feels better" or the life-threatening crises are over. I have seen many patients develop permanent nonfunctional contractures during a week of crisis because rehabilitation was associated with an active treatment program and put low on the agenda. In acute cases, the rehabilitation team should be called in on the second day solely *to prevent contractures*. Generally this can be done in a relatively painless manner. The effort to prevent orthopedic sequelae is worthwhile because, after the medical crises are over, the wrist-drop, foot-drop, loss of neck mobility, and hip, knee, and elbow flexion contractures become the focus of extensive rehabilitation and orthopedic measures. Some people live a lifetime with contractures that developed during a few days of hospitalization when they were children.

Positioning in bed and during activities is critical for children with arthritis. Positioning is the same as for adults except that it needs to be much more aggressive and must encompass school and play activities. This is discussed further when specific joint involvement is considered.

When joint contractures develop from dry synovitis, they can be extremely difficult to correct because the joint remains painful. Therapists at Children's Hospital in Los Angeles have found aggressive treatment with serial casting to be successful, especially in the wrist, knee, and ankle. The delicate digit joints, however, are difficult to correct when painful. There is so little understanding of this form of joint involve-ment that it really does not have a name beyond the vague reference of "dry" in contrast to a 'boggy" joint. It is referred to in review articles by pediatric rheumatologists and orthopedists, but there is no further description of the specific pathology in the literature. Surgeons report that surgical correction of contractures resulting from dry synovitis produces poor results and should be a measure of last resort, if done at all.

Pain Perception and Cooperation (Compliance)

The presence or absence of pain can have a significant impact on patient cooperation with treatment and recognition or acceptance of the condition. For example, if a child has a painful wrist, it is fairly easy to get the child to wear an orthosis if it alleviates the pain. If there is no pain nor any immediate benefit, the child may perceive the orthosis only as a hindrance.

Older children often have significant psychological denial and fear regarding their illness; the lack of pain may encourage this denial or make it difficult for them to perceive the importance of various rehabilitative measures. *It is critical to understand how the child perceives his or her illness, joint involvement, and therapy program, so that guidance and instruction can be geared toward these perceptions.* Chapter 15 outlines the child's perception of his or her illness as conceptualized through the development of cognition.

Pain and Joint Assessment in Children

In adults, pain is the prime criterion for determining synovitis or active joint involvement. In children, five separate criteria must be used to assess active joint involvement:

1. Pain at rest, with motion, and with palpation (tenderness)
2. Swelling with or without pain
3. Limited joint motion with or without tenderness
4. Joint stiffness in the morning or after prolonged positioning

5. Muscle weakness, which may precede limited motion, pain, or joint symptoms

JOINT INVOLVEMENT

Radiographic Changes

The most striking difference between adult and juvenile radiographs is the amount of cartilage present in the immature skeleton. Cartilage is not visible on x-ray film, thus creating an impression of open space. In fact, *the term "joint space" means cartilage* in reference to a radiograph. Thus, if inflammation has damaged a person's cartilage, the negative space between the bones on x-ray film will be diminished, and the patient is described as having "narrowed joint space on x-ray."

The epiphyseal plate also shows as a negative space on radiographs and separates the epiphysis from the shaft of the bone. Overgrowth and premature closure of the epiphysis and resultant bone length alteration are readily visible on x-ray film. In addition, the epiphyses may appear "cupped" on film, apparently owing to intra-articular pressure from inflammation. Localized altered bone length is common in pauciarticular JRA.[24]

In the younger child, the cartilage is so thick that early or mild cartilage damage does not show on radiographs. Also, because the cartilage is very thick, it may take years for the inflammation to reach the bone; therefore, bone erosions are not common in young children. Radiographic evidence of moderate to severe destruction, which would be clearly evident in an adult or older child (ages 14 to 16), may be absent or long delayed in the radiographs of a younger child.[25] In other words, the comment that "x-rays do not show any joint

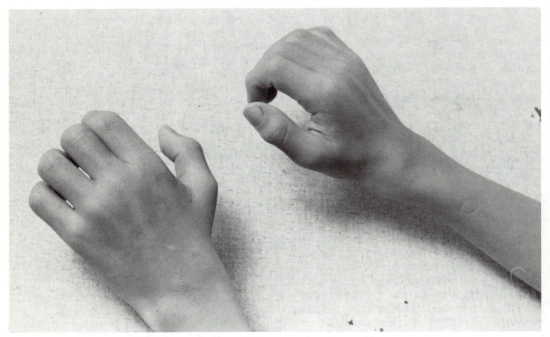

Figure 14–1. Classic hand involvement of polyarticular JRA. The hands in this photograph are in full active extension; full flexion is also limited. Note partial loss of wrist extension, flexion contractures of all digit joints, swelling over dorsal-radial aspect of wrist, ulnar deviation at wrist, and normal MCP alignment. Wrist flexor tenosynovitis prevents distal excursion of the flexor tendons, contributing to digit contractures. Severe swelling from digital tenosynovitis blocks PIP-MCP flexion, further contributing to loss of digit flexion. All DIP joints are severely involved. Note severe synovitis of thumb IP and MCP joints, typical of JRA.

erosions" does not have much meaning in relation to a young child and is more significant in relation to an older child. Persistent disease in a younger child may result in generalized growth retardation affecting the entire skeleton.

Periostitis (inflammation of the periosteum membrane covering the bones) of the phalanges in the hand and foot is common in association with severe digital flexor tenosynovitis characteristic of polyarthritis in association with either systemic or polyarticular-onset JRA. It produces thickening of the cortical bone, which fills in the natural concavity of the shafts of the phalanges, creating a "rectangular" appearance to the phalanges.[25]

Diffuse demineralization **(osteoporosis)** is a common finding in areas of persistent arthritis. Structural changes, as a result of progressive disease, such as joint subluxation, dislocation, and bony fusion are clearly evident on radiographs.[25] When a joint stops moving—that is, becomes ankylosed—a radiograph is the only means to distinguish between fibrous and bony ankylosis.

Hand and Wrist Involvement

When we refer to the typical adult RA hand, we describe the most common severe sequelae possible; for example, "radial drift of the wrist with metacarpophalangeal (MCP) ulnar drift and volar subluxation." But many people with RA never develop this particular pattern. It is the same with JRA. The classic "JRA hand" refers to the most common severe sequelae seen in children with *young-onset, polyarticular disease* who have persistent full-hand involvement. But, like adults, children can have a wide range and degree of involvement (Figs. 14–1 to 14–3).

In the child the pattern of involvement is related to age and maturation of the epiphyses at onset. Patterns also correlate to subtypes that affect specific age groups. Children who develop polyarticular RF-positive JRA *after the age of 12* can develop hand patterns identical to those of adult RA. In fact, some refer to this subset as "adult RA with childhood onset." Table 14–2 summarizes Chaplin and co-workers' radiographic review of 414 children with

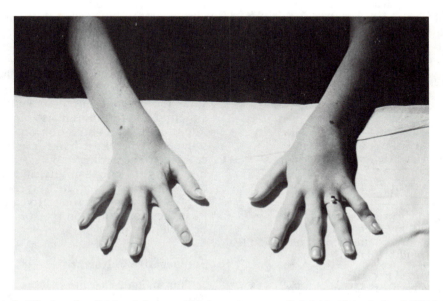

Figure 14–2. The hands of this adolescent girl demonstrate radial drift of the index MCP joints secondary to fixed ulnar deviation of the wrist. The normal alignment of the index finger is 20 degrees of ulnar deviation, so neutral alignment seen in her left hand represents 20 degrees of radial drift deformity. Her right index MCP is in 5 degrees of radial deviation, representing 25 degrees of deformity. Note classic wrist flexion deformity and severe PIP involvement.

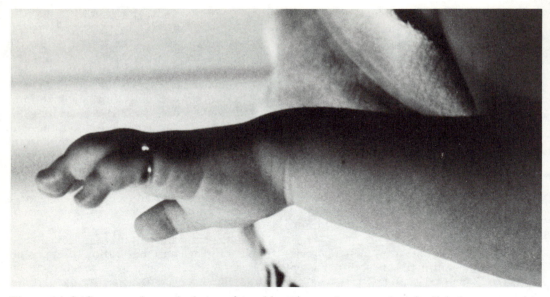

Figure 14–3. Severe volar and ulnar wrist subluxation and severe chronic digital tenosynovitis. When PIP contractures occur first, they encourage MCP extension and consequently a loss of MCP flexion. Swelling from digital tenosynovitis blocks flexion, further contributing to the loss of MCP flexion.

polyarticular-onset or systemic-onset (poly-articular-subset) JRA documenting age-of-onset related patterns.[26] Table 14–3 compares the classic hand patterns of adult and juvenile RA. Table 14–4 outlines the key sequelae of joint and tendon involvement in JRA.

Table 14–2 Polyarticular JRA: Age of Onset and Hand Deformity Patterns

Age of Onset	Hand Deformity Patterns
0–4	Ulnar wrist deviation
	DIP involvement
	Flexion contractures of the DIP, PIP, and MCP joints
5–12	Varied pattern
	Ulnar wrist deviation is greater than radial wrist deviation
	Radial MCP drift
13–15	Same patterns as those in adults

(Data from Chaplin and co-workers.[26])

Total hand involvement is common to children with polyarticular involvement, either polyarticular or systemic-onset. However, one subgroup, children with seropositive polyarticular-onset, can have more aggressive arthritis and deformities similar to adult RA as described above. Children with seronegative polyarthritis tend to have similar hand involvement despite the type of onset—polyarticular or systemic. These children also have a higher rate of remission and fewer long-term consequences; therefore, hand involvement is categorized according to polyarticular sero-negativity or seropositivity and pauciarticular involvement (which is always RF negative). Because seronegative polyarthritis is the most common type of JRA it will be reviewed first.

Seronegative Polyarthritis

This includes children with polyarticular-onset who have a negative RF (seronegative course) and those with systemic-onset and a polyarticular course.

Wrist. The wrist is the most common—and often the first—site of involve-

Table 14–3 Comparison of Common JRA and Adult RA Hand Patterns

Young-onset Polyarticular JRA	Adult RA (RF+)
WRIST	
Loss of extension (flexion contracture)	Loss of motion all planes with motion in midrange
Neutral to ulnar fixed deviation	Radial drift (ulnar drift can occur)
Carpal tunnel syndrome very rare	Carpal tunnel syndrome common
Severe intercarpal synovitis leading to spontaneous ankylosis	Minimal to moderate intercarpal synovitis leading to laxity and ulnar translocation
Severity and incidence of synovitis and flexor and extensor tenosynovitis are about the same for both.	
MCP JOINTS	
Radial drift (if wrist is in ulnar drift)	Ulnar drift
Flexion contractures	Volar subluxation
Periostitis (metacarpals)	Periostitis not significant
Children tend to have greater loss of MCP motion, more severe flexor tenosynovitis, and less intrinsic tightness compared with adults.	
PIP JOINTS	
Flexion contractures	Boutonnière or swan-neck deformities (flexion contractures possible)
Periostitis	Periostitis not common
Children tend to have greater loss of PIP motion.	
DIP JOINTS	
Severe synovitis	Minimal synovitis
Flexion contractures secondary to synovitis	DIP contractures secondary to restricted FDP excursion
THUMBS	
Severe IP synovitis	Minimal to moderate IP synovitis
Severity and incidence of synovitis in the thumb MCP joint appear about the same for both groups.	

ment.[26] It is associated with a fairly rapid loss of wrist extension and can progress to a flexion contracture and volar subluxation. **Limited wrist extension** may be the first sign of wrist involvement. It is not clear why there is such a rapid loss of extension, but the following factors may contribute to the process:

1. Wrist flexor tenosynovitis is a common, often painless, condition that is difficult to palpate or to detect visually. It can go undetected, producing flexion deformities of the wrist and fingers by restricting tendon excursion, resulting in the use of tenodesis action at the wrist to open the fingers.

2. Early, possibly painless, intercarpal synovitis could go undetected and cause an early loss of extension and radial deviation.[27]

3. In the presence of joint swelling and increased intra-articular pressure, the body assumes the posture that minimizes joint pressure and pain. In the wrist this is zero degrees of flexion and 10 degrees of ulnar deviation. Consequently, children use their hands in this position of comfort.

4. Pain in the wrist is theorized to elicit reflex inhibition of the wrist extensor and radial deviator muscles and stimulation or spasm of the wrist flexion and ulnar deviation muscles[28] (similar to that seen in the knee[27]).

Flexor tenosynovitis of the wrist is very common. It is typically painless without heat but can present with both pain and

Table 14–4 Joint and Tendon Involvement in JRA: Key Sequelae

WRIST FLEXOR TENOSYNOVITIS

Painless:	ROM lag in digits
	Decreased wrist mobility
	Loss of FDP and FDS distal excursion results in MCP or PIP flexion contractures
	Loss of FDP and FDS proximal excursion results in MCP, PIP, or DIP extension contractures
Painful:	All of the above plus pain severely limits use of the hand

DIGITAL FLEXOR TENOSYNOVITIS

Painless:	ROM lag
	Encourages MCP or PIP flexion contractures
	Swelling results in loss of MCP flexion
	Triggering
	Tenosynovium binds profundus and sublimis together
Painful:	All of the above plus pain severely limits use of the hand (rare)

WRIST EXTENSOR TENOSYNOVITIS

Painless:	No functional problems
	Possible long-term damage to tendon
Painful:	Limits use of the hand (not common)

WRIST CARPAL SYNOVITIS

Usually painful:	Swelling or pain promotes use in a flexed position resulting in loss of extension
	Flexion deformity results in decreased function
	Inhibits extensor muscle strength
	Volar subluxation

MCP SYNOVITIS

Usually painful:	Vulnerable to deviation deformity
	Pain severely limits function
	Loss of motion

PIP SYNOVITIS

Usually painful:	Flexion contracture
	Loss of extension—decreased function promotes loss of MCP flexion
	Damages lateral and central slips of EDC tendon resulting in extensor lag

DIP SYNOVITIS

Usually painful:	Loss of flexion
	Stiffness, contracture in slight flexion

warmth. It is difficult to detect because the carpal tunnel is deep, and swelling may not be visible or palpable. In fact, the only signs of this problem may be a "lag" in digital flexion or extension as a result of swelling blocking proximal or distal excursion of the flexor tendons.[28] For example, if **excursion in a distal direction is limited,** there will be a lag in PIP or MCP extension with the wrist in neutral, i.e., the MCP or PIP joints, or both, may appear flexed and unable to straighten. However, when the wrist is flexed, the digital joints have full extension. This tenodesis action is indicative of binding or constriction of the flexor tendons in the carpal tunnel secondary to flexor tenosynovitis. **Limitation of proximal excursion** as a result of carpal tenosynovitis is reflected in a lag in digital flexion; that is, passive flexion will be greater than active flexion. Flexion contractures of the digits or wrist may make it impossible to test for tendon excursion. The importance of testing for tendon excursion is to determine whether it impairs active motion, for it is this consequence that can lead to joint contractures.

When ROM lag in either direction occurs in all four digits, it is indicative of **carpal flexor tenosynovitis,** even in the absence of pain, swelling, or warmth. If ROM lag occurs in one or two digits, it may be due to **digital tenosynovitis.** If ROM lag is not corrected with measures to decrease swelling and to free the tendon (i.e., ice or corticosteroid injection*), this problem alone will result in digital contractures. (Heat is contraindicated because it increases swelling.) I have seen it happen in 3 weeks in an adult, and it can happen faster in children. The issues and processes around tenosynovitis are the same for both adults and children. (See section on tenosynovitis in Chapter 19 on hand assessment.)

Dorsal tenosynovitis is easily visible because it is covered by the thin dorsal skin and retinaculum. In children it may appear as a U-shaped swelling that conforms to the tendon sheaths underlying the third and fifth dorsal wrist compartments. This is also typically painless. If pain is present, it is often due to the underlying carpal synovitis. Because the retinaculum has extensibility and the tendons do not travel through a rigid tunnel, swelling does not cause binding of the tendon or ROM lag. **Rupture of the extensor tendons** is rare in children but may occur with long duration of wrist inflammation. The tendons rupture as a result of attrition over rough carpal bones. The pathomechanics are the same as for adults (see Chapter 19).

Carpal tunnel syndrome (CTS) is very rare in JRA.[29] In one review of 100 children with JRA, signs and symptoms of CTS were completely absent.[29] This is an interesting phenomenon, considering that relatively minor swelling in the carpal tunnel can cause binding of the tendons.

In adults, **wrist synovitis** primarily affects the radiocarpal, radioulnar, and trapeziometacarpal joints occasionally resulting in fibrous ankylosis but rarely bony ankylosis. In children, all of the carpal articulations can have severe synovitis, and spontaneous bony ankylosis of the radiocarpal, intercar-

pal, and carpal-metacarpal joints is common.[31] In some children **intercarpal ankylosis** can result in compensatory carpal-metacarpal hypermobility. Radiocarpal synovitis can also result in **overgrowth of the radial head,** which increases the distal volar-ulnar slope and contributes to the appearance of swelling on the radiodorsal side of the wrist (see Fig. 14–1). (In adults, swelling is greater on the ulnar side.)

When inflammation occurs before the age of 16 or when closure of the epiphyseal plates is premature, growth of the long bones can be altered. In the JRA hand this typically results in **shortening of the ulna** in relation to the radius.[26] In some cases, discrepancy in the length of these bones appears to encourage ulnar deviation and subluxation of the carpus, which can dislocate ulnarly with the hand resting at a sharp (70° to 90°) angle on the forearm, creating what is known as the **"ulna bayonet deformity."**[26] (When the bones mature, this condition can be corrected by a bone graft and wrist fusion.) There is a specific radiographic image that heralds the beginning of this deformity, called **glissement carpien,** in which the carpus as a whole rotates between the radius of metacarpals.[26] However, the influence of a shortened ulna is not clear-cut. Some children with significant shortening of the ulna have radial deviation, but others have no deviation. So it appears that shortening of the ulna is *associated* with an increased incidence of ulnar deviation of the hand but that there is no evidence of a cause-and-effect relationship.[26] Another factor to consider is that early fibrosis of the carpal ligaments can reduce the impact of biochemical forces toward ulnar deviation and, conversely, children with ligamentous laxity could be more prone to the deviating forces.[26] In addition, pain, swelling, intra-articular pressure, and associated extensor/radial deviator muscle inhibition and flexor/ulnar deviator muscle spasm can create an overpowering flexor imbalance in the presence of a normal-length ulna. The angle of wrist deviation has a direct influence on deviation deformity in the MCP joints. Ulnar deviation of the wrist can result in radial drift of the MCP joints, and radial deviation of the wrist as seen in some older children and adults can result in ulnar drift of the MCP joints.

---

*Corticosteroid injections are used more frequently for adults than for children.

Metacarpophalangeal Joints. In adults the MCP joints have the greatest frequency of severe synovitis. In children the PIP joints have the greatest frequency of severe synovitis, followed by the MCP and distal interphalangeal (DIP) joints.[29] Some children appear to have milder or less evident MCP disease in comparison with adults with RA even though many have severe MCP synovitis. The presence of MCP flexion contractures does not necessarily mean they have severe MCP synovitis. Children can also develop severe MCP contractures secondary to flexor tenosynovitis.

As noted in Table 14–2, children with young-age onset (under age 10) JRA tend to develop **MCP flexion contractures.** Once this occurs, ulnar or radial drift is not likely, because of fibrosis of the collateral ligaments and capsule. In an adult, an MCP flexion contracture would most likely be due to MCP synovitis and intrinsic muscle tightness. In a child, wrist tenosynovitis, preventing distal tendon excursion, or severe swelling associated with digital flexor tenosynovitis may contribute along with MCP joint synovitis to maintain the joint in a flexed posture and resulting contracture.

In young children, prolonged positioning of the joints in flexed position as well as hyperemia associated with inflammation distorts the growing cartilage, resulting in **enlargement of the bone ends.**[26] Significant **loss of MCP flexion** is a common finding in JRA. It can be due to (1) severe flexor tenosynovitis, blocking flexion; (2) PIP flexion contractures, encouraging an MCP hyperextension deformity and extension contracture (this may appear as a loss of flexion rather than as an extension deformity); (3) wrist flexion encouraging MCP extension; and (4) joint synovitis and swelling (see Figs. 14–1, 14–3, and 14–4).

If a child *does not* develop an MCP flexion contracture, the MCP joints may be influenced by the position of the wrist. Ulnar deviation of the wrist can result in radial drift of the MCP joints.[26] (Keep in mind that normal alignment of the index MCP is 20 degrees of ulnar deviation.[32] So neutral alignment represents 20 degrees of pathological radial drift, and 5 degrees of radial drift represents 25 degrees of malalignment.) This is most common when the onset of JRA occurs between the ages of 5 and 12 years (see Fig. 14–2).

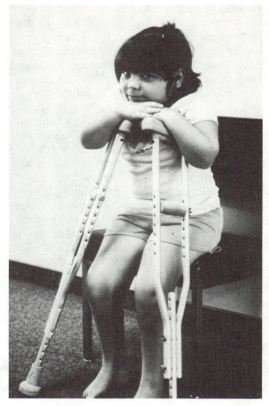

Figure 14–4. This child demonstrates the position of comfort that contributes to flexion deformities. Note neck, elbow, and wrist flexion posture (and MCP extension) as well as ankle plantar flexion because the seat is too high.

Proper positioning during leisure, sleep, school, and play activities is critical to preventing dysfunctional contractures. Children need chairs proportional to their size to allow good back support, arms to facilitate push-off, and a height that allows them to keep their feet flat on the floor. Chairs that meet these criteria should be provided at home and in the clinic.

Periostitis of the metacarpals is frequently seen and appears associated with intense inflammatory activity. One report links it with rapid progression of the disease at the joint nearest to the site of periostitis. The periostitis tends to resolve, leaving the bone slightly thickened.[26]

Proximal Interphalangeal Joints. Synovitis of the PIP joint is generally associated with **digital flexor tenosynovitis,** producing a characteristic wide swelling over the proximal phalanx and tapering over the mid-phalanx.[29] Swelling in the tendon sheath can prevent joint flexion or limit tendon excursion, resulting in a loss of joint mobility. The bone ends are also subject to distortion and enlargement, and periostitis over the proximal phalanx is common.[26]

Flexion contractures or loss of extension of both the PIP and DIP joints are the most common deformity, especially in young-onset JRA. **Boutonnière deformities** are the second most common.[26,29] Occasionally a digit with a PIP flexion contracture will progress to boutonnière deformity over time. Swan-neck deformities are rare because of the high incidence of PIP flexion contractures and MCP extension contractures with loss of MCP flexion.[29,33] (See Chapter 19 for a discussion of swan-neck pathodynamics.)

Tenosynovium in the sheath can result in binding or **adherence of the sublimis tendon** to the profundus tendon, impairing tendon gliding and reducing active flexion. By itself this can result in a joint contracture. Testing to isolate the sublimis tendon should be a part of all hand evaluations (see Chapter 19). Sometimes exercises that isolate the sublimis tendon can break up the adhesions. (This is the same method as used to isolate the tendon to determine muscle strength: Passive restriction of *all* finger joints in zero extension except the finger being tested; then active PIP flexion only of the test finger. Full PIP flexion indicates the sublimis is not adhered to the profundus.)

Distal Interphalangeal Joints. Aggressive DIP joint disease is characteristic, with the joints becoming stiff quickly in a slightly flexed position. In the absence of DIP synovitis, the DIP joints can become stiff because of wrist flexor tenosynovitis restricting proximal profundus excursion. The lack of full active flexion each day simply results in stiffness, then fibrosis. It is critical that patients with tendon involvement and ROM lag be taught PROM to prevent secondary contractures.

Seropositive Polyarthritis (Polyarticular-Onset Juvenile Rheumatoid Arthritis, Seropositive Course)

This subtype resembles adult RA, but joint destruction tends to progress more rapidly. Children who develop this subtype after age 12 tend to have a pattern of hand involvement similar to that seen in adult RA; that is, greater MCP synovitis, MCP volar and ulnar subluxation, and intrinsic tightness.[29] However, if these children develop ulnar deviation of the wrist, they will *not* develop ulnar drift of the MCP joints characteristic of adult RA (see Tables 14–2 and 14–3).

Children between 9 and 16 years of age are affected by this subtype. The younger the age of onset, the more vulnerable the hand is to localized growth alterations. Shortening of the ulna is common with sequelae, as described above.

Dr. Ansell[29] describes two frequently seen patterns: "The characteristic involvement is the radioulnar joint, with index and middle MCP joints followed fairly rapidly by PIP joint involvement; subsequently MCP joints of the ring and little finger and ulnar deviation at this level tend to occur very rapidly."

Carpal fusion is common, and extensor and flexor tendon ruptures as well as symptoms of CTS are seen more in this group than in the others.[29]

Pauciarticular Arthritis (Pauciarticular-Onset Juvenile Rheumatoid Arthritis)

Subtypes I and II. Unilateral wrist or hand involvement is not associated with these subtypes, but occasionally a patient may have wrist or single-digit joint synovitis.

Subtype III. The wrist is reported as the third most frequently involved. A single PIP joint with associated flexor tenosynovitis is also common. Dr. Ansell[29] reports "about 40 percent of these children progress to involvement of 5 or more joints; and half of this group develop over the years a severe, widespread, but often asymmetric, polyarthritis. Some of the more bizarre deformities of the hands with a mixture or overgrowth and undergrowth of the digits and asymmetrical bony enlargement are seen in this group."

Therapy

Wrist

When you first treat a child with wrist involvement, there is a hierarchy of biomechanical concerns that need to be addressed.

1. Prevention of flexion contractures in a nonfunctional position

The first and most important goal in hand management is the prevention of dysfunctional wrist flexion contractures. Children can develop aggressive wrist disease with rapid loss of ROM. It may not be possible to prevent the loss of motion, but it is possible to prevent fixed flexion deformities. A position of function that considers both current and future potential for ankylosis must always be promoted. In cases of severe rapid destruction, the carpal bones will fuse in the position supported by the orthosis. If it is apparent that wrist ankylosis is inevitable, the goal is to have the wrist become ankylosed in neutral (0 degrees extension) and 10 degrees ulnar deviation. Neutral is considered the optimal position for self-care and overall function for an ankylosed or fused wrist. When ankylosis is not the immediate issue, it is recommended that the wrist be held in 10 to 20 degrees of extension. (The concept of 30 degrees extension as the position of function is useful in the paralyzed hand, but it is not appropriate for the wrist with arthritis. See Chapter 23 for rationale for positioning.)

In the acute stage of inflammation, Children's Hospital of Los Angeles recommends a rigid circumferential (gauntlet) wrist immobilization orthosis. This type of orthosis is preferred over a volar or cockup design because it gives radial and ulnar support and restricts extension, providing almost complete immobilization of the radiocarpal joint. High-temperature polyethylene is used (see Appendix 3) because it is thin and durable and thus allows a minimal amount of plastic in the palm. Polyethylene is excellent if you have the time and equipment to work with the material; otherwise, excellent circumferential splints can be made from Aquaplast (coated) orthotic material, intermediate ($\frac{3}{32}$ inch) for older children and thin ($\frac{1}{16}$ inch) for younger children (see Chapter 23 for further details). They should wear the orthosis day and night except for hygiene and during ROM exercises or application of thermal (usually ice) modalities. The goals for this type of orthotic treatment are to reduce pain, flexor muscle spasm, and inflammation; to promote use of the hand while the wrist is at rest; and to prevent use in a flexed position. If the wrist extensors are weak, grade 3.5/5 (fair +) or less, an orthosis is necessary because the muscles will not be able to support the wrist in an extended position against gravity, especially if there is spasm of the flexor muscles and pain. (See Chapter 21 for methods of grading muscle strength.) After the acute stage, wearing schedules for rigid gauntlet orthoses are decreased during the day and alternated with flexible wrist gauntlet orthoses.

As with any orthosis, it is important to consider the effects on adjacent joints. The body works as a synchronous unit; **immobilization of any joint will place compensatory stress on adjacent joints.** In the case of the wrist, the larger, elbow joint seems to be able to absorb the stress without a deleterious effect. The smaller, more fragile MCP joints are not quite as fortunate and can be damaged by compensatory stress and the fact that the plastic in the palm makes part of the hand anesthetic. Therefore, the only part of the palm with sensation during grasp is the part over the MCP joints, further altering the amount of force applied on the joints to hold on to something.

In adults, the effect of wrist immobilization on the MCP joints is often increased inflammation and pain, symptoms that enable the patients to evaluate the impact of the orthosis. These are also symptoms that they are generally willing to report. In adults, it is also common to have solely MCP joint involvement without flexor tenosynovitis. In the child with wrist and MCP joint involvement, the impact is not as clear-cut. It is complicated because the child may not perceive a change in symptoms. Marcy Atwood has *not* found it to be a particular problem in her patient population at Children's Hospital; I (J.M.) used bilateral polyethylene gauntlet orthoses on an 8-year-old boy with a 1-year history of wrist synovitis with no apparent MCP involvement. After 2 days of use, all his MCP joints were inflamed. That was in 1975 and I have not used rigid daytime orthoses on children with MCP involvement since. I use flexible gauntlet orthoses during the day and rigid orthoses at night unless lateral stability, severe flexor spasm, or imminent ankylosis is an issue. Although I can cite a single dramatic example, Marcy's experience is more representative of JRA treatment.

There are many **factors that could account for children's responding differently from adults to orthotic wrist immobilization. First,** the child may not be able to do a lot of grasp activities with swollen painful digits, especially strong grasp. **Second,** the demands on hand function for a young child are very different from those for a homemaker with RA. **Third,** the swelling from the tenosynovitis alters the biomechanics of the MCP joint in relation to the orthosis. The impact that wrist immobilization has on the flexor tendons is not known and is not evident clinically; it may not have a negative effect. **Fourth,** children have a perception of pain different from that of adults. We determine the effects of orthoses on adults in large part by their subjective assessment and reporting of symptoms. This is often not appropriate in children, and it is often difficult to assess the signs of inflammation such as swelling, especially in a chubby hand. **Fifth,** if the child has limitations in MCP joint motion at the onset of orthotic use, the collateral ligaments and volar plate will be tight (fibrosed) and the cartilage will be distorted in comparison with an adult joint, which will significantly alter the biomechanics of the joint. And last, the physiology of growing tissue in children is very different from that of the adult in ways we are only beginning to understand; consider the fact that CTS common in adults is essentially nonexistent clinically in children.

In summary, rigid gauntlet orthoses are a valid and recommended approach to management of wrist synovitis as long as there is close follow-up to determine whether the orthosis is exacerbating MCP joint involvement. If it is, then a more flexible gauntlet orthosis should be used. (See Chapter 23 for further discussion.)

ROM exercises for the wrist should include both active and active-assisted exercises in all planes, including circumduction in both directions. ROM exercise needs to be appropriate for the degree of inflammation present and nonstressful to the joint during active inflammation. Emphasis is placed on maintaining range in extension and radial deviation.

2. Reduction of inflammation, using thermal modalities and orthoses, joint protection, and relaxation techniques

Inflammation (with or without swelling) is the source of pain, muscle spasm, and limited motion. For acute joint inflammation or tenosynovitis, cold modalities (ice packs, ice massage, contrast baths, or wraps) are the treatment of choice because cold reduces swelling. (See Chapter 1 for referenced guidelines.) For spasm of the flexor muscles, ice pack applications to the belly of the muscle has been the most helpful modality. The packs are used for 20 to 30 minutes and can be applied while an ice pack is applied around the joint. On rare occasions, ice can create a rebound spasm phenomenon. If this occurs, contrast wraps may be more successful. After the ice is removed, the forearm is supported and the wrist is moved through full ROM during the period of muscle spasm inhibition achieved by the use of the ice. Inhibiting the flexor muscle spasm also allows a better isometric/isotonic contraction of the extensor muscles.

Joint protection techniques are also employed for children, following the same general principles as those for adults. However, the operationalization of these principles must be viewed in the context of different joint pathology and developmental concerns. In general, the major concerns of joint protection for children with JRA are

1. Avoidance of compressive forces on the joints
2. Avoidance of holding the fingers and wrists in a flexed position for prolonged periods
3. Avoidance of resistive activities while the wrist is in a flexed or ulnar deviating position

For children, emphasis is placed upon not only performance of planned or volitional tasks (e.g., getting up from a chair or unscrewing containers) but also on protection of joints during "unplanned" play occurrences, such as falling, sliding, or being pushed. Therefore, the use of orthoses is conservatively advocated to protect the child from outside trauma during play. Specific teaching is recommended to instruct the child in proper techniques for carrying items, rising from chairs, and using tools.

Some techniques can be introduced as

early as age 3. The most effective methods for teaching joint protection to children are individual sessions, demonstration, role playing, and comparisons of the correct and incorrect procedures. Videotapes have been very successful as well. When a question arises as to the appropriateness of sports that place significant stress on the joints (e.g., volleyball, tetherball, tennis, or baseball), consideration must be given to the importance of that activity to the child, as well as to the stage of his or her disease. At an acute or subacute stage, the above-mentioned sports are not recommended. Children will usually concur that the activity causes pain. When the disease is chronic, participation must be judged on an individual basis and the joint should be protected. Ideally, therapists should suggest appropriate new activities to replace the potentially damaging ones if the child is willing. The need to pace activities is not as important in children, inasmuch as most, especially younger ones, will nap in the afternoon.

Relaxation techniques are effective and most easily taught to school-age children and adolescents. Guided imagery and visual imagery have been helpful with adolescents. The relaxation technique of concentrating on one word or syllable (e.g., the word *one*) is also helpful as a method of relaxation. Although it is a simple technique, the adolescent must have adequate levels of concentration and desire. Follow-through is increased if the techniques can be taught in such a way that the child can perceive the results. Progressive relaxation (Jacobson technique), involving alternate tensing followed by relaxing of each body part, is *not recommended*, especially with muscles around painful joints. Deep breathing can be successfully taught to very young children. The "ragdoll" or "letting your [part] go to sleep" game is a quick method for helping a child relax for a specific procedure.

3. Assessment (analysis) of the relationship of proximal joint (neck, shoulder, elbow) involvement to functional use and positioning of the wrist

Limitations or altered alignment of the neck, shoulder, or elbow can have a dramatic impact on the functional use of the wrist (and consequently the hand) and positioning of the hand during activities. To understand this phenomenon, sit straight in a chair, elbows at side, hands pronated in front of you. Now throw your dominant shoulder forward, and notice the movement and position of your dominant hand. With your shoulder forward, pretend to do a handwriting task. Note the alignment of your elbow and wrist and the increased ulnar deviation. Most children do not have their shoulder so far forward, but limited motion or muscular splinting around the shoulder alters the biomechanics of the upper extremity and can influence deforming forces at the wrist. Exercises for the proximal joints should be selected with consideration of the impact their alignment has on distal biomechanics.

4. Assessment of the effects of wrist alignment, bone growth changes, and functional use of the digits and thumb

The relationship of the wrist to the digits is truly a unique one, in part because the tendons that cross the wrist also cross all the digit joints, so alteration of the alignment and functioning of the wrist has a direct impact on the biomechanics of the digits. In addition to a specific musculoskeletal assessment, observation of the child's hands during functional tasks can provide valuable information. Marcy Atwood suggests the following questions to guide observations[34]:

1. What is the habitual position of the hands?
2. How are the hands held in the lap?
3. What is the position of the wrist when performing power grip? (20 degrees of extension, neutral, or flexion?)
4. Is there guarding of the wrist, fingers, during play? during rising from a seat? (For example, does the child push off of the seat with flexed MCP joint instead of bearing weight on the heel of the hand with wrist in extension?)
5. What type of grasp or prehension is habitually used? (Is lateral pinch substituted for pincer grasp?)
6. Are there any muscle substitution patterns?

Functional limitations arise from the purely biomechanical changes caused by positioning. When hands are positioned and used in a flexed position, finger flexors are at a biomechanical disadvantage to reduce force generated during grasp. Therefore, grip strength may be weakened not only because of actual muscle weakness or pain but also because of the wrist positioning. Often grip strength can be improved by strengthening wrist extensors and finger abductors and improving alignment while also adhering to measures to decrease inflammation.

Prolonged positioning in the flexed position can result in distorted growth of the bone ends. Thus the flexed position or position of comfort may be counterproductive to normal development; for example, a child may crawl on the elbows to prevent putting pressure on wrist joints or may use the wrists in flexion (at 7 months the wrists should be used in extension). These abnormal positions can become integral in the child's movements. Protection and positioning should facilitate normal movement patterns. If the habit has been established, the therapist should facilitate appropriate kinesthetic/proprioceptive feedback in the antideformity positions.

5. Strengthening of extensor muscles

Strengthening the wrist extensors and radial deviators is essential for maintaining wrist mobility and preventing flexion contractures. The extensor muscles weaken very quickly with active disease, because of several factors: (1) joint pain (and increased intra-articular pressure) reflexively facilitates the flexor muscles and subsequently inhibits the extensors; (2) the child guards and uses the joint in flexion, resulting in disuse weakness in the extensors; and (3) if the extensor muscles remain at an extended length, a strong extensor contraction is difficult to facilitate.[35]

In the acute stage, wrist extensor strength should be maintained without stressing the joint. Isometrics should be performed in conjunction with an active range of motion (AROM) warm-up (see Chapter 27 for discussion). Functional electrical stimulation has been used extensively in quadriceps extensor strengthening with good success. Its use for *wrist extensor* strengthening has met with limited clinical success. This modality needs more research to prove its efficacy in hand therapy with JRA. Care must always be taken to instruct the child to isolate the wrist extensors during exercises, because children tend to extend the wrist using the long finger extensors.

In the nonacute stage, resistive isotonic exercises can be performed provided that the weight is positioned proximally to decrease torque on the wrist joint. Exercises should be performed several times a day to prevent weakening. Strengthening of the wrist flexors is generally not necessary. Before initiating exercise or activity, muscle facilitation techniques such as brushing or tapping are recommended. For example, having the child "paint" or "rain" on his or her arm over the extensor muscle belly promotes this contraction. Note that the effect lasts only for as long as the stimulation takes place (in some cases, for 20 to 30 seconds longer), so exercise or activity must immediately follow if it is to be effective.

Activities following the exercises are important for increasing strength while using the outcome as a motivator. Activities also promote good patterns of use under supervision. See Table 14–5 for wrist and finger activities for the child with JRA, and refer to the discussion of play in Chapter 15.

6. Correction of wrist flexion contractures

Preexisting flexion contractures or those resistant to more conservative orthotic techniques may require repeated applications of cylinder casts. These casts are applied for 48- to 72-hour periods, during which the child is encouraged to strengthen the extensor musculature through activity and isometric exercises. When the cast is removed, ice packs may be used to decrease any flexor muscle spasming and/or joint swelling. Extensor exercises are performed and a new cast is put on at the straighter angle achieved by the combination of treatments.[35] Gentle traction with gentle passive range-of-motion (PROM) exercises is applied, being careful that equal pressure is applied to all carpals and that extreme pressure is not exerted on the flexor muscles while the cast is being applied. (See Appendix 5 for procedures for serial casting.)

When the maximal gains have been achieved by the serial casts, orthoses are used to maintain the position of the joint. They are used in combination with appropriate exercises to strengthen the muscles around the joint and to restore balance between the flexor and extensor muscles. Joints may require orthoses for months after the casting has been terminated. If the orthosis is not combined with appropriate exercise, severe muscle atrophy can result.[35,36]

After reduction of long-term contractures, a wrist orthosis must be worn for 6 months to 1 year, until collagen has

Table 14–5 Wrist and Finger Activities for the Child with JRA*

Finger Activities	Wrist Activities
TODDLER	
Play patty-cake	Jack-in-the-box (check direction of wrist rotation)
Experiment with shaving cream on window	Build with building blocks
Stack blocks, assorted size objects, into piles	Hide 'n'-seek—pull off blankets to find objects
Pat pictures—point to pictures	Musical instrument (guard against flexion)
Use finger paints	Cymbals with aluminum plates, drums upside down, and tambourines
Help dust or polish furniture (with extended fingers)	Lace cards or cloth book
Water play	Activities positioned at shoulder height to encourage wrist extension
Stick pregummed dots, squares, and triangles on paper	
Pick up large puzzle pieces or rings, put in box or puzzles	
PRESCHOOL	
Geometric design games	Finger paint
Parquetry blocks	Shadow images in front of projector
Paste with extended fingers	Knead bread dough with heel of palm
Sandbox play—run extended fingers through sand, pat to make towers	Hand puppet play
Flip paper balls with finger (thumb) to target	Water play—splash soap suds in water
Glue pictures on paper or wall	Experiment with shaving cream on window
	Build building with blocks
	Play dough
	Dust furniture
	Play Hungry Hippo
SCHOOL AGE	
Play cat's cradle	Erase chalkboard
Fold paper—make airplanes and origami figures	Roll clay—knead coils with heel of hand
Hold paper flat while drawing	Wire maze with handle
Use sock finger puppets	Play with jacks
Roll clay into coils	Wash dishes
Sanding	Build sand castles
Decoupage	Built-up checkers (check for correct wrist extension)
Toy typewriter	Ball push—use light beach ball
Electronic games that can be operated with heel of hand	
SCHOOL AGE/ADOLESCENT	
Table games	Beat weaving—various looms
Cards	Knead dough with extended wrist
Apply make-up with extended fingers	Sanding (use block to extend fingers)
Marionettes	Decoupage
Typing	Cooking
Album collections—paste leaves or stamps in a book	Wipe tables
Macrame—with fully extended fingers	Smooth covers on bed
Collage (gluing)	Drafting—hold paper with extended wrist
Clay figurines	
Sewing—hold down pattern pieces	
Finger weaving loom	
Drafting—hold paper with extended fingers and wrist	

*Activities are grouped by the age you start the activity. Most can be extended to older ages.
(Compiled by Marcy Atwood, MA, OTR.)

elongated and remodeled to this new length. AROM must be done to maintain flexion.

Fingers and Thumb

Concerns and issues in treatment of the fingers and thumb parallel those in the wrist and will be discussed together.

1. Prevention of deforming positions

Flexion contractures of MCP, PIP, and DIP joints are most effectively treated by prevention and early aggressive use of orthoses.

Acute Phase. During the acute phase, severely inflamed or painful MCP joints are positioned in slight flexion (20–30°) to prevent the tendency toward flexion and to decrease pain and inflammation. (The classic functional position of 40° MCP flexion is not appropriate for children with full hand involvement.) This is accomplished with application of a full-hand orthosis or a modified gauntlet orthosis with a metacarpal volar support bar. Orthoses are worn when the hands are not in use. (In times of acute pain, children will even request or apply orthoses themselves.) For hand use with MCP joint involvement, a soft gauntlet with MCP joint support allows full finger use. As with the wrist, care must be taken to examine the effects of the orthosis on the adjacent PIP joints. Because a position of MCP joint extension encourages PIP joint flexion, if the PIP joints are involved, the application of the gauntlet with the volar MCP joint support may exacerbate the PIP joint synovitis and flexion posture. Alternating joint exercise, orthoses, and protection during activities helps decrease this effect. After the acute phase, full-hand resting orthoses are worn at night to prevent insidious loss of ROM and to prevent tightening of flexor tendons or the volar capsule. Because bilateral full-hand orthoses worn at night do not allow *any* functional hand use—such as pulling up covers or drinking water—the full-hand orthoses are usually worn every other night on alternate hands. A wrist gauntlet orthosis is worn on the other hand.

The development of PIP joint flexion contractures can often be prevented if the PIP joint is positioned in extension during the acute stage. A ring-finger splint, a dorsal or volar cylinder splint, or a half-cylinder splint can be made. However, orthoses must fit carefully to be effective. To this end, one must consider the following: (1) fluctuating synovitis may cause the splint to become too loose or too tight, so the fit must be closely monitored; and (2) on small children, the lever arms of the volar orthosis may be too short to maintain the joint in extension effectively. Therefore, an orthosis may have to be extended into the hand or combined with a full-gauntlet orthosis. This principle also holds true for immobilization of DIP joints during the acute phase of the disease. Finger orthotics are worn day and night except when they interfere with essential hand use.

Chronic Phase. Measures to decrease flexion contractures during the chronic phase are more difficult. Furthermore, a long-standing PIP joint synovitis may result in loss of the lateral bands or central slip, creating an extensor lag even if the contracture is reduced.

Serial ring and cylinder orthoses are initially used to decrease contractures, combined with gentle manual passive stretch and thermal modalities (warm water). Use of custom-made dynamic PIP joint extension orthoses has been found effective when consistently monitored to apply an appropriate amount of stretch. These must be followed by use of static finger orthoses to maintain gains. Commercial dynamic orthoses have had limited success, because of patient complaints of too much pressure on the proximal and middle phalanges. For adolescents capable of self-monitoring, however, these may be an option. Finally, serial casting of PIP joints has shown good results for long-standing contractures of the soft tissue; however, the functional restriction of wearing follow-up static orthoses of the PIP joint can hinder compliance and diminish long-term gains in ROM.

Marcy Atwood's experience has shown that flexion contractures approaching 0 to 30 or 35 degrees can be reduced and range can be maintained. Flexion contractures of 35 degrees or more are more difficult to reduce because the supporting structures have been elongated (overstretched). Intraarticular corticosteroid injections have been found beneficial for reducing the swelling and preventing distention and damage to the extensor structures secondary to chronic synovitis. In the chronic phase, finger splints are worn at night to prevent progressive loss of range.

2. Reduction of inflammation by using thermal modalities and orthotic joint-protection and relaxation techniques

The use of ice in the form of cold packs to reduce inflammation is *not* recommended because it may decrease peripheral circulation. However, "playing" or finding toys in ice chips, crushed ice, or frozen peas has been suggested.

See the recommendations made earlier for joint protection, relaxation techniques, and the use of orthoses to reduce inflammation. Again, caution must be used in monitoring the fit of finger orthoses (see earlier recommendations).

3. The relationship of proximal joint involvement to functional use

Local immobilization of MCP and PIP joints will have concurrent effects on both joints as well as on DIP joints. Immobilization of MCP joints in extension encourages a position of PIP flexion; immobilization of PIP joints in extension can exert more flexion force on MCP joints and encourage DIP flexion, while preventing full excursion of the flexor tendons. Chronic positioning and use of MCP joints in flexion, in conjunction with PIP joint immobilization, may also contribute to tightening of volar capsule and intrinsic muscle tightness of MCP joints.

4. Assessment of the effects of alignment and bone growth changes on functional use

Hyperemia to PIP joints resulting in bony overgrowth of PIP joints and severe cartilage destruction can decrease joint space in PIP, MCP, and DIP joints. Joint space narrowing may prevent full flexion as well as extension ROM. These sequelae can also occur in the thumb.

Involvement of finger and thumb joints that decreases ROM obviously affects the ability to expand grasp. Severe flexion contractures of MCP or PIP joints, or both, can greatly interfere with spherical grasps or expanse of prehension needed for grasping a cup or a carton, or for handling a large ball. Decreased flexion of PIP joints prohibits the small cylindrical grasp needed to brush one's teeth, to hold a brush, or to stir a wooden spoon. The effects of MCP joint

subluxation, as seen in RF-negative polyarticular JRA, are similar to those of adult-onset RA and can be reviewed in Chapter 19.

Boutonnière deformities may be seen in older children. Flexion of the PIP joint encourages the loss of MCP flexion by necessitating MCP joint extension or hyperextension to bring the fingertip out of the way, allowing an object to be grasped or the palm to be placed on a flat surface. The PIP joint contracture may be a nonreducible soft tissue contracture, or it may be unstable as a result of damage of the collateral and/or extensor support structures. Inability to flex the DIP joint reduces the ability for precision prehension. There have been reports of reducing these deformities by use of an extension cylinder or trough orthosis. Either way, it is important to catch deformities early; that is, before loss of extension is 20 degrees or more and static extension positioning of the PIP joint is so dysfunctional that it is tolerable only on one or at most two digits at a time. (See Chapter 19 for treatment of boutonnière deformities and references.)

5. Strengthening of the hand

As with the wrist, establishing a balance between the flexor and extensor musculatures is key to maintaining alignment and optimal functioning.

Guidelines for strengthening the hand include the following:

a. Strengthening activities can be started after an acute episode has subsided. Strengthening can be done in the presence of chronic or low-grade inflammation, as long as the activity does not cause pain and compress the joint.

b. Facilitation techniques and active ROM warm-up exercises should precede resistive exercises or activities. For example, active finger abduction or finger wall walking should be done before such strengthening activities as spreading fingers in clay, finger painting, or working against resistance in weaving (see Table 14–5).

c. Strengthening the muscles throughout their available range is more effective than strengthening in a single static position. This may be done with a single isotonic exercise or with several activities that apply resistance in various positions.

d. The joint must be supported and aligned during strengthening exercises.

e. Resistance will be graded according to strength while permitting full ROM.

For most children the finger extensor muscles (extensor digitorum communis, indicis proprius, and extensor digiti quinti), abductor muscles (interossei dorsales and abductor digiti minimi), and the PIP extensors (interossei and lumbrical muscles) tend to need the most strengthening. Activities that can strengthen these muscles include (1) active finger extension exercises and games, such as cat's cradle and adapted checkers; (2) activities that maintain fingers in extension while holding items flat; and (3) crafts, such as macrame and weaving, in which the weft is packed with the backs of the fingers (see Table 14–5). Theraplast exercises are beneficial for all hand activities; make sure that the resistive qualities are appropriate for the patient. These exercises will ensure that strengthening of specific muscles is accomplished.

Strengthening of the hand intrinsic muscles to improve function of MCP joint flexion and PIP joint extension can be accomplished in two ways: (1) by applying resistance distal to the PIP joint during active PIP extension while the MCP joint is maintained in full flexion; (2) by strengthening the interossei by resisting the MCP joint in abduction and adduction. These motions can be incorporated into play or game activities.

Thumb strengthening focuses on the extensor muscles, particularly the extensor pollicis brevis, abductor, and opposition muscles. (*Note:* It is important to keep in mind that the extensor pollicis brevis muscle is often a very weak or ineffective extensor in normal hands.) Specific exercises need to isolate the problem area. However, opposition strengthening can be incorporated into crafts, games, or computer operations. Monitoring of opposition is critical to make sure flexion or adduction is not occurring as a substitution.

6. Maintenance of active finger flexion

Despite the emphasis on extension, maintenance of full AROM for the flexor digitorum superficialis (FDS) and profundus (FDP) muscles is critical. These mus-

cles need to be isolated and individually exercised to prevent the formation of adhesions. The isolation technique is the same as that for individual muscle testing. Full excursion of the flexor tendons is determined by comparing active flexion with passive flexion. A lag in active flexion indicates that something is impairing proximal excursion of the flexor tendons. Impairment of the FDP muscle is usually first evident in diminished active DIP joint flexion. If the FDS muscle is blocked, the resting posture of the PIP joints tends to be in greater extension (if there are no PIP joint contractures), and active PIP joint flexion is diminished. However, in the early stages the FDP muscles may substitute for the FDS muscles.

For the thumb, the flexor pollicis longus muscle should have active exercise, especially if the interphalangeal (IP) joint is hyperextended. Even in chronic stages, resistive exercises to flexor groups are not usually recommended, because decreased grip strength may be caused by (1) wrist position in flexion; (2) tenosynovitis, which has weakened flexors; (3) pain; or (4) decreased abduction strength, which prevents firm stabilization of the ulnar side of the hand.

7. Correction of deformity

When there is a fixed limitation in a digit joint, the source of the limitation needs to be determined before treatment can be given. If the MCP joints are limited in flexion because of swelling and tenosynovitis, heat and joint mobilization will not help; in fact, heat will make the swelling worse. Treatment needs to be directed toward decreasing swelling and inflammation.

As long as the disease is active in a digit joint, it is almost impossible to reduce a contracture; however, a contracture can be prevented from getting worse. If the synovitis subsides and the joint is stiff, warm water, gentle mobilization, and gentle sustained passive stretch with a Coban wrap or a dynamic orthosis can be effective for increasing ROM. In the event that the MCP joints seem to be losing flexion disproportionate to the amount of swelling present, or if it appears that they are becoming stiff because of inadequate flexor tendon function, gentle PROM is indicated. Another alternative for increasing active MCP joint flexion is to splint the PIP joints in extension for a time—for example, for 30 to 90 minutes—during activities involving active hand use. This increases flexion force at the MCP level.

Surgery

If synovitis in the PIP or MCP joints is aggressive and nonresponsive to medical and occupational/physical therapy measures over a 12- to 18-month period, a synovectomy may be considered if the joint cartilage is well preserved.[37] The waiting period for performing a synovectomy in children is longer than that for adults because of the higher rate of remission in children.[37]

Synovectomy of the wrist is rarely indicated because there is a high rate of ankylosis resulting in a pain-free, stable wrist. Consequently, when there is severe wrist involvement, the approach is to provide an orthosis to maintain positioning so that ankylosis, if it occurs, is in a functional position.[4,5] Tenosynovectomies and tendon repairs are not commonly done in children but can be done successfully if indicated.

Once the child's epiphyses close, all the surgeries performed on an adult can also be done on the child, if necessary. In a child with severe destructive arthritis, early fusion or closure of the involved epiphyses is common, so frequently, surgery *does not* have to be delayed until maturation. Children with young-onset polyarticular disease and a more typical "JRA hand" (see Table 14–3) may benefit from surgeries such as wrist fusion, thumb IP and MCP joint fusion, finger PIP fusion, MCP capsulotomy, tenosynovectomy, and tendon repair or transfer.[31,38] Children with late-onset polyarticular disease who develop deformities similar to those of adult RA may benefit from MCP arthroplasty, PIP fusions, and tendon surgery. PIP implant arthoplasty is rarely done because the medullary canals are often too small for the prostheses.[38] The unavailability of implant small enough to accommodate small medullary canals can also be a restriction to other implant arthroplasties; for example, MCP, wrist, shoulder, hip, and knee joints.

The postoperative management of hand surgery is the same for children as that outlined for adults in Chapter 29.

Cervical Spine Involvement

Spinal arthritis in JRA occurs primarily in the cervical spine, typically involving the C-2, C-3, and C-4 posterior diarthrodial joints (apophyseal joints).[39] It typically spares the thoracic and lumbar spine, but in rare cases inflammation may extend distally to the midthoracic level.[40] In the early stages, the main problem is spasm of the neck muscles (**muscular splinting**) in response to pain, thus limiting neck motion.[39] Extension is lost first, followed by rotation and lateral flexion, which can occur very rapidly.

Occasionally neck involvement takes the form of torticollis. If neck mobility cannot be maintained in therapy, the apophyseal joints, vertebral bodies, and muscles will become fibrosed, resulting in a stiff neck with extremely limited ROM. This can extend from the occipital skull to C-7[40] (x-ray film shows loss of cervical lordosis). In severe cases, the affected joints may progress to bony fusion. The damage to the capsule and ligaments may result in laxity and neurological sequelae, although neurological involvement is rare in children, compared with that in adults.[39] Subluxation is very rare; when it occurs, it is between C-1 and C-2, similar to that in adult RA.[41] In some cases, it is possible for the eroded apophyseal joints to become **eburnated** (dense and hard, like ivory) and to retain mobility.[39]

In children, growth failure may occur at the vertebral plate or ring epiphyses leading to vertebrae with normal height but narrow width of the vertebral body and discs. This is a radiographic hallmark of juvenile-onset cervical spine arthritis.[25,39] Loss of neck mobility limits the child's visual range and necessitates turning of the entire trunk as well as hip and pelvic rotation to see objects to the side. It can make prone activities difficult, and can interfere with reading the blackboard in school and with driving for adolescents. Loss of visual range may pale in priority to the consequences these children may experience in ambulation and hand function, but it can have a profound impact on the developmental process with respect to self-confidence, balance, sense of security, and motor competence in space; if one cannot see an object to the side, one is less inclined to reach for it.

Safety is a critical issue. The child may not notice a potential danger while riding a tricycle, and an adolescent, while driving a car. If the vertebrae become ankylosed, a fall could put the child at high risk for a cervical fracture. If there is a cervical subluxation, a car accident or sudden jolt could put this person at risk of a cervical cord injury.

In the past, loss of neck extension has made intubation for general anesthesia difficult. The new fiberoptic technology is making this task easier; however, it is still a major consideration as these children reach maturity and become candidates for joint reconstruction.

Therapy

In the texts and articles on JRA (especially the early ones), pictures show children with such severe loss of neck extension that the neck is contracted in flexed position and the children have to look up to see straight ahead (Fig. 14–5). This is a result of late medical and rehabilitative intervention or lack of attention to proper positioning during active cervical involvement; for example, sitting supported in bed with pillows behind the head holding it in flexion. When it is not possible to resolve the neck involvement with medications or therapy, and stiffness or ankylosis seems inevitable, it is critical that positioning day and night is evaluated and designed to ensure alignment in the optimal functional position. It is important to maintain the natural lordotic curve of the cervical spine whenever possible.[42] The concepts of positioning for children are the same as for adults; that is, cervical pillows or rolls should support neck muscles in good alignment and should not be used to maintain the head in flexion. For children the pillows have to be smaller, and it may take more creativity, ingenuity, and patience to create

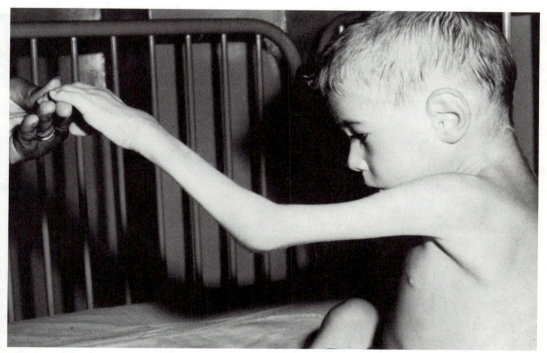

Figure 14–5. Classic systemic-onset polyarticular JRA. This child demonstrates the classic appearance of the child ill with severe systemic symptoms, including joint synovitis and limitations; sad, anxious expression; and severe weight loss that exaggerates the amount of joint enlargement. Note neck flexion contracture and classic wrist and digit limitations. This child also has severe hip, knee, and plantar ankle contractures. The severity of his limitations are due in part to the lack of preventative rehabilitative measures early in the course of his illness.

a positioning strategy that will work or one that the child will tolerate or cooperate with. This must be done for sleeping as well as for playing and for sedentary activities such as reading and watching television. Children with mild or early involvement are encouraged to lie prone on the floor to watch television in order to encourage neck extension. (This is also helpful for stretching the anterior chest and hip flexor muscles.)

A soft cervical collar may be used during specific prolonged activities, such as reading or playing computer games, not as a treatment but as a postural reminder to encourage optimal alignment. The collar requires the child to adapt the activity (e.g., the height of the book or game) to accommodate the straight neck rather than to keep the neck in flexion to accommodate the activity. The soft collar may also be used at night as a lordotic support.

Physical therapy includes heat or cold modalities, massage, relaxation techniques, extensor muscle strengthening, posture exercises, AROM, and deep-breathing techniques.[43] All these should be structured into games and activities as much as possible and should be implemented early.

Soft collars primarily provide postural feedback to encourage alignment. They also keep the neck warm and may help decrease pain and spasm. However, they do not immobilize or support the head. Children with cervical involvement need to be observed closely. If they lose extension rapidly and appear to be at risk for developing a flexion contracture, a semirigid, custom, Plastazote collar with a mandible cup to support the head should be considered to prevent a flexed posture. (This can be made in occupational therapy.) Sometimes the course of cervical arthritis is so virulent the therapeutic goal is to encourage stiffness in optimal functional alignment.

In the clinic common reference is made to "immobilizing the neck" in a collar. The implication is that this is the same as "splinting the wrist" and that the therapeutic benefits are the same. They are *not* the same thing. Soft collars, and to a greater degree semirigid collars, *only restrict motion; they do not immobilize.* Semirigid collars, or rigid collars with a mandible support, can provide some partial support for the

weight of the head, thus reducing some stress to the neck muscles; they can block forward flexion but do not stop rotation. The only way to immobilize the cervical spine is with halo traction. If the child has cervical subluxation, with or without neurological symptoms, soft collars offer no protection in the event of a sudden jolt. Semirigid collars with a chin cup provide a bit more support. The importance of neck positioning for children when they are at school or doing homework cannot be overemphasized, because most academic activities encourage neck flexion, shoulder protraction, and relaxation of the scapular muscles. A static posture of this type can encourage tightening of the anterior muscles, overstretching, and weakening of the posterior neck and scapula muscles.

Spine and Posture

Although the mid-thoracic, low-thoracic, and lumbar spine generally do not develop arthritis, they can develop compensatory deformity in response to a variety of joint limitations. Exercises and positioning to prevent and to correct postural distortion are a critical aspect of therapy for children with arthritis. Listed below are the common secondary distortions and the related primary joint involvement.

1. Scoliosis can result from leg length discrepancy (even small amounts), asymmetric hip flexion, or adduction contractures that restrict or alter unilateral pelvic alignment. The effect of asymmetric hip contractures on the spine is accentuated during prolonged sitting (e.g., in a wheelchair). (Custom seating should be considered in this situation.) Long-standing torticollis can also result in a compensatory thoracic scoliosis.[44]

2. Lordosis (sway back) frequently develops when the body compensates to stand straight in the presence of hip flexion contractures. Infrequently it can result from neck flexion contractures that require spinal extension to allow vision straight ahead.

3. Rounded or protracted shoulders may result from anterior muscle or trunk flexor guarding secondary to shoulder synovitis or sternocostal pain. Also, the psychological responses to pain—fear, sadness, and depression—invoke a flexed posture. Both situations reflect a neurological response that *facilitates* the flexors and *inhibits* the spinal extensors.

4. Limited thoracocostal and sternocostal mobility may result secondary to shoulder or neck pain that elicits guarding in the anterior shoulder/thoracic muscles as well as the posterior shoulder/thoracic/spinal muscles. It may also result from persistent pain, fear, and depression, which encourage shallow breathing as well as anterior muscle tightness.

To understand some of these relationships, pretend you have a very stiff, painful neck. Now stand (if you are sitting) and walk across the room, all the time guarding your painful neck. Notice the posture of your shoulders, elbows, low back, hips, and knees; also your gait, breathing, and rib cage excursion. After that try to walk fast, continuing to guard your neck, and notice the function of the other joints.

Therapy

Treatment to counteract the effects of compensatory posture and muscular guarding includes exercises and positioning techniques that lengthen the muscles facilitated during pain.

In physical therapy this may include scoliosis exercises, pelvic tilt progression, extensor muscle strengthening, anterior/flexor muscle stretching, Williams flexion exercises, chest excursion, and diaphragmatic breathing.[43]

One of the best methods for counteracting the prolonged facilitation of the anterior/flexor muscles is with posture exercises, deep relaxation, deep breathing, and laughter. All these should be incorporated into the child's daily routine.

Positioning at night is critical. Ideally, children with neck involvement should have a small, custom-made cervical pillow that supports the lordotic curve but does not flex the neck.[42] The softness and support of a mattress and warmth of the coverings can have a major impact on sleeping posture. If a child (or adult) is warm, he or she tends to sleep in a more open, extended position, whereas coldness encourages "huddling." Sleeping bags may be an effective, fun solution for children, because they are very efficient in retaining body warmth.[45] The mattress should have firm support but have at least a couple inches of foam on the top, either built into the mattress or added under the sheet. The soft, top layer reduces pressure on bony prominences, and it can feel very "comforting," which encourages relaxation and sleeping in an open posture. If the bed is used for prone activities, the top, soft surface will increase comfort and encourage compliance. If the child has nocturnal incontinence, it is best to cover the foam or mattress with one or two layers of very thin, supple plastic (not heavy stiff plastic) that does not inhibit the foam contouring. *All materials used must meet the fire safety code for children.* Materials should not be used unless their fireproof qualities are known. Retailers or manufacturers of products will have this information.

Temporomandibular Joint Involvement

The temporomandibular (TM) joint is formed by the condyle of the mandible and the mandibular fossa of the temporal bone. The joint is divided by a fibrocartilage disc forming two synovial-lined cavities. The joints are unique in that they are the only bilateral joints that work in symmetry or unison. This is quite a feat, or demand, considering the asymmetry of our bodies.[46]

Involvement of the TM joint is very common in polyarticular JRA. It can be mild and resolve, or it can result in premature closure of the mandible epiphyses and a short jaw, referred to as **micrognathia.** This creates malocclusion problems as well as cosmetic concerns.

If the inflammation stops and the TM joint limitations continue to cause pain or functional problems, there are surgical options available, including implant resurfacing of the condyle.[46] However, children with severe JRA have so many major problems that TM joint involvement tends to take a low priority. There is very little written in the JRA literature on TM joint arthritis and nothing written on long-term outcome of TM joint limitations.

Therapy

The TM joint allows opening and closing of the jaws, protrusion and retraction of the mandible, and lateral displacement of the mandible. A ROM program for a stiff jaw should include all these motions. For the most part, mobility is measured by the distance between the upper and lower incisors during maximal mouth aperture. The aperture norms for children depend on their age; the norm for adults is 5 to 6 cm.[46,47]

Evaluation of jaw mobility should be a part of the rehabilitation evaluation. At the first sign of pain or limitation, thermal modalities and ROM exercises should be introduced. The mouth aperture can be measured and marked on an index card for the patient or parent to use as a guide for measuring maintenance of mobility. During active involvement the aperture should be monitored daily. The child needs to achieve maximal range, as indicated on the card, once a day to maintain mobility. If the child is unable to achieve the range, a washcloth soaked in hot water and wrung out can be applied to each TM joint, and then gentle stretching exercise performed. This may help increase range sufficiently. For acute inflammation, ice packs may be needed. Relaxation techniques can also be helpful especially if unconscious muscular guarding is occurring.

Shoulder Involvement

The shoulder tends to be involved in children with severe polyarticular arthritis. Loss of movement may be the only sign of early involvement; pain may or may not be present. Mild swelling is difficult to detect in the shoulder, occasionally subacromial bursitis or bicipital tendonitis is the presenting problem.[48] In severe cases active glenohumeral abduction and internal rotation may be the first limitations noted (see Fig. 14–5).

The main cause of severe shoulder limitations is that early shoulder involvement is ignored because early synovitis does not necessarily limit function. The patient, family, and health care team are often focusing their attention and energy on hand and lower extremity joints that are posing a serious threat to function. This is certainly understandable, but it is early detection and *maintenance* of normal ROM that is the key in preserving shoulder function. We need approximately 90 degrees of shoulder flexion for most functional activities. Typically, the child (or adult) will be so focused on the hands, feet, or knees that he or she will not notice or call attention to the shoulder until he or she has difficulty reaching up (around 110 degrees); by that time they have lost 60 degrees of motion. At this stage, there is additional pain from adhesions, contractures set in, and recovery becomes difficult, if not impossible.

Therapy

Active shoulder ROM exercises should be included in all general therapy programs. It is critical that the exercises are performed to the child's full ROM, because losses of range can occur insidiously. When shoulders are actively painful, both heat packs and ice massage are effective, although effectiveness varies among individuals. Active range should be maintained in the acute stage. Codman's (pendulum) exercises can be performed in the gravity-dependent position to eliminate joint stress following thermal modalities. Isometric exercises can then be applied manually to shoulder flexor, abductor, and extensor muscle groups. While exercising to improve internal rotation, which is commonly decreased, make sure that there is no substitution of pectoral muscles. The pectoral muscles often become tight, because of several factors: neurological facilitation secondary to pain, fear, and depression; decreased reaching and mobility; fatigue, which encourages poor posture; and shallow breathing. Each of these factors encourages a chronic posture with shoulders protracted and the accompanying weak scapular musculature.

At the acute stage, self-care activities that require shoulder motion or sustained shoulder use that generates pain are not encouraged (unless it is very important to the adolescent). Gentle PROM exercise following deep relaxation techniques is critical for maintaining shoulder mobility during active inflammation. Active exercises that incorporate all motions can also be effective, especially if they are done slowly and incorporate active relaxation of the shoulders (when possible). These typically include exercises such as "towel and dowel," arm circles, "fountains" (bring palms together in front of body, raise above head and spread arms out to side), "superman" (lie prone, begin with arms at side and raise to front over head), "birds" (grasp hands behind neck, move elbows back as far as possible), and "wood chopper" (bring hands together overhead with elbows straight and "chop" straight down).

Once acute inflammation has subsided, exercises to increase ROM can be started. Gentle passive stretch can be applied at the end of range during exercise. Mobilization with gentle traction techniques can be performed to decrease adhesions while gaining range. During this procedure care should be taken to support the arm while moving slowly and holding at the end of the range position for a count of 7 or more. Another method for improving ROM is the "hold-relax" method of facilitation, performed by maximally contracting muscle groups against resistance, then relaxing while stretch is applied. This can increase range while isometrically contracting groups.

Muscle strengthening is critical to maintaining gains in range. Strengthening methods will include increasing the amount of time spent in an activity for endurance, proprioceptive neuromuscular facilitation (PNF) techniques, manual resistance, and applying weights at the proximal arm during therapeutic activities. Activities for ROM and muscle strengthening are many and varied. To increase purely range, wall walking can be performed for flexion and abduction while marking gains for motivation. Any game, dollhouse, or toy can be positioned at a height and distance to increase shoulder flexion range. Macrame hung from a pole, upright weaving, wall murals, bunting, easel painting, basketball, darts, and swinging a jump rope will encourage shoulder flexion and rotation while strengthening the triceps as well (Fig. 14-6).

Once the extent of permanent range limitations is determined, assistive devices are introduced but only as needed (see Chapter 25). The most common devices to increase

functional shoulder range are the dressing stick, long-handled shoe horn, back scrubber, and lengthening adaptations for combs or brushes. The environment (e.g., bedroom) can be arranged so as to enhance the child's functional capacities when range is a problem. Shelving, dresser heights, light switches, and door handles can all be positioned at the appropriate height, eliminating the need for further equipment in these areas (see Chapter 15 for adaptive devices for children). A problem of decreased shoulder muscle strength is the relative unavailability of lightweight and appropriately proportioned commercial adaptive devices for children. Beauty supply stores and general merchandise stores often carry plastic tool items.

In cases of bicipital tendonitis, a pillow to position the arm in abduction or slight flexion may help to increase comfort for sleep. Physical therapists at the Children's Hospital of Los Angeles have found transcutaneous electrical nerve stimulation (TENS) used at night helpful for reducing severe shoulder joint pain.

Surgery

Most cases of acute or severe shoulder synovitis or subacromial bursitis respond to corticosteroid injection therapy.

In rare, severe cases a synovectomy might be considered. In general, however, shoulder surgery is uncommon in children. When bone maturation has occurred, a total shoulder arthroplasty may be considered. This may be done for intractable pain or severe functional loss. Postoperative management is the same as that outlined for adults in Chapter 31.

Procedures such as manipulation under anesthesia, immobilization at 90 degrees, humeral osteotomy, glenoid osteotomy, and arthrodesis are occasionally done in Europe but essentially are not being done in the United States.

Elbow Involvement

The elbow joint is created by the articulation of the humerus with the ulna and radius (humeroradioulnar joint). The elbow joint capsule also encloses the proximal radioulnar joint; so synovitis of one joint af-

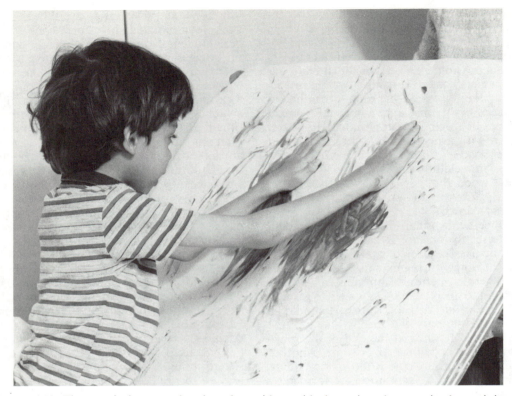

Figure 14–6. Finger painting on a slant board provides an ideal creative, therapeutic play activity to increase shoulder flexion and elbow, wrist, and finger extensions. The angle of the easel also can be adjusted to encourage neck extension and endurance. As with all activities, the therapist must observe and supervise the child to avoid substitution patterns that could prevent achievement of therapeutic goals; for example, substituting spinal extension for shoulder flexion, as this little boy is beginning to do.

fects both, even though they are considered two separate joints.

The capsule is loose and weak anteriorly and posteriorly but reinforced on the sides with strong ligaments.[49] *Swelling of the elbow joint is most easily visualized and palpated over the triangular area between the olecranon, radial head, and lateral epicondyle.*

The elbow joint is considered a compound joint that functions as a hinge joint, providing flexion and extension. The proximal and distal radioulnar joints are pivot joints that rotate in unison to provide supination and pronation.[49] Forearm rotation can be limited by damage to either the proximal or distal radioulnar joints. Supination usually becomes more limited than pronation. The joint responsible for the limitation can usually be identified by the

presence of pain at the end of range. For example, if a child in the test position for forearm rotation (elbows at side) demonstrates limited supination or pronation, ask the child if he or she has pain over the proximal or distal radioulnar joint. The site of pain indicates the restricting joint.

The elbow essentially shortens and lengthens the upper extremity and provides for placement of the hand in space. One of the more obvious primary functions is to bring the hand in contact with the face for feeding, hygiene, and so forth. When the elbow develops chronic synovitis, extension is usually lost first. An adult or child can lose up to 30 degrees of extension before there is noticeable interference with function. With a loss of 30 to 45 degrees of extension, the limb becomes noticeably shorter and the child may have difficulty reaching the feet, for example, in dressing. A loss of 45 to 90 degrees will restrict push-off leverage for standing up from a chair and interfere with dressing. A 90-degree contracture will seriously impair function, especially perineal care, and lower extremity dressing; it will also necessitate trunk flexion to accomplish desk activities. The loss of flexion can also seriously impair function. The extent of this is dependent on the status of other joints: If children have normal neck and shoulder function, they may be still able to feed themselves with an extension contracture of 90 degrees. The more limited a child's elbow, the more the child substitutes with neck flexion to accomplish feeding tasks. This, in fact, can put a considerable strain on the cervical spine.

Therapy

Reduction of Inflammation

Cold packs are the treatment of choice for active inflammation and reduction of spasm in the biceps and brachioradialis muscles.

Elbow orthoses can help prevent or correct a contracture, but they do not play much of a role in controlling inflammation because they are difficult—if not impossible—to wear during the day. Elbow sleeves may provide some warmth and comfort during functional activities or at night.

Prevention of Contractures

In the early stages of involvement, cold packs, ROM, and triceps-strengthening exercises may be sufficient to maintain mobility. If contractures occur, a volar, thermoplastic elbow orthosis may be used during the day as a means of applying sustained PROM for 1 hour (one to two times a day) or at night to stretch the elbow. For children with polyarticular JRA, orthotic treatment for the neck, wrists, and knees usually takes precedence over the elbows. (It would be easier to have a child get into a head-to-toe, bivalved body cast, then wear orthoses for all involved extremity joints.) However, if a child's wrist/hand is stable, use of an elbow orthosis may be possible for a few nights or may be alternated with the wrist orthosis.

If children's elbows hurt them at night or when they try to move around in bed, padded elbow sleeves can be helpful (Diamond or Heelbo brand). Lambswool cuffs should be avoided because elbow flexion is required to keep them in place. The sleeves are less cumbersome and have the added advantage of keeping the elbow warm at night.

Strengthening Extensor Muscles

Strengthening of elbow extensors (triceps) follows the basic principles of providing AROM warm-up and facilitation techniques (brushing or tapping the muscle belly) prior to strengthening. Strengthening is best accomplished through first isometric exercise against gravity, followed by activity. To strengthen the triceps against gravity, the child needs to be prone and close enough to the edge so that the forearm can flex and extend. Children can perform repetitions of AROM followed by manual resistance. For children with pauciarticular involvement it may be more comfortable to lean forward or to lean over a table so that the trunk and upper arm are parallel to the floor. Isometric contractions should be held for a count of 6. If strengthening needs to be done in an upright position, the arm should be supported at shoulder height on a table with a towel under the upper arm. To encourage a strong contraction, children can be directed to try to touch the table with the back of the hand, or to squish a noisy squeeze-toy with the forearm in extension.

Activities to encourage extensor strengthening can be integrated into other (particularly shoulder) activities. Careful positioning and the use of full available ROM are the key. Furthermore, it is important that the elbow be extended against gravity, so as not to strengthen the biceps inadvertently. For example, bunting a beach ball with a lightweight bat can provide full elbow extension range while increasing endurance of the triceps through repetitive activity. Wrist weights can be added to the forearm for more resistance. Other activities would include volleyball with a beach ball (protecting the wrist if needed), sanding wood on an incline, painting on an easel with an outstretched arm, and activities positioned so that the arm is extended during use. While hand weights are effective for exercising triceps with the shoulders abducted to 90 degrees or extended to maximum range, the weights should be cuffed (or strapped) through the hands or strapped to the forearm so that the child does not have to grip the weights statically (and there is no stress to the wrist).

Supination and pronation ranges are difficult to increase simply through activity. AROM exercises for forearm rotation should precede therapeutic activities. Screw driving (if fingers are not involved), turning pages, turning over blocks, pouring liquid, or flipping cards are among activities to encourage rotation. Limitations in pronation can seriously hinder tool use, typing, or keyboard capabilities. It will be important to practice these activities to discover whether effective use can be facilitated through exercise or whether the activities will require adaptation. Finally, the general upper extremity ROM exercises as discussed in therapy for the shoulder will also benefit strength and range of the elbow extensors.

When severely limited elbow ranges (either flexion or extension) limit self-care, modifications most commonly used are those to lengthen the utensils or to alter their shape. For example, severely decreased elbow flexion may necessitate use of a straw for drinking and extended handles for eating or applying makeup. A one-handed shower hose or extended sponge can be used for washing the face and upper body. Decreased elbow extension may require larger sleeves for dressing and front-opening shirts, as well as extended-handle equipment for donning shoes and socks. Reachers, if the grip area is small enough, can assist in obtaining items out of one's range.

Surgery

Synovectomy for aggressive elbow synovitis is not common but is an appropriate consideration if all other measures have failed. Occasionally it is combined with a radial head excision.[50]

Elbow contractures up to 40 degrees are generally not surgically corrected. If a child develops severe bilateral contractures that prevent feeding, self-care, or ambulation, a soft tissue release should be considered during childhood and a total elbow replace-

ment should be considered after epiphyseal closure.[37] In Europe, a procedure called a **resection arthroplasty** has been done successfully with children. It involves a limited excisional arthroplasty and covering of the end of the humerus with skin from the abdomen or fascia from the iliotibial band.[50]

Hip Involvement

In the early stages synovitis of the hip may be painless, or children may not refer to the pain if other joints are more troublesome. Either situation may allow a contracture to develop undetected. A slight hip flexion contracture may be compensated for with increased lumbar lordosis, making the contractures less noticeable. Careful physical examination of the hip motion is crucial in children whether they complain of pain or not, inasmuch as swelling is not easily palpated.

The most common limitations are flexion and adductor contractures secondary to pain and spasm of the psoas and adductor muscles. Internal rotation also may occur and is frequently associated with contracture of the iliotibial band.[37]

Lateral subluxation of the hip joint is a feature of disease in younger children, who maintain the immature configuration of the femoral neck. This is in contrast to protrusio acetabuli seen in older patients with hip involvement. With early and very acute hip synovitis there is more likely to be loss of adduction, whereas with more chronic disease abduction is lost.

Children with hip pain and flexion contractures begin walking with compensatory knee flexion and ankle plantar flexion. They can develop secondary pain and/or contractures in the back, knee, and ankle even if there is no arthritis in these joints. Therefore, a child with only hip arthritis needs an exercise and positioning program for back, knee, and ankle joints.

Granberry and Brewer[51] describe three patterns of destruction in the hip: (1) the most common, generalized joint space narrowing with cystic erosion and loss of anatomical congruity *without* significant anatomical displacement; (2) gradual lateral subluxation associated with significant generalized disease and proliferative synovitis in conjunction with adductor spasm and contracture. This is a serious problem, and these children need close follow-up for early detection of adductor spasm/contractures and concomitant abductor weakness. An active physical therapy program should include relaxation and stretching of the adductors and strengthening of the gluteus maximus and medius muscles. (If conservative measures fail, an adductor tenotomy and casting in abduction may provide a solution.) (3) Progressive medial migration (arthrokatadysis) is the least frequent pattern and is seen in some children with severe systemic-onset JRA. This occurs in response to aggressive synovial destruction of the cartilage and bone rather than muscular imbalance. There are no surgical solutions for this problem; the child is kept as active as possible and total hip arthroplasty is done at skeletal maturity.[51]

A unique phenomenon affecting the hips in children is the restoration or regeneration of the articular surface with fibrocartilage. It does not occur in all children but can occur even in severely damaged joints once the synovitis is controlled. When this occurs, children have improved hip joint function, and radiographs show widening of the hip joint spaces (cartilage increase), improved subchondral mineralization, filling in of subchondral cysts, and smoothing of the articular margins.[52] The potential for this repair has a direct impact on therapy. The molding and adequacy of the repair are influenced by the mobility of the joint, inasmuch as symmetric pressure may influence the concentricity of the opposing surfaces. Mobility and especially weight-bearing forces have been shown to improve cartilage repair.[53] *Consequently, immobilization can encourage cartilage degeneration.* Bernstein and colleagues,[52] who first reported on six children with this type of hip restoration, report that, beyond control of the synovitis, the common factor in the treatment of all six children was an emphasis upon increasing musculature, increasing ambulation, and avoiding wheelchair use.

As a result of these reports, non weight-bearing is still advocated for the acutely inflamed joint; but as soon as inflammation is controlled, ambulation is encouraged even though some inflammation is present. The incidence of fibrocartilage restoration in children is not known. It is believed that the synovitis must be brought under control for it to occur and that exacerbations of disease can destroy any repair that has already taken place.[52]

Nonambulation because of lower extremity arthritis is considered justification for hospitalizing a child for intensive physical therapy; nonambulation encourages joint degeneration, osteoporosis, hip, knee, and ankle contracture as well as compromised cardiopulmonary capacity—not to mention the psychological and social consequences of wheelchair use.

One 12-year-old, who had bilateral 90-degree hip and knee flexion contractures from wheelchair use since age 8, brought this point poignantly home following bilateral total hip and knee replacement when she exclaimed, "I can see my toes!"

Therapy

Physical therapy strengthening of hip extensors, abductors, and external rotators in conjunction with decreasing flexion contractures is the cornerstone of treatment. Walking in the pool and swimming can help relax musculature and decrease pain. Ice is generally not used because the joint is so deep. As in other areas, isometric exercise and AROM exercises are performed at the acute stage. Walking is encouraged early, grading endurance through the course of treatment. Bicycling and swimming provide good hip extension through strengthening. Abduction and external rotation exercises must usually be specifically prescribed.

Strengthening is accomplished through manual resistance, increasing endurance in walking and pushing objects, such as chairs, for added resistance. Graded inclines and stair climbing are introduced once motion, strength, and stability in all lower extremity musculature are ready or supported.

Prevention of Contractures

Children with painful or limited hips tend to avoid standing and ambulation activity so that their hips are in a flexed posture almost entirely throughout the day and night. Positioning to create a balance between flexion and extension posture is key to maintaining hip alignment and extension mobility. (Ultimately this can prevent secondary back, knee, and ankle problems.) This can be accomplished in a variety of ways.

1. Prone-lying. This includes prone on the floor, prone table, or hard bed for reading, homework, television, or activities. This is excellent for maintaining or increasing extension. At home, proning for younger children can be on a padded coffee table (for small children a padded ironing board on the bed or floor may work). These surfaces allow the feet to hang over the end. A wide strap holding the hips to the board can help provide specific stretch to the hip flexors. Precautions: increasing lumbar lordosis and pressure on ankles in plantar flexion.

2. Buck's traction (distal traction applied to a long leg orthosis with patient supine). This is used at night or during rest periods,[36] especially when hip flexion contractures are more than 20°. If there are severe knee contractures, a split mattress may be necessary in order that the knee can be in flexion while the hip is pulled in extension. Traction is also beneficial for reducing muscle spasm. This process is also used to correct contractures. With outrigger attachments, Buck's traction can also be used to increase hip abduction and external rotation. Precautions/contraindications: low back pain, stress on lordosis, pulmonary problems, high fever at night, spinal compression fractures, and gastric reflux.[36]

3. Supine stretch (extension of one hip, with the knee flexed, and slight flexion of the other hip with the leg suspended in a sling while the child is supine on a guerney). Supine stretch is indicated to increase hip extension by stetching the rectus femoris, to increase flexion by raising the suspended leg, or to decrease hamstring tightness. To be effective, the back must be flat on the guerney (in a pelvic tilt) with the extended hip and flexed knee secured with a strap.

4. Tilting (standing on a tilt table with back straight, and hips and knees secured in extension). Tilting is used to increase weight bearing to promote bone deposition, facilitate extensor musculature (gluteus maximus and quadriceps), decrease orthostatic hypotension, and as an alternate position to sitting. Tilting is indicated both for children who are nonambulatory or who are walking minimally, and for children needing a change of position. Children can eat, read, do homework, or play while tilting. To be effective for weight bearing, the tilt table must be at least 75° upright.

5. Prone standing (patient is prone on a guerney that is tilted upright). The indications and use of prone standing are similar to tilting. However, this position is often more amenable to function and promotes neck extension and scapular cocontraction.

The key to a successful positioning program is designing creative and engaging activities to increase tolerance to the positioning methods. The methods must be consistently reinforced.

In addition to positioning, strengthening of the hip extensors and abductors (in the presence of adduction contractures) is essential to preventing contractures.

Reduction of Inflammation and Spasm

The hip is different from other joints in that it is deep and surrounded by large muscles. Therefore it is not really possible to alter the temperature of the hip joint with superficial heat or cold. In the hip thermal modalities play a more important role in reducing muscle spasm and extra-articular pressure on the joint. For this purpose heat is generally the most beneficial. Other modalities and processes such as TENS, neuroprobe, ultrasound, mobilization, and diathermy, as well as visual imagery, and conscious relaxation may also be beneficial in reducing muscular tightness, spasm, and pain.[44] As noted above, traction too may help achieve this goal.

Strengthening Program

In physical therapy, strengthening the hip extensor and abductor muscles with special emphasis on the gluteus medius is essential to maintaining hip function and gait. The program should incorporate PNF techniques as well as resisted exercise. Additionally, strengthening should be a part of a pool exercise program in order that muscles can be exercised without weight bearing.[35,44] Exercises need to be incorporated into the child's daily routine several times a day. For example, bicycling (or tricycling) can be used to strengthen the hip extensors.

Range of Motion Program

The goals of therapy are to maintain hip extension, abduction, and rotation (opposite any existing rotary limitation). Also, whenever ankle/foot orthoses are used in bed, their impact on the knee and hip must be considered, because ankle placement can influence hip rotation. For some children, especially with late onset, the position of comfort is with the hip externally rotated. Ankle orthoses or positioning boots encourage this position and must have a lateral rotation stop-bar (attached to the heel) to prevent external rotation. Children with a tendency toward internal rotation need a medial rotation stop-bar.

Posture throughout the day needs to be assessed and included in treatment planning. It is important that recommended positions do not increase lordosis.

Surgery

If the hip joint cartilage is well preserved and hip contractures do not resolve with occupational/physical therapy measures, soft tissue release may be considered, but it does not have a high success rate. The most common procedure is an adductor and psoas tenotomy with postoperative immobilization in extension and abduction.[54] A femoral osteotomy may prove beneficial for some of these children.

If the cartilage is destroyed, options in the past have been a total hip replacement (THR) or a fusion. Hip fusions were sometimes preferable in a child whose other joints were not very involved. These children often became so active once the troublesome joint was replaced that the prostheses became loose, requiring a difficult replacement. As the child became older, the fusion could be replaced with a THR. The concerns regarding durability and loosening of the cemented prosthesis, infection, and skeletal growth are the same as described for the knee. There is information available regarding long-term use of a total hip cemented prosthesis. For example, it is reported that the rate of wear on the plastic acetabular component is 0.2 mm per year, giving a total effective life of 20 to 25 years for the component.[55] This raises serious questions about the risk of replacement surgery when necessary and the long-term effects of plastic and metal debris within the joint caused by wearing of the prosthesis.[55]

The cementless total hip prosthesis may provide a solution to the above problems and become the treatment of choice even for younger children. The indications and postoperative management of THR are the same as outlined for adults in Chapter 33.

Knee Involvement

The knee is frequently affected early in the disease. Even the initial visit may reveal a knee contracture. Flexion contractures are the most common problem and can occur secondary to hip or foot involvement as well as primary knee synovitis[51] (see Fig. 14–7).

Because knee swelling and pain increase intra-articular pressure, and a flexed position maximizes the articular space and reduces this pressure, children (and adults) tend to keep their knees flexed throughout the day and while in bed.[56,57] In addition, spasm of the hamstrings and tensor fascia lata may occur in response to the knee pain, reinforcing the flexed position, encouraging valgus deformity, and making it difficult to passively range the knee.[27] Maintaining constant flexion encourages weakness and atrophy of the quadriceps muscle, further reducing ability for active extension. Adhesions and fibrosis of the posterior capsule can occur fairly rapidly, preventing extension and contributing to posterior subluxation. Lack of extension is the critical problem; but loss of flexion can also occur secondary to an effusion restricting motion or fibrosis of the quadriceps expansion.[51]

Another possible contributing factor to knee flexion deformities is leg length inequality resulting from accelerated or retarded growth of the long bones as a result of the inflammatory process interfering with adjacent epiphyseal development.[39] Increased blood flow (hyperemia) associated with inflammation usually causes increased bone growth initially, but later on it can cause early closure of the epiphysis and decreased bone length. Therefore, in younger children bone length tends to be

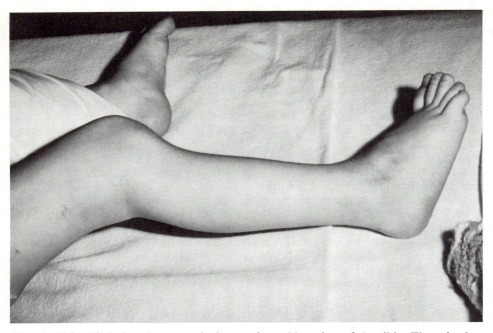

Figure 14–7. This child's leg shows marked posterior subluxation of the tibia. There is also ankle and forefoot swelling and loss of ankle dorsiflexion.

accelerated, whereas in older children bone growth is reduced. The inequality of length will encourage the longer leg to remain flexed during ambulation or weight bearing. This problem can usually be prevented with a heel lift. It is recommended that leg lengths be kept equal in a growing child.[51] Even less than a half-inch difference in leg lengths is considered significant in a toddler. If the length inequality cannot be corrected with shoe adaptions, epiphyseal stapling can be done to stop bone growth temporarily although this is rarely done. (See discussion of surgery, below.)

If a flexion contracture is not corrected early, the loss of normal articular motion reduces pressure on the anterior parts of the femoral and tibial growth plates and accelerated growth occurs, increasing the flexion deformity. Eventually fibrosis and deterioration of the cruciate ligaments will allow subluxation and incongruity of the weight-bearing surfaces.[42]

Valgus deformity is also common. However, it is important to keep in mind that the normal knee is in slight valgus, so weight-bearing forces on a swollen knee will encourage deformity in this direction. An early valgus deformity may be masked by a flexion contracture. Changes in the growth plate, especially acceleration of growth of the lower femoral epiphysis on the medial side, can contribute to this problem. Valgus deformity is also encouraged by an adduction contracture of the hip, which is common in children. Weight bearing on a valgus deformity encourages lateral subluxation of the knee.[42]

Radiographs of a knee with an established valgus and flexion deformity typically reveal narrowing of the lateral "joint space" (loss of cartilage), erosion of bone in late or advanced cases, collapse of the lateral tibial plateau, and elongation of the medial ligament of the knee. In some children, fibrosis or bony ankylosis may result.[42]

Knee deformity also may be secondary to hip arthritis. In the adult, the most common hip deformity is flexion, adduction, and external rotation (the position of comfort). In the child, flexion, adduction, and internal rotation are more common. Internal rotation of the femur creates secondary external torsion in the tibia in an attempt to keep the axis of movement of the ankle in line with forward movement. This is the same situation seen in children with persistent anteversion of the femoral neck.[42]

A common finding and one that must continually be observed for in children with hip arthritis is contracture of the iliotibial band. When this occurs, it results in flexion, internal rotation, and valgus deformity of the knee. Ideally this is caught early and resolved in physical therapy with a stretching program.[37]

Less frequently knee deformity can be caused by arthritis in the foot. Foot pain with ambulation causes the foot to be held in eversion and valgus, creating an external rotation force on the developing tibia and ultimately torsion. However, it is uncommon to have severe foot involvement without any knee involvement.

Therapy

Prevention of Flexion Contractures

Some children with knee synovitis can maintain knee extension with a closely monitored, home ROM program that includes proper positioning during activities. But children who cannot be monitored closely at home, or those who have any loss of active or passive knee extension, should have a long-leg knee orthosis to wear at night because it is much easier to prevent a contracture than to correct one.

There are several types of orthoses and considerations for each. If there is any hint of ankle involvement (with or without pain), the knee orthosis or cast should include the ankle. Knee orthoses that end proximal to the ankle encourage plantar flexion contractures or may cause pain and stiffness in the ankle.

Posterior Knee–Ankle Orthosis. For children it is preferable to make these out of lightweight material such as Hexilite casting material or low-temperature thermoplastic (for smaller children). Plaster shells work in an emergency or for short-term treatment but are often too heavy for children to apply and to remove, and they make it difficult for them to move in bed. Lighter materials tend to encourage acceptance of this treatment by both parents and

children. Tips on fabrication include the following:

1. The most common error made is making the proximal end too short. The proximal end needs to come to approximately 2 inches below the groin or underwear line in order to balance the long lever force distal to the knee. When the proximal end is too short, the force of the leg will cause the proximal end to "dig in."

2. The central strap should be wide, have a lambswool pad, and go directly over the knee, snug enough to prevent the knee from flexing out of the shell. If there are problems with the strap slipping, a circumferential Ace wrap may provide the best solution. If the child has a marked flexion contracture or spasticity and cannot be held comfortably in a posterior shell, bivalved Hexilite or fiberglass casts with strap closures may have to be used.[36] These will distribute the pressure over the length of the leg.

3. During the application of the orthosis with the knee in maximal extension, care must be taken to apply extension pressure gently and proximally to the joint to reduce the risk of posterior tibial subluxation.[35]

The orthoses are worn at night as long as there is active inflammation or tenderness. Prevention and management of knee contractures must include extensor muscle strengthening, activity positioning, inflammation and spasticity control, in addition to orthotic treatment.[44]

Reduction of Inflammation and Spasm

The knee joint is believed to be the most frequently involved joint in JRA. Although the reason for this is not known, it is theorized to be due in part to its being the largest joint in the body with the greatest amount of synovium, making it vulnerable to the inflammatory process. It is also subject to long lever and torque forces, making it vulnerable to stress, strain, and trauma.

When swelling is present, ice packs and contrast wrap modalities are the treatment of choice to reduce inflammation in the joint and spasm of the knee flexors. Treatment for both is done at the same. If stiffness is the main problem, heat may be more beneficial.

Strengthening Program

The forces that weaken the extensor muscle, neurological inhibition, disuse, and flexed posture, are powerful and ever present throughout the day during active inflammation.[35] To counteract these forces, extensor strengthening, facilitation, and positioning must be done throughout the day. Ideally, the exercise must be simple enough to be used frequently through the day and incorporated on a habitual basis.

Strengthening exercises for the quadriceps muscles should place special emphasis on the vastus medialis and the last 30 degrees of extension.[44] Electromyographic biofeedback can be a very helpful tool for teaching children, especially ages 4 to 10, the process of strong contractions. Children are very responsive to making lights go on and bells ring. The creative applications are endless. Children can sit on the floor and run electric trains and toys with quadriceps contractions. The therapists at Children's Hospital of Los Angeles are finding functional electrical stimulation an important adjunct for restoring quadriceps muscle strength along with PNF techniques.[44]

Tricycles are recommended as a means of mobility for young children because they strengthen the knee and hip extensors in a non-weight-bearing position. The goal to move about motivates children to persevere in this type of exercise.

Range-of-Motion Program

The ROM program for children focuses on maintaining extension and regaining flexion. Regaining extension is a separate process of correcting a contracture.

Maintaining extension is done through (1) night orthoses; (2) strengthening exercises; (3) positioning; (4) modalities to reduce hamstring spasm; and (5) working daytime knee orthoses. (Passive extension has to be done carefully to avoid subluxation of the tibia.)

Regaining flexion is done through (1) modalities to reduce spasm of the rectus femoris muscle; (2) facilitory/inhibitory techniques; (3) PNF techniques (e.g., contract–relax); and (4) continuous passive motion

(CPM).[44] (Strengthening of the flexors is generally not done.)

Correction of Contractures

Flexion contractures (less than 45 degrees) that are resistant to the above measures can often be corrected with serial casting.[35]

At Children's Hospital of Los Angeles the following procedure for serial casting is used.[35] The casts are applied for a 48- to 72-hour period, during which the child is encouraged to strengthen extensor musculature actively through ambulation and exercise. When the cast is removed, ice packs may be used to decrease flexor spasm and joint swelling. Extensor exercises are performed to facilitate extension, and a new cast is put on at the new level of maximal extension. The best long-term results are achieved when the serial casting is continued until full extension is achieved. Sometimes intra-articular corticosteroids are used to help achieve this goal. When the maximal gains have been achieved by the serial casts, custom-molded polyethylene knee orthoses are worn at all times except during therapy, exercise, and bathing. Wearing is gradually reduced as quadriceps strength is regained. This may take a long time—often a year. The orthoses are used in combination with appropriate exercises to strengthen the muscles of the joint and to restore a flexor-extensor muscle balance. Actively inflamed joints may require orthotic treatment for months after the casting has been terminated. Some knee flexion is lost but eventually returns. If the orthotic treatment is not combined with appropriate exercise, severe muscle atrophy can result. (See Appendix 5 for the procedure for serial casting.)

Surgery

Surgery for the knee includes the following:

1. Epiphysiodesis by stapling. This procedure involves surgical stapling across the growth plate to arrest growth of the longer bone.[37] It results in delayed, rather than immediate, arrest, and it is reversible if desired. It is typically done at the distal femur, or proximal or distal tibia. It is done on both sides of the bone, but if angular deformity is a problem there is a potential for correcting it with asymmetric stapling.[37,54] The indication for this procedure is 7 cm of leg length difference.[54] Stapling is not recommended to correct inequality of leg length when overgrowth is produced by unilateral inflammatory disease of the knee, inasmuch as this discrepancy tends to diminish after a synovectomy or when the arthritis goes into remission.[54]

2. Soft tissue release. This is indicated if the flexion deformity is due to soft tissue tightness, joint space is well preserved, and there is no angulation deformity.[37,54] The two common releases are (1) iliotibial band fasciotomy[58]; and (2) posterior release, which includes hamstring lengthening and capsulotomy with or without release of the posterior cruciate ligament.[54]

3. Osteotomy (supracondylar). Osteotomy is performed only when there is fixed flexion and angulation deformity.

4. Synovectomy. Indications are persistent synovitis nonresponsive to medical management of at least 18 months' duration.[37] The knee is the most frequent site of synovectomy.[59] The best results of this surgery are in the child older than 7 years with monoarticular or pauciarticular disease and well-preserved joint space.[37] Postoperative management is the same as that for adults.

5. Hemiarthroplasty. For selected patients, a hemiarthroplasty using the McKeever metallic implant is an option. It has less risk because there is only one uncemented component.[37]

6. Total knee replacement. Total knee replacement (TKR) is considered only after all other conservative occupational/physical therapy measures have been tried and other surgical possibilities have been tried or ruled out. Generally, the surgery is delayed until bone maturation has occurred. Occasionally the surgery is done on a young adolescent (the youngest has been age 12) when it is deemed that prolonged nonambulation will be more detrimental to the patient than the risk of reducing skeletal height.[37,55] This surgery is still controversial for adolescents and young adults, inasmuch as there are still a lot of unanswered questions regarding long-term fixation of components, wear and fatigue strength for materials (metal debris), and delayed infection, especially for people on steroids.[55] The chances for long-term success of the TKR are best in adolescents or young adults with polyarticular disease, because their small stature and restricted activity place the least wear on the prosthesis. The surgery often improves their ambulation status from "assisted" or "dependent" to "household" or "community ambulator."[37] The decision for surgery is more difficult in young adults, especially male, with monoarticular disease because the surgery will restore function to nearly normal, and the normal activity of the teens and twenties will place high stress on the prosthesis. This is especially true if the patient has denial about the disease or a strong desire to forget about the arthritic episode in his or her life.

Like adults, young people have to be willing and able to follow through with a painful and active postoperative regimen. Ipsilateral hip flexion contractures need to be resolved, too, before knee surgery, otherwise they will encourage knee flexion deformity. Likewise, ankle and foot involvement to prevent ambulation need to be resolved prior to knee surgery. The upper extremities must also be capable of using axillary or platform crutches during the postoperative rehabilitation program.[55] If hand surgery is needed, it is staged after knee surgery because the stress of crutch ambulation could destroy the hand repair.

Ankle and Foot Involvement

In the child with JRA, severe inflammation can occur in the forefoot, hindfoot, and ankle. The midfoot, which provides a kinematic bridge between the hindfoot and forefoot, tends to become stiff and fibrosed secondary to immobility and functional problems incurred in the other regions of the foot and ankle. These regions are reviewed here in ascending order because involvement frequently starts in the forefoot and moves proximal; and accommodation of forefoot pain creates the deforming biomechanical forces that can act upon the hindfoot and ankle and ultimately the knee and the rest of the body. The feet are our foundation, and like a building, any shift in the foundation is going to have an impact on the standing structure.

Forefoot

The forefoot consists of the metatarsal and phalangeal bones and their interconnecting joints.

Potential sequelae of synovitis in the MTP and IP joints are enumerated and discussed below.

1. Pain and swelling typically elicit spasm of the long toe flexors that can result in contraction of the muscles and ultimately in phalangeal joint flexion deformities. The avoidance of bearing weight on a painful joint elicits hyperactivity of the long toe extensors, which can result in a hyperextension deformity of the MTP joints. The result of both of these processes is the typical claw toe deformity.

Children try to reduce painful weight bearing by avoiding "push off" and develop what is described as a flat-footed "plodding gait" or "calcaneal gait." (To understand forefoot mechanics, try walking without putting pressure on the MTP heads. Notice the activity of the long toe extensors. This should make the biomechanics for both MTP subluxation and varus deformity more clear.) It is the phenomenon of spasticity and *avoiding pain* that produces the initial major deforming forces in the forefoot and midfoot. It is not uncommon to find children who deny having foot or toe pain yet who walk with a plodding gait in an unconscious effort to avoid pressure on the MTP joints. Secondary problems, such as atrophy in the underused muscles and tightness or contractures in the overused muscles, perpetuate the deformity.

2. The large toe tends to develop a valgus deformity, similar to that seen in adults. This can occur in children without arthritis as a result of altered body mechanics. The large toe does not usually claw.[60] If the large toe IP is inflamed, the child may develop hallux rigidus, which can interfere with roll-off.

3. The metatarsal epiphyses tend to develop prematurely and then close early, distorting the metatarsal heads and creating growth defects in the shafts. These differential growth lengths may cause pressure problems.[54]

4. The metatarsal heads splay and migrate plantarward, irritating and inflaming plantar bursae, creating callosities. During evaluation, the presence of plantar callosi-ties over the metatarsal heads is usually indicative of MTP subluxation.

5. In addition to clawing, the IP joints may dislocate or become ankylosed.

Tendon and Bursa Involvement

In all forms of JRA, tenosynovitis is common either with or without pain. It may be in a single tendon (e.g., the tibialis posterior) or it may affect all the tendon sheaths around the ankle. The paratenon (fatty and areolar tissue around the tendon) and bursae associated with the Achilles tendon are common sites of involvement in patients with ankylosing spondylitis.[43]

Hindfoot

The hindfoot consists of the talus, calcaneus, and the navicular bones that create the subtalar, talonavicular, and calcaneocuboid joints.

Potential sequelae of synovitis are the following:

1. Loss of inversion or eversion.
2. Varus deformity (more common in children). This necessitates weight bearing on the outer border of the foot. This typically results from avoidance of pressure on painful MTP or subtalar joints during ambulation.[54]
3. Valgus deformity (more common in adults). This can result from:

   A. Mechanical forces of weight bearing on the medial collateral, calcaneonavicular, and talocalcaneal ligaments weakened by synovitis. Another contributing factor is the biomechanical forces created by avoidance of full weight bearing on painful MTP joints.[54]

   B. Accommodation or knee valgus deformity and malalignment.

   C. Advanced sequela of peroneal muscle spasm (peroneal spastic flatfoot) with concomitant weakness of the posterior tibial muscle.[51]

   D. Swelling and inflammation of the medial compartment of the hindfoot.

   E. Rupture of the posterior tibialis tendon.

Ankle Joint

The ankle refers to the talocrural joint formed by the articulation of the talus, distal tibia, and fibula. This joint makes dorsiflexion and plantar flexion possible. (Inversion and eversion occur in the subtalar joint.)

Potential sequelae of synovitis are outlined below.

1. Synovitis that results in loss of ROM.

A. Plantar flexion contracture. Loss of dorsiflexion or ability to bring the foot to neutral will seriously impede ambulation. This results from improper positioning in bed or wheelchairs and during sedentary activity. Ankle contractures can also be encouraged by knee flexion contractures. This problem is completely preventable. See treatment below.

B. Dorsiflexion contracture. Loss of plantar flexion is less common but can occur, and it occurs more frequently in JRA than in adult RA.[61] When this occurs, the child is unable to "push off" during ambulation, creating an abnormal gait and distorting total body mechanics. (To understand this deformity and how it affects gait, try walking while maintaining slight dorsiflexion in one foot. Note knee and hip mechanics and ipsilateral arm motion.)

2. The ankle without synovitis may become painful secondary to mechanical stress from abnormal knee or foot alignment.[54]

3. Avascular necrosis of the talus is not common but can occur.[54]

Therapy

Forefoot and Hindfoot

In the forefoot the primary goals of therapy are *reduction of MTP inflammation, pain, and deformity.* This is done by reducing weight-bearing forces on the joint by redirecting the forces of push-off proximal to the joint with use of (1) metatarsal pads (inside the shoe) for early, mild, or isolated joint inflammation; (2) metatarsal bars (outside the shoe) effective when the MTP joints are the only foot problem; (3) soft or rigid custom-molded orthosis (this is an arch support with metatarsal pad) that may be made thicker to account for leg length discrepancy or wedged to correct a varus or valgus hindfoot (soft orthoses are generally used because they are more effective for forefoot problems than rigid ones); and (4) rocker soles may be helpful if the above treatments are not effective in relieving

pain.[61] The cavovarus foot also may need lateral soles and stretching exercises.

When these devices are effective, one hopes to see reduced pain with ambulation, improved push-off, reduced or relaxed ankle/toe dorsiflexion, increased walking endurance, and, ultimately, reduced inflammation as a result of reducing stress to the joint.[36]

The most effective cold modality for the feet is contrast baths, but it is difficult to get children to cooperate with this procedure, especially if they have polyarticular disease. Cold is more often used on the tendon sheaths and subtalar joint, where it can be applied with a pack. But, again, cooperation with all cold modalities is difficult.

Prevention of Toe Flexion Contractures

Inflammation of the MTP joints (by itself without any other involvement) can elicit spasm of the long toe flexors. When this occurs, the toes are flexed, and they may appear contracted with limited PROM. Toe flexion places the MTP joints in hyperextension. This, combined with overuse of the long toe extensors to avoid putting pressure on the joints during ambulation, produces the characteristic claw toe deformity. (It may also develop in the reverse order: MTP hyperextension puts stretch on the long toe flexors, resulting in IP joint flexion contractures.)

Restoration of toe mobility is possible when toe ROM is combined with modalities and massage to release the spasm in the associated muscles. The deforming influence of the extrinsic flexor/extensor muscles on the MTP joints occurs early in the inflammatory process. Consequently, *AROM* and *PROM* should be done daily and if—or when—the toes begin to lose mobility, treatment should be directed to reducing spasm or tightness in the extrinsic toe extensor/flexor muscles. When the phalangeal joints are inflamed, as is typical in polyarticular JRA, toe ROM is often best accomplished in a Hubbard tank or bathtub.

Reduction of Subtalar Joint Inflammation

The subtalar joint is primarily responsible for inversion and eversion. The most effective treatment for reducing inflammation is use of a rigid custom-molded heel-cup orthosis (e.g., UC-BL foot orthosis). If the forefoot is involved, the orthosis can include a metatarsal pad. It also can be wedged to correct for hindfoot valgus (and rarely varus). The heel-cup restricts inversion and eversion and thus reduces stress to the subtalar joint[61] (Fig. 14–8). It does not limit the ankle joint and, in fact, may aggravate inflammation in this joint by restricting motion in an adjacent joint.

If the heel-cup is effective, one would hope to see one or more of the following results: (1) an increase in stride length, push-off, velocity of ambulation, ambulation endurance; (2) improved lower extremity alignment; and (3) decreased foot and/or ankle pain. These orthoses can be used in-side athletic shoes, sneakers, and sturdy loafers after the manufacturer's liners are removed. The child often needs a shoe one size larger. Ankle tenosynovitis is very common in conjunction with subtalar and/or ankle joint inflammation. All these conditions may be responsive to cold modalities prior to ROM or exercises.

Reduction of Ankle Inflammation

If the ankle is the only joint involved, as may be seen in pauciarticular JRA, a below-the-knee custom-made, thermoplastic orthosis should be used at night to immobilize the joint and to maintain alignment while sleeping.[36] If the inflammation is severe, an ankle–foot orthosis may be indicated for daytime use to restrict ankle

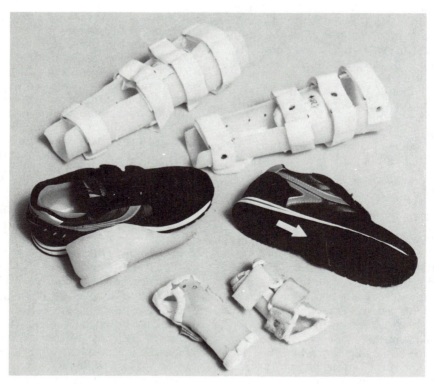

Figure 14–8. These orthoses are made of high-temperature polyethylene. At the top of the photograph are knee orthoses to maintain extension when the child is not ambulating. In the middle is a heel cup orthosis that stabilizes the subtalar joint; it can be designed to correct hindfoot alignment, support the arch, and reduce pressure on the MTP joints. The arrow on the right shoe points to an external MTP bar that shifts weight-bearing pressure proximal to the MTP joints. At the bottom are circumferential wrist orthoses for a 3-year-old child. Materials, such as Aquaplast, that allow smoother edge finishing, do not require moleskin covering of the edges. Moleskin should be avoided whenever possible because it is difficult to clean and requires frequent changing.

motion and stress to the joint. The staff at Children's Hospital in Los Angeles rarely recommends these orthoses because they can promote plantar flexor muscle atrophy and decrease ankle ROM.[36] Physical therapy must address this if the ankle–foot orthosis is used.

The ankle–foot orthosis also may be used to correct hindfoot and forefoot malalignment by reducing persistent peroneal or posterior tibialis spasm or marked muscle imbalance when they are nonresponsive to a heel-cup orthosis.[36]

Prevention of Ankle Contractures

Plantar flexion contractures are the most dysfunctional.[21] If moderate or severe, they can prevent ambulation. *Most of all, they are preventable.* These contractures develop because of (1) lack of proper positioning (orthoses) at night or during bedrest, especially during acute illness; (2) sitting in a wheelchair, stroller, or chair without sufficient foot support so the feet dangle in plantar flexion (see Fig. 14–4); or (3) secondary to a knee flexion contracture or ambulating on crutches with the knee flexed. Children who are nonambulatory with or without ankle involvement are at high risk for developing plantar flexion contractures. Therapists should monitor positioning of the ankle especially during occupational therapy, activity therapy, or proning activities.

In children who are ambulating it is common to see dorsiflexion contractures caused by chronic spasm of the ankle dorsiflexor muscles (tibialis anterior, extensor hallucis longus, extensor digitorum longus, and peroneus tertius).

Any child with stiffness in the ankle because of either synovitis or tenosynovitis should have positioning in bed, during sedentary activities, in chairs, wheelchairs, strollers, or car seats adapted to keep the foot in neutral to avoid plantar flexion because these are the children at risk for developing foot-drop contractures. These children need a blanket cradle to keep sheets and blankets from pulling the feet into plantar flexion, and adaptations on wheelchairs in order that the child's foot is in neutral while sitting. Also, knee orthoses for use while the child is in bed should encompass the foot to prevent plantar flexion

forces and discomfort from prolonged plantar flexion positioning even if the ankle itself is not inflamed.

Strengthening, Range of Motion, and Correction of Ankle Contractures

In physical therapy, strengthening procedures for the ankle are aimed at preventing atrophy of the posterior or anterior calf musculature and preventing plantar flexion or dorsiflexion deformities. AROM exercises are performed throughout all ranges; manual resistance is applied to weakened musculature. Plantar flexion and dorsiflexion motions can be exercised through bicycle or tricycle riding. Subtalar motions generally necessitate specific AROM exercises, with care taken to make sure the ankle is in correct alignment. In cases of severe spasm of peroneal musculature, ankles have been serial casted to decrease the spasm. Children's Hospital of Los Angeles has also had success in improving longstanding subtalar malalignment by serial casting toward a neutral position. Correction of the subtalar contracture must always be followed by use of UC-BL foot orthoses; correction of ankle contractures should be followed by use of ankle–foot orthoses and continued strengthening. As stated earlier, proper positioning in bed and during tilting and sitting is necessary for preventing plantar flexion contractures. The foot should be supported in neutral position at all times. This is accomplished through foot supports, ankle–foot orthoses, and bivalved casts.

MORNING STIFFNESS

Morning stiffness has the same significance in JRA as it does in adult disease; that is, it is a generalized stiffness throughout the body felt upon awakening. Its presence and duration are associated with the activity of the disease. Morning stiffness is clearly a significant problem in children with polyarticular involvement. This stiffness increases the difficulty of voluntary motion and may cause the *child to refuse to use the hands or even to ambulate.* Evaluation of this phenomenon and patient/family education on how to accommodate or to reduce morning stiffness is a part of the therapy for these children. Children with pauciarticular arthritis also have morning stiffness, but it may not be a chief complaint and often needs to be specifically asked about. (For assessment of morning stiffness, see Chapter 18.)

Therapy

If children have a significant duration of morning stiffness (1 to 3 hours), independence in their morning self-care skills— feeding, dressing, and bathing—needs to be assessed with regard to early morning performance as well as to how they perform throughout the day.

Older children often find an electric blanket a helpful adjunct; some turn it on high before they get out of bed to "help thaw out." I've known children of all ages, even college students, who found it helpful to sleep in sleeping bags, which keep the warmth in and simplify bed making in the morning.

It is generally recommended that children take a 20-minute warm bath and do basic limbering exercises in the morning before going to school. Care should be taken to ensure adequate warmth in the room during and after the bath. The temperature of the bath water can be adequately maintained by a continuous small stream of warm water.[35] (Young children require continuous supervision.) After the first 5 to 10 minutes, active exercises are encouraged for all joints. If the neck is particularly stiff, a small towel can be rung out in warm water and wrapped around the neck. This may mean the child has to get up extra early to accomplish this. Because mornings are generally a hectic time in most families, both patients and parents are appreciative of any suggestions the therapist can offer to smooth out the transition from bed to school.

Children with JRA have so much pain and stiffness that it is often difficult for them to distinguish between the two. If the main problem is stiffness, motion tends to make it better. If the main problem is pain (inflammation), motion *may* make it worse.

For example, consider Jonathan, a 12-year-old boy with active arthritis in both wrists and both knees. His wrists were incredibly stiff in the morning, and trying to move through the stiffness to do wrist exercises was distressful for him. He discovered that dribbling a 10-inch rubber ball loosened up his wrists and made them feel better. So this became part of his morning routine. It worked for him because his main problem was stiffness. Had his main problem been pain and inflammation, bouncing the ball probably would have made it worse. Each child's home program clearly has to be matched with his or her individual needs and interests.

COMPLIANCE

Compliance, or patient cooperation, in therapeutic regimens is critical for successful management of JRA and is often the major challenge in delivering therapy. Several factors complicate the task of attaining full cooperation or follow-through from the child: (1) the need to integrate regimens into the family's routine; (2) the child's desire for novelty and control; and (3) difficulty for the child in understanding the need for ongoing exercise despite adequate functioning. (This last factor is often closely associated with psychological denial.)

Litt and Cusky have studied children with JRA in regard to compliance with medical regimens and physical therapy.[62] They found the following positive correlations with compliance: (1) adolescents with more internal control orientation and higher self-esteem, (2) previous hospitalization for the disease, (3) recommendations for thermotherapy, and (4) parents' perception that the exercise was effective. The main negative correlation was among parents who reported "difficulty getting through the day." These parents tended to be older and had children with other significant health problems.

Variables of socioeconomics, patient education, age, and sex have been investigated in other populations with no conclusive evidence. However, the following five components have been suggested to assist the patient and family in compliance.

1. Specific, written instructions should be at the level of understanding and in the language of the patient and family.

2. A simple program should include a maximum of five to seven exercises.

3. Parent and patient should understand the relation of exercise, activity, or orthosis to disease.

4. Therapeutic regimens must be consistent with family life-style, and it helps to actually schedule what time an activity will be performed.

5. Child and parent should be motivated with a positive age-appropriate reinforcer for the child (e.g., stickers for a toddler, trips to a movie for an older child).

6. Activities should be changed periodically to prevent monotony.

DRUG THERAPY

Medications are chosen on the basis of severity of the systemic and articular manifestations rather than disease classification.

Aspirin and Nonsteroidal Anti-inflammatory Drugs (NSAIDs)

The initial drug of choice may be either aspirin or another NSAID. Two NSAIDs are current approved for children: naproxen (Naprosyn) and tolmetin (Tolectin).[5] Of the two, naproxen is sometimes preferred because it is given in two doses per day, rather than three or four doses per day as tolmetin is. Dosage can be a critical factor influencing patient and parent compliance. For example, naproxen can be taken before and after school and therefore reduces the stigma of taking medications at school.[5] Naproxen is also available in a liquid form, which makes it easier to give to small children.

Only two NSAIDs are approved for children, although pediatric rheumatologists in major research treatment centers have experience using other NSAIDs with children. All the NSAIDs work with about the same efficacy, but children react differently to each of them. Trial and error is the only method available to match the child with the drug. There are no predictive indicators.

Some of the NSAIDs have properties that encourage their selection[63]:

1. The propionic acid derivatives (ibu-profen, naproxen, and fenoprofen) may be more effective in reducing fevers.

2. Clinoril (sulindac) causes less renal toxicity and is the drug of choice if a child has renal disease.

3. In young children with systemic disease, drugs with a short half-life, such as ibuprofen, may be preferable because they can be given more frequently, offering more control over the inflammation. In older children, a drug with a longer half-life, such as naproxen, would be preferable because it is given less frequently and is thus likely to increase compliance.

Sucralfate (Carafate), one of a new group of drugs, coats the stomach and creates a barrier to protect the stomach from NSAID irritation. Sucralfate is taken one half hour before the NSAID.

Most children are responsive to one of the NSAIDs. If after a (approximately) 1-month trial period the patient's symptoms are not reduced to a well-controlled level, a different NSAID should be tried.

Aspirin is generally well tolerated by children if it is taken with meals. It is typically given in four divided doses of 80 mg per kg of body weight each day.[64] The main side effects of aspirin and other NSAIDs are gastrointestinal symptoms in the form of "stomach upset." Younger children do not complain of tinnitus from toxicity as older children and adults do, but they can develop metabolic acidosis or hyperpnea.[5] Another serious potential side effect is liver toxicity (hepatotoxicity). Children on aspirin therapy, therefore, need careful monitoring. There have also been a few reports of Reye's syndrome (acute encephalopathy and fatty infiltration of the liver and other organs) in children with JRA on aspirin therapy who incidentally developed a viral infection, especially chickenpox.[65,66] For all of these reasons, some physicians prefer to use an NSAID, but aspirin is still considered a mainstay drug of choice.

Gold

At Children's Hospital of Los Angeles, intramuscular gold is the preferred second-line drug for children who do not respond adequately to NSAIDs alone. Adding a second-line drug is indicated when (1) x-ray findings show diminished joint space or joint erosions in older children, (2) there is loss of ROM, (3) an increased number of joints are involved, or (4) ambulation is reduced and the patient is becoming bed bound.[63]

Gold is administered initially in weekly injections (1 mg per kg) for 5 months to 1 year; the frequency of injections is then changed to once every 2 weeks and eventually every 3 weeks. A complete blood count (CBC) and urinalysis are done before each injection. Gold is rarely administered to children on a monthly basis as it is to adults. In pediatrics, children who need it only once a month are probably doing well enough to be taken off the medication. In contrast to adult management, children are not kept on disease-modifying drugs (DMDs) forever. For example, if a child has no evidence of active disease for 6 to 12 months, medication is generally discontinued.[6]

Auranofin (oral gold) is used on an experimental basis and is not officially approved for children. Auranofin is sometimes used when parents refuse to allow their child to receive injections. Some children who do well on the intramuscular gold also do well on the oral gold, which is easier to take and less expensive to administer. For these reasons, children may be switched to Auranofin.[67]

Other Second-Line Drugs

Plaquenil and D-penicillamine play the same role in the management of disease in children as they do with adults. Plaquenil may be tried before gold because of the easier method of administration. It is frequently the second DMD to be used.[67]

Low-dose intermittent (weekly) methotrexate is proving successful with children as it has with adults and is frequently the second or third choice of DMD. Penicillamine is now seldom used with children (and adults) because it has greater toxicity than low-dose methotrexate. However, it may provide an option if all other DMD have failed.[67]

Corticosteroids

Oral corticosteroids are not given to children except in extreme situations, such as when cardiac involvement is life-threatening, or when all other medications and therapy have failed and corticosteroids would allow the child to be ambulatory rather than bed bound.

Low daily doses are the most common form of administration. Occasionally intermittent high-dose intramuscular injections followed by low-dose oral corticosteroids may be used as a method for controlling severe disease without the effects of chronic corticosteroid use. For children, the physical and psychological effects of being bed bound are worse than the effects of the corticosteroids, which can suppress growth as well as cause Cushing's syndrome and osteoporosis.[5,67] (See Chapter 3 for a detailed discussion of the side effects of corticosteroids.)

Intra-articular cortiscosteroid injections do not have a deleterious systemic effect and are safely used in children of all ages. But no more than three injections should be given in the same joint during a 1-year period. The only residual effect may be asymptomatic calcium deposition at the injection site.

Corticosteroids are also used in eyedrops for iridocyclitis. If used over a prolonged period, these can result in corneal cataracts and have been associated with glaucoma.[67]

REFERENCES

1. Brewer, EJ, et al: Current proposed revision of JRA criteria. Arthritis Rheum 20(Suppl 2):195–199, 1977.
2. Glass, D, Kitvin, D, and Wallace, K: Early onset pauciarticular JRA associated with DRw5, iritis and antinuclear antibody. J Clin Invest 66:426, 429, 1980.
3. Gewanter, HL, Royhmann, KJ, and Baum, J: The prevalence of juvenile arthritis. Arthritis Rheum 26:599, 1983.
4. Stillman, JS, and Barry, PE: Juvenile rheumatoid arthritis: Series 2. Arthritis Rheum 20(Suppl 2):171–175, 1977.
5. Kredich, DW: Chronic arthritis in childhood. Med Clin North Am 70(2):305–322, 1986.
6. Petty, RE: Epidemiology of JRA. In Miller JJ III (ed): Juvenile Rheumatoid Arthritis. PSG, Littleton, MA, 1979.
7. Jacobs, JC: Pediatric Rheumatology for the Practitioner, Springer-Verlag, New York, 1982.

8. Alepa, FP: Juvenile rheumatoid arthritis. Primary Care 11(2):243–258, 1984.
9. Schaller, J: Juvenile rheumatoid arthritis: series I. Arthritis Rheum 20(Suppl 2):165–170, 1977.
10. Cassidy, JT: Juvenile rheumatoid arthritis. In Kelly, WN, Ruddy, S, Harris, ED, and Sledge, CB (eds): Textbook of Rheumatology, WB Saunders, Philadelphia, 1981.
11. Baum, J, and Gutowska, G: Death in JRA. Arthritis Rheum 20(2):253–255, 1977.
12. Jacobs, J: Juvenile rheumatoid arthritis. In Downey, JA, and Low, NL (eds): The Child with Disabling Illness: Principles of Rehabilitation. Raven Press, New York, 1982.
13. Shaller, J, and Wedgewood, RJ: Juvenile rheumatoid arthritis: A review. Pediatrics 50(6):940–953, 1972.
14. Alepa, FP: Juvenile rheumatoid arthritis. In Riggs, GK, and Gall, EP (eds): Rheumatic Diseases—Rehabilitation and Management. Butterworth & Co, Boston, 1984.
15. Ansell, B: Chronic arthritis in childhood. Ann Rheum Dis 37:107–120, 1978.
16. Ansell, BM: Juvenile chronic arthritis with persistently positive tests for rheumatoid factor. Ann Pediatr (Paris) 30:545, 1983.
17. Chylack, LT: The ocular manifestations of JRA. Arthritis Rheum 20(2):217–223, 1977.
18. Schaller, JG: Iridocyclitis. Arthritis Rheum 20(2):227–228, 1977.
19. Ball, J: Enthesopathy of rheumatoid and ankylosing spondylitis. Ann Rheum Dis 30:213–223, 1971.
20. Beales, JD, Keen, JH, and Lennox Holt, PF: The child's perception of the disease and the experience of pain in juvenile chronic arthritis. J Rheumatol 10:61–65, 1983.
21. Laaksonen, AL, and Laine, V: A comparative study of joint pain in adults and juvenile rheumatoid arthritis. Ann Rheum Dis 20:386, 1961.
22. Scott, PJ, Ansell, BM, and Huskinsson, EC: Measurement of pain in juvenile chronic polyarthritis. Ann Rheum Dis 36:186, 1977.
23. Varni, JW, and Jay, SM: Biobehavioral factors in juvenile rheumatoid arthritis: Implications for research and practice. Clinical Psychology Review (in press).
24. Ansell, BM, and Kent, PA: Radiological changes in juvenile chronic polyarthritis. Skeletal Radiol 1:129–144, 1977. (This journal reviews radiology by subtypes.)
25. Forrester, DM, Nesson, JW, and Brown, JC: Radiology of Joint Disease, ed 2. WB Saunders, Philadelphia.
26. Chaplin, D, Pulkki, T, Saarimaa, A, and Vainio, K: Wrist and finger deformities in juvenile rheumatoid arthritis. Acta Rheum Scand 15:206–223, 1969.
27. deAndrade, JR, Grant, C, and Dixon, ASJ: Joint distensions and reflex muscle inhibition in the knee. J Bone Joint Surg 47A:313, 1965 (also see Chap 1 of this text).
28. Nalebuff, EA, and Potter, TA: Rheumatoid involvement of tendon and tendon sheaths in the hand. Clin Orthop 59:147, 1968.
29. Ansell, BM: Juvenile arthritis. Clin Rheum Dis 10(3):657–672 (review), 1984.
30. Granberry, WM, and Mangum, GL: The hand on the child with juvenile arthritis. J Hand Surg 5:105–113, 1980.
31. Nalebuff, EA, Yerid, G, and Millender, LH: Incidence and severity of wrist involvement in juvenile rheumatoid arthritis. J Bone Joint Surg 54A:905, 1972.
32. Flatt, AE: The Care of the Rheumatoid Hand. CV Mosby, St Louis, 1974.
33. Nalebuff, EA, and Millenter, LH: (1) Surgical treatment of the swan-neck deformity in rheumatoid arthritis and (2) surgical treatment of the boutonniere deformity in rheumatoid arthritis. Orthop Clin North Am 6:733–764, 1975. (This review contains classification of these deformities.)
34. Outline Assessment of JRA Wrist and Hand. Handout from Children's Hospital of Los Angeles, Division of Physical and Occupational Therapy (revised by Marcy Atwood, May 1982).
35. Mehn, J, Hanson, V, and Isaacson, J: Management of Contractures of Juvenile Rheumatoid Arthritis. Handout from Children's Hospital of Los Angeles, 1981.
36. Lower Extremity Splints/Orthoses Used in Juvenile Rheumatoid Arthritis. Outline of treatment from Children's Hospital of Los Angeles, Division of Physical Therapy and Occupational Therapy, April 1985.
37. Scott, RD, and Sledge, CB: The surgery of juvenile rheumatoid arthritis. In Kelly, WN, Harris, ED, Ruddy, S (eds): Textbook of Rheumatology, ed 2. WB Saunders, Philadelphia, 1985.
38. Ansell, BM: Juvenile arthritis. Clin Rheum Dis 10(3):657–672, 1984. (This article reviews hand involvement.)
39. Bywaters, EGL: Pathology of juvenile chronic polyarthritis. In Arden, GP, and Ansell, BM (eds): Surgical Management of Juvenile Chronic Polyarthritis. Grune & Stratton, New York, 1978.
40. Hensinger, RN, et al: Changes in the cervical spine in juvenile rheumatoid arthritis. J Bone Joint Surg 68A(2):189–198, 1986.
41. Bywaters, EGL: Pathologic aspects of juvenile chronic polyarthritis. Arthritis Rheum 20(2):271–276, 1977.
42. Jackson, R: The Cervical Syndrome, ed 4. Charles C Thomas, Springfield, IL, 1977.
43. Physical Therapy in JRA. Outline of treatment from Children's Hospital of Los Angeles, Division of Physical and Occupational Therapy.
44. Svantesson, H, Marhaug, G, and Haeffner, F: Scoliosis in children with juvenile rheumatoid arthritis. Scand J Rheum 10:65–68, 1981.
45. Brewer, EJ: Reduction of morning stiffness and pain using a sleeping bag. Pediatrics 56(4):621, 1975.
46. Kent, JN, Carlton, DM, and Zide, MF: Rheumatoid disease and related arthropathies. II. Surgical rehabilitation of the temporomandibular joint. Oral Surg 61(5):423–439, 1986.
47. Friedman, MH, and Weisberg, J: Application of orthopedic principles in evaluation of the temporomandibular joint. Phys Ther 62:597, 1982.
48. Arden, GP: Upper limb problems. In Arden, GP, and Ansell, BM (eds): Surgical Management of Juvenile Chronic Polyarthritis. Grune & Stratton, New York, 1978.
49. Norkin, C, and Levangie, P: Joint Structure and Function. FA Davis, Philadelphia, 1983.

50. Arden, GP: Upper limb problems. In Arden, GP, and Ansell, GM (eds): Surgical Management of Juvenile Chronic Polyarthritis. Grune & Stratton, New York, 1978.

51. Granberry, WM, and Brewer, EJ: The combined pediatric-orthopedic approach to the management of juvenile rheumatoid arthritis. Orthop Clin North Am 9(2):481–507, 1978.

52. Bernstein, B, Forrester, D, Singsen, B, et al: Hip joint restoration in juvenile rheumatoid arthritis. Arthritis Rheum 20(5):1099–1104, 1977.

53. Jacobs, JC, Dick, HM, Downey, JA, et al: Weight bearing as a treatment for damaged hips in juvenile rheumatoid arthritis [letter]. N Engl J Med 305(7):409, 1981.

54. Swann, M: Management of lower limb deformities. In Arden, GP, and Ansell, BM (eds): Surgical Management of Juvenile Chronic Polyarthritis. Grune & Stratton, New York, 1979.

55. Sledge, CB: Joint replacement surgery in JRA. Arthritis Rheum 20(Suppl 2):567–572, 1977.

56. Eyrin, EJ, and Murray, WR: The effect of joint position on the pressure of intra-articular effusion. J Bone Joint Surg 46A:1235, 1964.

57. Jayson, M, and Dixon, SJ: Intra-articular pressure in RA of the knee. III. Pressure changes during joint use. Ann Rheum Dis 29:401, 1970a.

58. Vanace, PW: Yount fasciotomy in the treatment of progressive knee deformities. Arthritis Rheum 20(Suppl 2):575, 1977.

59. Granberry, WM: Synovectomy in juvenile rheumatoid arthritis. Arthritis Rheum 20(Suppl 2):561–564, 1977.

60. Inman, VT: Hallux valgus: A review of etiologic factors. Orthop Clin North Am 5(1):59–66, 1974.

61. Wood, B: The painful foot. In Kelly, WN, Ruddy, S, Harris, ED, and Sledge, CB (eds): Textbook of Rheumatology. WB Saunders, Philadelphia, 1981.

62. Litt, IF, Cuskey, WR, and Rosenberg, A: Role of self-esteem and autonomy in determining medication compliance among adolescents with juvenile rheumatoid arthritis. Pediatrics 69(1):15–17, 1982.

63. Bernstein, B (Head, Division of Rheumatology, Children's Hospital of Los Angeles): Personal communication, September 24, 1987.

64. Baum, J: Aspirin in the treatment of juvenile arthritis. Am J Med 74(6a):10–15, 1983.

65. Remington, PL, Shabino, CL, McGee, HC, et al: Reye syndrome and juvenile rheumatoid arthritis in Michigan. Am J Dis Child 139:870–872, 1985.

66. Rennebohm, RM, Huebi, JE, Daugherty, CL, and Daniels, SR: Reye syndrome in children receiving salicylate therapy for connective tissue disease. J Pediatr 107:877–880, 1985.

67. Bernstein, B: Juvenile rheumatoid arthritis. In Moss, JA, and Stiehm, ER (eds): Pediatric Update. Elsevier, New York, 1986, pp 201–213.

ADDITIONAL SOURCES

Allen, RC, and Ansell, BM: Juvenile chronic arthritis—Clinical subgroups with particular relationship to adult patterns of disease. Postgrad Med J 62(731):821–826, 1986 (review).

Allin, RE, and Lawton, DS: The Management of Ju-venile Chronic Polyarthritis. The Association of Paediatric Chartered Physiotherapists, 1977. (Order from Physiotherapy Department, Brays School, Brays Road, Birmingham, B 26 1 NS, England.)

Baldwin, J: Movement in the hands of children with arthritis. Physiotherapy 61(7):208, 1975.

Calabro, J, et al: Juvenile rheumatoid arthritis: A general review and report of 100 patients observed for 15 years. Semin Arthritis Rheum 5(3):257–298, 1976.

Cherry, DB: Review of physical therapy alternatives for reducing muscle contracture. Phys Ther 60(7):877–881, 1980.

Coley, IL: The child with JRA. Am J Occup Ther 26(7):325–329, 1972.

DeBenedetti, C: Juvenile rheumatoid arthritis. Compr Ther 2(10):53–62, 1976.

Donovan, WH: Physical measures in the treatment of juvenile rheumatoid arthritis. In Miller, J (ed): Juvenile Rheumatoid Arthritis. PSG Publishing, Littleton, MA, 1979.

Fink, CW, Ansell, BM, and Wood, PHN: Juvenile arthritis in England—A long-term follow up. Arth Rheum 23:673, 1980 (abstract).

Garcia-Morteo, O, and Maldonado-Cocco, JA: Rehabilitation of severe hip damage in juvenile arthritis. Arthritis Rheum 26(6):815, 1983.

Hanissian, AS: Pediatric Rheumatology Case Studies. Medical Examination Publishing, 1979.

Hollister, JR: Immunosuppressant therapy of juvenile rheumatoid arthritis. Arthritis Rheum 20(Suppl 2):544–547, 1977.

Horn, J, and Glickman, L: Toe splint. Phys Ther 63(5):677–678, 1983.

Juvenile rheumatoid arthritis. Patient Care 11(10), 1977.

Levinson, JE: The ideal program for juvenile arthritis. Arthritis Rheum 20(Suppl 2):607–610, 1977.

Licht, S (ed): Arthritis and Physical Medicine. Waverly Press, Baltimore, 1969.

Management of Juvenile Rheumatoid Arthritis—A Handbook for Occupational and Physical Therapists. (This handbook is available from La Rabida Children's Hospital and Research Center, Rheumatology Department, E 65th Street at Lake Michigan, Chicago, IL 60649.)

Miller, JE (ed): Juvenile Rheumatoid Arthritis. PSG Publishing, Littleton, MA, 1979.

Moore, TD (ed): Arthritis in Childhood: Report of the Eightieth Ross Conference in Pediatric Research. Ross Laboratories, Columbus, OH, 1981.

Nicholas, JJ, and Ziegler, G: Cylinder splints: Their use in the treatment of arthritis of the knee. Arch Phys Med Rehabil 58:264–267, 1977.

Nicholas, JJ, et al: Splinting in rheumatoid arthritis. II. Evaluation of lightcast II fiberglass polymer splints. Arch Phys Med Rehabil 63:95–96, 1982.

Ozel, AT, and Kolke, FJ: Rheumatoid arthritis in children. Minn Med 60(9):637–639, 1977.

Person, DA: Juvenile rheumatoid arthritis: Diagnosis and medical management. AORN J 44(3):428, 1986.

Rosenberg, AM: Uveitis associated with juvenile rheumatoid arthritis. Semin Arthritis Rheum 16(3):158–173, 1987 (review).

Sapega, AA, Queendenfeld, TC, Moyer, RA, and Butler, RA: Biophysical factors in range of motion exercise. The Physician and Sports Medicine 9(12):57–65, 1981.

Scull, SA, Dow, MB, and Athreya, BH: Physical and occupational therapy for children with rheumatic diseases. Pediatr Clin North Am 33(5):1053–1077, 1986.

Taylor, N, Sand, PL, and Jebson, R: Evaluation of hand function in children. Arch Phys Med 54:129–135, 1973.

Surgery

Ansell, BM, and Swann, M: The management of chronic arthritis in children. J Bone Joint Surg (Br) 65(5):536–543, 1983.

Arden, GP: Surgical treatment of juvenile rheumatoid arthritis. Ann Chir Gynaecol 198:103–109, 1985.

Colville, J, et al: Total hip replacement in juvenile rheumatoid arthritis. Analysis of 59 hips. Acta Orthop Scand 50(2):197–203, 1979.

Garcia-Morteo, O, Maldonado-Cocco, JA, and Babini, JC: Ectopic ossification following total hip replacement in juvenile rheumatoid arthritis. J Bone Joint Surg (Am) 65(6):812–814, 1983.

Greaves, JD: Endotracheal intubation in Still's disease. Br J Anaesth 51(1):75–76, 1979.

Green, WT, Jr: Orthopedic overview of juvenile rheumatoid arthritis. Pediatr Ann 5(4):82–94, 1976.

Herring, JA: Destructive arthritis of the hip in juvenile rheumatoid arthritis. J Pediatr Orthop 4(2):259–261, 1984.

Lachiewicz, PF, McCaskill, B, Inglis, A, Ranawat, CS, and Rosenstein, BD: Total hip arthroplasty in juvenile rheumatoid arthritis—Two- to eleven-year results. J Bone Joint Surg (Am) 68(4):502–508, 1986.

Morgensen, B, Svantesson, H, and Lidgren, L: Surface replacement of the hip in juvenile chronic arthritis. Scand J Rheumatol 10(4):269–272, 1981.

Ranawat, CS, Bryan, WJ, and Inglis, AE: Total knee arthroplasty in juvenile arthritis. Arthritis Rheum 26(9):1140–1144, 1983.

Roach, JW, and Paradies, LH: Total hip arthroplasty performed during adolescence. J Pediatr Orthop 4(4):418–421, 1984.

Ruddlesdin, C, Ansell, BM, Arden, GP, and Swann, M: Arthritis of the hip in children. Lancet 2(8501):260, 1986.

Ruddlesdin, C, Ansell, BM, Arden, GP, and Swann, M: Total hip replacement in children with juvenile chronic arthritis. J Bone Joint Surg (Br) 68(2):218–222, 1986.

Scott, RD, Sarokhan, AJ, and Dalziel, R: Total hip and total knee arthroplasty in juvenile rheumatoid arthritis. Clin Orthop Jan–Feb (182):90–98, 1984.

Simon, S, et al: Leg length discrepancies in monoarticular and pauciarticular juvenile rheumatoid arthritis. J Bone Joint Surg 63A(2):209–215, 1981.

Singsen, BH, et al: Total hip replacement in children with arthritis. Arthritis Rheum 21(4):401–406, 1978.

Swann, M: Juvenile chronic arthritis. Clin Orthop (219):38–49, 1987.

Psychology

Beales, JG, Holt, PJ, Keen, JH, and Mellor, VP: Children with juvenile chronic arthritis: Their beliefs about their illness and therapy. Ann Rheum Dis 42(5):481–486, 1983.

Beyer, JE, and Byers, ML: Knowledge of pediatric pain: The state of the art. Children's Health Care 13:150–157, 1985.

Katz, ER, Varni, JW, and Jay, SM: Behavioral assessment and management of pediatric pain. Prog Behav Modif 18:163–193, 1984 (review).

King, K, and Hanson, V: Psychosocial aspects of juvenile rheumatoid arthritis. Pediatr Clin North Am 33(5):1221–1237, 1986.

Litt, IF, Cuskey, WR, and Rosenberg, A: Role of self-esteem and autonomy in determining medication compliance among adolescents with juvenile rheumatoid arthritis. Pediatrics 69(1):15–17, 1982.

Perrin, EC, Ramsey, BK, and Sandler, HM: Competent kids: Children and adolescents with a chronic illness. Child Care Health Dev 13(1):13–32, 1987.

Rapoff, MA, Lindsley, CB, and Christophersen, ER: Improving compliance with medical regimens: Case study with juvenile rheumatoid arthritis. Arch Phys Med Rehabil 65(5):267–269, 1984.

Wynn, K, and Eckel, E: Juvenile rheumatoid arthritis and home physical therapy program compliance. Physical and Occupational Therapy in Pediatrics 6(1):Spring, 1986.

Chapter 15

Developmental Assessment and Integration

MARCY ATWOOD, M.A., O.T.R.

The child with juvenile rheumatoid arthritis (JRA) has developmental needs similar to those of other children. To appreciate the complexities of development, the therapist must maintain a broad, creative mode of thinking that encompasses biological, psychological, social, and cognitive areas in the present as well as along a continuum of skill attainment. The occupational therapist's unique perspective ensures that this developmental and biomechanical approach is carried throughout all rehabilitation efforts.

To assess the degree to which the child is able to perform age-appropriate activities, the therapist must be familiar with (1) basic principles of development and assessment, (2) fundamental developmental sequences, and (3) developmental norms in neuromotor, psychological, social, and cognitive areas. To assist the synthesis of this information, a summary description of four developmental stages (toddler, preschool, school-age, and adolescent) has been created to show the impact of JRA on the child's overall development (Table 15–1). This information will assist the therapist in setting realistic expectations for the child's skills and behavior. *Before* conducting a developmental assessment, therapists should be knowledgeable about JRA and the nature of the child's specific joint involvement. This will allow the therapist to focus on the evaluation and to formulate a plan that integrates developmental concepts with physical remediation. At the end of this chapter is an outline for an occupational therapy assessment of children and adolescents with arthritis (Table 15–8), which integrates assessment of development, occupational role, and physical and psychological status as described in this chapter and Chapters 14 and 16. Chapter 17 presents three case studies that illustrate this type of integrated assessment and treatment.

DEVELOPMENTAL PERSPECTIVES

Development proceeds in a hierarchical fashion, which means that successful accomplishment of basic skills is necessary for competency at higher levels. All children follow similar sequences as determined by a delicate balance of neuromotor maturation and environmental challenge. Most theorists believe that there is a particular stage of development in which learning in response to the appropriate stimuli is easier than at other times. This is called a **critical** or **sensitive period.**[1,2] Consequently, if a particular skill is introduced too early, the child may become frustrated; if introduced too late, that skill may be more difficult to learn. For example, training a child to tie shoes at age 3 may result in failure, because fine motor coordination is not yet advanced; toilet training at age 1 to 1½ years is futile without sphincter control, which occurs around age 3. Conversely, learning a new language is much easier for young children than for adults, according to this concept. Thus, the timing and content of environmental stimuli play an integral part in development.

All systems develop interdependently and parallel to each other, more or less. However, in children with chronic diseases, a "scattering" of skills or uneven development is not uncommon. The child with JRA is no exception. While cognitive skills may be at one level, disease-imposed limitations (decreased range of motion, strength, or pain) may delay gross motor development and decrease opportunities for social and environmental exploration. These factors, coupled with parental overprotection, may contribute to delayed self-care and social skills. Each child will pose a different set of problems and challenges. The therapist's task is to ascertain the child's strengths for adaptively accomplishing age-appropriate skills.

DEVELOPMENTAL ASSESSMENT

The developmental theories presented here represent four areas that are most directly affected by the disease process: neuromotor, emotional, social, and cognitive development. These theories provide a developmental framework for understanding the child and applying this knowledge to treatment. Before interpretations regarding age level can be made, one must consider the standardization of assessment procedures, variability in age ranges, and the fact that the child may temporarily regress during periods of acute illness.

In the clinic setting, the therapist may not have time to perform a full developmental assessment. However, screening can be performed with a few basic tools and good observational skills. If major deficits are detected in the screening, further evaluations should be performed. The screening should include a developmental history (either by the physician, nurse, or occupational therapist), which assesses environmental factors that may have influenced development; that is, stresses or other illnesses, prenatal factors, the child's rate of development, familial patterns, and history of developmental milestones. Parents' descriptions of the child's behaviors can supplement those behaviors that the examiner may not observe directly.[1]

Guidelines for Assessment Process

Cooperation of the child during the evaluations is necessary for gaining an accurate picture of the child's skills. To promote optimal results during evaluations, while also promoting a positive experience for the child, the following recommendations are suggested:

1. Scheduling. The initial evaluation should be scheduled at the patient's best time for increased alertness and mobility— preferably not in the morning or after blood tests! Although you will need a full account of morning stiffness and the associated functional limitations, the initial evaluation preferably should assess full available range of motion (ROM), manipulative hand skills, strength, and functional status (developmental/psychosocial).

2. Preparation. Gathering toys and tools or arranging the room prior to the assessment encourages an organized, relaxed flow to your evaluation. This is particularly important if the patient is highly distractable. Also, an organized approach encourages both the parents' and the child's trust and confidence in the therapist.

3. Rapport. The time should be taken to establish rapport with the patient before the physical assessment. A toddler can be invited to play with toys or assessment tools while the therapist observes, plays with the child, or interviews the parent. A school-age child or adolescent may be interviewed about personal interests, school activities, or daily routine prior to the "hands-on" assessment. In all cases, the therapist must be sincere, and the patient must trust the therapist.

4. Instruction. After explaining the nature of occupational therapy, the therapist should prepare the patient for each part of the evaluation by explaining what tools will be used and what will be done. Children usually benefit from a demonstration prior to assessment. They may want to try out the tool on you or the parent. (Do whatever is necessary to put the child at ease!) As is evident, your flexibility will make all aspects of evaluation easier.

5. Therapist flexibility. During the physical and joint assessments, standard positioning is certainly optimal for accuracy in measurements; however, you may need to adapt the evaluation to the cognitive level or behavioral tolerance of your patient.

Example 1. The standardized supine position for assessing upper extremity passive range of motion (PROM) is very threatening to a toddler (especially one in pain!). If the child cannot be calmed by your entertaining diversions (toys, books, or songs), a more accommodating position may have to be assumed for a general picture of the child's physical status (e.g., being seated or in a parent's arms).

Example 2. Directions for manual muscle testing are difficult for toddlers to understand. You may need to alter directions ("hold like a statue," "be a strong man," "don't let me push it down"), or demonstrate muscle testing on parents.

Example 3. Pain in children can translate into an aversion to being touched. You may then have the option of assessing only functional strength or ROM (e.g., observation of the child playing with toys in an antigravity position to indicate at least 3.5/5 or fair+ strength or better). *Note:* Young children are experts at compensating for limited joint range or strength by using other body parts. At some point, then, it will be necessary to gain an accurate picture of specific joint movement as well as total functional use.

6. Observations. Keen observations are an essential part of the pediatric evaluation and will often yield as much information as standardized procedures. By observation, one can note the functional range of joints, which joints are guarded or avoided, the child's interaction with the environment (passive or eager involvement), energy level, and problem-solving and risk-taking skills.

7. Demonstration. Finally, whenever possible, the patient's demonstration of self-care skills is preferable to an interview. If a parent has been habitually performing personal-care duties for the child, neither parent nor child may have an accurate picture of the patient's capabilities.

When demonstration is not possible, an interview with directed questions, such as "Can you tell me how you put on your shirt?" can yield information regarding difficulties and may alleviate discrepancies between parent's and child's reporting. A cautionary note regarding pain: As stated, a parent's interpretation of the child's pain may be more severe than the child's perception. It is helpful to view the functional limitations pain imposes through context of the typical day. An hour-by-hour accounting of the daily routine provides a picture of the play–rest–work balance, energy for social interaction, sleep patterns, interests, and responsibilities.

In summary, at all costs, try to gain the child's confidence. You will undoubtedly be following the individual for a long time and will want to initiate a trusting experience.

DEVELOPMENTAL SEQUENCES

Neuromotor Development

Neuromotor development refers to the maturation of the nervous system and parallel acquisition of control over the muscular system.[1] In other words, the development of motor skills is dependent upon the physical maturation of the nervous system and its response to environmental stimuli. Reflexes dominate early patterns of movement until increased strength and voluntary control expand an infant's capabilities. Neuromotor development is nearly complete at 2 years of age and becomes more

precise through practice by 6 years of age.[1] In effect, the nervous, muscular, and cognitive systems develop simultaneously to create a developmental process that is greater than the sum of its parts. The human integrates, organizes, and adaptively responds to environmental demands.

A formal developmental assessment (such as the Gesell or Bayley) may not always be necessary; however, knowledge of the patient's developmental level is essential for well-integrated therapy. The following discussion provides a brief picture of gross motor, fine motor, and adaptive developmental and self-care sequences (Table 15–2). For an informal assessment of developmental status, the therapist can refer to Tables 15–1, 15–2, 15–3, and 15–4 as general guides to developmental sequences. Although JRA is rarely detected before 6 months of age, previous stages will be included to understand this sequence.

Gross Motor Development

The following sequence refers to milestones as determined by Gesell[1,2] (see Table 15–2). Gross motor development begins with movement patterns *in utero*. The newborn emerges with a complete lack of head control, assuming positions of full flexion (prone) and extension (supine). Patterns of movement are largely dominated by reflexive movements. Although they appear aimless, these movements integrate the sensory experiences so that the child pays attention to visual, kinesthetic, and auditory sensory stimuli. As early as 3 months of age, the child has established increased head control but needs support in a sitting position. From a prone position, the child lifts the head off the floor while leaning weight on the forearms; from a supine position, the child is able to move the arms and to swipe at objects.

By 5 to 6 months, the infant can sit unsupported, which facilitates purposeful reaching. The baby can bear weight on his or her legs while being held in a standing position, and can smoothly roll from prone to supine and reverse. The infant now creeps bearing weight on hands and abdomen off the floor. At 9 months the infant crawls, creeps, and begins to pull to standing. The baby then cruises with support of

(*Text continues on p. 201*).

**Table 15–1 Effect of Juvenile Rheumatoid Arthritis on Selected
Developmental Tasks***

Developmental Tasks	How They Are Normally Accomplished	Restrictions due to Severe Polyarticular JRA	Therapeutic Intervention to Facilitate Development
TODDLER (Ages 1–3 Years)			
Gaining sense of control over self and environment†	By increasing motor development By increasing mobility By exploring surroundings	Impaired motor development Lack of mobility Decreased opportunity for exploration Treatments that restrict normal movement (splinting, casting, positioning)	Enhance strength and coordination Therapy on scooter (prone) board, platform swing, or large Swiss ball to enhance equilibrium Place objects within reach during positioning procedures and during parallel play
Differentiating self from others	By actively moving through space By manipulating objects By interacting with people	Decreased active movement in all planes Decreased interaction with other children Less chance for reaching, manipulating objects	Treat with or near other kids Place objects within available reach Therapy that incorporates varied movements
Gaining confidence through internal feedback from movement†	Through positive internal feedback from movement and balance	Normal feedback, which gives a positive sensation of movement, is masked by pain and stiffness Stiffness and joint limitations and decreased strength may diminish balance, which further decreases positive feedback and confidence	Help alleviate pain Provide for mastery of physical tasks Incorporate movement activities that do not cause pain (pool, prone balancing on a large Swiss ball or platform swing)
Increasing one's concept of cause-and-effect relationship	By playing and exploring	Possible decreased exploration resulting from static positioning	Position educational toys in reach while tilting (e.g., pull toys, busy box) Integrate causality into therapy choices
PRESCHOOL (Ages 3–5 Years)			
Increasing awareness of self in relationship to others†	By experimenting with spatial relationships, objects, and people through play	Decreased body schema awareness Decreased opportunity for novel experiences Decreased interaction with others	Attend therapy with others Water play with others Tactile stimulation to increase self-awareness Explore a variety of new textures, toys, people, and settings

Table 15–1 Effect of Juvenile Rheumatoid Arthritis on Selected Developmental Tasks* (*Continued*)

Developmental Tasks	How They Are Normally Accomplished	Restrictions due to Severe Polyarticular JRA	Therapeutic Intervention to Facilitate Development
Playing cooperatively Learning social roles†	By children working together By increasing verbal communication By observing adult routines	Decreased socializing; isolation	Play with others in therapy Attend a preschool program Role model (e.g., model parents, teachers, and therapists in grooming and household chores) Encourage games with siblings
Learning a sense of self-identity† Imitating play	By watching others By acting out episodes; using imagination through play	Not always able to learn full extent of their own limitations or assets because of overprotectiveness or lack of successful experiences	Play house on tilt table Clean kitchen Dress up Experience new toys or situations
Taking responsibility for self; developing self-care habits†	By learning to dress, to feed, and to write for self By watching and imitating others By using others as role models	Decreased independence secondary to time limitation and functional inabilities	Reinforce participation in ADLs Reinforce education of parents Pick up toys after self Clean kitchen
Acquiring motor skills	By playing; experimenting with body in space Through mastery of one skill (which encourages further skill development)	Decreased potential for overall movement Increased fear of falling when balance reactions are not strong	Use platform swing/ bolster to place children in alternate planes; encourage varied nonhabitual movements Encourage participation in appropriate physical play activities (e.g., ball, social games, walking) Pool activities

SCHOOL AGE (5–11 Years)

Learning physical skills necessary for school, games (throwing, kicking, writing, using tools)	By learning through school activities By learning through practicing in gym class, recess, and after-school games	Missed schoolwork Decreased joint mobility Pain limits type of activity and involvement Decreased energy for after-school games, sports	Increase basic skills; physical coordination; balance through craft, games, and activities that do not stress affected joints

Table 15–1 Effect of Juvenile Rheumatoid Arthritis on Selected Developmental Tasks* (*Continued*)

Developmental Tasks	How They Are Normally Accomplished	Restrictions due to Severe Polyarticular JRA	Therapeutic Intervention to Facilitate Development
Becoming a contributing member of society; feeling useful†	By making presents for parents in school By performing chores By receiving positive feedback from parents and authority figures for task accomplishment	Decreased attendance at school or social groups Limited opportunity to master a skill Excluded from chores Decreased self-esteem and confidence	Make gifts or provide a service to others Help clean equipment Experience success (e.g., mastery at a hobby) Do chores at home
Mastering tasks that contribute to self-identity†	With paper and pencil activities at school with others By competitive games, sports By exploring and trying new interests and hobbies By using adults as role models	Limited opportunity for competition Limited chance for exploration of interest or skill Limited exposure to new experiences and people	Use mildly competitive games during therapy (beanbag, Velcro darts) Encourage trying new crafts or cooking Provide novelty whenever possible Encourage assessment of personal strengths and limitations
Getting along with peers; receiving peer approval to validate self-concept†	Through group involvement By belonging to groups By feedback from family peers, and teachers	Limited involvement with groups Limited social interaction	Treat in groups whenever possible
Developing morals and respect for others	Through parents, school, and peer groups	Lack of participating in performing chores Limited involvement with helping and caring for others Limited responsibility for self	Encourage responsibility for self (dressing, treatment, chores, time) Make child accountable for behavior (be consistent in follow-through with consequences for behavior)

Table 15–1 Effect of Juvenile Rheumatoid Arthritis on Selected
Developmental Tasks* (*Continued*)

Developmental Tasks	How They Are Normally Accomplished	Restrictions due to Severe Polyarticular JRA	Therapeutic Intervention to Facilitate Development
Achieving independence	By crossing the street, playing next door with neighbors, dressing self, taking the bus, choosing games, making own purchases, ordering things by mail	Increased dependence on parents Often restricted to home Need assistance in self-care Decreased decision making	Encourage patient to make decisions Give choices when possible Encourage ADL independence Encourage activities outside the home (e.g., Brownies, Cub Scouts, visit friends)

ADOLESCENCE (12–18 Years)

Separating from parent or adult†			
a. Emotionally	By developing constructive channels for emotional release By developing coping mechanisms By spending more time with peers By making decisions for self By taking responsibility for self (i.e., behavior) and belongings (e.g., car)	Limited physical mobility Limited constructive channels for emotional release Overprotection by parents Exclusion from medical and physical management decisions Limited responsibility for self and belongings	Encourage ventilation of feelings in group activities or individual settings Role play uncomfortable situations Explore self-help techniques for pain Make responsible for expressions of anger, discuss methods for handling frustration
b. Physically	By learning to cook, to budget, to drive, and to care for self	Dependence on others for self-care and living skills	Train patient to be independent in self-care or direct others in his care Increase ability to make decisions (e.g., choices in treatment activities, times) Incorporate independent living, personal safety, money management, and problem-solving skills into treatment goals

Table 15–1 Effect of Juvenile Rheumatoid Arthritis on Selected Developmental Tasks* (*Continued*)

Developmental Tasks	How They Are Normally Accomplished	Restrictions due to Severe Polyarticular JRA	Therapeutic Intervention to Facilitate Development
Developing a positive self-concept: accepting one's physique	By increasing awareness of one's body and establishing a good body image By acquiring knowledge of one's assets and liabilities (by exposure to varied experiences) By receiving reinforcement through peer groups, family, and school	Possible deficit in body awareness and body image Poor sense of identity (assets and abilities) because of limited exposure Lack of positive social reinforcement because of decreased social contact (e.g., peers, school)	Train patient to be aware of body: know one's joint ranges, draw onself: label parts that are strong, painful, and so forth Perform exercise in front of mirror, massage body, experience different planes of movement Enhance appearance: groom daily, know proper care, consult with cosmetologist, discuss flattering styles, and so forth Achieve competence in work and hobby during group and individual sessions Request feedback from others regarding performances

*Developmental tasks as described by Erickson[9] and Havighurst.[10]
†Most affected areas of maturity
Compiled by Marcy Atwood, MA, OTR.

Table 15–2 Development Norms: Gross Motor, Fine Motor, Adaptive and Language Skills

Gross Motor	Fine Motor-Adaptive	Language
NEWBORN TO 3 MONTHS		
Lifts head when in prone position momentarily Lies with head to one side (tonic neck reflex) Head lag when pulled from supine to sitting Makes swimming movements when in prone position Head erect with bobbing in vertical position Sits with back rounded when supported Raises chest when in prone position—usually supported on forearm	Sucking, rooting, and Moro reflexes present Palmar and plantar grasp reflexes present Does not reach for object but holds object when placed in hand for a moment Random movement of arms Follows moving object to midline Holds hands in front of self, plays with hands Reaches for or bats at shiny objects Brings hands to mouth Holds rattle for brief time Movements are symmetric	Cries when hungry and uncomfortable Responds to moderate sound by ceasing activity or widening eyes Makes small throaty sounds Pays attention to speaking voice

Table 15–2 Development Norms: Gross Motor, Fine Motor, Adaptive and Language Skills (*Continued*)

Gross Motor	Fine Motor-Adaptive	Language
3 TO 6 MONTHS		
Symmetrical body posture	Palmar grasp disappearing	Coos and gurgles
Holds head steady	Holds hands open	Very "talkative"
Lifts head and shoulders up 90 degrees	Moves arms at sight of toy	Laughs out loud
Tries to roll from back to side	Hand-to-mouth movements	Vocalizes displeasure
Tonic neck reflex disappears	Reaches for objects beyond grasp	Babbles
Supports some weight on legs	Whole hand grasp of moderate sized objects	Shows displeasure with crowing
No head lag when pulled to sitting	Holds object in each hand briefly	
Moro reflex disappears	Raking grasp	
Sits propped		
Neck righting reflex developing		
Turns over both ways		
May pull self to sitting		
Stepping reflex disappearing		
6 TO 9 MONTHS		
Head precedes body when pulled to sitting	Bangs two objects together	Makes two syllable sounds
Sits alone leaning on arms	Transfers toys from hand to hand	Says *Ma Ma* and *Da Da* without meaning
Plays with feet	Reach and grasp is direct	Imitates expressions
Bounces when in standing position	Beginning pincer grasp	Sounds stand for things
Sits alone steadily	Holds own bottle	Responds to adults' emotional tone
Hitches	Puts nipple in and out at will	Cries when scolded
Crawls	Feeds self cracker	
Creeps	Rooting, sucking, and plantar grasp reflexes disappear	
Gets to sitting position		
Parachute reflex developing		
9 TO 12 MONTHS		
Sits steadily	True pincer grasp	Says one or two words appropriately
Does not like to lie down except when sleepy	Picks up small objects	Knows own name
Pulls self to standing	Can release a toy	Uses jargon
Creeps well	Can hold and mark with crayon	Communicates with self and others
Cruises		Recognizes *no, no*
Stands erect with help of mother's hand		Speech development slows with onset of walking
Walks with help		
Can sit down without help		
Landau reflex developing		

**Table 15–2 Development Norms: Gross Motor, Fine Motor, Adaptive and
Language Skills (*Continued*)**

Gross Motor	Fine Motor-Adaptive	Language
1 YEAR OLD		
Walks alone—wide-based gait	Builds tower of 2 to 4 blocks	Uses jargon
Walking improves, becomes form of play	Throws objects	Names familiar pictures or objects
Creeps up stairs	Opens boxes	Vocalizes wants
Runs—seldom falls	Pokes fingers in holes	Points to desired objects
Pulls toy behind	Turns pages of a book	Knows about 10 words
Walks backward	Differentiates between straight and curved lines	Uses short phrases
Climbs steps or upon furniture	Throws ball	Points to several body parts
Seats self on small chair	Scribbles vigorously	
	Grasps spoon, takes to mouth but spills food	
2 YEAR OLD		
Steady gait	Builds tower of 5 to 8 blocks	Has about 300 words
Walks up and down stairs—both feet on one step	Can make cubes into a train	Uses pronouns
Runs—fewer falls	Can open door by turning knob	Jargon disappears
Walks on tip toes	Imitates vertical strokes	Makes 3 to 4 word sentences
Can stand on one foot alone	Uses spoon with little spilling	Does not readily ask for help
Can ride a tricycle	Manipulates play material	Enjoys hearing stories
Throws ball overhand	Can drink from small glass held in one hand	
3 YEAR OLD		
Jumps with both feet	Builds tower of 9 blocks	Knows nursery rhymes
Jumps off bottom step	Imitates building of bridge	May count to 10
Goes upstairs with alternate feet	Copies circle—imitates cross	Names one color
Rides tricycle	Cuts inaccurately with scissors	Uses pronouns
Throws ball without losing balance		Asks questions
4 YEAR OLD		
Balances one foot 4 to 8 seconds	Imitates gate of blocks	Questioning
Hops on one foot	Copies cross	Follows directional cues: over, under, up, down
Walks on heels	Cuts accurately with scissors	Tells tall tales
Goes downstairs on alternate feet	Works simple puzzles	Names two colors
Skips on one foot		Repeats 3 digits
Throws ball overhand with some direction		

Table 15–2 Development Norms: Gross Motor, Fine Motor, Adaptive and Language Skills (*Continued*)

Gross Motor	Fine Motor-Adaptive	Language
	5 YEAR OLD	
Climbs purposefully	Makes gate from model	Gives age
Runs upstairs and downstairs quickly	Copies square and triangle	Compares 2 items
Tries to skip with alternate feet	Colors, staying in lines	Distinguishes day and night
Uses good posture stance	Works puzzles with several parts	Repeats 4 digits
Balances on one foot for 8 seconds		Obeys 3 commands
Hops in place 7 times		Names 4 colors
Throws ball overhand with fair direction		
Bounces and catches ball with both hands		
Uses hands and arms to catch ball		
	6 YEAR OLD	
Balances on one foot for 10 seconds	Copies triangle	Repeats 5 digits
Jumps 8 inches with both feet together	Hammers vigorously	Knows number of fingers
Tries to walk heel to toe	Plays organized table games	Names weekdays
May ride bike	Likes art forms	Right from left
Learns to pitch underhand	Prints first name	Counts 13 pennies
Uses hands to catch ball	Copies printing ABC	
	7 YEAR OLD	
Rides bicycle within limits	Plays table activities	Continues development in reading, writing, and verbal skills
May jump rope	Adept at art forms	
Walks heel to toe	Copies diamond	
Accurately pitches underhand	Prints full name	
Successfully throws overhand with direction		
Uses hands to catch ball		
Learns to bat ball		
	8 YEAR OLD	
Rides bicycle longer distances	Copies geometric patterns	Continues development of reading, writing, and verbal skills
Plays active games without difficulty	Smooth eye–hand coordination	
Jumps rope	Likes creative construction	
Jumps with both feet together 12 to 14 inches	Plays table games	
Team play		
Good eye–motor control		
Skilled performance		

Ages 0 to 2 years from Evans, Marilyn and Hansen, Beverly. *Guide to Pediatric Nursing.* New York, Appleton-Century-Crofts, 1980.
  Ages 3 to 8 compiled by Marcy Atwood, MA, OTR.

Table 15–3 Ages for Self-Care Skill Acquisition

Acquisition of Hygiene Skills

12 months	Cooperates in washing and drying hands
18 months	Washes and dries hands
24–36 months	Washes and dries face with assistance
24 months	Knows hot and cold faucets
36 months	Turns faucets on and off
24–50 months	Washes and dries hands and face without help
36 months	Blows nose on request
24–36 months	Brushes teeth with help
32–48 months	Blows nose independently
60 months	Brushes teeth without help
5–8 years	Bathes without help
6–8 years	Brushes and combs hair with supervision
6 years	Cleans nails
6 years	Shines shoes

Acquisition of Toileting Skills

12–15 months	Indicates wet or soiled pants
12 months	Approaches bathroom willingly
12–18 months	Sits on potty with assistance
12–24 months	Verbalizes toilet needs
18–24 months	May be toilet regulated by adults
24–36 months	Knows difference between bowel and bladder and communicates the difference
24–36 months	Anticipates need to eliminate on time during day
24 months	Pulls down pants for toileting
30 months	Approaches toilet when prompted
31–48 months	Cares for self at toilet; requires help in wiping
42 months	Pulls up pants
44 months	Goes to toilet alone
60 months	Totally cares for toileting needs, including flushing toilet, washing and drying hands

Acquisition of Undressing Skills

12–18 months	Takes off hat, shoes, socks
18–24 months	Unzips zipper
24–36 months	Undresses except for fasteners
24–36 months	Undresses without help
24–36 months	Unbuttons
48 months	Unzips back zipper and undoes buttons

Acquisition of Dressing Skills

7–12 months	Cooperates in dressing
16½–18 months	Places hat on head
22–26 months	Puts shoes on partway but may put on wrong feet
24–30 months	Pulls on shorts
18–48 months	Zips large zipper (first uses zipper pull)
33–38 months	Puts on coat, dress, shirt, shoes, and socks with supervision
33–38 months	Dresses with supervision
36 months	Knows front from back
24–36 months	Buttons large buttons
33–36 months	Does snaps
48 months	Puts on socks without help; discriminates front from back of clothes
18–66 months	Identifies shoe with correct foot
5–6 years	Ties shoes; buttons small buttons
	Dress and undress completely; simple meal preparation

Table 15–3 Ages for Self-Care Skill Acquisition (*Continued*)

Acquisition of Feeding Skills

3 months	Sucks food off spoon
3½–4½ months	Recognizes bottle visually
4–5 months	Pats bottle, both hands, while feeding
4½–5½ months	Places both hands on bottle
5½–9 months	Holds own bottle
6½–12 months	Drinks from held cup or glass
7–9 months	Feeds self cracker or cookie
9–12 months	Finger feeds
12–18 months	Uses spoon, with spilling
12–18 months	Drinks from cup with spilling, unassisted
15 months	Leaves dish on tray
18 months	Sucks from straw
18 months	Hands back dish to adult
18 months	Lifts and returns cup to tray
20–30 months	Holds small cup in one hand
22–25 months	Unwraps food
19–36 months	Uses a fork
24–30 months	Feeds self, little spilling
30–36 months	Pours liquid from container
30–48 months	Uses napkin
31+ months	Serves self with little spilling
36–72 months	Pours from pitcher
43–72 months	Prepares dry cereal
48 months	Holds spoon with mature grasp
55–60 months	Uses knife to spread
55–84 months	Fixes a sandwich
67–96 months	Cuts with a knife
79–90 months	Uses proper utensil with different foods

Compiled by Laura Vogtle, OTR, from the following instruments:
  The Vineland Social Maturity Scale
  The Brigance Inventory of Early Development
  The Learning Accomplishment Profile
  The Early Learning Accomplishment Profile
  The Hawaii Early Learning Profile
  The Developmental Profile (Alpern-Bowle)
  Norms from *Developmental Diagnosis*[2]

furniture. The child's strong drive toward moving and spinning toys will help motivate the child to walk.

By 13 to 14 months, the infant has taken his or her first steps with a broad-based support. The child is an energetic bundle who gains increasing confidence through positive feedback from movement. Equilibrium continues to be refined to allow going upstairs at 15 months, running and walking backward by 2 years, and balancing on one leg by 3 years. The child will experiment with the body in various planes of movement, such as jungle gyms and swings. The ability to balance and to use opposite sides of the body alternately allows the toddler to skip and to ride a tricycle by 4 years (see Table 15–2).[1,2] In the upper extremity, the 4-year-old child demonstrates the ability to throw and to catch using a stable, proximal basis of support. By 4 years old, the child's solid base of locomotion enables exploration of the environment for the purposes of learning, manipulation, and interacting socially.

In the young child with JRA, gross motor delays or temporary regressions are not uncommon. Ankle, knee, or hip pain may cause an avoidance of weight bearing in standing positions. Shoulder, elbow, and wrist pain may decrease the infant's desire to creep. In both instances, the attainment of higher-level skills, such as balancing, walking, and running, may be delayed along with a thwarted desire for active exploration. While therapy will encourage creeping and upright locomotion, the involved joints must always be considered and protected. (See the section on therapy through play and activity in Chapter 16). In addition, activities that incorporate movement in various planes of motion should be gradually introduced to promote postural security.

Fine Motor Development: Manipulative Skills

Manipulation is a primary means by which an infant explores the environment. Obviously, hand use is dependent not only upon the skill to grasp but also on the acts of reaching an object and perceiving it accurately. The interdependency of gross motor, fine motor, and visual perceptual development is demonstrated.

Erhardt's work[3,4] on the development of prehension using a neurodevelopmental approach expanded upon the previous work of Gesell[2] and Halverson.[5] In addition to recognizing the sequence of neuromotor readiness, Erhardt postulated that prehension development follows the progression of upper extremity weight bearing, which allows for elongation of flexor musculature and permits increased sensory input (tactile proprioceptive) to the hand. She stated that skills are completed by 15 months and refined through learning and practicing (at play, at school, and in self-care) up to 6 to 7 years.[3,4]

At birth, the infant holds the hands in a tight fist, grasping reflexively at anything he or she contacts. By 3 to 4 months, the infant begins to establish voluntary control over this grasp and holds, shakes, and rattles objects in an ulnar grasp (the object is held in the ulnar palm, thumb adducted). At 4 to 5 months, sitting frees the infant to explore objects further. Now using the entire hand with an expanded visual field, the infant begins to transfer objects, looking from one to the other. While the infant begins to creep at 6 to 7 months, weight is distributed on radial surface hands. This readies the neuromotor system for a radial palmar grasp (object in radial side of hand). The infant can reach more directly with advanced perception and shoulder control. At 7 to 8 months, opposition emerges that promotes manipulation of more pliable materials and finger feeding. The inferior pincer grasp (thumb abducted on radial side of index distal interphalangeal joint) precedes a precise pincer and develops at the same time as voluntary release begins. Control moves distally, and precision is enabled with increased differentiation of parts of the hand. The last skill to develop is forearm control. Writing and feeding provide practice and further refine forearm coordination. Maturation of prehension and distal upper extremity control occurs at 4 or 5 years of age when the child begins to use patterns of writing and feeding prehension similar to an adult pattern.[4] In general, fine motor and adaptive development does not tend to be delayed as long as the child with JRA is provided with environmental stimuli and toys.

Self-Care Skill Development

Self-care skills are described specifically because of the tendency for children with severe JRA to fall behind in this area. Factors attributing to this disruption or delay initially may be pain, immobilization, or parental overprotectiveness. Often children have performed a skill prior to the onset of JRA but regress during the time of acute disease activity (which is to be expected). Once the disease is controlled, however, the children (1) may have forgotten how to execute the task, (2) are not in the habit of performing the task, or (3) enjoy receiving attention from parents. This cycle reinforces dependency, and the sick role reinforces passivity and lowered expectations for the child's performance. Therefore, the importance of *participation* in self-care cannot be emphasized enough. Realize that while participation in self-care is basic to autonomy, participation can refer to actual task execution or to instructing someone to help the child with severe limitations. The latter requires teaching the child to instruct others. Parents can be prompted to focus their attention on reinforcing this independence.

Performance of self-care is dependent upon opportunity, motivation, and practice. Self-care skills can be introduced gradually as early as 1 year with washing and drying hands[2] (see Table 15–3). The child at 1 year cooperates with dressing by positioning body parts in anticipation of the task. At about 15 months to 2 years, the child begins to remove socks, shoes, and then clothes independently. As the child becomes more coordinated, he or she learns to put clothes on independently, differentiating front from back by 4 years. Between 4 and 5 years, a child can dress and undress except for small buttons, ties, and laces. At 5 or 6 years, a child demonstrates the coordination and motor planning necessary to tie shoes. By 5 years the child handles all aspects of toileting and begins to participate in grooming (using a comb and shampoo). The child from 5 years old on will additionally begin to style hair and bathe independently.

Self-care independence is expanded to meal preparation and the performance of chores or responsibilities for the school-age child and adolescent. These activities are essential to a child's self-worth. The child learns to make a sandwich or toast and to pour liquid. Simple chores include making the bed, cleaning the room, setting the table, or managing pets and plants. Later, the adolescent contends with shaving, makeup, and more complicated dressing (e.g., stockings). He or she now prepares a complete meal and accepts (theoretically) further responsibility for clothes management, housework, and shopping. For any adolescent, these chores are not usually met with enthusiasm! Tables 15–3 represents the major self-care areas with corresponding ages, compiled from a range of assessments, including Doll's *Vineland Social Maturity Scale,*[6] Brigance's *Brigance Diagnostic Inventory of Basic Skills,*[7] and Coley's *Pediatric Assessment of Self-Care Activities.*[8]

Socioemotional Development

Erikson's basis for socioemotional development proposed that individuals progress through eight stages from birth to adulthood that incorporate a widening range of personal and social relationships.[9] At each stage, the individual is met with certain psychosocial problems that must be resolved. These resolutions are positive or negative and may have long-standing implications for other areas of psychosocial

Table 15–4 Erikson's Eight Stages

Stage (Approximate Age)	Developmental Tasks
1. Oral (0–1)	Trust versus mistrust
2. Early childhood (1–2)	Autonomy versus shame, doubt
3. Play (3–5)	Initiative versus guilt
4. School	Industry versus inferiority
5. Adolescence	Identity versus identity diffusion
6. Early adulthood	Intimacy and solidarity versus isolation
7. Young and middle adulthood	Generativity versus self-absorption
8. Later adulthood	Integrity versus despair

development. For example, in Erikson's first stage, trust versus mistrust, the child depends on consistent attention for establishment of feelings of security, safety, and trust in the caretaker. Any lack of attention in this area may foster the development of mistrust, which will interfere with other psychosocial areas (i.e., intimacy, self-worth, and autonomy) (Table 15–4). The reader is encouraged to consult the references to gain a more indepth understanding of this area.

PSYCHOSOCIAL DEVELOPMENT

Research Related to Juvenile Rheumatoid Arthritis

Developmental tasks, as defined by Havighurst,[10] are those elements or behaviors an individual learns at a certain time in life that are the basis for happiness and success in later challenges. These tasks are the culmination of physical maturation, social adjustment, and the emergence of personal values. As in neuromotor development, performance in basic skills is requisite to achieving higher-level competencies. The literature in this field suggests that a chronic disease such as JRA can disrupt the accomplishment of these tasks by affecting self-esteem, sense of identity, autonomy, and future goal orientation.[13-16] Data, however, are not conclusive. Gliedman and Roth[11] put forth that the socialization process for children with chronic disabilities is different from that for able-bodied children. These children, therefore, follow a different developmental continuum than their peers. Because this theory has not been fully investigated, our discussion will assume that children with JRA are expected to perform the same skills as those without JRA in order to function as members of our society. Remember that the adaptive nature of humans will allow these tasks to be accomplished in many different ways. Research related to psychosocial issues will follow a discussion of psychosocial development.

Table 15–1 was established as a working tool to examine the effect of JRA on psychosocial development. The chart depicts selected developmental tasks most readily affected by JRA, but not exclusively. Therefore, it should be used more as a problem-solving guide than as a history of milestones. The tasks for toddlers reflect primarily Erikson's theory. Tasks for school-age children and adolescents reflect Havighurst's developmental stages.

Havighurst's depiction of developmental tasks is easily applicable to clinical settings. He creates six age periods and assigns 6 to 10 tasks for each age period in his model of developmental tasks.[10] The first developmental tasks of infancy and early childhood are concerned with mastering basic motor skills, communication, body control, learning simple concepts of social conscience and physical reality, and relating emotionally to oneself and others. In middle childhood, the child learns more advanced physical skills and develops a "wholesome" attitude toward the body. The child relates to peers and begins to identify with a masculine or feminine social role model. The middle-aged child further establishes a conscience and attitudes toward social groups, while achieving personal independence. In adolescence, more time is spent with peers, establishing mutual relationships and intimacy, and identifying with social ideas. Adolescents achieve emotional and physical independence and begin to plan for their future occupation. The adolescent has developed a set of values based on family and social influences and is increasingly responsible for his or her behavior. The capacity for abstract and future thought is demonstrated in the developmental tasks of adolescence.

Studies of psychosocial functioning of children with JRA have revealed no conclusive evidence regarding the presence of a "JRA personality" or definite psychosocial limitations.

In their review of psychosocial factors in JRA, Hanson and King[12] were unable to identify a personality profile after the onset of the disease. Early references to depression, withdrawal, hostility, and inability to express anger in the literature emanated from studies that were not controlled and did not represent a cross-section, or a uniform sampling, of all children with JRA. Hanson and King[12] noted that many of the features previously ascribed to a "JRA personality" are *reactions* to any chronic disease that would influence personality structure and social adjustment.

Problems with adjustment to JRA in relation to its severity have been studied in comparison to healthy children and to children in other chronic disease groups. Rimon and Kroll found *emotional* and *behavioral* problems—depression, anxiety, feelings of being different from other children, increased irritability, social withdrawal, overdependency, and disturbed relationships with other people—in children with JRA that did not necessarily correlate to the severity of the illness.[13] McAnarney's study[14] comparing psychosocial adjustment between healthy children and children with JRA found more emotional problems in the children with JRA. This study further revealed that children with less visible disability had more psychosocial difficulties. This finding was significant in relation to poor school adjustment, negative self-concept, and difficulty in personal adjustment. McAnarney explained this with Baker's theory of marginality: "If a child does not appear to be ill or different from his peers, normal behavior is expected of him."[14]

Kellerman and colleagues[15] conducted an extensive study on psychological functioning on 800 adolescents of varying diagnoses. They found that psychosocial maladjustment is not an inevitable result of chronic disease. Aspects of self-esteem and anxiety for adolescents with JRA compared favorably with those for healthy adolescents. However, in this study, adolescents with JRA did exhibit specific problems. They perceived less control over health than did adolescents with other disabilities and the healthy group. They also reported more illness and treatment-related disruption of body image. Lastly, Wilkinson[16] descriptively reported concerns of the adolescent in Great Britain with JRA: social isolation, decreased opportunity for sexual contact, parental dependency, and fear of the future. On the brighter side, outcome studies of social functioning of young adults with JRA found marital status, education, and employment comparable with those of their siblings and peers.[17]

Relationship of Physical Limitations to Psychosocial Development

This section highlights psychosocial evaluation and treatment considerations in consideration of physical limitations.

In the toddler with JRA, decreased mobility and decreased opportunities for varied experiences can thwart activities that promote acquisition of developmental tasks (see Table 15–1). For example, gaining a sense of autonomy over oneself and control over one's surroundings is a hallmark of children at this age. In the toddler with young-onset polyarticular JRA, weight bearing on knees and ankles may be particularly painful. Negative sensory feedback from all movement that incorporates weight bearing may inhibit the child from actively exploring the environment; the child may avoid changing positions because it induces pain or weakness. This avoidance of new situations, from lack of control over oneself and the environment, can generalize into overall decreased self-confidence or decreased risk-taking behavior. Play in various planes on gross motor equipment promotes acquisition of good balance reactions and positive feedback from movement.

Preschoolers are discovering how they fit into this world; to do this they must develop an awareness of themselves (their bodies) and their relation to others. This comes through play with other children and

adults. If the child's joints are particularly painful, he or she will not want to be touched or moved, and ultimately will not establish a clear perception of where and how each body part functions. The child may not know his or her full capabilities. A 10-year-old boy with severe polyarticular JRA stated, "Gee, I didn't know my body could do that!" when working on a large Swiss balance ball during an activity. Body awareness is integral to later development of self-concept. To encourage body awareness, a child can experiment with varied textures in therapy and working in these various planes of movement.

For preschoolers, nursery school encourages cooperative play and socialization outside the home. In the hospital, treatment groups can also facilitate the socialization process. As stated, self-care is very important and encouraged. Although the child with JRA may spend more time performing and learning self-care, the child must learn at an early age the habits involved in self-care. Most children are able to brush their teeth, comb their hair, and take off some clothes even when severely involved (see Chapter 16).

The school-age child strives to prove himself or herself as a respected member of society and thus wants to be productive and involved with friends. A child now experiments with many sports, hobbies, and crafts. Feedback from authority and peers helps formulate the self-concept. Because the school environment normally provides the arena for these experiences, a child who is frequently absent due to illness or physical limitation must use other avenues for accomplishment. At home, community groups (Brownies or Scouts), and peer play provide interaction and skill development. In therapy, assisting with chores, making articles for others, and treatment in groups are important. The necessity of the child's taking responsibility for his or her own actions (physical care and emotional outbursts) cannot be stressed enough. The child must be accountable to himself or herself and should begin to make his or her own decisions if the child is to perform responsibly later (see discussion on school in Chapter 16).

Adolescence is characterized by solidifying identity and establishing independence. These tasks can be in conflict with the child's present status if much dependency and social isolation has taken place previously. Earlier tasks culminate in adolescence as the individual continues to develop personal strengths and stronger social intimacies and becomes more future oriented in career decisions. Although society pressures adolescents to plan their futures, those who have not participated in earlier decision making may be ill equipped at this stage to make these major decisions. Therapy can facilitate the process by having the adolescent begin to make choices.

Control is important for the child at each stage, but it is manifested more obviously in the adolescent's struggle for independence. Careful measures in listening, compromising, planning, and education can prevent manifestations of independence that result in noncompliance with medications, orthoses, and exercise. Treatment should allow as many options as possible (e.g., scheduling times or activity choices); however, the limits of acceptable behavior and consequences to these actions must be clear.

Tips for Treating Adolescents

1. Be open and direct about both behavioral and task oriented expectations. Don't assume the adolescent will do any task unless explicitly stated.
2. Be consistent in treatment times and reinforcements.
3. Give the adolescent control whenever possible. Let the adolescent choose the activity and treatment times. Avoid power struggles by compromising if the situation warrants it.
4. Set goals and a weekly schedule together.
5. Hold the adolescent responsible for knowing his or her own physical status, home program, arriving to therapy on time, and pain management.
6. Listen. Acknowledge the adolescent's beliefs, feelings, and concerns.
7. Make sure activities and rewards are meaningful.
8. Acknowledge the adolescent's uniqueness and importance.
9. Discover the adolescent's interests. Ensure success and competency in one avocation.
10. Show you really care. (Don't divide your attention among other children during individual treatment; stop by just to say "Hello.")
11. Give the adolescent some personal time during the day.
12. Know yourself and your personal biases. Be able to laugh at yourself.
13. Teach to the adolescent's level.
14. Treat adolescents in groups. Enlist peers to facilitate adjustment problems.
15. Prepare the adolescent for program changes and procedures (particularly younger children).
16. Have adolescents assist in teaching others and organizing events.
17. Hold them responsible for a daily productive chore (e.g., care of the hospital pet, daily filing, stuffing envelopes).
18. Hold adolescents responsible for behavioral outbursts. Let them be aware of your feelings and how their actions affect others.

Treating the adolescent can be the most rewarding experience . . . but it won't be the easiest!

COGNITIVE DEVELOPMENT AS RELATED TO CONCEPT OF ILLNESS, EDUCATION, AND THERAPY

Piaget's work on cognitive development provides the basis for the cognitive framework presented.[18] Although no deficits in cognitive development are reported resulting directly from JRA, it is relevant to discuss cognitive development in children as it relates to the educational approach in occupational therapy, compliance in treatment, and the child's perception of the disease. Piaget describes **cognitive development** as a process of organizing our perceptions of the environment and integrating these perceptions into behaviors in terms of past and present experiences and adapting present behaviors to new situations. Piaget conceptualizes cognitive development into four states characterized by qualitatively different cognitive structures that shift from primitive egocentric reasoning to more logical abstract processes (see the section on therapy through play in Chapter 16). This sequence of cognitive development is believed to parallel the child's perception of disease[19] and has been used as a basis for formulating medical educational programs.

It is important to understand that a child's age-related level of cognition and understanding of disease-related issues may not always be at the same level. (Table 15–5 outlines the cognitive developmental stages as related to control, concept of illness, and pain perception. Table 15–6 identifies the implications for therapy of these stages. Table 15–7 outlines children's responses to illness-related questions.) Discussions of education refer to the child's comprehension and recommendations for teaching strategies. Remember that the parent and child must be included in educational sessions in order to improve treatment compliance, lessen anxiety, and stop "magical" thinking.

The following discussion will briefly explain three cognitive stages, beginning with the preoperational stage, and then relate these concepts to the child's perception of disease, compliance, and education.[20]

Preoperational Stage

General Comprehension

The child of 2 to 7 years of age develops the ability to use symbols (words or mental images) to represent, or relate to, objects or events. Thinking, however, is based on only one static perception of an experience

---

Table 15–5 Cognitive Developmental Stages as Related to Control, Concept of Illness, and Pain Perception

I. **Preoperational: Ages 2–7 years**
  A. General Comprehension
    1. Reason based on one's *immediate* experiences
    2. One perceptual focus
  B. Locus of Control: primarily *external*
  C. Concept of Illness
    1. Defines illness according to its *direct* effect on them
    2. Believes initially that illness is caused by external events, later believes illness is the result of one single event
    3. Relates illness to body changes according to *visible, external* cues (e.g., swelling, deformity)
II. **Concrete Operational: Ages 7–12**
  A. General Comprehension
    1. Begins to think *logically*
    2. Thinks *concretely*
    3. Thinks in two dimensions
  B. Locus of control: shifts from *external to internal*
  C. Concept of illness
    1. Defines illness by *concrete* signs and symptoms
    2. Understands that *illness is located inside* body
    3. Believes that self is responsible for health and illness (e.g., illness as punishment for actions or result of contact with contaminant)
III. **Formal Operational: Ages 12 and Older**
  A. General Comprehension
    1. Uses abstract thought
    2. Considers alternatives
    3. Predicts future implications
  B. Locus of Control: more internal
  C. Concept of Illness
    1. Defines illness as internal pathology
    2. Understands that illness has multidimensional causes
    3. Understands individual differences, severity, and consequences
    4. Appreciates psychological components of disease

Compiled by Marcy Atwood, MA, OTR.

Table 15–6 Cognitive Developmental Stages: Implications for Therapy

I. **Judging Disease Activity**
   A. Preschool (young) children depend on observations (guarding) and exhibit external cues (e.g., "swollen" knee or change in physical activity).
   B. School-age children equate body change with disease but do not always correctly interpret pain.
   C. Adolescents relate pain to activity or arthritis and can judge a continuum of activities.

II. **Compliance**
   A. Preschool children require a consistent schedule or routine based on visible body changes.
   B. School-age children understand simple cause-and-effect relationships and recognize short-term gains in activity.
   C. Adolescents relate illness to pathology and equate long-term gains to prevention.

III. **Reinforcement**
   A. Preschool children require external reinforcement (e.g., stickers, rewards, praise).
   B. School-age children begin to respond to internal reinforcement (charts, calendar, praise related to gains) and short-term gains.
   C. Adolescents need more internal rewards (e.g., independence, responsibility, praise for making good decisions or reaching physical goal) and long-term rewards.

Compiled by Marcy Atwood, MA, OTR.

Table 15–7 Children's Responses to Illness-Related Questions at Different Ages

Age (Years)	Responses
If a child does get sick, how can he or she get better again?	
5–7	Stay warm . . . get lots of rest
	Eat foods that are good for you
	Take medicine
9–11	Take the right medicines that can fight off the germs
	Do what the doctor says; you do different things for different sicknesses
13–15	Medicines help the body repair itself
	Eating good foods gives your body extra energy to fight off germs
How do children get sick?	
5–7	By going out in the rain without boots
	From other people
	Eating bad foods or poisons
9–11	From breathing in sick people's germs
	From germs getting inside your chest
13–15	By eating something that is a poison to your body so your heart doesn't work right
	Certain germs might get in your bloodstream and mess up the muscles and things
How can children keep from getting sick?	
5–7	Eat good foods . . . get lots of rest
	Take the medicines you're supposed to
	Stay away from sick people
9–11	Get shots to build up your tolerance to germs
	Eat vitamins so you can fight off germs
13–15	Take good care of yourself so your body will be strong enough to fight off the sickness
	Good foods nourish the fighting cells so they'll kill germs if they get inside you

(From Perrin, EC, and Perrin, JM: Clinician's assessment of children's understanding of illness. Am J Dis Child vol 137, Sept 1983, with permission.)

and is regarded only in the *immediate* presence. It is largely illogical. Piaget's classic conservation experiments demonstrated this single perceptual focus. In comparing equal quantities of water in unlike containers (short, wide, tall, or thin), the quantity is judged unequal when regarded from the single perspective of height.[18]

A child's sense of immediacy is demonstrated in cause-and-effect relationships; children believe that when two events occur in succession, the first has caused the second.[18] Finally, children do not differentiate between internal and external perceptions. They perceive thoughts as reality; body functions are related to only that which is visible.[19,21]

Concept of Illness

Children explain—identify—their illness according to its direct impact on them. "Arthritis makes me stay in bed." "Arthritis is not being able to walk." To the child, the etiology is based on one external event that may have occurred simultaneously with, or just prior to, the onset of JRA. Thus, a child whose onset of JRA occurred following unacceptable behavior may interpret arthritis as a punishment. To the child, symptoms of arthritis are perceived through external, visible cues such as swelling or redness.

Education

Potter, Potter, and Roberts[22] demonstrated that although younger children feel "more vulnerable to the disease," their general comprehension can be improved when information is presented in a global, nonspecific manner. Education is important because most children believe they get better by passive healing (staying inactive or in bed) and that any treatment that is painful is bad. When a 5-year-old Spanish-speaking boy was receiving gentle passive stretch to decrease long-standing proximal interphalangeal joint (PIP) flexion contractures, he asserted to his therapist, "I'm teaching you new words, and you're hurting me!" For him, an educational program included showing him *his* range gains after therapy and demonstrating functional uses of increased ROM. One should avoid ex-

planations that may have unintended or fearful imageries for the child.

Implications for Therapy

The child needs to see immediate results of performance in therapy, particularly associated with increased function (through play). For example, a young child can perceive orthotic positioning as bad because it restricts mobility; it is often not *until* the child can use the affected extremity *more* effectively, or *as* effectively, in play that he or she can perceive the positive aspects of orthotic treatment. For reinforcement a child will respond best to immediate external rewards such as stickers, small toys, and verbal praise. The child will also respond to exercises or education that is integrated into a dramatic story with himself or herself as the key character. (Refer to the section on therapy through play and activity, Chapter 16.)

With daily repetition, a child can learn and demonstrate a simple home program. This should be begun while the child is in the hospital (as it should for adults). *Emphasize what is right, NOT what is wrong, because the child cannot reverse logic.*

Concrete Operational Stage

General Comprehension

With the acquisition of concrete operations the child's imagery becomes less static and guided by perceptions.[19,20] The child now perceives two dimensions to situations and events, which allow him or her to *compare, to contrast, and to comprehend* changes. Although reasoning now encompasses simple logic, it is still based on the child's *own concrete* experience. It is no accident that as logic develops, formal school education commences. As the child begins to separate internal from external concepts, he or she can begin to understand internal body parts and view the associations between health, behavior, and disease (see the discussion on compliance in Chapter 14).

Concept of Illness

Children 7 to 11 years of age perceive arthritis according to its concrete, immediate manifestations. Most children identify and describe arthritis by the symptom: "Arthritis is painful. It gives me fevers. It makes my knees stiff." They are beginning to understand that illness is located inside the body, but they have little concept of internal pathology. Furthermore, they are concerned with the disease only as it affects them now and are not concerned with long-term implications.

Children believe that the cause of illness is contact with a germ (contaminant) or the consequence of engaging in a "morally bad" act. As they are gaining increased control over themselves, they may implicate themselves as the cause of the disease. In a positive light, they now see the relation between exercises and activities that lead to health and illness (see Table 15–7).

Education

The child now benefits from specific, yet simple, logical explanations of the disease. Use of comparisons, transitional sequences, simple diagrams, and demonstrations are particularly helpful. A notebook consolidates information for the child and promotes responsibility, likened to school work.

With increased cognition in linguistics, metaphors can help illustrate difficult concepts because these children can generalize from their experiences.

Children can associate several different symptoms as belonging to the same disease (fevers or swelling), although they still need structured guidelines for compliance regimens. Questions should be asked to delineate clear comprehension and avert any magical thinking.

Implications for Therapy

These children benefit from recognition of short-term gains in activity with clear associations between their actions and gains in therapy: "Therapy will let you ride a bike with your brother." "You can walk through Disneyland with your family." "Hand orthoses will let you play computer games better." This reinforces responsible behavior and promotes the maturation of an internal locus of control. Rewards should be more internally and motivationally related. (Provide a calendar for the child to mark the days of good performance and to chart

progress.) These children do need strict guidelines regarding what time to practice exercises, for how long, and for what purpose. They benefit from playing games with other children.

Formal Operational Stage

General Comprehension

The ability for abstract thought and conceptualization crystallizes during adolescence. "The adolescent can imagine the possibilities inherent in a situation, develop hypotheses concerning what might occur, and make interpretations based on his reasoning."[20] The adolescent is concerned with future implications.

Concept of Illness

The adolescent will perceive arthritis as a state of internal pathology with manifestations existing both visibly and invisibly. He or she will identify illness as an unseen process that involves sequences of multiple steps with long-term consequences. The multidimensional aspects of an illness, which include the effects of stress and emotions on physical symptomatology, can now be appreciated. It is necessary that education is accurately provided. Adolescents without correct information on the disease may create a more devastating picture in their minds than really exists.

Implications for Treatment

Adolescents are more future oriented and can equate present compliance with long-term outcomes. Education becomes very important in order for them to make informed decisions. They can understand treatment aspects of the disease over which they have control and can benefit from understanding the relationship of attitude and life stress to health, and the options of pain control measures, relaxation techniques, and psychological support.

EFFECTS OF HOSPITALIZATION ON A CHILD

Adults undoubtedly feel a loss of control and depersonalization during a hospitalization stay, but the effects on a child can be ultimately more traumatic. Wolff[23] discussed three factors that may cause emotional disturbances during a hospitalization: (1) the age of the child, (2) personality and previous living experience, and (3) treatment procedures imposed. It is suggested that children ages 2 to 4 years are the most sensitive to parental separation and show the most disturbed behavior. Infants under 7 months of age show minimal reaction to separation from parents; above this age, separation behavior will vary to 2 years of age.[24]

The stress of both an acute illness and an unfamiliar environment commonly precedes a temporary regression in development, particularly personal behavior. The last skills to develop will be the first to disappear temporarily. For example, the school-age child may revert to thumb sucking or hugging a teddy bear. These effects on the child's behavior, participation in treatment, activity level, and perception of pain may be minimized if recognized.[24]

Initially, the greatest sources of anxiety may not be directly disease related. A fear of what is happening and separation from parents and family will often provoke feelings of anxiety. Careful *preparation* for procedures—such as play therapy, using dolls, role playing, and *education*—will significantly minimize this fear and increase cooperation. Secondly, inclusion of family and friends in treatment (either by personal contact, calling, letter writing, or making items) helps decrease the child's feeling of being punished or abandoned. It is important to impress on the child that he or she is not being punished for arthritis.

Behaviorally, the acutely ill child may be demanding, accusatory, and very labile. His or her desire to participate in self-care or in therapies (play *or* exercise), or to socialize with other children is at a low level. Responses such as "you're killing me, leave me alone" are not uncommon. Attention span, concentration, creativity, and the ability to make choices from multiple options all typically decrease. To reengage the child in activity, surround him or her with personal belongings and decorate the room with his or her projects or favorite posters. Activities should be short term, and fewer activity options should be presented. Children should eat and socialize with others whenever possible.

The child hospitalized for long-term rehabilitation also needs the same preparation and contact with family; however, this child also needs more long-term involvement in activities to continue to be motivated and to prevent becoming preoccupied with himself or herself.[24] Learning a hobby (or longer-term craft) is beneficial; participation in planning group activities (puppet shows, carnivals) maintains motivation. Children need entertainment to which to look forward (e.g., family visit, lunch, or a project), and, importantly, they need to feel productive and that they are contributing to others. Helping clean up or making presents for significant others or for hospital staff addresses this need. Finally, while in the hospital, children should get dressed, try to keep similar habits as at home, and participate in daily routines so as not to assume the passivity of a sick role. See Table 15–8 for an outline of an occupational therapy assessment.

Table 15–8 Outline for Occupational Therapy Assessment for Children or Adolescents with Arthritis*

I. **History**
   A. Age, sex, school grade, ethnicity
   B. Diagnosis
   C. Medical history; previous admissions, surgeries, and therapy
      Chief complaint (reason for present admission)
   D. Medications; side effects
   E. Precautions
   F. Morning stiffness
   G. Activity level
II. **Assessments Used for This Evaluation**
   A. Specific tools; standardized or informal assessments
   B. Time of day
   C. Persons present

Table 15–8 Outline for Occupational Therapy Assessment for Children or Adolescents with Arthritis* (*Continued*)

III. **Response to Testing**
   A. Attitude, cooperation, emotions, affect, attention span
   B. Pain tolerance
   C. Parents' observations, comments, requests, complaints, concerns
IV. **Upper Extremity Joint Status**
   A. Joint status: joint pain, swelling, tightness, spasm, crepitus, deformity, subluxation, contracture
   B. ROM: active and passive
   C. Muscle strength
      1. Individual manual muscle test (MMT) for hands
      2. Group MMT for wrists, elbows, shoulders, forearms
   D. Influence of postural reflexes
   E. Quality of movement
      1. Ease, fluidity, guarding, habitual patterns of use
      2. Influence of pain: avoidance of using body parts because of pain
      3. Asymmetry in motion; tone imbalances
   F. Manipulative skills
      1. Dominance
      2. Prehension types; expanse of prehension; substitution patterns
      3. Grip/pinch strength—note position of wrist during grip
      4. Coordination: fine motor, gross motor
      5. Performance in tool use (e.g., scissors and tableware)
      6. Performance in fine motor skills (e.g., buttons, fasteners)
V. **Occupational Role Performance**
   A. Activities of daily living
      1. Self-care: feeding, dressing, hygiene, grooming, bathing transfers
      2. Daily schedules
         a. School—transportation
         b. Home—chores, responsibilities, family time, homework
         c. Therapy—outpatient or home
         d. Clubs/community involvement
         e. Work/rest/play balance
   B. Personal and emotional
      1. Age, living situation, siblings, general affect, general appearance
      2. Activity level and degree of involvement in age-appropriate activity
      3. Self-esteem
      4. Body image
      5. Knowledge of strengths and weaknesses
      6. Emotional control
   C. Understanding of disease
   D. School
      1. Degree of involvement
      2. Academic status—ability to keep up routines
      3. Problems (architectural barriers, psychosocial)
      4. PE classes
   E. Basic independent living skills
      1. Concentration, attention span
      2. Motivation, locus of control, emotional control
      3. Decision making, problem solving
      4. Time management
      5. Meal preparation, responsibility for self, social skills, shopping, laundry, transportation, money management, use of community resources
   F. Relationships
      1. Type
         a. Family: parents, siblings, extended family
         b. Peers—school/home
            School/community authority figures
         c. Hospital personnel
      2. Dyad versus group

Table 15–8 Outline for Occupational Therapy Assessment for Children or Adolescents with Arthritis* (*Continued*)

    G. Avocational interests/play
       1. Quality of play or leisure activity (individual/group; active/passive); degree of competency
       2. Strong versus casual interests
       3. Interests states versus activities performed
    H. Vocational development
       1. Academic strengths
       2. Career goals
       3. Knowledge of work world (job exploration, work values)
       4. Prevocational skills
       5. Part-time jobs
       6. Resources
       7. Avocational strengths and range of experiences

VI. Sensory-Motor Screening
    A. Visual perception
    B. Tactile perception
    C. Proprioception
    D. Motor skills

VII. Developmental Screening
    A. Gross motor
    B. Fine motor, approach, grasp, and release
    C. Adaptive
       1. Upper extremity skills, influence of use
       2. Organization of behavior
       3. Attention span
       4. Relation to cognition
    D. Language screening
       1. Receptive and expressive language
       2. Nonverbal communication
    E. Personal social
       1. ADL, including adaptive equipment
       2. Interaction with therapist, family, peers
       3. Type of educational and/or school program, accomplishments, problems
       4. Daily schedule, play behavior, and so forth
       5. Emotional and psychological status

VIII. Orthoses/Adaptive Equipment
IX. Home Programs
X. Child or Adolescent's Goals for Therapy
XI. Summary
    A. Assessment
       1. Summary of evaluation results
       2. Impact of physical limitations on development or occupational role performance
       3. Developmental deficits: scattered or generalized lag
       4. Assets and liabilities
    B. Problem list
    C. Goals: short and long term

XII. Recommendations and Plans
    A. Duration and frequency
    B. Treatment activities
    C. Nursing consultation
    D. Home program
    E. School recommendations
    F. Parental instructions
    G. Discharge planning

*See Chapter 17 for examples of this type of assessment.
Compiled by Marcy Atwood, MA, OTR, and Jeanne Melvin, MSEd, OTR.

REFERENCES

1. Illingworth, RS: The Development of the Infant and Young Child. Churchill Livingstone, New York, 1983, pp 120–162.
2. Gesell, A, and Amatruda, CS: Developmental Diagnosis. Harper & Row, New York, 1969.
3. Erhardt, RP, et al: A developmental prehension assessment for handicapped children. Am J Occup Ther 35:237–242, 1981.
4. Erhardt, RP: Developmental Hand Dysfunction: Theory, Assessment, Treatment. Ramsco Publishing, Rockville, MD, 1982.
5. Halverson, HM: An experimental study of prehension in infants by means of systematic cinema records. Genetic Psychologic Monographs 10:107–286, 1931.
6. Doll, EA: Vineland Social Maturity Scale: Condensed Manual of Directions. American Guidance Service, Circle Pines, MN, 1965.
7. Brigance, AH: Brigance Diagnostic Inventory of Basic Skills. Curriculum Associates, Woburn, MA, 1977.
8. Coley, IL: Pediatric Assessment of Self-care Activities. CV Mosby, St Louis, 1978.
9. Erickson, EH: Childhood and Society, ed 2. WW Norton & Co, New York, 1963.
10. Havighurst, EJ: Developmental Tasks and Education, ed 3. David McKay, New York, 1972.
11. Gliedman, J, and Roth, W: The unexpected minority: Handicapped children in America. Harcourt Brace Jovanovich, New York, 1980.
12. King, K, and Hanson, V: Psychosocial aspects of juvenile rheumatoid arthritis. Pediatr Clin North Am 33:1221–1237, 1986.
13. Rimon, R, and Kroll, F: Psychosomatic aspects of juvenile rheumatoid arthritis. Scand J Rheum 6(1):1–10, 1977.
14. McAnarney, ER, Pless, IB, Satterwhite, B, and Friedman, SB: Psychological problems of children with chronic juvenile arthritis. Pediatrics 53:523–528, 1974.
15. Kellerman, J, Zeltzer, L, Ellinberg, L, Dash, J, and Rigler, D: Psychological effects of illness in adolescence. I. Anxiety, self-esteem, and perception of control. J Pediatr 97:126–131, 1980.
16. Wilkinson, VA: Juvenile chronic arthritis in adolescence: Facing the reality. Int Rehab Med 3:11–17, 1981.
17. Miller, JJ, Spitz, PW, Simpson, U, and Williams, GF: The social function of young adults who had arthritis in childhood. J Pediatr 100:378–382, 1982.
18. Piaget, J: The Child and Reality: Problems of Genetic Psychology. Grossman Publishers, New York, 1973.
19. Perrin, EC, and Gerrity, SP: Development of children with a chronic illness. Pediatr Clin North Am 31:19–30, 1984.
20. Bibace, R, and Walsh, ME: Development of children's concepts of illness. Pediatrics 66:912–917, 1980.
21. Whitt, JK, Dykstra, W, and Taylor, CA: Children's conceptions of illness and cognitive development. Clinical Pediatrics 18:327–339, 1978.
22. Potter, R, Potter, PC, and Roberts, MC: Children's perceptions of chronic illness: The roles of disease symptoms, cognitive development, and information. J Pediatrics Psychology 9:13–27, 1984.
23. Wolff, S: Children under Stress. Penguin Press, London, 1969.
24. Banus, BS: The Developmental Therapist. Charles B. Slack, Thoroughfare, NJ, 1971.

ADDITIONAL SOURCES

(See additional sources in Chapters 14 and 16)

Fassler, J: Helping Children Cope: Mastering Stress through Books and Stories. The Free Press, New York, 1978.
Greene, J, Walker, L, Hickson, G, and Thompson, J: Stressful life events and somatic complaints in adolescents. Pediatrics 75(1):19–21, 1985.
Miller, J: Coping with Chronic Illness: Overcoming Powerlessness. FA Davis, Philadelphia, 1983.

Chapter 16

Treatment Considerations

MARCY ATWOOD, M.A., O.T.R.

This chapter highlights intervention strategies that help integrate the range of concerns that need to be addressed in children with juvenile rheumatoid arthritis (JRA). Provided here is an overview of (1) play and the selection of therapeutic activities appropriate to developmental and physical requirements; (2) adapted equipment to improve function in self-care, play, and school activities; (3) the challenges school poses and effective transition from hospital to community; and (4) family and adolescent psychosocial adaptation to chronic disease. Chapter 17 presents three case studies that illustrate the practical integration of motor, cognitive, and psychosocial assessment as delineated in Chapter 15, with treatment strategies discussed in this chapter.

THERAPY THROUGH PLAY AND ACTIVITY

Play is the primary means of developing a child's ability to use tools while establishing language and social skills. Theorists have approached play through many disciplines, including anthropology, psychology, sociology, and biology. Mary Reilley,[1] however, was the first to approach play through occupational therapy as its own major construct that "organizes human behavior and is the basis for adult competence." Reilly's theory is based on a system of "appreciative learning," whereby curiosity directs a child's exploration, and rules or tools of mastery give meaning to environmental interactions. Rules further govern the limits of behavior.

Florey,[2] Michelman,[3] and Takata[4] operationalized Reilly's theory to provide usable schemes of activity selection. Florey classified play according to various behaviors exhibited in human and nonhuman interactions. Takata integrated concepts of Piaget, Erikson, and Florey in a sequence of age-related epochs that focused on representative elements (materials, actions, people, and settings) for each epoch. (These epochs will be discussed later.) Michelman elaborated on Florey and Takata's concepts of constructive play and studied the development of children's creative interests.

As a general introduction, play integrates and organizes our basic senses into patterns of behavior that become more complex in response to environmental demands. Inasmuch as the environment is the stimulus for challenge, the child is self-directed in promoting his or her own development.[1] For example, a child's gross motor skills will become more refined by playing hopscotch; cognitive skills will develop through playing mailbox with plastic mail pieces in a variety of shapes; social skills are fostered through playing games. Play is unique in that it allows the child to develop basic skills without negative consequences. It is later when skills are consolidated (as in a vocation), that the child will be responsible for the outcome.

Anthropologists suggest that play in children and adults promotes flexibility in behavior that facilitates adapting to new situations and solving problems.[4] Because those with rheumatic disease are continually adapting to some aspect of the disease, the ability to play would appear to benefit the adaptation process.

In children with arthritis, joint limitations, pain, and decreased energy can potentially limit the child's ability to explore. Therefore, the play environment must come to the child. It is entirely possible that the therapist and family can arrange the environment so that the child can have these explorative opportunities. When Kielhofner and colleagues[5] studied environmental factors conducive to play in the hospital, they found that those conditions that challenged the player (while keeping the consequences of play safe) and provided social support could increase and elicit play.

The following discussion will guide the therapist in understanding stages of play and in selecting and adapting an activity. Tables are provided that compile Takata's epochs with practical activities for children and adolescents with arthritis (Table 16–1). Those particularly beneficial for elbow, wrist, or finger extension are noted as examples.

Play Development

Sensory/Motor Epoch

In the first two years, play is oriented toward the senses and those activities that produce a cause and effect on the child and the environment. The child repeats these ef-

Table 16–1 Play Epochs: General Principles and Practical Games Appropriate for the Child with Polyarticular JRA*

Typical Behavior	Fine Motor and Constructive Abilities	Gross Motor Coordination and Strength	Social-Cultural Skill Development	Imagination, Imitation, and Dramatization
AGE 0–2 YEARS				
Sensory-Motor Epoch: Emphasis on Independent Play and Exploration, Expressed through Trial and Error				
Solitary play	Simple cause and effect	Reaches, pushes, and pulls	Relates to parents and immediate family	Imitates new sounds
Enjoys different sensory experiences	Touches, mouths, throws, bangs, and shakes	Changes positions often	Develops body awareness	Learns songs
Repeats actions for practice	Likes bright colors	Creeps on all fours, stands, falls, and climbs	Develops object permanence	Recognizes self
	Repeats actions	*Examples:*	*Examples:*	*Examples:*
	Examples:	Cradle gyms	Anticipation games:	Cuddles toys
	Rattles wrist bells	Reaches for dangling toys or busy box	Pop-up toys	Rattles bells
	Pushes balls	Wades in pool	Pats picture books	Plays with see-me mirror
	Pats and points to pictures	Uses scooter board (lies prone)	Pats see-me mirror	Parent-child singing games
	Finger paints with pudding	Rolls and picks up balls	Plays peek-a-boo	
	Uses busy box	Swings brightly colored ribbons	Plays pat-a-cake	
	Plays with musical toys	Rocks toys	Applies lotion to body	
	Uses stacking rings	**Note:** Splints should protect wrists while the child uses the scooter board.	Plays with dolls	
	Water play: washes toys, splashes water, makes bubbles			
	Fingers parts of crib mobile			
AGES 2–4 YEARS				
Symbolic and Simple Construction Epoch (Preoperational): Emphasis on Parallel Play, Beginning to Share, Symbolic Play Expressed in Simple Context and Simple Constructional Use of Materials				
Increased interest in activity	Combines and takes things apart	Learns rules of motion	Learns simple action–reaction events	Make-believe friends
Increased attention span	Learns spatial relationships	Runs, jumps, balances, drags, dumps, and throws	Enjoys parallel play	Imitates adults
"Quiet play"	Empties and fills, scribbles, squeezes, and pulls	Explores environment	Learns to share and to take turns	Uses imagination in story telling
Learns basic gross motor coordination	Learns material management	*Examples:*	Demonstrates possessiveness of toys	*Examples:*
Scares easily	*Examples:*	Crawls through barrels	*Examples:*	Recites nursery rhymes
	Pats stickers on paper	Throws beanbags	Follow the leader	Dusts furniture
	Plays with dolls	Plays action games and sings songs	Hide and seek	Plays house
	Uses puppets with extended fingers	Rides prone on scooter board	Plays house with puppets and pets	Dresses up
	Sandbox—makes buildings with extended fingers	Slides		Plays musical toys
	Fingers sand to find hidden objects	Plays with water toys		Plays with miniature cars and animals
	Makes playdough pancakes	Swings prone on platform swing or large balls		Tea sets
	Masks	Walks in sandbox or grass		Story telling
	Fingerpaints	Uses wheel toys		Creates simple masks
	Smears pudding on tray			
	Applies shaving cream on wall or glass			

Table 16–1 Play Epochs: General Principles and Practical Games Appropriate for the Child with Polyarticular JRA (*Continued*)

Typical Behavior	Fine Motor and Constructive Abilities	Gross Motor Coordination and Strength	Social-Cultural Skill Development	Imagination, Imitation, and Dramatization
AGES 4–7 YEARS				
Dramatic, Complex-Constructive, and Pregame Epoch (Preoperational): Emphasis on Cooperative Play, Dramatization of Reality, Purposeful Use of Materials for Construction, and Building Habits of Skill and Tool Use				
Stubborn, rebellious, or cooperative Highly emotional: swings from one extreme to the other (either loves or hates people or things) Responds *negatively* to pressure More sensitive to reactions of adults Needs assistance to complete tasks Talks constantly Loves novelty	Likes simple construction Uses simple tools Makes useful objects Learns concept of quantity versus quality Wants products saved *Examples:* Pasting with extended fingers Fingerpaint with flat hand Traces with open hand Uses puppets Makes playdough figures Makes paper dolls and airplanes—folds with fingers extended Creates masks and paper-plate decorations or tambourines	Masters basic forms of locomotion Practices "daredevil" stunts Increases physical space and freedom Dance, hop, balance games *Examples:* Plays ring toss Rolls ball (both hands) Catches/throws Tricycles Dances Balance games—Simon Says Relay races Obstacle courses Rhythm games	Takes on social roles Cooperative and crowd play Enjoys speed/timing Often disagrees *Examples:* Leads games (Simon Says) Cleans up Makes items for others	Imitates what occurs in real life Involved in fantasy: costume and props Recognizes music *Examples:* Incorporates exercises into a story or theme Elaborates stories Plays house, doctor, or grocery store
AGES 7–12 YEARS				
Games Epoch (Concrete Operational): Emphasis on Appreciation of Friendship and Cooperative Play, Enhanced Constructional and Sport Skills with Rule-Bound Behavior, Competition, Decision Making, and Responsibility for Actions				
Sensitive to praise, blame, and failure Moody, complaining Impatient with self Gains great satisfaction from achievement Begins to think logically and concretely Sets high goals for self	Games with rules Smooth fine-motor coordination Complex projects Collecting/swapping Seasonal interests Precision in tool use *Examples:* Paper weavings Paste scrapbooks or collages Craft sets Paper airplane Simple sewing Block printing Dominos Flick paper balls into "goal" Clay coil or pinch pots Macrame Clay and bead jewelry	Refines skills for performance Combines skills Competition *Examples:* Kite flying Basketball (protect wrists) Bicycle Ball games Swimming Dance lessons Social sports: Fishing Miniature golf Velcro darts Volleyball tournaments using a beach ball	Making rules with peers Competition and compromise with peers Interested in collecting, swapping Group projects *Examples:* Organized groups or play, particularly with possessions (e.g., Brownies, stamp collecting) Building play houses Make own games	Hero worshipping Confidence in acting Plans social events *Examples:* Creative drama Play acting Magic tricks Music, dance lessons Parties

Table 16–1 Play Epochs: General Principles and Practical Games Appropriate for the Child with Polyarticular JRA (*Continued*)

Typical Behavior	Fine Motor and Constructive Abilities	Gross Motor Coordination and Strength	Social-Cultural Skill Development	Imagination, Imitation, and Dramatization
AGES 12–16 YEARS				
Recreation Epoch (Formal Operations): Emphasis on Both Team Participation and Independent Action Expressed in Organized Sports, Interest Groups, and Hobbies During Leisure Time				
Participates in long-term projects	Develops craftsmanship and special talents	Team sports	School, neighborhood, extended community involvement	Special interest groups for dancing, singing, discussion
Enjoys helping and teaching others	Knowledge of design, color	Individual precision sports (tennis or golf)	Team sports	Collecting
Likes to make useful articles	Hobbies	***Examples:***	More time spent with peers	Social role models
Wants recognition for uniqueness	***Examples:***	Frisbee	Visiting friends	Teaches others
Directs hobbies and skills toward a career	Tie dye—press palms together	Darts	Organized group altruism work	Special classes (art, photography, mechanics)
Compromises	Baking	Ring toss	Peer group belonging or opposite sex	
Wants expectations clear	Kneading dough with heel of palm	Badminton	***Examples:***	
	Decoupage: sanding with block	Fishing	Weekend trips	
	Drafting on incline table	Biking	Personal competency in skills or hobbies	
	Typing: position correctly	Walking	Seeks social rewards	
	Gardening	Low-impact aerobics	Dating	
	Origami	Social dance	Clubs	
	Playing musical instrument		Sells hobbies	
	Sewing, pattern making with extended fingers			

*The activities selected as examples are recommended for children with JRA to provide active use of upper extremity extensor musculature and full ROM. Involved joints should be protected from compressive forces. Table-top activities should be positioned at shoulder height.

Note: Children with mild or absent upper extremity involvement have a broader range of activities from which to choose.
Chart adapted from Takata, N.[4]
Compiled by Marcy Atwood, MA, OTR.

fects over and over to reproduce the patterns and outcome. The child attempts trial-and-error problem solving but still remains keyed into one perceptual focus: Play is primarily self-centered and individualistic.[4]

Symbolic and Simple Constructive Epoch

As verbal and coordination skills rapidly progress, the child interacts with the immediate social environment. The child now uses symbols to represent situations or objects. This pretend play helps organize past experiences and newly learned symbols.

Children will now play alongside one another (parallel play).[4]

Dramatic, Complex Constructive, and Pregame Epoch

A child's social arena widens to include other people outside the immediate family. The child plays with two or more children, shares tools, and begins to imitate people and situations. Through drama, the child begins to assume a social role and views himself or herself as distinct yet related to others. The child is fascinated by novelty and simple constructional activities.[4]

Game Epoch

A child's curiosity about the real world extends outside the family boundaries as the child enters school. The child becomes fascinated by how things work and the rules that govern play. Involvement in a close friendship facilitates learning cooperation prior to entering the world of competition. Imaginative play incorporates hero worship.[4]

Recreation Epoch

All previously learned skills are mastered and incorporated into a diversity of activities that allows the adolescent to develop personal competencies. Heterosexual group activities promote social cooperation. Interest in altruism and more involved constructive projects reigns high.[4]

ACTIVITY SELECTION

The selection of activities strikes a delicate balance in integrating biomechanical factors with individual preferences and developmental challenges (Fig. 16–1). Prior to initiating therapeutic play, one must determine the physical gains needed, then critically analyze the biomechanics of activity choices. Done jointly with the patient, this can be a valuable lesson in education and joint protection. Most activities can be adapted to promote physical gains (Fig. 16–2). To select and to perform an ac-

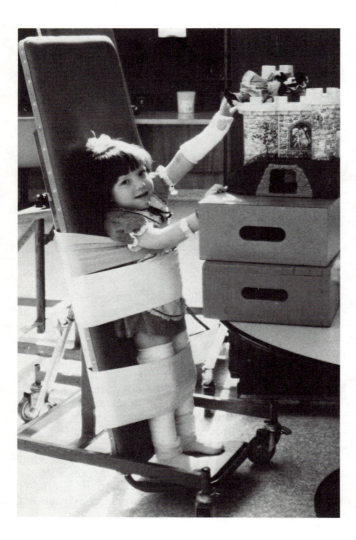

Figure 16–1. Combined biomechanical and developmental treatment. This child demonstrates tilting, a positioning method that allows *active* play to be therapeutic for improving function of the shoulders, elbows, and fingers during serial casting of the wrist and knees.

The use of a tilt table provides several advantages. It stabilizes the trunk to prevent spinal extension as a substitution for limited shoulder flexion; it encourages hip extension and neutral ankle positioning during therapy; and it requires weight bearing to facilitate bone mineralization.

This activity (acting out a play based on a medieval castle and dolls) provides imaginative, age-appropriate play, yet it is effective in providing active finger and elbow extension as well as increasing shoulder flexion and upper extremity endurance. The child was encouraged to select the play activity of her choice to increase her sense of control, help develop her decision-making skills, enhance her self-esteem, and encourage cooperation in therapy. Activities that are fun help elicit the child's full participation and cooperation in therapy.

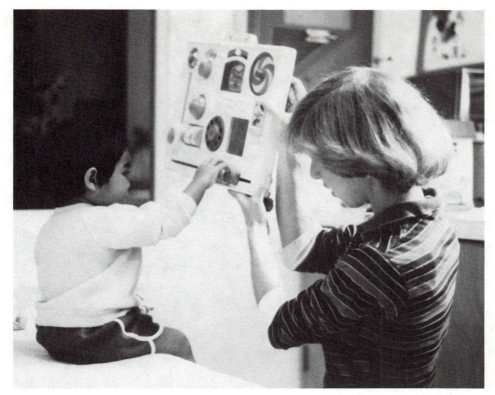

Figure 16–2. For young children, play activities can be designed and positioned to help develop basic perceptual and fine-motor skills while improving active finger ROM and shoulder ROM and endurance.

tivity, a logical process should proceed. The therapist should determine the following:

1. The child's physical needs
2. The child's cognitive level
3. His or her interests and experiences
4. Clinic resources
5. Biomechanics involved in the activities of interest (activity analysis)
6. Adaptations for the activity
7. Alternate choices

Remember to offer choices, because this promotes the child's and adolescent's decision making. When the child or adolescent embarks on a new hobby, make sure that this hobby can be continued realistically at home.

Adaptation of Activity

The principles of joint protection will apply to all activities (see Chapter 24). For the child with JRA the most important principles include

1. Avoiding activities that are statically positioned in flexion
2. Incorporating full range of motion (ROM) into the activity
3. Moving during activity at least every 20 minutes
4. Exercising extensor muscles
5. Avoiding compression on involved joints
6. Protecting involved joints
7. Avoiding long sedentary periods
8. Avoiding activities that incorporate repetitive wrist flexion or deviation in the direction of the deformity (this means avoiding ulnar deviation for some and radial deviation for others) (see section on Hand Involvement in Chapter 14)

Positioning of activity is the prime means of adapting an activity (Fig. 16–3).

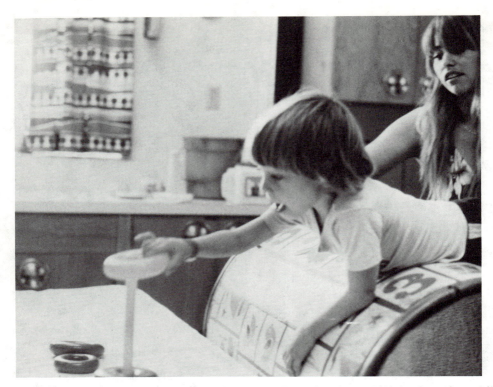

Figure 16–3. This child is playing a competitive game of stacking rings while the therapist stabilizes his feet. The use of a barrel allows movement and function in a different positional plane. This helps compensate and correct for the debilitating effects restricted movement has on equilibrium, balance, and sensory integration. This type of activity in the prone position helps strengthen neck, back, and hip extensor muscles as well as shoulder flexor, elbow, and wrist extensor muscles. It also has the advantage of being a bilateral activity.

Planning Activities for Children

Toys can be placed within a child's reach to increase endurance, range, and exploratory play. Tools can be adapted; for example, using a sanding block, enlarging handles, and adapting computer joysticks. (See the following section on adapted devices and methods.)

If the activity is on target, the child will be happily engaged and self-directed. However, this is not always the case! When children are sick, they will be irritable, short tempered, less creative, and less attentive (as we all are). (See Chapter 15, the section entitled "Effects of Hospitalization on a Child.") They may regress temporarily to previous stages of play but should be engaged, nevertheless.

Whenever a child has an unsuccessful experience with an activity, you need to ask

Table 16–2 Planning Activities for Children

Activity Level Too High	Activity Level Too Low
Typical Behavior	*Typical Behavior*
Gives up	Rushes through activity
Frustrates easily	Makes mistakes
"I don't want to do it."	Finishes early
"This is boring."	Distractable
"I'm never going to use this."	Low attention span
"I can't."	Not interested
Therapist does entire thing	Not concerned with end product
"See, I told you I couldn't do it."	
Unsuccessful end product	

the question, Why didn't it work? If the activity is on target, the child will be involved at least for an age-appropriate length of time. Often our initial throughts are that the child is uncooperative, spoiled, or not motivated. Although resistive behaviors can be signals of depression, they usually indicate that the activity is not appropriately targeted for the child. Most children can become interested in something once short-term success is demonstrated and if they are gently prompted into participation. Table 16–2 describes some behavioral manifestations of activity programs that seem unsuccessful.

ADAPTED DEVICES AND METHODS

Adapted devices accomplish the same purpose in children as in adults, that is, (1) to reduce pain and to preserve joint integrity by minimizing stress, and (2) to increase the patient's independence. (See Chapter 25 for a detailed discussion on assistive equipment for people with arthritis.)

In children, adaptive devices are prescribed less frequently than for adults and only when alternative positioning techniques still prohibit performance of a task. In general, the fewer devices the better. Some children feel more disabled and different from their peers when using the equipment. Furthermore, they complain that the equipment is burdensome when spending the night at a friend's house. These are important considerations; however, modifications are invaluable when independence is facilitated.

The scope of adaptive equipment in children includes self-care items, ambulation and positioning aids, as well as play and vocational modifications (Fig. 16–4). To determine the need for adaptive equipment, the therapist must consider the patient's level of independence (from the activities of daily living evaluation) and the need for joint protection. (See Chapter 24 for further considerations.) Recommenda-

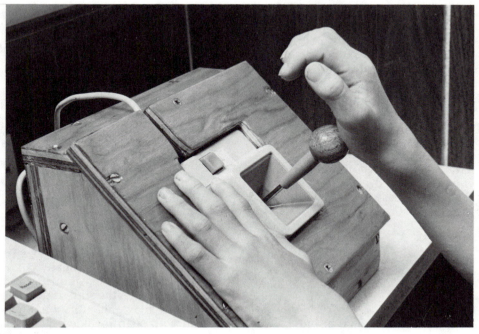

Figure 16–4. This custom-made stand allows a computer joy stick to be positioned at a specific height and angle to allow use of the stick with the wrist in extension. The enlarged handle allows operation with the palm, eliminating stress to the fingers and thumb. This is in sharp contrast to the tight cylinder grip required on vertical joy sticks.

tion and training for adaptive equipment are usually initiated at the rehabilitative phase and treatment. During acute disease activity, use of equipment may tire the patient and aggravate the inflammatory response. Also, losses in ROM, strength, or endurance may be temporary and thus not yet warrant training with assistive devices.

Once the need for adaptive equipment is determined, the patient's long-term use of the aid is dependent upon (1) the child's acceptance, (2) the child's efficient use of equipment (i.e., can the child use the equipment independently within a realistic time period?), and (3) financial status. To enhance compliance and responsibility for himself or herself, the child should participate in this problem-solving process.

Generally, adaptations include modifications of the environment, the item, or using additional equipment to perform the task. Most adaptive equipment for children includes measures to

1. Decrease weight of the item
2. Extend a handle (to increase reach)
3. Alter handle grip
4. Decrease resistance (or strength) needed for the process
5. Alter the shape of equipment already in use
6. Use of backpacks instead of shoulder bags

Commercially available equipment for adults usually does not suffice for children, because it is usually too long, too heavy, or incorrectly scaled for children. Thus, therapists and parents must summon all creative instincts to fabricate or to find alternative solutions to these problems.

The following discussion summarizes the most frequently used adaptive devices or modifications. Please refer to Chapter 25 for a discussion of household and driving devices.

Self-Care

Dressing

The child's clothes should be loose fitting for the easiest application and optimal comfort. Shirts with Dolman or raglan sleeves with a V-shaped or boat neckline are recommended. Front buttons can be al-tered by elastic thread or replaced by Velcro closures to decrease the resistance needed in buttoning (Fig. 16–5). Dresses with a drop waistline are now currently in style and are very practical to don. Pants and skirts with elastic or drawstring waistband are saviors for children and parents. Loops can be sewn to inside seams for easier use with a dressing stick. Putting on socks and shoes presents a challenge to the child with hip, knee, and ankle flexion limitations. Sock cones can be used for the child with sufficient grip to pull a sock over the cone (plastic) and sufficient plantar flexion to point the toes into the sock. However, many children are unable to complete this task. A movable piece at the bottom of the sock cone must be incorporated to rotate the equipment into flexion. (See the section on resources in Chapter 25.) Cotton/polyester socks are suggested because they expand yet retain shape. A list of the most commonly used adaptions follows.

Long-handled dressing stick
Long-handled shoehorn
Coat hanger inverted lengthwise, using hook end to pull up pant loops
Dressing clips
Velcro closures
Rivets in Velcro shoe strap to be used with dressing stick
Sock cone (make with x-ray film—plastic is too stiff)
Wide strapping attached to back side of shirt used to remove shirt over head
Hooks placed in the child's room at shoulder height (to push strap over shoulder) and at waist height (to help pull pant loops over hips)
Elastic belts
Clasp buckle
Clip-on tie
Zipper pull

Hygiene

Washing one's face is usually not a problem with a properly positioned washbasin or a stool to reach the sink. If needed, wash mitts are available that allow full finger extension with soap included in the sponge. To brush the teeth, foam padding can increase brush diameter, or an electric toothbrush can be used if cleaning is not effective. Adaptations must take the weight of

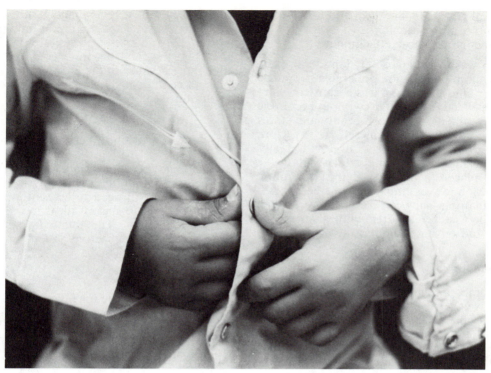

Figure 16–5. This child's hands demonstrate deformities typical of the child with polyarticular JRA. Limited dexterity and two-point tip prehension require that activities be performed with a lateral pinch. The manner in which he is using his thumbs in this activity is contributing to an instability and hyperextension deformity. A thumb interphalangeal stabilization orthosis (see Chapter 25) would stabilize his thumb and improve his prehension strength and control.

the handle into account. Some toothpaste now allows dispensing with minimal thumb opposition, which is easier to use than applying pressure to squeeze the tube.

Toileting

Toilet safety bars and elevated toilet seats are reliable assists for patients with lower extremity limitations. Problems persist, however, in locating or fabricating effective aids for children to wipe themselves. Adult commercial aids are too large in grip size and length. Clinic adaptations often do not allow for sanitary effective cleaning or removal of paper. Children's Hospital of Los Angeles has fabricated two alternative designs in the clinic. One is coiled wire (dipped in plastic coating) around which paper is wrapped, used, then knocked against the toilet side for removal. The other is a Polyform "stick" with a pyramid-shaped piece of Polyform attached to

one end. This end is used for cleaning; the shape of the "stick" can be bent to facilitate the child's reach. Some children will need a bed urinal or pan for middle-of-the-night emergencies. Toileting hygiene in school or public facilities must also be taken into account. Lastly, a bidet can be attached to a toilet for cleansing without the necessity of paper. This is less often used in the population of children at Children's Hospital of Los Angeles. (Refer to Chapter 25, "Assistive Devices.")

Bathing

Step-in showers are the most practical method for most children; however, most tub showers can be adapted for safety of child and parent. Safety is a prime prerequisite for all recommended adaptations. Most commonly used adaptations are

Tub mat nonstick surfaces

Wall grab bars—vertical and horizontal
Tub chair or bench
One-handed hose attachment

To wash in the shower, long loofa pads with cloth handles are preferable to sponge material for backs and legs because they are more effective (abrasive) without becoming heavy when wet. Most beauty-aid stores carry these. To dry oneself, a terrycloth bathrobe or poncho or a towel with a handle is suggested. Some adolescents have also placed a heater in the bathroom. Safety, however, must be considered. Additionally, a shower cap or shower screen can be used for children while shampooing to avoid getting soap into the eyes.

Grooming

Combs and brushes can be attached to lightweight handles fabricated of orthotic thermoplastic material (Hexalite or Polyform) or Alumafoam. The handle shape will most likely be altered to accommodate ROM. Children find that headbands are the easiest for holding hair back (followed by cloth-covered rubber bands and clips), but many opt for a "perm" and a short haircut that eliminates the need for constant attention and blow dryers. Whatever they decide should be supported. Makeup and shaving can be accomplished with long-handled equipment. Aerosol deodorant is difficult to adapt; however, deodorant sticks or roll-on deodorants add some extra length to reach armpits. Other adolescents attach the deodorant stick to a bedpost and simply abduct their arms to slide the deodorant stick underneath.

Feeding

Adaptations are usually needed when the child has not enough strength to cut food, to hold a cup, or to extend the neck to drink from a cup. The knives and built-up utensils described in Chapter 25 for adults can suffice. Some children, however, find plastic knives easier to use. To drink, straws or cups with a part of the top edge scooped out aid independence for limited neck mobility or upper extremity strength. As the child raises the cup during drinking, the scooped-out edge provides clearance of the nose. Finally, if the child takes a long time to eat

because of difficulty managing the food, one must consider the texture of food (is it too tough?) and size of pieces (are they too large?). If the food becomes cold and unappetizing because of the length of time requried to eat, a warming plate may provide a solution.

Avocational Activities

Many safe and appropriate toys exist that can be used for children with physical limitations. You will need to assess the child specifically and to suggest ideas to the parent or adolescent. The following adaptations have proven effective.

Crafts

Large plastic needle for sewing
Adapted handles for paintbrushes
Vices to hold items to table
Sewing frames
Pegboards for ease in storing tools
Adapted scissors
Inclined table
Adaptations for sewing-machine controls

Games and Sports

Control adaptations for electric train set, computer
Holders for drum sets
Table for water games
Big Wheels
Swing made of wooden crate padded with foam
Sandbox raised on a platform or table
Padded slide
Magnetized checkers

Writing or Drawing

(See also the section, below, "Daily School Activities—Solving Problems.")

SCHOOL INVOLVEMENT

Involvement in school is vital to all children's cognitive, psychosocial development, and the child with JRA is no exception. Although school ultimately promotes a sense of accomplishment and self-worth, it also promotes informal social learning. Social learning involves relating to authority, beginning to incorporate social values and rules into behavior systems, accepting increasing responsibility, and, most importantly, interacting with peers. Hence, every effort should be made to promote participation with a positive experience.

Many children will need only minor adjustments in school programs and physical education activities, or perhaps only permission to take medications. The more severely involved children will require a coordinated effort between health professionals and educators for maximal participation.

Factors that may impede attendance in school are decreased ability to ambulate, decreased endurance throughout the day, presence of systemic symptoms, pain, stiffness, and *fear*. Some degree of fear is inherent in every child's return to school. Whether fear of being knocked down, fear of teasing, or fear of the unknown, this emotion must be acknowledged and discussed. Methods to avert fear may simply be discussion, role playing potentially fearful situations, or visiting the school prior to resuming attendance.[6]

This section presents an outline of federal laws relating to handicapped children in school settings, present key factors implementing therapeutic adjustments for school, and specific recommendations for common school problems.

Public School Mandates

In 1975, the Education of Handicapped Children Act was established by Congress (PL 94-142). It required all schools to provide the necessary modifications for a handicapped child to receive an appropriate education "in the least restrictive setting." Although these terms lend themselves to individual interpretation, the act has had significant impact in provision of services for children ages 3 to 21 years with JRA. Basically, public school districts must provide services that are necessary for education (i.e., education for any child that has special needs); these services are not necessarily instructive in nature. "Related services" include those that increase that child's capabilities to participate in any educational program. Therapy and transportation are examples of services that improve children's capabilities.

A regular classroom is by far the best choice for most children with arthritis. It offers optimal intellectual stimulation and benefit of peer interaction. Adaptations can usually be provided with prearrangement. Schools for orthopedically handicapped children are not the best for children with JRA, inasmuch as many children in these classrooms have delayed or limited intellectual capabilities. (The majority of children will benefit from a full grade-level program.)

Home tutors are available if the child is recovering from a prolonged exacerbation or surgery necessitating more than a 2- to 4-week absence. As soon as possible, the child should be encouraged to return to school.

Part-time attendance is beneficial directly following hospitalization or an exacerbation and can usually be arranged to accommodate endurance. Missing the afternoon or even the first two morning periods is preferable to not attending at all. Lastly, a hospital teacher or supplemental homework can keep the child up to grade level during a hospitalization.[6]

School Communication and Placement

Most schools and teachers will comply with requests for adaptations if communication has been *clear, direct,* and *timely.* This is essential. The occupational therapist may need to communicate with the school nurse, adaptive physical education teacher, and classroom teacher, depending on the clinic structure and role of the therapist in individual facilities. A phone call and written information (pamphlets, too) facilitate understanding the request based on the disease. Parents and patients should initiate this process, with the therapist providing specific information. Content of communication should contain the child's physical status, functional limitations, needs during school, and recommendation for solutions. Make your plans collaboratively with educators and school nurses. (They know their setting best.)

Daily School Activities—Solving Problems

The school checklist (Table 16–3) has proven to be a particularly useful tool to identify school problems with the child and to find solutions. This can be used in the clinic or taken home for the parent and child to fill in. Many solutions relate to adaptive equipment and joint protection techniques (Fig. 16–6), as outlined in the appropriate chapters. The following is simply a problem and solution list that follows the school checklist categories.

Table 16–3 Checklist for Students with JRA

The following is a list of problems that some students with JRA have at school. Remember, every student has different problems. In order to help you, we need to know what your specific problems are. So read the list and check off those problems that apply to you. Then return the list to your doctor or any of the rheumatology team members.

Your name: _____ Date: _____

School: _____ City: _____ Grade: _____

_____ 1. Getting to school is difficult for me.
_____ 2. I have to wait for the bus or my ride outside, sometimes in the cold.
_____ 3. I get stiff when I have to sit too long.
_____ 4. I'm stiff in the morning, even after I take a warm bath.
_____ 5. I'm stiff in the morning, but I don't have time to take a warm bath before school.
_____ 6. My hands hurt when I write.
_____ 7. I can't write fast enough during tests or when taking notes.
_____ 8. Writing on the chalkboard is difficult for me.
_____ 9. I have trouble raising my hand to ask or to answer questions.
_____ 10. I sometimes forget to take my splints to school.
_____ 11. I don't have the special equipment at school that I need, such as splints, a tilt board, a wheelchair.
_____ 12. It's hard for me to take off my coat, boots, or shoes.
_____ 13. It's hard for me to turn door handles or to open my locker.
_____ 14. It's hard for me to carry my books or lunch tray.
_____ 15. I have trouble eating at school.
_____ 16. I have trouble using the bathroom at school.
_____ 17. I don't have enough time to change classes.
_____ 18. My classes, the bathroom, or the cafeteria is too far away for me.
_____ 19. Staircases are a problem for me.
_____ 20. I have trouble with fire drills or earthquake drills.
_____ 21. I have trouble changing my clothes in PE class.
_____ 22. I have trouble taking a shower in PE class.
_____ 23. I don't have time to exercise at school.
_____ 24. I'm too tired after school to exercise at home.
_____ 25. PE is too much for me.
_____ 26. My school day is long, and I'm very tired when I get home.
_____ 27. I need a rest in the middle of my school day.
_____ 28. I have trouble standing in long lines, like in the cafeteria.
_____ 29. I have trouble doing all of my homework on time.
_____ 30. I can't keep up with the other students in my schoolwork.
_____ 31. I'm absent from school a lot (1 week or more is "a lot").
_____ 32. My school makes me keep my medicine with the school staff.
_____ 33. I sometimes forget to take my medicine at school.
_____ 34. I feel different when I have to go to the office for my medicine.
_____ 35. Some of the other students make fun of my arthritis.
_____ 36. I don't know how to talk to my classmates about my arthritis.
_____ 37. My teacher doesn't understand my arthritis.
_____ 38. My teacher babies me.
_____ 39. My teacher forgets that I have arthritis.
_____ 40. Other _____

From Children's Hospital of Los Angeles. Revised 1986, with permission.

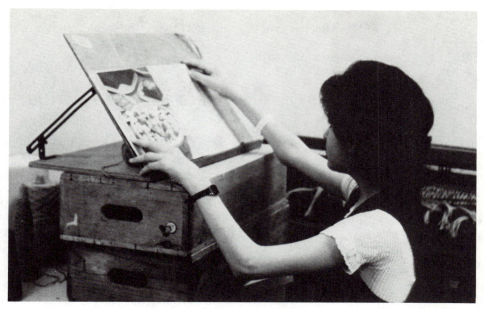

Figure 16–6. Positioning of reading materials to prevent flexion positioning of the neck is critical, especially inasmuch as reading is often a prolonged activity. At school or at home an inexpensive wire bookstand can be set up on top of a stack of books.

Transportation

Try to arrange to have the child picked up last on the bus route. This provides the child with extra time to dress and less time to sit on the bus.

Stiffness

(Refer to section on morning stiffness in Chapter 14.)

Before School
- Use electric blanket at night or take a 20-minute warm bath.
- Wear thermal underwear, or warm the clothes in the dryer prior to donning.
- Shower and dress in a warm bathroom.
- Use terry cloth robe.

During School
- Move around in class to pass out/collect papers, erase chalkboard, do errands.
- Sit in back of class so one can stand unobtrusively when joints start to become stiff.

Hand Manipulation Problems

(Refer to Chapter 24, "Joint Protection and Energy Conservation Instruction," and Chapter 25, "Assistive Devices.")

All adult joint-protection principles will apply except those favoring ulnar deviation at the wrist.

Handwriting

Pain
- Hold pencil between index and third fingers, and oppose with the thumb.
- Extend fingers every 10 to 15 minutes.
- Use built-up handles, felt-tip pens, and soft lead pencils.

Cannot Write Fast Enough
- Use dictaphone to give answers to a test instead of writing them.
- Tape lectures.
- Request extra time to complete task.

Cannot Write with Splints on
- Remove for writing.
- Use cock-up instead of gauntlet splints.
- Replace thenar piece with a foam strip.

Writing Workload
- Type homework with an electric type-writer or computer.
- Adjust homework assignments with teacher.

Carrying Difficulty

- Carry lunch tray with both hands, under tray, close to body. Use a tray of lightweight material.

Books
- Use backpack with straps on both shoulders.
- Obtain an extra set of books—one for home, one for school.
- Ask a friend to help carry heavy or bulky items.

Using Bathrooms

- Leave early from class with a friend to help carry belongings.
- Bring foldable adaptive equipment for hygiene and grooming.
- Elastic waistbands make it easier to remove clothes.

Mobility

Trouble Passing Between Classes
- Leave 5 minutes early or have a friend accompany the child during class changes.
- Try to arrange classrooms close to each other.

Physical Education
- A prescription for the child's involvement in adaptive physical education (PE) is essential. The therapist should write out a program to incorporate into PE if the child is unable to participate in the activity being performed.

Other Problems

- Can't give money to cashier: Put money on tray.
- Can't raise hand to answer question: Hold up pencil to answer question.
- Use book holder to keep book at a good angle to reduce neck pain.
- Lockers, door handles, faucets, flip-top cans, cereal boxes, milk containers, drinking from a cup: Commercially bought adaptive equipment can be useful for these special items. Please refer to self-help catalogs.

THE IMPACT OF JUVENILE RHEUMATOID ARTHRITIS ON THE FAMILY

Comprehensive treatment for JRA places multiple demands on all family members. Therefore, their adjustment to the disease and the changes in family members' roles must be considered. A family's adjustment to the disease is dependent upon several factors. Previous experiences with illness and crisis, family values, and flexibility in life-style influence adaptations.[7] A negative adjustment is one in which hostility and anger are directed at the child and health professionals. The further a disease progresses, the more responsibility is placed on the family. More hostility can result. A positive adjustment is one in which the parent is motivated to participate in therapy, follow through with home recommendations, and encourage the child to be as independent as possible.[8] A positive adjustment will take time to occur. It is facilitated by support from team members and coherence within the family. Before reaching the stage of acceptance, however, it is common that parents go through stages of acceptance as described by Kübler-Ross.[9] Parents may exhibit denial by endlessly searching for an alternative diagnosis or cure; they may vent anger at other family or health care team mambers; parents may blame "ineffective" treatment for their child's condition; or parents may assume an overassertive role in determining which therapies are necessary for their child. Although parents are encouraged to participate in therapy, they must be advised and educated carefully about treatment principles. For many parents, the most destructive emotion is guilt.[8] The belief that they somehow caused the illness can result in an overprotectiveness that limits a child's independence.

To facilitate positive adaptation for the family, identification of the emotions and the actions that accompany these emotions should be communicated between the parent and child.[8] For example, a parent's *fear* of the child harming himself or herself by falling may result in the parent prohibiting the child from riding a bike or playing outside. The child may interpret this worry as strict disciplinary or punitive measures. Discussion of these concerns with the health care team can frame the need to protect joints in a more realistic manner. To enable a smoother adjustment to the disease, the therapist may participate more specifically in the following ways.

1. Understand the child's and parents' perceptions of the disease. Ask them directly how they perceive various issues. Provide educational materials for accurate information about the disease. The family and child's lack of information about the disease may cause anxiety. Play therapy, role playing, and informal discussion will help understanding.

2. Understand the family's life-style (specific schedules, interests, family members' roles, and other family commitments). This will make clear

    a. The child's level and type of activity prior to the illness,

    b. Alterations in the family's life-style resulting from the disease,

    c. The increased demands placed on each family member (e.g., helping with self-care, driving to appointments, and bringing the child to school)

A discussion of how the family's life-style has changed and what will be the priorities for treatment will help families plan and adapt to a new schedule.

3. Discuss the parents' reactions to the illness. To some parents, the disease has shattered their hopes of a perfect child.

4. *Do not forget the siblings.* Encourage parents to spend time with the child's siblings. Siblings can easily suffer from lack of parental attention and become resentful of their added responsibility in household chores. Include siblings in home programs (play) to emphasize their importance in the treatment process. The occupational therapist or another professional on the rehabilitation team should interview the siblings to understand their feelings about the illness and their concerns about their brother or sister with JRA.

5. Emphasize the need to discipline the child with JRA as one would discipline other siblings. It is important for normal psychosocial growth.

6. Help the family find ways that they can show affection and have fun with their child!

7. Point out the need for the parents to consider their own needs for emotional support and "time off" vacations. Suggest involvement in parent support groups or individual counseling (if appropriate) to help resolve their emotional conflict about the illness.

Children's emotions need to be validated; however, they need to understand the limits of acceptable behavior. Parents do need to spell out these limits as they would for other children. Finally, parents need to give the child control over compromise situations when possible. This will enable psychological growth and decrease struggles for power.

Once open lines of communication are established, the parents and children's expectations for therapy and medical treatment should be discussed to eliminate unrealistic expectations and frustrations between the child, family, and health care team.

PROMOTING SELF-ESTEEM IN THE CHILD WITH JUVENILE RHEUMATOID ARTHRITIS

A critical determinant of adjustment to a chronic disease is the establishment of a clear self-concept and good self-esteem.[10] **Self-concept** describes an individual's view of himself or herself. In *A Dictionary of the Social Sciences,* Kuhn defines self-concept as "an individual's view of one's identity, a notion of one's interests and aversions, a concept of one's goals and successes in achieving them, a picture of the ideological (world view) frame of reference through which one views himself or herself and other objects, and some kind of self-evaluation."[11] This definition gives one an idea of the complexities involved in forming one's self-concept. **Self-esteem** is simply one's feelings about one's self-concept, the judgment one places on oneself, and the approval or disapproval of one's capacities. Self-esteem helps formulate one's perception of one's abilities to succeed;[12] therefore, one can have an accurate or inaccurate self-concept and a positive or negative self-esteem. An accurate self-concept is really the basis to positive self-esteem and is fostered inherently throughout all of occupational therapy intervention. A more thorough understanding of the components can enrich the treatment experience.

Body image is one component of self-concept that is addressed in occupational therapy. It is the very core of one's knowledge of the physical self and the core of personal control. Body image encompasses not only one's appearance but also postural cues, tactile impressions, degree of functional effectiveness, and social reinforcement.[13] A patient's knowledge of body image can be advanced during treatment by performing exercises in front of a mirror and holding the patient responsible for knowing his or her own ROM measurements. The use of lotion to massage all body parts, and actually drawing or labeling body parts marking areas of pain, makes the child much more aware of physiological and anatomical associations. If a child has not had opportunities to experience various planes of movement and postural sensations, this sensory input can be provided by swings, balls, or platform. My experience has shown that many severely involved children are fearful to engage in new experiences, or new activities that challenge their balance. If the child does not feel he or she has control over postural reactions and cannot trust what his or her body might do, the child may experience a general insecurity when introduced to new situations.

Appearance is obviously important to a majority of adolescents, who strive to be accepted by their peers. To a severely involved adolescent, acknowledgment and enhancement of physical assets are vitally important. For example, the therapist should emphasize positive aspects of physical appearance (e.g., hair, facial features, and nails) and encourage proper care for each care area. Consultations in makeup, grooming, and color coordination have been motivators to the female adolescent struggling with her own self-acceptance.[14]

Another aspect of self-esteem is the concept of control (initially discussed in psychosocial section). Control over oneself begins early and needs to be fostered at each stage (refer to the developmental task chart, Table 15–1). Inasmuch as a child with arthritis may be dependent on others for medical care, personal care, and even emotional security, control must be introduced in increments that will enhance personal responsibility. The child's participation in choosing treatment times, activities, clothes to wear, and decision making enhance control.

Competence in some avocational or academic activity can positively affect self-esteem. Although children gain increasing competence and establish personal strengths in a hobby or craft, they also need a realistic appraisal of themselves in comparison with others. Pezzuti[10] describes this comparison of self with others as a process of self-concept. Family and therapist can help validate a child's assets. The formulation of one's ideal self and achievement of this ideal are often a difficult process for the adolescent, which will require familial and peer support.

Family support and significant adults are said to influence the child's self-esteem broadly.[10] Acceptance by teachers and positive feedback from these relationships influence the child. Clearly defined limits of behavior and the endorsement of these limits positively affect self-esteem and a child's self-respect.

Finally, functional effectiveness, or degree to which a task is competently performed to the adolescent's expectations, contributes to self-esteem. Participation in self-care and independent living skills—such as cooking, money management, time management, problem solving, and personal safety—can increase self-reliance. Working in groups can reinforce the adolescent's competency socially. Group work can also help identify personal strengths and values through conversations with others.

REFERENCES

1. Reilly, M (ed): Play as Exploratory Learning: Studies in Curiosity Behavior. Sage Publications, Beverly Hills, 1974.

2. Florey, L: An approach to play and play development. Am J Occup Ther 25:275, 1971.

3. Michelman, SM: Play and the deficit child. In

Reilly, M (ed): Play as Exploratory Learning: Studies in Curiosity Behavior. Sage Publications, Beverly Hills, 1974.

4. Takata, N: Play as prescription. In Reilly M (ed): Play as Exploratory Learning: Studies in Curiosity Behavior. Sage Publications, Beverly Hills, 1974.

5. Kielhofner, G, Barris, R, Bauer, D, Shoestock, B, and Walker, L: A comparison of play behavior in hospitalized children. Am J Occup Ther 37(5):305–312, 1983.

6. Health Professionals Guide to Teaching Patients and Family with Juvenile Rheumatoid Arthritis—School Section. Arthritis Foundation, Atlanta, 1987.

7. Power, PW, and Del Orto, A: Role of the Family in the Rehabilitation of the Physically Disabled. University Park Press, Baltimore, 1980.

8. Health Professionals Guide to Teaching Patients and Family with Juvenile Rheumatoid Arthritis—Family Section. Arthritis Foundation, Atlanta, GA, 1987.

9. Kübler-Ross, E: On Death and Dying. Macmillan, New York, 1971.

10. Pezzuti, L: Self-concept/self-esteem development: Its relevance to occupational therapy. Occup Ther Health Care 2(3):41–48, 1985.

11. Gould, J, and Kolb, W (eds): A Dictionary of the Social Sciences. Free Press, New York, 1965.

12. Coopersmith, S: The antecedents of self-esteem. WH Freeman & Co, San Francisco, 1967.

13. Schilder, P: The image and appearance of the human body. The International University, New York, 1950.

14. Atwood, MJ: Occupational therapy intervention for the adolescent with juvenile rheumatoid arthritis. Occup Ther Health Care 2(3):109–126, 1985.

ADDITIONAL RESOURCES

Professional Resources

Beales, G: Juvenile arthritis—the "whole child" approach. Nursing (Oxford) 3(31):908–909, 1984.

Bibace, R, and Walsh, ME: Development of children's concepts of illness. Pediatrics 66:912–917, 1980.

Blom, GE, and Nichols, G: Emotional factors in children with RA. Am J Ortho Psychiatry 24:101–104, 1953.

Brewster, AB: Chronically ill hospitalized children's concepts of their illness. Pediatrics 69:355–362, 1982.

Coley, IL: Pediatric Self-Care Evaluation. CV Mosby, St Louis, 1978.

Eissler, RS, et al: Physical illness and handicap in children. Yale University Press, New Haven, 1977.

Ettinger, RL, Lancial, LA, and Peterson, LC: Toothbrush modifications and the assessment of hand function in children with hand disabilities. J Dentistry Handicapped 5(1), Fall 1980.

Ferris, J, and Fujishige, C: Do you have a child with JRA in your class? For a free copy, write to the Arthritis Center of Hawaii, 347 North Kuakini St, Honolulu, HI 96817.

Henoch, MJ, Batson, JW, and Baum, J: Psychosocial factors in juvenile rheumatoid arthritis. Arthritis Rheum 21:229–233, 1978.

Herstein, A, Hill, RH, and Walters, K: Adult sexuality and juvenile rheumatoid arthritis. J Rheumatol 4:35–39, 1977.

Hill, RH, et al: Juvenile rheumatoid arthritis: Follow-up into adulthood—medical, sexual and social status. Can Med Assoc J 114:789–794, May 8, 1976.

Kellerman, J, Zeltzer, L, Ellenberg, L, Dash, J, and Rigler, D: Psychological effects of illness in adolescence: Anxiety, self-esteem, and perception of control. J Pediatr 97:126–131, 1980.

Knoll, F: Children with JRA: Social and development problems. New York Chapter of the Arthritis and Rheumatism Foundation, 1958.

Llorens, L: An evaluation procedure for children 6–10 years of age. Am J Occup Ther 21:64, 1967.

MacBain, KP, and Hill, RH: A functional assessment for juvenile rheumatoid arthritis. Am J Occup Ther 26(16):326–330, 1973.

Miller, JJ III, Sjpitz, PW, Simpson, U, and Williams, GF: The social function of young adults who had arthritis in childhood. J Pediatr 100(3):378–382, 1982.

Morse, J: Aspiration and achievement. A study of 100 patients with JRA. Rehab Lit 33(10):290–303, 1972.

Pennington, V, and Sharrott, G: The developmental tasks of adolescence and the role of occupational therapy. Occup Ther Health Care 2(3), Fall 1985.

Price, A: Juvenile rheumatoid arthritis and occupational therapy. Am J Occup Ther 19(5):249–254, 1965.

Rapoff, MA: Helping parents to help their children comply with treatment regimens for chronic disease. Issues Compr Pediatr Nurs 9(3):147–156, 1986.

Rennebohm, R, and Correll, JK: Comprehensive management of juvenile rheumatoid arthritis. Nurs Clin North Am 19(4):647–662, 1984.

Silva, JM, and Klatsky, J: Body image and physical activity in recreation for the disabled child. In Bernhardt, DB (ed): Recreation for the Disabled Child. Haworth Press, New York, 1985.

Singsen, BH, Johnson, MA, and Bernstein, BA: Psychodynamics of JRA. In Miller, J (ed): Juvenile Rheumatoid Arthritis. PGS Publishing, 1979.

Taylor, J, Passo, MH, and Champion, VL: School problems and teacher responsibilities in juvenile rheumatoid arthritis. J Sch Health 57(5):186–190, 1987.

Travis, G: Juvenile rheumatoid arthritis. In Travis, G: Chronic Illness in Children, Its Impact on the Child and Family. Stanford University Press, Palo Alto, 1976.

Wolff, S: Children under Stress. Lane Press, London, 1969.

Play Theory and Programs

Azarnoff, P, and Flegal, S: A Pediatric Play Program: Developing a Therapeutic Play Program for Children in Medical Settings. Charles C Thomas, Springfield, IL, 1975.

Chance, P: Learning through Play. Gardner Press, New York, 1979.

Ellis, MJ, and Scholtz, GJL: Activity and Play of Children. Prentice-Hall, Englewood Cliffs, NJ, 1978.

Frost, JL, and Klein, BL: Children's Play and Playgrounds. Allyn & Bacon, Boston, 1979.

Hoyme, K: Play Activities for Parents of Children with Juvenile Rheumatoid Arthritis. Order from Patient Education Center, North Carolina Memorial Hospital, Manning Drive, Chapel Hill, NC 27514. Cost: $1.

Kielhofner, G, Burke, JP, and Igi, CH: A model of human occupation. Part 4. Assessment and intervention, Am J Occup Ther 34:657, 1980.

Levy, J: Play Behavior. John Wiley & Sons, New York, 1978.

Lindquist, I: Therapeutic use of play. Pediatrician 9(3–4):203–209, 1980.

Moersch, MS: Training the deaf-blind child, Am J Occup Ther 31:425, 1977.

Morris, AG: Nationally speaking: Parent education in well-baby care: A new role for occupational therapist. Am J Occup Ther 32:75, 1978.

Newman, J: Swimming for the junior arthritic child. In Newman, J (ed): Swimming for Children with Physical and Sensory Impairments: Methods and Techniques for Therapy and Recreation. Charles C Thomas, Springfield, IL, 1976.

Parent, LH: Effects of low-stimulus environment on behavior. Am J Occup Ther 32:19, 1978.

Robinson, AL: Play: The arena for acquisition of rules for competent behavior, Am J Occup Ther 31:248, 1977.

Takata, N: The play milieu: A preliminary appraisal. Am J Occup Ther 25:281, 1971.

Wehman, P, and Abramson, M: Three theoretical approaches to play: Applications for exceptional children. Am J Occup Ther 30:551, 1976.

Wehman, P, and Marchant, J: Improving free play skills of severely retarded children. Am J Occup Ther 32:100, 1978.

Parents' Resources

Bogin, M: The Path to Pain Control. Houghton-Mifflin, Boston, 1982.

A Consumer's Guide to Mental Health Services. 20 pages. National Institute of Mental Health, 5600 Fishers Lane, Rockville, MD 20857.

Coping with Lupus. 244 pages. Avery Publishing Group, Wayne, NJ.

Coping with Stress. Pamphlet. Available from the Arthritis Foundation, 1314 Spring St, NW, Atlanta, GA, 30309, (404) 872-7100. Catalog #9326.

Dennis the Menace—Coping with Family Stress. 14 pages. Available from Miss Kay Hults, Field Enterprises, Inc., PO Box 19620, Irvine, CA 92664.

Epstein, GJ: Help Yourself to Chronic Pain Relief. The Manchester Group Ltd, Seattle, 1981.

Florence, D, Hegedus, F, and Reedstrom, K: Coping with Chronic Pain. Sister Kenny Institute, Minneapolis, 1982.

A Guide to Managing Stress, 1985. 15 pages. Krames Communications, 312 90th St, Daly City, CA 94015-2621, (415) 994-8800.

Help for Your Troubled Child. 24 pages. For sale by Public Affairs Pamphlets, 381 Park Avenue South, New York, NY 10016, (212) 683-4331. $1.00; bulk discounts available.

Helping Children Face Crisis. 24 pages. For sale by Public Affairs Pamphlets, 381 Park Avenue South, New York, NY 10016, (212) 683-4331. $1.00; bulk discounts available.

How to Get Unstressed: The Bare Facts. 14 pages. For sale from the Wisconsin Clearinghouse, University of Wisconsin Hospitals and Clinics, 1954 East Washington Ave, Madison, WI 53704, (608) 263-2797. $1.00; bulk discounts available.

How to Handle Stress: Techniques for Living Well. 28 pages. For sale by Public Affairs Pamphlets, 381 Park Avenue South, New York, NY 10016, (212) 683-4331. $1.00; bulk discounts available.

Plain Talk About the Art of Relaxation. 2 pages. Single copy free from the Public Inquiries Section, Science Communication Branch, National Institute of Mental Health, Parklawn Building, Room 15C-17, 5600 Fishers Lane, Rockville, MD 20857, (301) 443-4513.

Plain Talk About Dealing with the Angry Child. 2 pages. Also available in Spanish: Charla franca: como tratar al nino enojado. Single copy free from the Consumer Information Center, Department M, Pueblo, CO 81009.

Taking Charge: Learning to Live with Arthritis. 24 pages. Available from the Arthritis Foundation, 1314 Spring St, NW, Atlanta, GA 30309, (404) 872-7100. Catalog #4221.

US Department of Health and Human Resources: Chronic Pain: Hope Through Research. National Institutes of Health, Bethesda, MD, 1982.

Ziebell, B: As Normal as Possible: A Parent's Guide to Healthy Emotional Development for Children with Arthritis. Order from the Arthritis Foundation, Southern Arizona Chapter, PO Box 43084, AZ 85733. Cost: $5.00.

Children's Resources

Don't Just Sit in a Big Green Chair. (For adolescents, with emphasis on sexuality issues, employment, fitness, and driving.) La Rabida Children's Hospital and Research Center Rheumatology Dept, E65th St at Lake Michigan, Chicago, IL 60649.

Falco, J, Block, D, Vostrejs, M, and Mergendahl, K: JRA and Me: A Fun Workbook. Arthritis Foundation, Atlanta, 1986.

Kapiolani Women's and Children's Medical Center: Let's Learn about JRA with Kela. Pediatric Arthritis Center of Hawaii, 1985.

Olson, M: How to Feel Better with Your Arthritis Pain and Stiffness. University of Cincinnati, Cincinnati, 1982.

Singsen, BH, et al: You Have Arthritis Coloring Book. Available from Pediatric Rheumatology Team, Health Sciences Center, University of Missouri, 807 Stadium Road, Columbia, MO 65212. Phone: 314-882-8738. $2.00 each.

Chapter 17

Evaluation and Treatment—Three Case Reports

MARCY ATWOOD, M.A., O.T.R.

The case reports presented here illustrate the practical application of the evaluation and treatment principles discussed in Chapters 14, 15, and 16.*

Jamie's case is presented first because it represents the typical complexity and challenge of treating a young child with severe polyarticular juvenile rheumatoid arthritis (JRA) and systemic involvement. Her case illustrates the importance of having children of this age participate fully in school and family activities. The specifics of hand assessment and treatment are emphasized. Three-year-old Amy, who has pauciarticular JRA, illustrates the integration and implementation of the developmental assessment in therapy. The case of Martha, a 17-year-old with polyarticular arthritis, portrays the necessity of emphasizing psychosocial concerns, self-image, and school and vocational planning for adolescents. Additionally, the conflicts that different cultural mores can have on children are represented.

An outline for organizing a comprehensive assessment of a child with JRA is presented in Table 15–8 in Chapter 15.

---

* Muscle grades are recorded both numerically as 0, 1, 2, 3, 4, and 5, and also using the corresponding grade levels of zero, trace, poor, fair, good, and normal.

CASE STUDY: JAMIE

History

Jamie is a 6-year-old girl with progressive systemic-onset polyarticular JRA since age 2. At initial onset, Jamie displayed wrist, knee, and small joint involvement that was controlled through orthotic treatment, home exercise, and medication (Naprosyn). At age 3½ Jamie developed flexion contractures of the left wrist, left knee, and bilateral index fingers that did not respond to conservative orthotic management. She was then hospitalized for serial casting and medical management. Jamie gained back lost range but opted to leave the hospital before her extensor musculature was strengthened enough to sustain the range. Her cooperation with the postcasting orthotic schedule and outpatient therapy was inconsistent. Hence, she never maintained full extension ranges. At age 4 Jamie showed progressing joint limitations in elbows, left hip, and subtalar joints. She was treated with gold, but that was discontinued after 6 months because there were no signs of response. She was again hospitalized to increase her functional status, undergo another round of serial casting, and determine therapeutic levels of other nonsteroidal anti-inflammatory drugs.

Jamie recently presented in the rheumatology clinic with a 2-week history of severe pain and progressive range limitations in her neck, left hip, and knee. She was unable to walk and displayed increased swelling and tenderness in wrist and finger joints. Jamie complained of morning stiffness for about 2 to 3 hours that was somewhat alleviated by a 20-minute bath. She had high spiking fevers in the afternoon and evening that were accompanied by an erythematous rash and exquisite joint tenderness. Jamie had little desire to eat or play with friends and was described as "cranky" by her mother, especially during her fevers. Following a medical evaluation, Jamie was admitted to the rehabilitation unit with team goals of stabilizing Jamie's medication and increasing her functional status (self-care and ambulation); increasing Jamie's range of motion (ROM) and muscle strength; teaching Jamie and her parents about arthritis; and providing an effective home program. Recent medications were low-dose prednisolone and Naprosyn as well as intramuscular methotrexate. It should be noted that Jamie had missed her methotrexate injections for 4 weeks prior to the clinic visit. On this dose of prednisolone she had not had a weight gain. She was rheumatoid factor negative.

Occupational and Physical Therapy Evaluation and Recommendations

Response to Evaluation

Jamie appeared to have an age-appropriate understanding of her disease ("Arthritis is something that makes it hard to walk, but ice makes my knee better.") and was aware of the reason for the hospitalization. Jamie was comfortable with the hospital routine but still became teary eyed when asked about her family, saying she missed her Mom. Jamie's complaints of pain appeared consistent with disease activity and degree of physical involvement.

Summary of Physical Findings

Joint Status
Upper Extremity
Neck. Extension, rotation, and lateral deviation were all moderately limited.

Head was positioned in slight flexion at rest and during activity.

Shoulders. Shoulder tightness was noted in the adductor and internal rotator muscles bilaterally although there was no complaint of pain upon movement. There were minimal range limitations (decreased 25 percent) bilaterally in abduction, flexion, and internal rotation. Shoulder strength was in the 3.5/5 to 4/5 (fair+/good) point range with the flexor muscles stronger than the abductor muscles.

Elbows. Synovial thickening was noted at the medial epicondyle but no tenderness was present. Jamie had bilateral elbow flexion contractures of 30 degrees and 25 degrees (right and left). Elbow ROM was 30 to 140 degrees on the right and 25 to 145 degrees on the left. Elbow flexor strength was 4.5/5 (good+); extensor strength was 3.7/5 (good−).

Forearms. There was no pain upon motion; ranges were minimally limited as follows: supination: 0 to 60 degrees right, 0 to 70 degrees left; pronation: 0 to 70 degrees right, 0 to 75 degrees left. Forearm rotation strength was 3.5/5 (fair+). Pronator muscles were stronger than supinator muscles.

Wrists. Wrists were subluxed bilaterally with visible swelling on the dorsal radial aspect of the wrist. The right wrist had more swelling and pain than the left wrist. The flexor carpi ulnaris and palmaris longus muscles were in spasm bilaterally. Wrists were positioned in 15 degrees of ulnar deviation and 10 degrees of flexion at rest. ROM was severely limited, more so in the right wrist than in the left wrist.

Wrist Range of Motion (in Degrees)

	Right	Left
Wrist flexion	10–45	0–40
Wrist extension	−10	0–5
Radial deviation	−15	0–10
Ulnar deviation	15–25	0–25

Strength in wrist extensor and radial deviator muscles was 1.5/5 (poor−) on the right and 3.5 (fair+) on the left; flexion and ulnar deviation were 4/5 (good).

Hands
Metacarpophalangeal (MCP) joints: Effusions were noted bilaterally in the index, middle, and little fingers. MCP flexion was

minimally limited; MCP hyperextension was severely limited except on ring fingers bilaterally. (Refer to measurements of hand ROM, below.) Strength in extensor digitorum communis was 3.5/5 (fair+); lumbricals and interossei were 3.5/5 to 3.7/5 (fair+ to good−) (palmar interossei were stronger than dorsal interossei).

Proximal interphalangeal (PIP) joints: The index and middle fingers had fusiform swelling, pain, and flexion contractures bilaterally. PIP flexion ranges were moderately decreased for index and middle fingers. Strength of the flexor digitorum profundus was 4/5 (good) and strength of flexor digitorum sublimis was 2 to 2.5/5 (poor to poor+). (See hand ROM for specific measurements.)

Distal interphalangeal (DIP) joints: Synovial thickening was apparent bilaterally on all fingers. Dip joints were positioned in flexion, although there were no flexion contractures and minimal range limitations. (See hand ROM for measurements.)

Hand Range of Motion (in Degrees)

Right	II	III	IV	V
MCP flexion	0–80	0–85	0–90	0–90
MCP hyper-extension	0–10	0–12	0–30	0–15
PIP flexion	10–80	30–70	0–105	0–110
DIP flexion	0–50	0–60	0–60	0–65
Left	II	III	IV	V
MCP flexion	0–83	0–87	0–90	0–90
MCP hyper-extension	0–12	0–15	0–30	0–12
PIP flexion	10–80	25–75	0–100	0–100
DIP flexion	0–55	0–65	0–60	0–65

Lower Extremity

Hips. Jamie complained of pain in her left hip. She had hip flexion contractures of 15 degrees on the right and 25 degrees on the left. (The right appeared compensatory to the knee contractures.) Hip flexion was within normal limits. Strength in the hip was 3.7/5 to 4/5 (good− to good) with hip flexors and adductors stronger than hip abductors and extensors.

Knees. There were painful effusions in both knees with spasm of the hamstrings and knee flexion contractures of 17 degrees (left) and 7 degrees (right). Knee extensor (quadriceps) strength was 3/5 (fair) and flexor strength was 4/5 (good).

Ankle and Subtalar Joints. The subtalar joints were painful and swollen with associated spasm of the peroneus longus bilaterally. Forefoot and hindfoot inversion ranges were severely limited bilaterally (0 range). Hindfoot eversion was limited on the left. Forefoot eversion was 0 to 20 degrees bilaterally. Ankle plantar flexion was 0 to 40 degrees bilaterally, and dorsiflexion was approximately 0 to 20 degrees bilaterally. Muscle strength was decreased as follows: Posterior tibialis, right 3.5/5 (fair+), left 3/5 (fair), peroneus longus and brevis were 4/5 (good) bilaterally.

Metatarsophalangeal (MTP) and interphalangeal (IP) joints appeared normal.

Posture. Jamie's posture typified that of many children with systemic-onset polyarticular disease. She showed round shoulders, increased lumbar lordosis, bilateral genu valgus, and bilateral hindfoot valgus with pronation. She guarded bilateral elbows and wrists in a flexed position.

Gait. In pre-swing there was decreased plantar flexion (decreased roll off) and decreased knee flexion. Decreased trunk rotation was noted throughout the gait cycle.

Functional Upper Extremity Use and Developmental Status

Gross Motor Coordination (Upper Extremity). Within normal limits as measured by Box and Blocks Test.

Fine Motor Coordination (Upper Extremity). Within normal limits as measured by the Southern California Sensory Integration Test of Motor Accuracy.

Manipulative Skills. Patient was right-hand dominant with an expanse of prehension 3½ inches on the right and 4 inches on the left (4½ to 5 inches is normal). She performed all prehension types: lateral pinch, 2-point tip, and 3-point pad; however, she typically substituted a lateral pinch for a 2-point pinch on the right due to pain in the index MCP and PIP joints. Although Jamie was able to paint and draw, she had pain in cutting with scissors and writing for long periods. Jamie was unable to cut food with a knife, turn a doorknob, open a safety pin, or fasten resistive buttons and snaps.

Note: Expanse of prehension, which reflects spherical grasp, is measured by picking up round wooden discs of increasingly larger diameter (1-, 2-, 3-, 3½-, 4-, 4½-, 5-inch diameters) with the tips of all digits abducted around the disc. A flexion contracture may decrease the "expanse of prehension" or spherical grasp, which would functionally limit tasks such as picking up a ball or large mug.

Grip Strength. Jamie's grip strength was severely decreased on the right side and moderately decreased on the left side. This was apparently due to decreased muscle strength as well as using and positioning her hands in flexion. She appeared to guard her wrists when rising from a chair by putting weight on clenched fists (rather than extended wrists). Decreased grip strength interfered with pulling up pants and with opening containers.

Note: Grip strength is measured using a sphygmomanometer for small children and those in the acute stage. The sphygmomanometer is sensitive in measuring changes, causes less pain upon measurement (with less resistance), and does not force the hand into a potentially harmful position. However, there are no norms for children. (See Chapter 21 for procedure.)

Occupational Role Behavior (Including Developmental Skills)

Self-Care. *Dressing:* Jamie was independent in donning an overhead shirt, T-shirt, and jacket, but she was unable to put on pants, socks, or shoes. *Bathing:* She had difficulty shampooing her hair and washing her lower extremities and back. *Grooming:* She was unable to comb her hair and put in barretts but was independent in washing her face and brushing her teeth. *Eating:* Jamie was unable to cut meat, pour milk, open small cellophane-wrapped packages, open jar tops, or push down the toaster. She had difficulty opening her hands around large cups due to contractured fingers.

Personal/Social. Jamie was a spunky 6-year-old girl in the first grade who attended school regularly, but who felt school was "boring." She appeared to get along with her classmates, but she rarely played with them outside after school. Jamie stated "I hate it! I can never run as fast as them and I'm always picked last for the relay race teams! Sometimes I don't think they even want me to play!" Her parents tried to assuage her frustration by enrolling her in swim classes and encouraging her to play with neighborhood children. Their efforts helped, but could not erase the damaging effects of the teasing from Jamie's peers who did not know her. Luckily, Jamie and her parents had a wonderful sense of humor that appeared to assist coping. When Jamie became upset and refused to eat, play, or wear splints, her mother would lovingly tease with her "poor, poor, Jamie . . ." and discuss funny responses for the kids' mean comments. Jamie and her family took frequent camping trips and vacations so that Jamie was exposed to as many opportunities and experiences as possible.

School. Jamie's school routine had been adapted for her needs prior to the increased disease activity. As stated, Jamie attended school regularly and was in the first grade. She participated in swimming, relay races, and dancing games (no jumping involved) and kept score for contact team sports. Jamie was driven to school because the long bus ride stiffened her neck and hips. She usually arrived at school late to avoid crowds. She had a friend who helped carry her lunch tray, and she wore her splints while writing. At recess Jamie usually went outside with friends but could not participate in "four square" (a hopping and bouncing ball game). She had two sets of books, one at school and one at home, and had no difficulty keeping up academically in school. She became stiff when sitting for longer than 30 minutes during class periods. For the past 2 weeks, Jamie had not attended school because of decreased ambulation and very low energy level.

Play. Jamie enjoyed riding her bicycle, swimming, playing ball outside, playing with dolls, and helping her mother. Jamie had two good friends who lived near her and understood that Jamie could not always keep up in *active* playing. Usually, however, Jamie played with her cousin or baby sister. Recently, she has had no energy for play activities or socializing.

Family. Jamie had a very supportive, intact family. Although her parents were concerned with promoting Jamie's independence, they had difficulty in setting limits on Jamie's behavior. They put very few demands on Jamie, tolerated her frequent outbursts, and did not have her routinely perform home chores. Jamie appeared to use her arthritis to get what she wanted (usually by complaining of pain). Although her parents recognized this, they did not know how to change this behavior. When Jamie's sister was born, Jamie became very jealous. Initially Jamie cried, was very demanding, refused to take medications, and continually removed her orthoses. A child psychologist was consulted and suggested that Jamie start to help care for her baby sister. He further suggested that the parents spend individual time with Jamie and give her more responsibility for home chores. He explained that it was important for Jamie's self-concept to contribute to the family's needs. Helping take care of the baby served as good role modeling and was helpful to the family. As Jamie's parents became more consistent in limiting temper tantrums, encouraging responsibility and praising her for independence in self-care, Jamie's behavior improved.

Equipment/Orthoses. Jamie had day wrist (gauntlet design) and finger orthoses, neither of which fit. She complained of pressure on the radial side of the right wrist orthosis (probably due to the increased ulnar deviation deformity in the right wrist) and redness through both web spaces. The lower extremity UC-BL foot orthoses and posterior night knee orthoses also did not maintain alignment due to the small size and change in joint status.

Jamie used a long-handled sponge, dressing stick, and shoehorn to assist with self-care.

Summary. Jamie was a 6-year-old female with systemic-onset polyarticular-course JRA who was in an acute stage of disease activity affecting both wrists, hands, knees, ankles, and left hip. She displayed moderate to severely decreased ranges in affected joints with 3.5/4.0 (fair+ to good) musculature throughout. Both wrists and left hip and left knee were particularly painful and swollen which had prevented Jamie from attending school for the last 2 weeks and fully participating in self-care or play with friends. Prior functioning indicated that Jamie had adapted her school and home environments to promote independence and optimal age-appro-

priate functioning. Her greatest limitations to functioning were decreased energy, ambulation, pain, and decreased functional hand use.

Goals for Occupational Therapy

1. Increase strength in shoulder and elbow extensor musculature to 5 (normal); maintain strength of wrist extensors and hand musculature.
2. Increase ROM in both shoulders and elbows by 10 percent; maintain ROM in wrist and hand.
3. Decrease inflammation of both wrists; decrease muscle spasm of right wrist flexors and ulnar deviators.
4. Increase functional hand use as measured by ability to button, cut with scissors, and open small, mildly resistive containers.
5. Prevent further finger flexion contractures.
6. Increase participation in self-care.
7. Increase participation in age-appropriate activities.
8. Teach principles of therapeutic management and joint protection to family and school personnel.
9. Coordinate outpatient therapy and follow-through of recommendations for school.
10. Help integrate patient's self-care, home program, and leisure time into family's schedule.

Occupational Therapy Treatment Plan

Therapeutic Exercise

1. Perform general active ROM for all upper extremity muscles and joints. Emphasize strengthening of *noninvolved* upper extremity musculature (remember to include scapular strengthening—"fountains," "superman," and so forth) and active ROM of *involved* musculature. Provide active assistive ROM for wrist and finger musculature with less than 3 (fair) strength. Isolate flexor digitorum profundus and sublimis for active ROM and active assistive ROM exercises. Integrate exercises into imitative games (e.g., "Simon Says") or imaginary play (e.g., animals), making sure Jamie uses full available ROM.

2. Provide facilitation techniques to wrist, finger, and elbow extensors (tapping, rubbing with lotion) prior to isometrics.

3. Perform isometric exercise (manual resistance) for elbow extensors, wrist extensors, radial deviators (while supported), finger extensors and intrinsics, and for forearm rotators to maintain extensor strength.

4. Pronate daily to decrease hip flexion contractures.

Orthotic Treatment

1. *Casting:* Because the right wrist is acutely painful and swollen and has flexor spasms, a plaster cast is recommended to decrease swelling and spasms. The cast should be applied and worn for 24 hours, followed by rigid wrist orthosis during the day.

2. *Daytime orthoses:* Fabricate and wear a rigid left daytime orthosis. Progress to a flexible orthosis much later when spasms have subsided and wrist extensor strength is improved. Wear a rigid right wrist orthosis following cast removal. Progress to a flexible leather orthosis if the orthosis can ensure proper fit to maintain the range. Remove for therapeutic exercise and activity.

3. *Nighttime orthoses:* Fabricate both left and right full wrist–hand orthoses. At night, wear left full wrist–hand orthosis and right daytime orthosis with finger splints. Alternate splint use nightly.

4. Fabricate cylinder finger orthoses for both index and third PIP joints. Finger orthoses should be used to tolerance and removed for activity and exercise. (MCP and DIP joint inflammation must be monitored carefully because immobilization of PIP joints can increase compensatory stress of these joints.)

5. *Serial casting:* Once the disease activity has subsided, serial casting to *increase* bilateral wrist ranges may be considered.

Therapeutic Activity

1. Lie prone on a hanging swing; pick up balls from one side of the room and throw them into a pail on the other side of the room. This will increase shoulder, elbow, and scapular strength and range while helping to decrease hip and knee flexion contractures in the prone position. Balancing on the swing provides additional, varied

sensory input and may contribute to enhanced postural security and body awareness.

2. Play doll house; place the doll house on a table at a proper height and distance so that wrists and elbows are used in extension and shoulders are used in flexion. This activity will increase shoulder and elbow endurance and maintain wrist strength while Jamie partakes in imaginary play.

3. Finger paint on mural paper placed on a wall or easel. Position the paper so that the wrist and fingers are used in extension. One-pound weights around the arms close to the shoulders can be added to progress strengthening. This activity increases shoulder, elbow, and scapular endurance and maintains wrist and finger active range and isometric strength. It allows Jamie to experiment with textures, express herself nonverbally, and enhance creative skills and fine motor coordination. Be sure to guard against lordotic posture.

4. Wash dishes or dolls in sink or basin with warm water. Warm water play can encourage full active ROM finger flexion and extension to maintain ranges.

5. Prepare (or unfreeze) cookie dough. Roll dough with extended wrists and fingers. Make round or flat balls. Decorate cookies with raisins or sprinkles using outstretched fingers. This will provide isometric finger extension strength and full use of PIP extension range. Distribute cookies to other children to encourage positive social feedback for Jamie.

6. Perform a puppet show. Use finger puppets for finger and wrist extension. This activity will encourage peer participation and dramatic play while isometrically strengthening fingers.

Activities of Daily Living

1. *Dressing:* Practice putting on pants first by propping feet on a stool or dressing on top of the bed. A reacher or dressing clips may be offered if Jamie is unable to reach her feet. Adapt clips if they are too resistive. A sock cone should not be used until inflammation in hands subsides.

2. *Bathing:* Offer Jamie a long-handled lightweight sponge to wash her lower extremities and back. Recommend rubber grips on the tub floor and grab bars on the walls for safety. Suggest a hand-held shower

for ease in washing hair, or a scrub brush in which soap is inserted.

3. *Eating and meals:* Cut meat for Jamie; transfer milk into smaller containers for easy pouring, use both hands to pour milk. Use a pencil or the entire side of hand to push down toaster. Arrange items that Jamie will need on a low shelf (e.g., peanut butter and jelly). Once symptoms have subsided, Jamie could cut softer food products with a plastic knife.

Education/Joint Protection

1. Have Jamie exercise and perform self-care in front of a mirror. This will encourage Jamie to see and appreciate her body. Discuss and acknowledge which joints are involved and the nature and extent of the pain. Discuss methods to alleviate pain at Jamie's level of comprehension.

2. Discuss the very basic principles of exercises with Jamie and her family (the necessity of strengthening extensors) and tendency of arthritis to favor flexion.

3. Demonstrate proper technique of carrying and lifting toys, opening containers, and using utensils. Adapt toy handles with a larger grip and foam padding. Play with toys (dolls) that do not have resistive pull-apart pieces.

Family Involvement

1. Invite the family to attend therapy. Demonstrate the exercises that will be included in the home program as well as other possible activities.

2. Plan a daily schedule with Jamie and her family that includes not only home exercise programs for occupational/physical therapy, but that also includes time for homework, family, and peer socialization. Discuss the priorities in occupational/physical therapy treatment. Make the home program short (no more than 5 exercises) and routinely vary the program to prevent boredom.

3. Prepare a calendar for Jamie to check off each day that she does her home exercise program and wears orthoses. Reward each successful week with something special (trip to the park, zoo, a special meal). Coordinate this with Jamie.

4. Encourage the family to help problem solve daily living tasks and think of new activities for therapy.

5. Encourage parents' consistency in chores and routines that will increase Jamie's personal responsibility. Reward good behavior.

Age-Appropriate Activity (Age 6)

1. In the hospital, plan group activities with other children (evening Disney movies, games, bake sales, magic shows, "volleyball" [beach ball] tournaments, and so forth); kids need to learn to organize, to work together, and to win and lose.

2. Encourage talking about school problems. Role play Jamie's response to kids who tease her.

3. Make sure Jamie eats all meals with other children.

4. Encourage Jamie to be responsible for some aspect of therapy or for straightening up her own room (putting away toys).

5. Allow Jamie choice in activities and emphasize *her* effect (positive or negative) on the outcome of the activities.

6. Encourage both exploration of many hobbies and competency in a few. Further, have Jamie make items for several other people. This will promote her social worth.

School

1. Additional information should be provided to teachers on Jamie's need to change positions frequently. It is recommended that Jamie be given responsibilities such as passing out papers, sharpening pencils, or helping erase the chalkboard to provide position changes less obviously. Further, teachers must know that Jamie needs to rest her fingers frequently and thus she may be slower in writing.

2. Recommend an alternate program for gym class when Jamie is unable to participate in class. (This is done in conjunction with physical therapy and the physical education teacher.)

Physical Therapy Program

1. Orthotic treatment
   a. UC-BL ankle–foot orthosis for daytime wear
   b. Circumferential knee orthosis for day use
   c. Posterior knee–ankle orthosis (plantar, Hexilite, or thermoplastic)
2. Therapeutic exercise to strengthen ex-

tensor muscles of the hips and to maintain strength in swollen knees and ankles; exercises to increase hip ROM and maintain knee and ankle range

3. Activities designed to increase overall endurance

4. Thermal modalities, particularly ice applications to decrease inflammation at knees and ankles

5. Pool therapy to increase strength and ROM throughout

6. Prone lying to stretch hip and knee flexors

7. Ambulation training and evaluation of Jamie using a bicycle with training wheels

8. Activities to improve balance, ease, and confidence in movement

CASE STUDY: AMY

History

Amy is a 3-year-old girl with *pauciarticular JRA* (rheumatoid factor negative). Onset of the disease occurred at age 2 with pain and limitation of motion in Amy's right wrist. Her mother reported that Amy avoided using her wrist in activities and rarely put weight on the wrist when playing. Amy was initially given a wrist orthosis and a home exercise program and treated with aspirin. In the following 6 months, she developed pain in the right knee, right ankle, and right foot. She was then given a more extensive home program to include the lower extremity and a posterior knee–ankle orthosis for the right lower extremity to be worn at night and during naps. Her aspirin was discontinued and she was changed to tolmetin. Amy was seen in the rheumatology clinic for her regular monthly check-up. Her mother reported that Amy continued to guard her right wrist during outside activities, but was resistant to wearing her wrist splint. She still had about 60 minutes of morning stiffness that was alleviated by a morning bath. She appeared to be "limping" more at preschool. Because Amy was significantly underweight for her age she was referred to a nutritionist.

Amy was referred to occupational and physical therapy for an updated evaluation and treatment recommendations.

Occupational and Physical Therapy Evaluation and Recommendations

Response to Evaluation

Amy played with the evaluation tools (goniometer and sphygmomanometer) on a doll prior to use in the evaluation. Amy denied having pain in her right wrist, knee, and ankle; however, she cried when ROM evaluations and joint examinations were initiated. Amy demonstrated age-appropriate responses to questions regarding her disease. She simply stated, "I just can't kick the ball." Her mother was present during all evaluation procedures.

Summary of Physical Findings

Joint Status
Upper Extremity
   Shoulders. No clinical findings; ROM was within normal limits bilaterally; strength was 4/5 (good), which is normal for this age.
   Elbows. No clinical findings; ROM was within normal limits bilaterally; strength was 4/5 (good) (normal for age).
   Forearms. Left forearm ROM and strength were within normal limits. Right ROM was minimally limited for age. Amy complained of right wrist pain at the end of rotation ranges. Right supination was 0 to 75 degrees; pronation was 0 to 60 degrees; right supinator and pronator strengths were 3.7/5 (good−).
   Wrists. Left wrist ROM and strength were within normal limits. The right wrist was swollen across the entire dorsum; however, Amy did not complain of pain upon palpation. There was spasm of the flexor carpi ulnaris and a tendency to hold the right wrist in a flexed and ulnarly deviated position. X-ray reports note diffuse demineralization, advanced carpal bone age, and beginning carpal subluxation on the right. Right wrist passive motion was severely limited in all ranges, extension (−5 degrees), radial deviation (0 to 5 degrees), flexion (5 to 15 degrees), and ulnar deviation (0 to 10 degrees), with pain at the end of range. These ranges represent insidious losses most pronounced in extension and radial deviation. Active wrist range showed a lag in extension and radial deviation. A muscle strength evaluation indicated that

the wrist extensors and flexor carpi radialis were 2.75 (fair−), and the wrist flexors were 3.5 (fair+) (with pain). These assessments were performed functionally during games and thus should be reassessed.

MCP, PIP, and DIP joints. There were no clinical findings. ROM was within normal limits. Strength was 4/5 (good) throughout all intrinsic and extrinsic hand muscles.

Lower Extremity

Hips. Left lower extremity ROM and strength were within normal limits. Amy had no complaints of right hip pain; however, she had a compensatory 10-degree right hip flexion contracture (10 to 130 degrees). Hip extensor and flexor musculatures were 4/5 (good) bilaterally; bilateral internal rotation and external rotation were 3.5 (fair+); bilateral abduction was 4− (good−).

Knees. An effusion of the right knee was present with marked swelling in the popliteal fossa and the prepatellar and suprapatellar bursae. The patella was ballotable but a fluid wave was not elicited. Crepitus occurred with patella mobilization. She displayed a 20-degree right knee flexion contracture and 125 degrees of knee flexion (145 degrees was normal for her). X-ray reports noted generalized osteoporosis and enlarged epiphysis of the right knee, as compared to the left knee, but no bony destruction or erosions in the right knee were reported.

Left knee extensor (quadriceps) strength was 4−/5 (good−), which is normal for her age. Right knee extensor strength was 2+/5 (poor+). Medial and lateral hamstring strength was 4/5 (good) on the left and 3−/5 (fair) on the right.

Ankles. Bilateral ankle plantar flexion was within normal limits (0 to 40 degrees); dorsiflexion was moderately limited on the right (0 to 10 degrees) but within normal limits on the left (0 to 25 degrees). Strength of the gastrocnemius and soleus musculature was 4/5 (good) on the left and 3/5 (fair) on the right.

Subtalar joints. Right subtalar joints were slightly swollen. Mild spasms of the peroneal muscles were noted with passive subtalar inversion. Right hindfoot inversion was 0 (left was 0 to 20 degrees); right hindfoot eversion was 0 to 12 degrees (left

was 0 to 15 degrees). The peroneus longus and brevis were left 4−/5 (good−), right 3.5/5 (fair+). The posterior tibialis was left 4−/5 (good−), right 3−/5 (fair−).

MTP and IP joints: Strength and ROM were within normal limits with no clinical findings.

Posture. Amy held the right knee in 25 degrees of flexion and the right ankle in 10 degrees of plantar flexion while at rest. The right forefoot showed increased pronation and the hindfoot showed valgus. The wrist was held in flexion and ulnar deviation.

Gait. Amy ambulated with her right knee and hip flexed. She had decreased heel strike on the right. Single limb stance was decreased on the right and increased on the left.

Developmental Status

Fine Motor Coordination. Amy's manipulative skills were at an age-appropriate level. She performed a precise 2-point pad, 3-point pad, and lateral pinch. Amy could scribble, stack blocks, and button large buttons. However, her grip strength was decreased on the right as compared to the left. She used her right hand in flexion.

Adaptive Skills. Amy was at a 36-month level in adaptive abilities. She could build a tower of 10 blocks, recognized geometric forms, and copied vertical and horizontal strokes (as tested by the revised Gesell Adaptive Scales).

Gross Motor Coordination. Amy was only slightly delayed in gross motor skills. She rode a tricycle, threw a ball overhand, and was able to climb stairs. However, she had difficulty in standing on one foot (either right or left), walking backwards, and running. Overall, she was much less active than most 3-year-olds, who love to climb and jump and involve the whole body in activity.

Personal/Social. Amy was able to perform age-appropriate dressing skills, such as pulling up pants and putting on her shirt and jacket. However, her mother tended to do these tasks if Amy was cranky or exceptionally stiff, or if the clothes were too tight.

Amy ate independently, although she sometimes had difficulty holding a full cup. She used a spoon and fork well. Amy was able to brush her teeth and wash her face and chest independently. She needed assistance with shampooing hair (appropriate for her age) and washing legs. Amy attempted to comb her own hair.

Amy went to the bathroom by herself, but she had recently had bouts of bedwetting at night.

Occupational Role Behavior

Self-Care. See Developmental Status, above.

Personal/Emotional. Amy was a sweet, shy 3-year-old girl who had always been compliant with evaluation procedures as long as her mother stayed close for reassurance. Amy's mother stated that since the onset of JRA Amy had been much less energetic and less inquisitive about her surroundings. She did not seek out *active* exploratory play and appeared more fearful of other children and pets. Her mother related that at times she had had difficulty giving and receiving affection from Amy, particularly when Amy was in pain. At these times Amy cried when touched yet wanted attention. Her mother had questioned the efficacy of her parenting and needed much positive feedback and suggestions from the staff. Although Amy enjoyed more sedentary activities, she was quite meticulous about her clothes and room and cleaning up after herself.

Play. Amy primarily played by herself at home and at the playground. She rode a Big Wheel and frolicked in the outdoor wading pool and sandbox. However, she tended to avoid jungle gyms, slides, and other apparatus that tested her balance. Amy liked playing with materials of different textures. She enjoyed dolls, finger painting, drawing, water play, and musical instruments. She also liked helping her mother with chores and taking care of her younger sister.

School. Amy attended preschool 3 days per week. The preschool teacher said that Amy had learned to take turns and will play with 2 or 3 other children when encouraged. She previously attended "mommy and me" gymnastic classes at the YMCA but had not returned since the onset of JRA. Both Amy's preschool teacher and parents agreed that Amy was now much less active at the playground, stayed closer to her mother or teacher, and was afraid to try new games unless coaxed by her father. Amy had fallen several times at the play-

ground when pushed by some other children. She had difficulty climbing the steps to a slide and holding on to a merry-go-round.

Family. Amy was the oldest of 2 girls (her younger sister was 18 months old). The family was intact. Her mother was a full-time homemaker and her father was beginning an engineering consulting business. Her parents had complied with all recommendations and had demonstrated good observational skills regarding Amy's joint status. However, they appeared to deny the permanence of Amy's disease ("When the disease ends, she'll be just fine—no contractures or anything."). They belittled any changes in her joint status ("She's fine, she is just having a little trouble using her right hand.") Neither had discussed their fears about Amy's future.

Equipment/Orthoses

1. Right rigid wrist orthosis
2. Right posterior resting orthosis for knee–ankle

Summary. Amy was a 3-year-old female with pauciarticular JRA since age 2. She had involvement of the right wrist, knee, ankle, and foot, which had progressed since the last visit. Physical examination showed swelling, muscle spasm, and severely decreased range and strength in her right wrist. Amy held and used her right wrist in a flexed and ulnarly deviated position but did not complain of pain. She had a 10-degree compensatory hip flexion contracture on the right but good strength at the hip. Right knee showed swelling, a 20-degree flexion contracture, and severely decreased knee extensor strength and decreased flexion. Subtalar motions were decreased in hindfoot eversion and inversion.

Developmentally, Amy displayed age-appropriate fine motor and adaptive skills although her grip strength was decreased. This limited some manipulative play and self-care activities. Decreased grip strength may have been due to pain, muscle weakness from disuse, and use of wrist in a flexed position. Amy could perform most self-care activities that did not require a strong grip or right knee mobility. She attended preschool and enjoyed playing outside; however, she had become less active, adventuresome, and inquisitive in the last year.

Goals for Occupational Therapy

1. Decrease right wrist inflammation and muscle spasm.
2. Promote functional hand use.
3. Maintain present strength and wrist range (then progress to increasing strength).
4. Protect right wrist during play.
5. Increase independence in age-appropriate self-care activities.
6. Maintain interest in age-appropriate activities.
7. Promote developmental skills through play activities.
8. Teach parents basic joint-protection and exercise principles.

Occupational Therapy Treatment Plan

General occupational therapy recommendations are to continue with a morning bath to alleviate morning stiffness and strive to maintain the strength range and use of the right wrist. Amy should perform all age-appropriate self-care activities (even if extra time is needed) and be encouraged to try other outside activities under the guidance of her parents. Amy should surely wear her wrist splint to school and when playing outside for protection. Friends should be encouraged to come to Amy's house to play. Amy should continue at preschool and attend swimming classes with her mother at the YMCA. Exercises should be done twice per day and reassessed at least every 2 weeks.

Amy's case clearly represents a challenge in clinical decision making. Although serial casts are usually applied when the disease is *less* active, for Amy conservative orthotic treatment has not maintained the range in her wrist. Her disease has continued to smolder and she has lost wrist range insidiously. The two options were: 1) to again try daytime orthoses (knowing that 3-year-olds do not always keep on orthoses all the time) or 2) serial cast the right wrist to gain back lost range. The serial casting treatment was chosen.

Serial Casting

Due to the severe (and progressive) limitation in right wrist extension, which was active but not acutely tender, serial casting would be indicated for the following rea-

sons: (1) to increase wrist extension range, (2) to prevent further soft tissue contracture, (3) to prevent overstretching of extensor musculature, and (4) to prevent habitual use in the flexed position. Ideally, the cast would be changed every 48 hours with isometric and extensor facilitation and active use between casting. Ice can be applied between casts if spasms persist. Casting would continue until there were no changes in 2 to 3 successive castings. At that point, a focus on strengthening and maintenance of range would commence. Casting could resume at a later date if increased gains were still believed possible. The last serial cast should be bivalved to wear at night. Gauntlet orthoses would follow casting. The program described next would follow the casting procedure.

Water Play to Relieve Morning Stiffness and to Exercise the Wrists

1. Play in water—smash bubbles; wash body parts and dolls to decrease stiffness.
2. Rub lotion on wrists and forearms (particularly right wrist extensors) to facilitate extensor musculature.
3. Flick water—make waves in the bathtub to exercise wrist extensors without resistance.

Therapeutic Exercise (for Wrist Extension Active ROM and Strengthening)

1. Wrist extension game: wave hello to doll, dog, Mom, Dad.
2. Keeping forearm on table, try to touch finger knuckles to Mom's hand held above Amy's hand.
3. Play motorcycle. Move wrists *back* as if to accelerate. Hold to a count of 7. Repeat 10 times.
4. Play "Simon Says," integrating wrist extension into games.
5. Have Amy move wrists into extension. Tell her to "hold like a statue" and give manual isometric resistance.

Therapeutic Activity (to Enhance Functional Hand Use and Maintain Extensor Strength)

1. Play with shaving cream on windows.
2. Play with dolls positioned on a table at shoulder height.

3. Finger paint on an easel.
4. Help Mom clean (dust) furniture.
5. Play volleyball with a beach ball, wearing wrist orthosis.

Orthotic Treatment

1. Wear rigid orthosis day and night while right wrist extensor strength is below 3.5 (fair+) and muscle spasm is still present. The orthosis should be fabricated in her maximal extension range. A flexible orthosis can follow the rigid orthosis when strength has increased and ROM has stabilized. However, the orthosis must fit correctly.
2. Wear the bivalve serial casts at night if orthoses do not appear sufficiently rigid to maintain gains.
3. Have Amy perform her favorite activities with orthosis on. This will enable her to know she can play while wearing orthoses.
4. Make an orthosis for the child's doll to encourage acceptance.
5. Decorate the orthosis with stickers.
6. Do not make the child wear the orthosis when eating if she doesn't want to.

Age-Appropriate Activities

Amy should be encouraged to play with simple constructive, perceptual toys (blocks, mailboxes with letters of various shapes and sizes), musical toys, and materials of various textures (pudding, play dough). To become more aware of her body, Amy can rub body parts with lotion or soap and name body parts as she does her exercises. Amy can also learn to "paint" or rub her dorsal forearm to facilitate extensor musculature prior to active ROM. To promote balance reactions, Amy can walk on grass or have therapy on a large Swiss ball or platform swing with supervision close by. Amy should play with or alongside peers whenever possible.

Joint-Protection, Relaxation, and Exercise Principles

The basic principles of avoiding static positions of wrist flexion and resistance in flexion can be taught to 3-year-olds through demonstration. Children can learn which motions are "good" and can be rewarded for remembering 2 to 3 exercises. The parents or another adult must be present to ensure proper positioning of the extremity. Three-year-olds can also be taught quick-relax methods that help decrease anxiety during casting, evaluation, or splinting procedures. The child is instructed to act like a rag doll, following the therapist's demonstration. If inflammation or spasms recur, ice (or frozen peas) can be applied circumferentially around the wrist and/or the flexor muscle belly.

Physical Therapy Program

1. Cold modalities to decrease inflammation at knee and ankle
2. Therapeutic exercise to strengthen extensor muscles of the hip, knee, and foot (plantar and dorsiflexors) and to increase active ROM of the lower extremity
3. Prone lying to decrease hip flexion contracture
4. Pool therapy to increase strength and active ROM
5. Orthotic treatment
   a. Serial casting of the knee
   b. Knee orthosis at night to maintain ROM gains
6. Functional electrical stimulation to quadriceps to maintain strength
7. Gait training

CASE STUDY: MARTHA

History

Martha is a 17-year-old Latin-American female who was diagnosed with polyarticular JRA at age 14 (rheumatoid factor positive). At initial onset, Martha had predominantly bilateral upper extremity involvement of the elbows, wrists, and small joints in her hands. At age 15, she developed pain and limitations in her ankles and toes with gait deviations. Martha was initially treated with aspirin and Nalfon; she was then quickly switched to a combination of Nalfon and prednisolone (a corticosteroid) because of the early progressive nature of the disease. On prednisolone she has maintained stability in strength, ROM, and functional status (self-care and ambulation) for the past year. She reports morning stiffness for only 10 minutes per day, which is alleviated by a bath or morning wake-up routine. She has not suffered from extreme lethargy or malaise and has not had low-grade fevers. She has reported gaining weight while on prednisolone (7 pounds in the last year) and sees the dietitian for balanced but low-calorie diets.

The physician's examination suggested that Martha's functional status could be improved with an outpatient strengthening program and by independent living skills program. Martha was referred to physical and occupational therapy for an updated evaluation, home programs, and recommendations for avocational and vocational planning.

Occupational and Physical Therapy Evaluation and Recommendations

Response to Evaluation

Martha is a very pleasant young lady who was cooperative during evaluation procedures and appeared reliable in describing past history. Martha demonstrated a basic understanding of her disease, but she had construed a frightful picture of joint pathology and disease progression. "It's like a fire going on inside your joints. When the disease is active, the fire burns the ends of your bones. That's why ice is important." Her understanding of her disease may be influenced by her family's traditional beliefs in Latin American folk medicine. Martha's pain responses were appropriate for the degree of joint involvement.

Summary of Physical Findings

Joint Status
Upper Extremity
Shoulders. There were no clinical findings except for tightness at the end of shoulder flexion and abduction ranges. (Pectoral muscles were tight.) ROM was minimally limited in flexion and abduction ranges, lacking 20 degrees of full range. Internal and external rotation was within normal limits. Shoulder strength was 4/5 (good) for shoulder flexion and 4−/5 (good−) for abduction and internal and external rotation. Martha fatigues during successive repetitions of muscle testing, maintaining moderate resistance during muscle testing for 2 repetitions only.

Elbows. Synovial thickening was noted around the medial epicondyle. Martha had elbow flexion contractures of right, 20 degrees, left, 30 degrees. Elbow flexor strength was 5/5 (normal); extensor strength is 4/5 (good).

Forearms. Crepitus occurred with forearm rotation. ROM was moderately limited in supination (0 to 50 degrees right, 0 to 45 degrees left) and pronation (0 to 60 degrees right, 0 to 55 degrees left). Forearm strength in supination and pronation was 4/5 (good).

Wrists. Synovial thickening was noted on the radial dorsum of the wrists bilaterally. Wrists were subluxed and positioned in 15 degrees of ulnar deviation at rest. There was no spasm in the wrist flexors although the flexor carpi ulnaris was tight (left more so than right). X-ray films show fusion of the lunate and capitate carpal bones with erosions at the distal end of the ulna and in the proximal carpal row. There was joint space narrowing of the radiocarpal joint. Wrist motion was severely limited in all ranges, as follows (in degrees):

	Right	Left
Wrist extension	0–15	0–10
Wrist flexion	0–30	0–25
Radial deviation	0–10	0–5
Ulnar deviation	0–15	0–20

Wrist extensor and radial deviation strength was 4−/5 (good−); wrist flexor and ulnar deviation strength was 4/5 (good).

Hands
MCP Joints: Both index and middle fingers showed chronic effusions and synovial thickening. Involved digits showed a significant loss in hyperextension as follows: right—II 0 to 15 degrees, III 0 to 10 degrees; left—II 0 to 12 degrees, III 0 to 15 degrees, with minimal to moderate intrinsic tightness; MCP flexion, however, was full throughout all MCP joints. X-ray films showed erosions of metacarpal heads of both index and middle fingers. There was mild intrinsic tightness of the index and middle fingers.

PIP joints: Synovial thickening and flexion contractures were noted only on right middle (15 degrees) and ring (17 degrees) fingers and left ring (15 degrees) and little (20 degrees) fingers. PIP flexion was limited to 90 degrees for involved digits. Otherwise PIP flexion range was 0 to 100 degrees. X-ray films showed diffuse generalized osteoporosis and joint space narrowing of involved digits.

DIP joints: No clinical findings. ROM was within normal limits.

Muscle Strength in the Hand. Muscle strength was generally 4/5 to 5/5 (good to normal) throughout.

Flexor digitorum profundus: 4 (good) throughout all digits

Flexor digitorum superficialis: 3.5/5 (fair+) in involved digits, 3.7/5 (good−) in uninvolved digits

Extensor digitorum communis: bilateral II, III—3.5 (good−); bilateral IV, V—3.5 to 4.5/5 (good− to good+)

Dorsal interossei: 4/5 (good) throughout

Palmar interossei: 5 (normal) throughout

Thumb flexors: abductors, opposers: 5 (normal) throughout

Lower Extremity

Hips. There were no clinical findings. ROM was within normal limits; strength was 4/5 (good) in hip flexors and rotators, 3.7/5 (good−) in hip extensors.

Knees. No clinical findings. Martha complained of arthralgias in her right knee after walking long distances. ROM was within normal limits; strength was 4.5/5 (good+) for quadriceps and 5/5 (normal) for hamstrings.

Ankles. No pain was noted although plantar flexion was minimally limited. Subtalar inversion and eversion were slightly limited bilaterally to 10 degrees and 15 degrees, respectively. There was synovial thickening around the lateral malleolus but no pain with palpation. Strength of tibialis anterior and posterior and peroneus longus and brevis was decreased to grade 3/5 (fair).

MTP. Martha has right hallux valgus. MTPs II and III show synovial thickening but no pain upon palpation; extension, abduction, and flexion were limited. Strength of the extensor hallucis and flexor hallucis longus was 2/5 (poor).

Gait and Posture. Martha showed a mild lordosis with a lateral trunk sway during gait. She did not push off during terminal stance, walked flat footed, and pronated her feet while bearing weight. She had a round-shouldered posture.

Functional Upper Extremity Use

Manipulative Skills. Martha was right-hand dominant. She demonstrated good functional use of all prehension types except those tasks that require significant strength. She was able to write, type, and fasten large buttons. However, she tired after doing any manipulative task for longer than 15 minutes. She could not open resistive containers or fasten heavy-duty snaps.

Fine Motor Coordination. Fine motor dexterity as measured by the Southern California Motor Accuracy Test was within norms for age. Gross upper extremity coordination, as measured by the Box and Blocks Test, was also within normal limits.

Grip Strength and Prehension Strength. These were moderately decreased for age. Wrists were positioned in neutral when grip was measured. (An extended position affords the best biomechanical advantage.) Grip strength, measured by a dynamometer, was right, 15 pounds, left, 12 pounds. Prehension strengths measured using a pinch meter were decreased for 2-point tip and 3-point pad pinches.

Occupational Role Behavior

Self-Care. *Dressing:* Martha was independent in donning loose-fitting overhead shifts, button-down shirts, pants, socks, and shoes. She needed assistance in putting on a tight shirt or dress and was unable to zipper or button back closures. Occasionally, she was unable to snap her pants but was able to fasten most buttons and snaps. *Light hygiene:* She was able to wash her face, brush her teeth, and apply deodorant independently. *Grooming:* Martha applied all makeup independently, but she tired easily when blow-drying, styling, and combing her hair. *Bathing:* Martha bathed and shampooed independently. She used a long-handled sponge to wash her back and legs because she tired from bending. Martha complained that she did not have the strength to scrub as strongly as she would like. *Eating:* Martha ate independently but required help with meal preparation (e.g., opening containers, pouring liquids, and transferring food from the counter to the table).

Personal/Social   Martha was a 17-year-old high school senior. Prior to the onset of arthritis, she was very active on her junior high school drill team and enjoyed horseback riding, shopping with friends, cooking, and attending church retreats. All these activities were curtailed by the onset of JRA. Although her disease was presently not active, Martha was unable to walk long distances (which limited mall shopping), and she did not have the energy for after-school and family evening activities. She did socialize with friends on weekends, attended school dances, and dated occasionally.

Martha frequently became frustrated with her physical limitations. Initially, she did not tell her friends about her JRA and tried to maintain her active pace at school. She became so completely exhausted that she slept every afternoon at home and was unable to participate in family chores, such as cooking, babysitting, and cleaning. Once she finally told her friends about her arthritis, she was able to slow her pace and could balance social and family activities much better.

Martha said that she sometimes felt very unimportant. She missed the social recognition she received from drill team activities. She excelled in school work, particularly languages and psychology, but got little reinforcement for her academic performance at home. Her family did not value education.

Presently, Martha was most concerned about her future employment opportunities, ability to bear children, and her appearance. On the prednisolone Martha had gained 7 pounds and still felt "not pretty" despite her careful efforts to enhance her appearance. She was unable to wear low-cut fashionable shoes or tight-fitting fashions.

School.   Martha did well academically. She was particularly good in languages, composition, and psychology. Although her grades reflected much hard work, they were not well rewarded at home. Martha's teachers knew she had arthritis and had made special arrangements for her when necessary. Martha was allowed extra time for essay tests, and she taped lectures when she could not keep up with note taking. Martha used a backpack to transport books and had a locker with the handle removed for ease in opening. Friends usually offered to take Martha's lunch through the cashier line so that she didn't have to carry the tray or wait in line. Since gym classes were not mandatory for seniors, Martha did not take gym.

Vocational.   Martha wanted to become a bilingual education teacher, social worker, or "something to do with children." Her previous desire to become a hairdresser or cosmetologist was thwarted when Martha's ankle and wrist involvement progressed to such a degree that prolonged standing and static flexed wrist positions caused pain. Although Martha's aspirations appeared realistic, her family did not fully support her desire to attend college before starting a family. She had been referred to vocational rehabilitation who had agreed to pay for her college education.

Independent Living Skills.   Martha took care of her personal belongings independently (although not to the meticulous degree she desired). She did laundry twice per week and alternated cooking with her sister. (Previously she performed these tasks daily.) Martha bought her own clothes and had a bank account. For transportation, Martha depended on her family and friends because she had difficulty boarding the bus. Martha would have liked to live on her own but was still physically and financially dependent on her parents.

Family.   Martha was the oldest of five siblings (2 girls and 3 boys). Her brother took care of children in the afternoon, and her father was a mechanic in a foreign car dealership. Martha had taken a strong role in helping raise her brothers and sisters and had helped her mother with many home chores. With the onset of Martha's arthritis, other family members have had to assume increasing responsibilities. Martha's parents were born and raised in El Salvador. They had very traditional Latin beliefs about women's role in the home as a support for the husband and a mother for the children.

Equipment.   Martha preferred to wear flexible wrist orthoses for writing at school and doing chores at home. She wore UC-BL foot orthoses in her sneakers.

Summary.   Martha was a 17-year-old high school senior of Latin-American background who was diagnosed with polyarticular JRA at age 14. Martha suffered rapid, destructive joint changes early in the disease course, but had maintained stable physical and functional status during the past year. Upon occupational therapy assessment, major physical problems included decreased shoulder strength and endurance, bilateral elbow flexion contractures, moderately limited forearm rotation, and severely limited but functional wrist ranges. Wrists were positioned and used in ulnar deviation. Bilateral index and middle MCP joints showed chronic effusions. All MCP joints had severely limited hyperextension but full flexion. She had PIP flexion contractures of the right III and IV fingers and left IV and V fingers. Although grip and prehension strengths were decreased, Martha's only self-care limitations were decreased speed in dressing and difficulty in grooming and fastening. Her major difficulties were in psychosocial areas of self-esteem, social isolation, and independent living skills. Problems in these areas were related to her poor body image, inability to continue valued activities, and decreased endurance to keep up with friends. She did appear to have good motivation and a strong familial support system; however, her Latin-American family's traditional views of the female role made it difficult for Martha to plan her future.

Occupational Therapy Treatment Plan

Short-Term Occupational Therapy Goals

1. Increase upper extremity shoulder, elbow, and wrist strength, emphasizing extensors.
2. Increase independence and rapidity of all self-care activities.
3. Maximize hand function by increasing manipulative strengths. Maintain present upper extremity ROM measurements.
4. Increase overall endurance (in conjunction with Physical Therapy).
5. Teach joint-protection and energy-conservation techniques.
6. Begin investigation of vocational options.
7. Investigate activities to help enhance self-esteem.
8. Facilitate competence in one avocational activity to enhance self-esteem.

9. Review accurate knowledge of disease course with Martha.
10. Encourage Martha to express her feelings and concerns about the arthritis.

Adolescent Outpatient Program

Measures to Alleviate Morning Stiffness. Take a warm bath for 20 minutes. Perform active ROM exercises for wrist, fingers, and ankles in tub.

Home Exercise Program
1. Warm-up with low-impact, slow aerobics that emphasize full ROM with slow rhythmical beat for upper and lower extremities. Use her favorite music. Build up to using ankle weight secured proximal to elbow.
2. *Isometrics*
   a. Elbow extension isometric exercises: Place towel roll under elbow and extend 20 times; hold to count of 7 after each repetition.
   b. Forearm rotation: Rotate forearm and hold at the end of the range.
3. Perform strengthening exercises for wrist extensors.
4. Perform hand active ROM exercises to finger and thumb abductors and extensors, flexor digitorum profundus, flexor digitorum sublimis, and thumb opposers. Perform exercises to reduce intrinsic tightness bilaterally in digits II and III.
5. *Thermaplast exercises* for hand intrinsics and extensors, thumb abductor, thumb extensor, and thumb opposer strengthening.
6. Therapeutic activities (1) to encourage strengthening of upper extremity extensors and shoulder musculature; (2) to maintain full active ROM of flexors; and (3) to increase prehension strengths. Integrate with chores and avocational choices:
   - Home chores: sweeping, dusting, washing dishes (be sure to pace herself)
   - Kneading dough with the heel of the hand
   - Macrame suspended at shoulder height (check for full finger ROM)
   - Pattern making—using wrists and fingers in extension
   - Clay: ceramic coil pots, ceramic pinch pots, ceramic sculpture
   - Decoupage

Self-Care Activities

1. *Grooming:* Try gradually to increase time spent in blow drying hair. If Martha is still unable to dry her hair because of decreased shoulder or hand strength, attach the blow dryer to a wall. As a last resort, recommend a permanent.

2. *Dressing:* Continue to dress independently. Use adapted equipment (zipper pull, dressing stick) only as needed. Adapt fasteners with Velcro only as needed.

3. *Bathing:* Use a loofa pad (for deeper cleaning with lightweight handles).

Independent Living Skills

1. *Home chores:* Martha is dependent in washing, meal preparation, and laundry due to decreased endurance. Teach her proper energy-conservation techniques to allow her to pace herself and execute tasks most effectively.

2. *Shopping:* Martha should continue to shop, but should go to selected stores so as not to fatigue completely from walking long distances. (Realize that "hanging out" with friends is more important than actual purchases.)

3. *Living independently:* Make Martha aware of financial resources to aid independent living (vocational rehabilitation). Arrange physical environment to facilitate independence.

Psychosocial Involvement

1. *Body image:* Reinforce careful grooming; encourage Martha in weight maintenance and reduction programs (refer to nutritionist); go shopping together to delineate which styles are the most flattering while also easiest to don. Increased strength and overall energy will generally enhance Martha's good sense about herself.

2. *Self-esteem:* Recommend helping choreograph drill team configurations; join the high school yearbook committee or debate club to feel "important" or as a "contributing" school member; appreciate reinforcement from school personnel (guidance counselors, teachers) and medical team for academic success; become confident and competent in one avocational activity; maintain some home responsibilities; refer Martha to a teen support group, if she is interested.

3. *Social interaction:* Make *sure* that Martha continues to visit and go out with friends.

School. Recommend adapted writing utensils for writing fatigue. Continue with frequent rest periods during writing and adaptive strategies for school. Use a backpack to carry books.

Vocational Planning. Observe and explore the various career paths in which Martha is interested (e.g., visit bilingual schools, social work settings, and nursery schools). This will give Martha a clearer picture of the physical requirements and daily responsibilities of these careers. Investigate continuing educational requirements of each career.

Joint Protection

1. Wear wrist and finger orthoses at night to help prevent further loss of ROM in wrists and fingers.

2. Wear orthoses during heavy work to protect wrists from outside trauma.

3. Teach joint-protection principles that apply to cooking, carrying books, doing chores, and choosing avocational and vocational activities.

Education

1. Draw, describe, and discuss the arthritis disease process. Have Martha reiterate her present understanding of the disease.

2. Review the most effective modalities to decrease joint pain for Martha.

3. Help her understand how exercise, relaxation, and having fun can help her systemic health and her arthritis. Include the family in this discussion.

Physical Therapy Plan

1. Orthoses: UC-BL foot orthoses to wear in sneakers. Attach toe separators to foot orthoses to maintain alignment of great toes.

2. Overall strengthening program to increase shoulder, scapular, wrist, and hip and knee extensor strength.

3. Specific therapeutic exercise to increase strength and ROM of ankle plantar and dorsiflexion, toe flexion and extension, and ankle inversion and eversion.

4. Thermal (heat) modalities to decrease knee arthralgias.

5. Therapeutic activities to increase endurance.

6. Gait training.

PART IV

EVALUATION METHODS

Part IV describes evaluation methods unique to the treatment of people with rheumatic disorders and the considerations necessary to apply general evaluative measures to this specific patient group.

Chapter 18 reviews the nuances of interviewing that need to be considered when evaluating a patient's medical history and medical treatment. Chapter 19, on hand pathodynamics and assessment, describes in detail the components that make up a comprehensive assessment for rheumatoid arthritis hand involvement. Chapter 20, on evaluation of ROM, has been revised and contains new material on the importance of evaluating and treating MCP hyperextension and evaluation of the complex motions of the thumb. Chapter 21, on evaluation of muscle strength, includes the latest research on standardization of grip and pinch strength measurement. Chapter 22, on evaluation of activities of daily living, includes new material on vocational assessment to determine the need for joint protection and energy conservation measures in the workplace. Since more women are remaining employed outside the home, vocational assessment has become an integral part of occupational therapy in rheumatology.

Chapter 18

Evaluation of Medical History and Symptoms

Interviewing patients about their diagnosis, onset of disease, medications, joint involvement, and systemic manifestations is critical to planning treatment and effective patient education. It is also essential to professionalism. The nature and extent of the interviewing will differ for outpatients and inpatients. For outpatients, it may be appropriate to ask what kind of arthritis they have to learn about their level of disease sophistication and the need for patient education. (I do this in my clinic by asking this question on the initial intake form each new patient fills out.) Inpatients might be unnerved by such a question, for they expect, or at least hope, that the members of the "medical team" are communicating among themselves and that the therapist knows about their problems before beginning treatment.

I have made changes in the way I document and report the medical history in my practice. I take an in-depth history and record it in my patient-care chart, but I no longer summarize the medical history in my reports to physicians as traditionally taught. I simply note in the report that the "medical history was reviewed." The concept of summarizing the medical history in the report was to let the physician know the medical information the therapist took into consideration before planning treatment. In an inpatient chart, the information is clearly redundant. In an outpatient report to a physician's office, the information is not helpful: it clutters the report and does not add anything. Because physicians (like everyone else) are overwhelmed with reading material, they prefer therapists' reports that are "lean and keen." So I generally try to adhere to this rule. However, occasionally, it is necessary to include data to serve as legal documentation rather than purely for patient-care communication.

For therapists new to working with or interviewing patients with arthritis, this chapter shares the nuances of interviewing that one learns from experience rather than from medical texts or departmental procedural guides. I have tried to focus on topics most relevant to planning effective treatment.

DIAGNOSIS AND ONSET

For outpatients, I find it quite helpful to ask the patient what his or her diagnosis is. It is quite revealing when a patient, under the care of an excellent rheumatologist, does not know what type of arthritis he or she has. This alerts me that possibly the patient is in denial about the illness and does not want to attend to the facts about it. Or it suggests that the patient gets so nervous or has so much pain that he or she cannot hear or retain verbal instructions. (As it is safe to assume that a rheumatologist is going to tell the patient a specific diagnosis.) This response can be a cue to the need to write out all instructions for the patient or send the patient a copy of my report to the physician, or both.

Determining "onset" sounds simple enough, but *in relation to arthritis there can be* **three "onsets": symptoms, diagnosis, and disability.** If you ask a patient, "When did you get rheumatoid arthritis?" or "How long have you had osteoarthritis?" he or she will most typically tell you the date the diagnosis was made. This may be close to or years after the onset of symptoms. It is actually the onset of symptoms that gives the most accurate picture of how much damage may have occurred in the joint. The onset of disability can also differ significantly from the onset of arthritis. For example, if you ask a homemaker disabled by arthritis in her knees, "How long have you had arthritis in your knees?" she may tell you 10 years, implying that she has been disabled for 10 years. In truth, she may have been disabled for only 1 year. With osteoarthritis, the reverse is more typical. Because people can have osteoarthritis for years without pain (only joint changes), they associate the onset of arthritis with the onset of pain. Thus, a woman with osteoarthritis of the basal thumb joint may tell you she has only had "arthritis" for 6 months, when in fact she has had it for 10 to 15 years without pain. (This can be pointed

out to the patient as at least one positive aspect of the situation.) Determining the onset of disability in specific joints helps provide a clearer picture of how the disease has affected the patient's life-style.

Questions you may want to ask about disease onset are as follows:

When were you diagnosed?
How long before that did the symptoms start?
How long has the arthritis in your joints limited your ability to do things?

JOINTS AFFECTED

During an initial evaluation, one of my procedures is to review all the joints that may be affected by the type of rheumatic disease that the person may have. Table 18–1 shows the **joint review** list I use for evaluating a patient with rheumatoid arthritis (RA). This is a brief, cursory assessment (interview and AROM demonstration only) to get a sense of the current and past involvement of each joint, which determines the scope of the treatment, the need for additional referrals (e.g., physical therapy or podiatry), and which joints need an in-depth evaluation. I use general, lay terms in the interview (e.g., "Do you have

Table 18–1 Joint Review for Diagnosis of Rheumatoid Arthritis*

Temporomandibular (TM) joints
Cricoarytenoid joints
Sternum
    Sternoclavicular joints
    Sternocostal joints
Neck
Upper back (to screen for fibromyalgia)
Lower back (for concomitant lower back pain, not RA)
Shoulders
Elbows
Wrists
Hands
Hips
Thighs (to screen for fibromyalgia)
Knees
Ankles
Subtalar joints
Metatarsophalangeal (MTP) joints

*Involvement of the joints listed above in RA is described in Chapter 6.

any problems with your jaw or neck?") and document the patient's own descriptors in the chart (e.g., "It is occasionally stiff." "It hurts only when I shake my hair dry in the morning."). I ask further questions as necessary to get as clear a picture as possible about joint involvement in terms of pain, swelling, warmth, stiffness, catching, limited range of motion, or deformity.

The brief joint review described above allows me to get a broad overview of the problem so that I can determine where to narrow my focus in treatment. I find this essential to effective treatment planning. If I start with narrow focusing on the hand or shoulder, I inevitably overlook critical elements in the patient's situation.

The joint review can be very helpful and serve as grounding for the patient. Frequently, a patient will state that he or she has "arthritis all over," but the joint review may actually reveal joints *not* involved. This situation often occurs with patients who have RA of the peripheral joints but not of the axial or central joints. These patients feel as if the pain is all over, but when you interview them closely, you find that they may not have any pain in the back, sternum, or jaw. Some patients may not have shoulder or hip involvement.

When people are in an emotional crisis and feel overwhelmed, they tend to generalize the problem. The joint review can be used as a psychological tool to help break up the huge generalized problem into specific manageable units. And finding out that some units are okay, not damaged, makes the entire problem more manageable.

Therapists can use the joint review most effectively if they know the typical patterns of joint involvement for each disease. This is outlined in each medical chapter in Part II.

MEDICATIONS

Fast-acting medications (e.g., aspirin and nonsteroidal anti-inflammatory drugs [NSAIDs]) and analgesics can alter patient performance on objective assessments, such as dressing time, grip strength, range of motion, and so forth, in as little as one-half hour. Therefore, it is important to note the name and dosage of the medication, and the frequency and regularity of the patient's intake, and to determine when medications have been taken prior to a physical evaluation.

For some reason, when you ask patients, "What medications are you taking for your arthritis?" they readily tell you about the anti-inflammatories but omit telling you that on an exceptionally bad day, they take 2 Darvon tablets or other pain killers before coming to the clinic. Sometimes patients take pain killers borrowed from a friend or prescribed for another problem and would prefer not to admit this. Sporadic use of analgesics can definitely skew objective assessments from one visit to the next.

The proper use of medications can make or break a therapy program. Consider the following examples of this.

Example 1

A patient with long-standing Kienbock's disease (avascular necrosis of the lunate) has secondary transcarpal arthritis and ruptured extensor tendons. After surgical removal of the lunate and tendon repair, the wrist is stiff. The therapy goal is to increase wrist range of motion to the preoperative range. The surgeon prescribed Motrin for the carpal arthritis. On the third therapy visit, there was no improvement in wrist motion and there was excessive muscular guarding, and the patient reported that she was having trouble using her hand because of the wrist pain. Initially, it appeared that the Motrin was not working, but further questioning revealed that the patient was not taking the medication as a therapeutic inflammatory measure (2400 mg per day) to reduce the arthritis but as a mild analgesic on an as-needed basis. Further interviewing revealed that the patient does not eat breakfast, eats only a light lunch, and does not drink milk because of lactose intolerance; therefore, she has difficulty taking the Motrin as prescribed with meals. If the pain is not resolved in the wrist, she will not be able to use it, and the contractures from postoperative immobilization will become permanent. The options are to change her eating habits or switch to a medication like Feldene, which only needs to be taken once per day to be therapeutically effective.

Example 2

I had instructed a patient with RA in an isometric strengthening program for her hands. The following week she reported that the exercises were making her hands worse, so she stopped doing them. But her hands have remained painful. The fact that her hands did not get better after stopping the exercises made me suspicious that the exercises were not the aggravating factor. Inquiry regarding her medications revealed that she had been on a new NSAID for 2 months with minimal improvement. She had other increases in systemic manifestations, but she was so sure that the exercises were the source of the pain that she had not made the connection that the NSAID she was taking was no longer working for her. It turns out that it was the fourth NSAID prescribed in a short period of time, and the trial-and-error approach to finding the right medication made the patient feel like a guinea pig. She did not want the latest medication to also fail. After acknowledging her feelings about medication trials and the importance of controlling inflammation so that she could benefit from exercise, the patient contacted her physician, who changed her medication. This time the medication worked fairly effectively, and the patient was able to do the hand exercise programs without any increase in inflammation.

The following are questions you may want to ask about medications:

Do you feel that the medications are working?
Are you taking them as prescribed?
Are you having difficulty taking them?
If there is a change in symptoms, is it related to a change in medications?

SYSTEMIC MANIFESTATIONS

Percentage of Good Versus Bad Days

Patients with intermittent or episodic arthritis often report that they have good days during which they can do all activities independently and bad days during which they cannot work or do housework. *If* it becomes difficult during the interview to assess the patient's functional ability, it is helpful to have the patient estimate the approximate number of days per month during which he or she has more problems than usual from the arthritis. This can be computed into an approximate percentage, if desired. In addition to a clearer picture of the patient's life-style and disability status, this information can provide a convenient quantitative means of relaying information to the physician or other therapist. For example, if the patient has 3 to 4 bad days a week, this is equal to being disabled approximately 50 percent of the time. Even though this person's arthritis is not constant, he or she would have difficulty maintaining a house or working full time. The need for work simplification and assistive devices is much greater for a patient with 50 percent disability compared with the need in a patient who may be limited only one day a week (14 percent).

Morning Stiffness

Morning stiffness is a term used to describe the prolonged generalized stiffness that occurs in association with the inflammatory polyarthritides (especially RA, juvenile rheumatoid arthritis, psoriatic arthritis, and ankylosing spondylitis) upon awakening. The stiffness tends to be generalized and may last for several hours and is indicative of systemic involvement. This contrasts with the stiffness of degenerative joint disease that is localized and occurs only in involved joints after inactivity and that disappears within one-half hour after moving the involved joint.

Morning stiffness is an objective indicator of the degree of disease activity present.[1,2] Patients with uncontrolled or untreated RA may have up to 5 hours of generalized stiffness in the morning. As the disease becomes controlled by medications or becomes less active, the duration of morning stiffness decreases and may only be 15 to 30 minutes long. Patients may have some degree of stiffness all day. This is usually due to swelling or inflammation of the joints. Morning stiffness is a distinct feeling of excessive stiffness that wears off at a given point. Patients will often describe the situation thus: "My morning stiffness wears off about 10:00 AM; then I have my regular stiffness the rest of the day."

Severity

Determining how morning stiffness interferes with or influences functional ability also needs consideration. Many patients feel stiff but are able to get around and to perform self-care functions, whereas others are totally dependent during periods of morning stiffness.

The ability to assess the duration effectively can facilitate occupational therapy treatment planning. Many patients are quite disabled by morning stiffness. If the patient has 3 to 5 hours of morning stiffness, he or she may need assistive devices to increase independence during this period. Consequently, functional ability may need to be assessed when morning stiffness is present and later in the afternoon after it has subsided.

Duration

The duration of morning stiffness is a common rheumatological assessment tool. It is calculated from the time the patient wakes up until the stiffness wears off. It is recorded in number of hours.[1]

Every patient with arthritis seems to have his or her own routine for limbering up in the morning. This needs to be taken into account when interviewing the patient. Some patients have established a pattern of waking up, taking medications, and then going back to sleep for a couple of hours until the stiffness wears off. Simply asking patients what time they get up and what time the stiffness wears off may not reveal the extra two hours of stiffness described in the above example.

The following questions are suggested for determining the patient's *duration of morning stiffness:*[3]

Are your joints usually stiff in the morning when you awaken?
What time do you usually awaken?
What time do you usually get out of bed?
Does the stiffness wear off? About what time? Or, What time does the *morning* stiffness wear off and do you have the regular stiffness?

It is also helpful to ask "Which joints are stiff in the morning?" If patients describe stiffness only in specific or isolated joints, then this is probably due to swelling and not generalized systemic morning stiffness.

Endurance

Easy fatigability is one of the complications of all systemic diseases. It is further enhanced by chronic loss of sleep (due to pain), diminished deep (stage 4) restorative sleep (see Chapter 5 on fibromyalgia), decreased muscle tone and strength, inactivity, poor or inadequate nutrition, and psychological factors such as depression (see Chapter 2). Fatigue associated with systemic disease varies with the time of day, whereas fatigue associated with depression tends to be more constant. Early afternoon fatigue (around 2:00 PM) is such a consistent finding that physicians frequently use the elapsed time between arising in the morning and the onset of fatigue as a parameter of disease status.

Assessment of Fatigue for Planning Treatment

For the purpose of planning treatment I find it helpful to determine the patient's *energy pattern.*[3] This would include the following interview questions.

Pattern or time of peak and low energy?
Time of day fatigue occurs?
Duration of fatigue?
How does the patient handle the fatigue? What does he/she do to improve endurance or reduce fatigue? For example, takes short naps or meditates, or just "pushes through the day."
What factors, besides illness, contribute to the patient's fatigue or endurance level?

Assessment of the patient's energy pattern and fatigue/endurance-related behaviors provides essential data for planning patient education with regard to energy conservation, exercise, rest, relaxation techniques, improving sleep patterns, nutrition, and psychological support for reducing depression. Awareness of the patient's energy pattern is also important when scheduling therapy appointments and making recommendations for the home program.[3]

AMERICAN RHEUMATISM ASSOCIATION (ARA) FUNCTIONAL CLASSIFICATION[4,5]

This general classification system was specifically designed for patients with rheumatoid arthritis but, because it is so general, it can be used with other rheumatic diseases.

Class I Complete functional capacity with ability to carry on all usual duties without handicaps.

Class II Functional capacity adequate to conduct normal activities despite handicap of discomfort or limited mobility of one or more joints.

Class III Functional capacity adequate to perform only a few or none of the duties of the patient's usual occupation or of self-care.

Class IV Largely or wholly incapacitated with patient bedridden or confined to wheelchair, permitting little or no self-care.

This classification is limited, in so far as it is general and can reflect only gross changes in the patient's progression or regression. However, it is often helpful in providing a quick overall gestalt of the patient's status. Therapists should be aware of this classification because it is used in research.

REFERENCES

1. McCarty, DJ: Clinical assessment of arthritis. In McCarty, DJ (ed): Arthritis and Allied Conditions. Lea & Febiger, Philadelphia, 1979, pp 131–149.
2. Polley, HF, and Hunder, GG: Rheumatologic Interviewing and Physical Examination of the Joints, 2nd ed. WB Saunders, Philadelphia, 1978.
3. Melvin, JL: Rheumatic Disease—Occupational Therapy and Rehabilitation. FA Davis, Philadelphia, 1977, p 94.
4. Rodman, GP, and Schumacher, HR (eds): Primer on the Rheumatic Diseases. The Arthritis Foundation, Atlanta, 1983.
5. Steinbrocker, O, Traeger, CG, and Batterman, RC: Therapeutic criteria in rheumatoid arthritis. JAMA 140:659, 1949.

Chapter 19

Hand Pathodynamics and Assessment

Boutonnière Deformity
Chronic Synovitis
Lengthening of the Central Slip
Volar Displacement of the Lateral Bands
Mallet Finger Deformity
Thumb Deformities—Rheumatoid
Type I—Flexion of MCP Joint with Hyperextension of IP Joint and Compensatory CMC Abduction ("Extrinsic Minus Thumb")
Type II—CMC Joint Subluxation (Adduction) with MCP Joint Hyperextension and IP Joint Flexion
Type III—MCP Lateral Deviation with CMC Joint Adduction
Type IV—MCP Hyperextension and IP Flexion (Normal CMC Joint)
Type V—Mutilans Thumb

MUSCLE INVOLVEMENT
Intrinsic Muscle Atrophy
Intrinsic Muscle Weakness
Abductor Pollicis Brevis
Dorsal and Volar Interossei
Abductor Digiti Quinti
Intrinsic Muscle Tightness

TENDON INVOLVEMENT
Tenosynovitis
Volar Wrist Tenosynovitis
Palmar Tenosynovitis
Digital Flexor Tenosynovitis
Dorsal Wrist Tenosynovitis
Trigger Finger
de Quervain's Tenosynovitis
Tendon Ruptures
Extensor Digiti Quinti (EDQ)
Extensor Digitorum Communis (EDC)
Extensor Pollicis Longus (EPL)
Flexor Pollicis Longus (FPL)
Flexor Digitorum Profundus
Flexor Digitorum Superficialis (FDS)

SKIN AND VASCULAR INVOLVEMENT
Skin Changes
Skin Ulcerations
Drug Reactions
Skin Tightness
Vasculitis
Telangiectasia
Palmar Eythema
Purpura
Keratoderma Blennorrhagica
Temperature Changes and Sweating
Raynaud's Phenomenon

NEUROLOGICAL INVOLVEMENT
Cervical Radiculopathy or Nerve Root Compression Syndrome
Entrapment Neuropathies
Median Nerve Entrapment
Carpal Tunnel Syndrome (CTS) Wrist Level
Median Nerve Entrapment in the Proximal Forearm

The key to effective management of the arthritic hand is early identification of pathodynamics that can cause secondary limitations and the prevention of those secondary limitations. It is generally not possible to prevent the primary disease, but the consequences of disease can often be controlled or reduced.

For example, it may not be possible to prevent tendon adhesions in the wrist due to tenosynovitis, but with early detection, it is often possible to mobilize the tendons and/or prevent digital joint contractures secondary to the restricted tendon function. Another example is joint stiffness secondary to digital flexor tenosynovitis. Again, it is not possible to prevent the tenosynovitis, but it is possible to prevent stiffness or to restore joint motion if stiffness results from flexor tenosynovitis. These are just two of many deformities that can be prevented with early detection and intervention. In order to detect early manifestations of disease and thereby have an opportunity for early intervention, a systematic and thorough hand assessment must be carried out.

Comprehensive hand assessment and treatment offer a major contribution to rheumatological rehabilitation. The occupational therapist with a knowledge of hand anatomy (Fig. 19–1), skill in functional analysis, and the ability to determine splinting and joint-protection interventions is in a unique position to provide this service. This chapter will review the assessment criteria for determining the status of anatomical structures and the common manifestations of arthritis in the hand. There is an emphasis on the pathology that can be altered by treatment and on secondary limitations that can be prevented.

This chapter can be used in sections to review specific phenomena, or it can be used in its totality as a description of a *comprehensive hand evaluation program.* The hand assessment form was developed to facilitate documentation and data retrieval and is included at the end of this chapter as an example of how these complex data can be organized in a medical record format. The grouping of arthritis manifestations on this form was based on the natural sequence of evaluation by the staff occupational therapists (at the former Robert B. Brigham Hospital). The same grouping or sequence is used in this chapter to review assessment criteria. Thus, arthri-

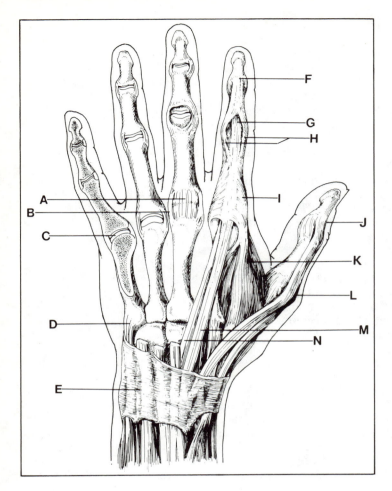

Figure 19–1. Normal hand structures are illustrated here: (*A*) joint capsule, (*B*) collateral ligaments, (*C*) hyaline cartilage, (*D*) insertion of the extensor carpi ulnaris tendon, (*E*) dorsal retinaculum, (*F*) distal attachment of the extensor communis tendon, (*G*) central slip of the extensor communis tendon, (*H*) lateral bands of the extensor communis tendon, (*I*) extensor hood mechanism, (*J*) insertion of the extensor pollicis longus tendon, (*K*) first dorsal interosseous muscle, (*L*) insertion of the extensor pollicis brevis tendon, (*M*) extensor communis tendon, (*N*) extensor indicis proprius tendon. (Adapted from Gatter, RA, and Andrews, R: Articular and Periarticular Diseases of the Wrist and Hand. Merck, Sharp, and Dohme, West Point, PA, 1972.)

tis manifestations are discussed in the following order: joint and soft tissue involvement, common hand deformities, muscle involvement, tendon involvement, skin and vascular involvement, and neurological involvement.

CONSIDERATIONS PRIOR TO HAND ASSESSMENT

Medications

The type of medication and dosage pattern used by the patient can significantly affect objective measurements and the accuracy of longitudinal assessments. The effect of the patient's medication regimen on functional ability should be determined prior to performing a hand assessment. Most patients can describe the effects the medication has on their mobility, pain, stiffness, and function.

Fast-acting medications (such as aspirin, nonsteroidal anti-inflammatory drugs [NSAIDs], analgesics) can create a day-to-day variability in performance. Slow-acting medications (e.g., gold, Plaquenil; see Chapter 3) can influence longitudinal assessments (i.e., re-assessments that may occur over a 1- to 3-month period). For example, some patients who take aspirin or another NSAID every 4 hours have greater stiffness at the end of the 4-hour cycle than 30 minutes after taking the medication. Patients on steroid medication every other day can have marked fluctuations in mobility, depending on what day of the cycle assessment is done. Also, some patients take an extra analgesic on "bad days," which can affect range of motion (ROM) and strength measures.

See Chapter 3, Drug Therapy, for additional information on classification of medication, side effects, and references; and Chapter 18 for examples of medications affecting hand therapy.

Neck, Shoulder, Elbow, and Forearm Involvement

There are several conditions in the proximal upper extremity that can cause deformity in the hand or alter hand function in some manner. When there is a marked or noticeable condition present, relevant information is usually conveyed in the referral to occupational therapy and included in the assessment. However, there may be minor conditions or disabilities that may have occurred in the past that can influence a detailed hand assessment and the treatment plan but that the physician did not consider important enough to note on the referral form. Additionally, in some clinics, the patient's chart, history, or assessment by the physician is not available at the time of the patient's therapy session. It therefore becomes the responsibility of each therapist to be knowledgeable of conditions in the neck and upper extremity that can influence hand function. Assessment of the proximal upper extremity prior to performing the hand assessment helps safeguard against accidental omission of one of these contributing factors and can provide information that may explain pathology seen in the hand.

In clinics in which the occupational therapist treats all upper extremity disorders, it is reasonable to perform an in-depth musculoskeletal evaluation of the neck and upper extremity prior to the hand assessment for arthritis. In clinics in which the physical therapist treats the neck and proximal extremity, it is more reasonable for the occupational therapist to perform a cursory proximal assessment and then refer the patient to physical therapy for a detailed assessment if significant problems are detected.

Methods for conducting a detailed musculoskeletal evaluation are available in several excellent texts.[1–4] The most common proximal conditions that can mimic localized hand problems and confound the hand assessment for arthritis are included here.

1. Cervical arthritis (RA or OA) producing nerve root compression. This can result in paresthesias and sensory loss along associated dermatomes and motor loss along nerve root patterns.[5] For example, compression at C-6 level can cause sensory loss on the volar aspect of the thumb, which may be confused with carpal tunnel syndrome. Sensory loss usually occurs before motor loss.

Patients with neck pain or stiffness may be candidates for instruction in joint-protection techniques and use of a cervical pillow. (See Chapters 24 and 28.) Treatment for cervical arthritis is described in Chapter 4 (OA), Chapter 6 (RA), and Chapter 14 (JRA).

2. Shoulder pain secondary to synovitis, tendonitis, or bursitis frequently refers to pain down the extremity. This usually occurs along the lateral border to the midarm or midforearm level. Occasionally it can extend into the palm.[6] In one clinical experience, a patient with RA related the pain in her palm to newly made wrist orthoses; however, there were no evident pressure areas. After several return visits and multiple splint modifications, an association was made with referred pain from severe ipsilateral shoulder synovitis. The patient was referred back to the rheumatologist, who injected her shoulder—and the palmar hand pain disappeared. The original orthosis had to be recreated.

Pain from the neck or shoulder is commonly referred to the mid-upper arm region (around the area of the deltoid insertion); to the lateral epicondyle; and to the mid-lateral forearm, but the referred pain can be anywhere along the lateral border. Referred pain from the neck or shoulder is likely when patients describe arm pain that does not seem to be associated with specific underlying anatomical structures. Another common source of referred pain is fibromyalgia. All therapists treating hands should be familiar with upper extremity involvement of fibromyalgia (see Chapter 5).

It is also possible for certain internal organs, such as the gallbladder, to refer pain *to* the shoulder. In these cases, the patient may complain of shoulder pain but have no clinical shoulder findings.[6] Shoulder pain may also limit the kind of exercises used for the hand, for example, isometric towel-loop exercises.

3. Abnormal spinal or shoulder alignment can distort wrist–hand mechanisms. In one case an elderly woman referred for de Quervain's tenosynovitis repeatedly denied any type of pinching activity that could be the aggravating source of the problem. Proximal analysis revealed that she had a severe spinal curvature with anterior displacement of her shoulder girdle, placing the arm in internal rotation and necessitating marked ulnar deviation of the wrist to write or do table-top activities. In order to prevent stress to her first compartment tendons, physical therapy was needed to improve shoulder alignment.

4. Reflex sympathetic dystrophy (shoulder–hand syndrome). This can occur in patients with arthritis. In the early stages it can be very mild. When this occurs, it typically results in diffuse unilateral hand pain that does not correlate with joint or tendon involvement. (This condition can also be bilateral.) Shoulder–hand syndromes can result in flexion deformities of the digits.[7] Occasionally, a patient with arthritis presents with residual contractures from a reflex dystrophy that resolved several years prior to the arthritis.[1]

5. Elbow synovitis commonly causes ulnar nerve entrapment, resulting in paresthesias, sensory loss, and eventually weakness in the ulnar innervated muscles distal to the forearm.[8] Weakness in 2-point pinch and mild clawing of the ring and little fingers are easily detected clinical signs.[9] Although rare, it is possible for elbow synovitis to cause compression (volar to elbow) of the posterior interosseous branch of the radial nerve, resulting in weakness of the thumb and finger extensors.[10] (A detailed review of other nerve entrapment syndromes is given in the section on neurological involvement in this chapter.)

6. Forearm rotation can be limited by synovitis at either the distal or proximal radioulnar joint, or both.[1] The patient generally feels pain in the joint that is causing the limitation at the end of the rotation.

7. Tennis elbow (lateral epicondylitis) and golfer's elbow (medial epicondylitis) are common conditions. These conditions often occur unrelated to their namesake sports. They are believed to result from occupational strain on the tendoperiosteal junction (enthesis) of the respective lateral or medial muscles. The characteristic symptom is pain over the lateral epicondyle when resistance is applied to the wrist extensors and pain over the medial epicondyle when resistance is applied to the wrist flexors.[11,12]

An activated trigger point in the extensor muscle group is a common symptom of fibromyalgia (see Chapter 5).

Diabetes

Diabetes, a common systemic disease, needs special consideration because it can cause a wide range of specific hand dysfunctions that can be confused with problems associated with an inflammatory arthritis. Diabetic hand dysfunction can include any of the following:

1. Tightening or thickening of the skin that appears like scleroderma and can lead to mild flexion contractures of all the digit joints (referred to as *limited ROM*)
2. Dupuytren's contracture, extending the length of the digit as well as in the palm
3. Trigger finger
4. Median and ulnar nerve entrapment (This can be very specific; e.g., of the median motor nerve to the abductor pollicis brevis.)
5. Peripheral neuropathy, mononeuritis multiplex
6. Raynaud's phenomenon
7. Pseudogout in the wrist; calcium pyrophosphate crystal deposition in the cartilage

(See section on diabetic hand involvement in Additional Sources at the end of this chapter for references.)

History of Hand Surgery or Trauma

Mallet finger and boutonnière, swanneck, and angulation deformities can result from trauma. Contributing factors in the patient's history should be ruled out before deformities are attributed to arthritis. It is also helpful specifically to ask the patient about prior surgery, trauma, or hand therapy. Many patients forget to mention these issues, which can influence a treatment plan.

JOINT AND SOFT TISSUE INVOLVEMENT

The following parameters are applicable to the wrist and individual digital joints.

Pain

For adults pain is a major symptom of both synovitis and OA. Therefore, the assessment of pain provides information about the severity of these two conditions. For synovitis, joint **pain during rest** (when the joint is not moving) indicates severe or acute inflammation, and the pain is a result of increased intra-articular pressure.[1] **Pain during motion but not at rest** indicates active but less acute inflammation. Patients with mild synovitis may only have **pain with lateral-medial compression of the joint** (i.e., they will report no pain with active motion, but when gentle compression is applied they identify pain in the involved joints).[1] In most cases, applying lateral-medial pressure is sufficient (Fig. 19–2). A more discriminating procedure in the proximal interphalangeal (PIP) and distal interphalangeal (DIP) joints is to apply medial-lateral pressure with one hand and then anterior-posterior pressure with the other hand. Extremely mild synovitis will be evident when this additional pressure is applied.[1] (Care must be taken not to apply pressure over a tender area such as an osteophyte.) Mild synovitis identified with compression is common in patients in whom medications are controlling the disease. Joint-protection methods may be appropriate for joints with mild synovitis; however, it is more difficult for the patient to perceive the benefits of the techniques if there is no sense of pain with active motion.

If children have pain with joint involvement the above assessment procedures apply to them. Some children do not perceive, experience, or report pain in the same manner as adults. These children can appear to have joint effusions without subjective pain. Understanding this aspect of children with arthritis is critical to successful evaluation and treatment of the hand. (See the section on pain in juvenile rheumatoid arthritis in Chapter 14.)

In the hand the process of **osteoarthritis (OA)**, that is, the cartilage wearing down, and secondary osteophyte formation is typically *painless*. The presence of pain with OA indicates inflammation. We do not know why inflammation occurs in some joints and not in others. One theory is that debris from cartilage damage and wear and tear irritates the synovial lining. (In the lower extremity joints, weight bearing creates additional forces that can stimulate subchondral pain receptors.) Another component of OA is the formation of bony cysts. These can be very tender or inflamed during formation, then painless as they ossify. The method of assessment and of defining severity of pain described above also applies to OA.

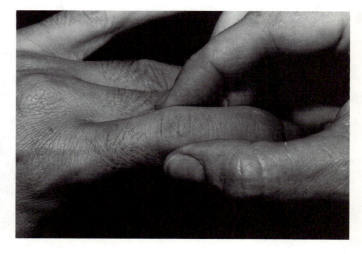

Figure 19–2. Palpation for mild synovitis is shown here. Support the patient's hand and apply firm medial and lateral compression as shown. When synovitis is present, tenderness will be elicited with this maneuver. Compare with a non-involved joint, if possible.

Pain can also inhibit muscle function.[13,14] Pain may be sudden, for example, when acute wrist or knee pain inhibits supporting muscles and the joint gives way. It may also be subtle and only reduce rather than completely stop muscle function. This may manifest as a sense of subjective weakness; for example, the patient will report that his or her hands are weak because he or she can no longer open jars or apply hard pressure. It is possible for true muscle weakness to be present with this same symptom, but for patients with painful hands, pain inhibition of muscle strength is the most common cause of this problem. Whenever a patient reports weakness it is important to determine if there is true muscle weakness, which will be clearly evident on a group or individual manual muscle test, or if pain during the activity is impairing muscle performance. If pain is the limiting factor, the treatment is often joint-protection instruction to eliminate the pain during the activity. If muscle weakness is present, strengthening exercises are indicated. Often this problem initially becomes evident during a grip strength test. For example, if a woman patient records a 20-lb grip and denies any pain in her fingers, wrist, or upper extremity during the test, it is likely that her grip is diminished due to true muscle weakness. (A group muscle test is indicated; however, it may not provide additional information because it is less sensitive than an objective grip gauge.) If in another situation, a patient records a 20-lb grip but reports pain in her fingers, wrist, elbow, or shoulder during the test, a manual group muscle test of the finger flexors is indicated. If the patient scores normal or 5 out of 5 on this test it is likely that the diminished grip is due to pain inhibition during the grip test rather than true muscle weakness. Whenever muscle strength is evaluated it is important to document the presence of pain anywhere in the upper extremity during the test, for pain invariably affects muscle performance.

Pain is usually identified as **articular** or **periarticular** (external to the joint). When it is periarticular, it is helpful to localize it to anatomical structures; for example, pain over the first dorsal interosseous muscle.

It is often very difficult for some patients to distinguish between pain and joint stiffness. If a patient reports pain that is disproportionate to the degree of joint involvement, careful interviewing may reveal that the patient is interpreting stiffness as pain.

Pain as a perception and pain as a function of disease activity (increased stimuli) can also be altered by environmental and psychological factors. Pain is affected by the circadian cycle, which reflects the concentration of humoral substances in the blood, such as cortisol, catecholamines, beta-endorphins, serotonin, and other substances. It can also be profoundly affected by depression, anxiety, lack of sleep (especially stage IV sleep), barometric pressure, humidity, and hot or cold environments.[15]

There have been multiple attempts to quantitate pain, primarily to provide objective measurements of drug effectiveness.[16,17] Having patients grade or indicate their pain on a visual analog scale (a line marked with increments ranging from mild to severe) has proven to be one of the most effective measures.[16] Mechanical devices that quantitate the pressure required to elicit pain (dolorimeter) have also been used.[18] These devices are useful in research but are not practical or helpful in a clinical hand assessment designed for treatment planning.

Synovitis

The synovial tissue is responsible for producing synovial fluid, which lubricates the joint, and for removing or draining the fluid. When the synovial membrane becomes inflamed it produces excessive amounts of fluid; the drainage mechanism becomes ineffective and the fluid becomes trapped in the joint capsule (an **effusion**). The swelling conforms to the shape of the capsule and is referred to as **fusiform swelling** (Fig. 19–3). (**Fusiform** means spindle-shaped, i.e., larger in the center and tapered on the ends.)[1] In rheumatology, *fusiform swelling* is a specific term, indicating synovitis or inflammation confined to the capsule. In the early stages of synovitis, the swelling is soft and fluctuant and is often described as boggy. The synovium is still thin and the joint is essentially full of fluid. As the synovitis becomes chronic, the synovial membrane proliferates and becomes thicker. The tissue may grow from 3 or 20 or more cells in depth. If the inflammation

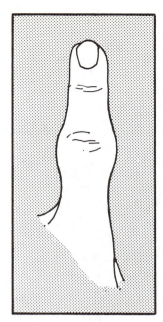

Figure 19–3. Fusiform swelling is illustrated here.

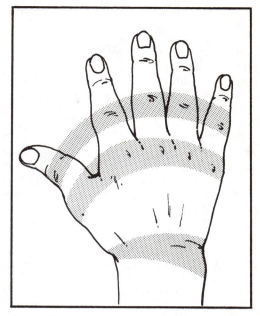

Figure 19–4. Common areas of synovitis in rheumatoid arthritis are shown as the shaded areas.

is not controlled by medication, pannus tissue begins to develop and fill the joint.[1] **Pannus** is a combination of synovial and granulation tissue. As the joint becomes filled with tissue it starts feeling firm rather than boggy, when compressed or palpated. In the advanced stages, the synovium may herniate dorsally through the joint capsule and can present as a hard, focal mass and is often mistaken for a subcutaneous rheumatoid nodule.[19]

The signs of inflammation are swelling, warmth, redness, or discoloration; and the symptoms are pain and decreased motion.[1] Typically, the **severity of inflammation** is described as **acute,** denoting a hot, swollen, painful joint with marked limitation of motion; or **active or subacute,** denoting a warm, swollen joint, with less than acute inflammation. (The term *active* is redundant in this instance, since all synovitis is active.) **Chronic and chronic-active** are terms used to describe low-grade synovitis that persists over time. There joints are warm and swollen, and generally this synovitis is present despite an optimal medication regimen.[17] The joints typically involved in early rheumatoid arthritis are shown in Figure 19–4.

Examples of clinical descriptions of syn-

ovitis include: "boggy swelling, localized to the metacarpophalangeal (MCP) joints"; "fusiform swelling of the PIP joints"; "synovial herniation over the dorsum of right and middle finger PIP joints"; and "active synovitis in all MCP joints and wrist."

Swelling

Swelling is one of the cardinal signs of inflammation in adults. In children it is also a cardinal sign but not an absolute one since some children develop **dry synovitis**—joint inflammation with tenderness and rapid loss of ROM but *no* swelling. This means that in adults you can rely on swelling as an indicator of inflammation but with children you have to assess joint motion, stiffness, and pain as prime criteria for synovitis as well as swelling. (See Chapter 14.) Swelling confined to the joint (fusiform) or tendon sheath indicates synovitis in these structures. (See sections on synovitis and tenosynovitis in this chapter).

Patients with severe or acute RA can also develop various patterns of **diffuse edema** in the hand. Periarticular swelling may be around the inflamed joints or throughout the dorsum of the hand.[1] The lymphatic system drains toward the dorsum of the hand, and it is theorized that interference with lymphatic drainage could be a factor contributing to diffuse dorsal edema.[20,21] Positioning at rest with the wrist flexed can also impair lymphatic return.[21] Bilateral diffuse swelling of the hands and feet should be brought to the attention of the referring physician, because swelling may occur with other types of systemic involvement such as congestive heart failure or renal failure. Medications such as NSAIDs and prednisone can cause fluid retention, further aggravating the swelling problem.

Patients with psoriatic arthritis or one of the other spondyloarthropathies often develop a characteristic firm swelling throughout the entire digit referred to as **sausage swelling** (Fig. 19–5). This diffuse swelling is attributed to a combination of

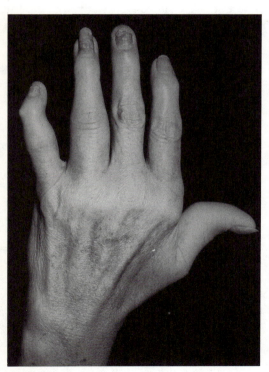

Figure 19–5. This woman has psoriatic arthritis with characteristic sausage swelling of the ring finger and classic psoriatic nail changes. Also, note the mild dorsal wrist swelling, the marked mallet deformity of the little finger, beginning mallet deformity of the index finger, and the enlargement of the thumb, typical of flexor tenosynovitis of the flexor pollicis longus sheath.

acute PIP (and possible MCP and DIP) joint synovitis and severe flexor digital tenosynovitis often accompanied by phalangeal periostitis. It is not known why people with psoriatic arthritis develop diffuse swelling in response to these conditions and patients with RA do not.[22]

One method of determining the degree of swelling is to **compare the dorsal skinfolds** of the edematous hand with those of the nonedematous hand. The skinfolds will be diminished if there is swelling. If the swelling is unilateral, it is helpful to compare side views of the digit with the contralateral digit by placing the palms together. Swelling of the digits can be quantitated by measuring the circumference of the fingers using a regular tape measure, a circumference arthrometer, or a jeweler's ring sizer.[21,22] The measurement can be taken over the PIP joint or over the proximal phalanx depending on whether the goal is to document synovitis or diffuse swelling. It is important that the measurement process be consistent and that the measurement device does not constrict or compress the swollen area.

If there is a need to quantitate edema throughout the entire hand, a circumference measure is not sufficient. The most effective means for measuring the total hand is by using water volume displacement, that is, submerging the hand in a tank containing a precise amount of water (a volumeter) and measuring the water displaced in a graduated cylinder.[21] This process is not commonly used with arthritis patients, but it can be very useful on certain occasions for documenting the effectiveness of treatment to reduce edema.

Subcutaneous (Rheumatoid) Nodules

Subcutaneous (rheumatoid) nodules are discrete tissue masses present under the skin, and occasionally in the skin, and are composed of fibrous and granulomatous tissue.[1] A subcutaneous nodule is one form of rheumatoid nodule that can occur in RA. (Rheumatoid nodules can also form in the lungs and eyes.) These nodules can be of any size, and it is not unusual to find them as large as 4 cm in diameter at the elbow. They can be freely movable or fixed

Figure 19–6. Subcutaneous rheumatoid nodules are most commonly seen over the olecranon and ulnar border of the forearm. They can also occur over the dorsum of the knuckles and in the palm. They are often associated with pressure irritation. They can occur over other regions of the body, for example, occipital skull, Achilles tendon, ischial tuberosity, and foot. (Photograph from American Rheumatism Association slide collection.)

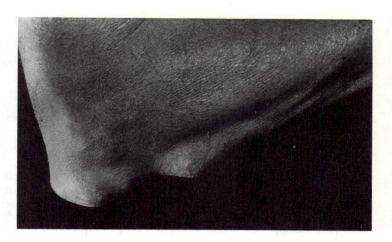

to other structures. Generally, they are not painful but can become tender if irritated by pressure.[19,23] Consistency varies from a soft, amorphous, fluctuant mass to a firm, rubbery lump firmly attached to the periosteum.

Subcutaneous nodules are commonly found over bony prominences exposed to pressure, for example, along the ulnar ridge or the forearm just distal to the olecranon process of the ulnar edge of the hand and wrist (Fig. 19–6). Occasionally they occur on the dorsum of the finger joints and less commonly on the palmar surface of the hand.[1] Nodules may arise over the bony prominence created by a subluxed joint, typically the thumb interphalangeal (IP) joint. (They also occur in other areas of the body, such as over the ischial tuberosities, occipital bone of the skull, and in the Achilles tendon of the heel). Some nodules appear to occur in response to pressure (microtrauma) or are aggravated and enlarged by pressure. However, others can occur in nonpressure areas.[23] Nodules that are related to pressure will diminish in size (or disappear) if the pressure source is eliminated (e.g., by using elbow pads or padding/adapting equipment). Nodules on the palmar surface of the hand appear to be particularly sensitive to pressure forces.

Subcutaneous nodules are associated with seropositive RA, and their presence indicates a more severe disease course.[1,23] They occur in both children and adults but are far more common in adults because the majority of children with juvenile rheumatoid arthritis (JRA) are seronegative for rheumatoid factor (RF). Since subcutaneous nodules have a prognostic significance, it is important that they be appropriately defined. In the hand, synovial hypertrophy or herniation is often mistaken for a nodule.[19] Also, Heberden's nodes are caused by bony proliferation and are completely unrelated to rheumatoid nodules. (In rheumatology, **nodes** and **nodules** are not interchangeable terms.) There is a rare condition called **rheumatoid nodulosis,** in which patients develop multiple nodules and have a positive RF but do not have arthritis.[24–26] Another condition, called **benign rheumatoid nodules** (pseudorheumatoid nodules or granuloma anulare), can occur in children and young adults but generally does not occur in the hands.[27–29]

To document a nodule, it is helpful to note consistency, sensitivity to pain, size, number, fixation, and location (e.g., "Patient has a single, firm, fully movable, nontender nodule about 0.5 cm in diameter, overlying the dorsum of the ring PIP joint"). Size can also be related in terms of a common object (e.g., pea size or golf ball size) or by diameter.

Synovial Cysts and Ganglion

A **synovial cyst** is formed by a herniation of synovial tissue. It appears as a soft enlarged mass (cyst) under the skin and is usually found overlying tendon sheaths. It is most commonly found over the dorsum of the wrist but can be found overlying any synovial joint.

A **dorsal wrist ganglion** is a synovial cyst that arises from the portion of the joint capsule that attaches to the scapholunate ligament. Dorsal ganglions can be primary and occur in people without any other form of arthritis. They may be asymptomatic or very tender during functional activities.[30]

Ganglions are very common, and the majority of soft masses over the dorsum of the wrist are confirmed as ganglions. But any mass should be carefully diagnosed, because a variety of uncommon conditions can have the appearance of a ganglion, including synovial cysts, anomalous extensor muscle bellies, lipomas, neuromas of the posterior interosseous nerve, dorsal exostoses, radial artery aneurysm, periarticular calcareous deposits, partial tendon rupture, sarcomas, and giant cell tumor.[31] Since it is often difficult to distinguish between ganglions, cysts, tumors, or synovium, it is preferable for the therapist to describe the location and size of the swelling or mass; for example, "Flattened, puffy enlargement over the dorsum of the wrist (about 3 cm in diameter)."

Osteophytes (Heberden's Nodes, Bouchard's Nodes)

OA involves two major processes: degeneration of the cartilage, and bone proliferation around the margin of the joint. In the digits, this bone growth takes the form of osteophytes. When osteophytes occur at the DIP joint they are referred to as **Heberden's nodes;** at the PIP joint they are referred to as **Bouchard's nodes** (Fig. 19–7). Osteophytes are also common around the thumb carpometacarpal (CMC) joint. They rarely occur at the MCP joint level.[32]

The presence of these osteophytes is diagnostic of DJD. The ability to assess os-

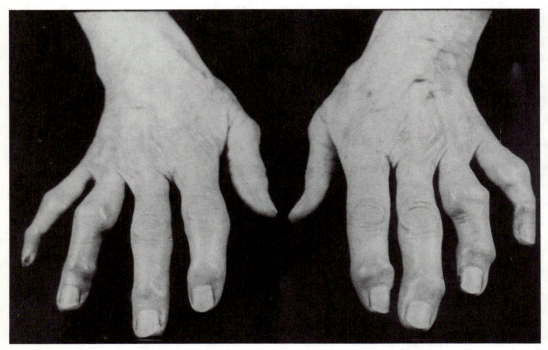

Figure 19–7. Osteophyte formation in the PIP joints (Bouchard's nodes) and DIP joints (Heberden's nodes) are characteristic of primary OA. These bony protuberances are hard to the touch and asymmetric, compared with synovitis, which is symmetric and boggy. Generally these nodes are nonpainful and noninflammatory. Occasionally patients like the one pictured here will have painful localized inflammatory episodes. Note the redness or discoloration over the DIP joints secondary to inflammation. She also has an angulation deformity of the right middle finger DIP joint and a mallet deformity of the right little finger. (From the Arthritis Teaching Slide Collection, Arthritis Health Professions Association, Arthritis Foundation, with permission.)

teophytes correctly can be a valuable aid to the therapist for treatment planning because osteophytes are a sign that the cartilage is damaged. Many patients have both OA and RA. Often the limitations in the joints with OA are greater than or disproportionate to the other joints and to the degree of inflammation present. The ability to determine the presence of OA (indicated by osteophytes) allows the therapist to determine if the limitation is due to OA or RA and to plan treatment appropriately. (See Chapters 4 and 6.)

Thumb Carpometacarpal Joint Arthritis

In the DIP and PIP joints, OA is generally easily recognizable by the presence of osteophytes. However, detection of early OA in the thumb CMC joint is often more difficult, since the structure of the joint and the overlying muscles prevents palpation or visualization of osteophyte formation.

Evaluation of OA of the CMC joint requires a separate assessment for several reasons. First, this joint may be the first joint to become symptomatic in OA. Patients with no previous history of arthritis may seek medical care for the sole complaint of CMC pain. This symptom can be quite limiting since the thumb accounts for 45 percent of hand function.[33] Second, this condition is often confused with de Quervain's tenosynovitis, particularly when the OA causes inflammation of the CMC joint with pain radiating into the wrist or forearm. These two conditions need to be differentiated, since their evaluation, treatment, and prognosis are completely different. Third, x-ray evidence of OA does *not* necessarily correlate with clinical symptoms. Patients can have minimal to absent x-ray changes and debilitating pain or the reverse—severe x-ray changes and no pain. It is not uncommon for some patients to progress to marked subluxation without pain.

Generally people do not seek treatment for OA of the thumb until it becomes painful. In some cases the degenerative process has been present but painless for years before the right combination of joint derangement, cartilage debris, functional stress, and immune system function allows inflammation to occur. As the OA progresses, osteophyte formation causes the joint to sublux, giving a squared-off appearance to the joint. "Squaring" of the CMC joint is considered a diagnostic sign of OA.[34,35]

Evaluation (Fig. 19–8)

The **grind test** is a specific procedure for localizing pain to the CMC joint.[1,35] To perform the evaluation, stabilize the patient's hand with your thumb over the CMC joint to palpate crepitus or subluxation. Then grasp the patient's metacarpal bone and approximate the joint; that is, press the head of the metacarpal into the trapezium and gently rotate the metacarpal in the joint. The test is positive for CMC involvement if the maneuver elicits pain or crepitus in the CMC joint.

Orthoses to immobilize the CMC joint are very effective for relieving symptoms

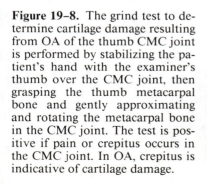
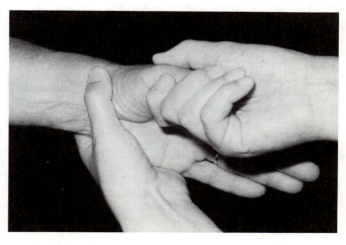

Figure 19–8. The grind test to determine cartilage damage resulting from OA of the thumb CMC joint is performed by stabilizing the patient's hand with the examiner's thumb over the CMC joint, then grasping the thumb metacarpal bone and gently approximating and rotating the metacarpal bone in the CMC joint. The test is positive if pain or crepitus occurs in the CMC joint. In OA, crepitus is indicative of cartilage damage.

and thus improving function.[35] (An orthosis for this condition is discussed in Chapter 23.) Orthoses are considered the treatment of choice for patients with short-term or sporadic episodes of pain or with pain related only to a specific task, such as writing or driving. They are also useful for patients who do not want surgery. Once the pain becomes unrelenting or nonresponsive to splinting, some form of arthroplasty should be considered.[35] (See Chapter 29, Hand, Wrist, and Forearm Surgery.)

When ROM measurement of the CMC joint is indicated as part of the preoperative and postoperative assessment, the following should be documented: abduction, adduction, flexion, extension, opposition, and retropulsion. (See Chapter 20 for a detailed description of the ROM procedure.) For general conservative orthotic management, documentation of pain and swelling is more important than determining ROM because treatment can improve pain and reduce inflammation, but there is no treatment for improving ROM or preventing progression of joint damage. Of course, one always hopes that control of the inflammation will slow down the progression of damage.

Crepitation

Crepitation refers to a grating, crunching, or popping sensation (or sound) that occurs during joint or tendon motion; it can be heard and felt (audible and palpable).[1] The cause or source can be bony, synovial, tendinous, or bursal. If it occurs in a joint, it is usually caused by roughened articular surfaces rubbing together and is indicative of cartilage damage.[36] In the hand it is very common to palpate crepitus over the volar aspect of the digit during flexor tenosynovitis. Crepitus, if present, can be heard or felt and is further documented by its location or by the motion that elicited it, or both.

Range-of-Motion Lag

Lag refers to a difference between active and passive ROM. It is not a specific pathological condition but a consequence of tendon damage, adhesions, or muscle weak-

ness. The determination of lag and its causal factor should be a specific focus of an arthritis hand assessment. Each of the factors listed here is discussed separately in this chapter.

Types of Lag and Possible Causal Factors

If passive extension is greater than active extension, evaluate extensor structures:

1. At the wrist: rupture or weakness of the wrist extensors; assess for tenodesis.
2. At the MCP joint: rupture, weakness, or displacement of the finger extensors; rarely, it is due to dorsal tenosynovitis blocking tendon motion. Entrapment of the posterior interosseous nerve (PIN) can cause extensor lag in the third and fourth digits.
3. At the PIP joint: elongation (overstretching) or rupture of the central slip.
4. At the DIP joint: partial or complete rupture of the distal attachment of the extensor communis tendon.
5. At the thumb IP joint: rupture of the extensor pollicis longus tendon at the wrist can reduce IP extension when the thumb is in extension. (When the thumb MCP joint is flexed, the intrinsic muscles provide IP joint extension.)

If passive flexion is greater than active flexion, evaluate flexor structures:

1. Flexor tenosynovitis at the wrist or digit level.
2. Flexor tendon rupture.
3. Trigger finger (nodule catching on the pulley mechanism).
4. Weakness, e.g., entrapment of the anterior interosseous nerve can cause flexion lag in the index finger and thumb.

Tenodesis, Extrinsic Tendon Tightness

Technically, the term **tenodesis*** means fixation of a tendon at a new point. For example, a tendon transfer involves a surgical tenodesis. Clinically, tenodesis action or

---

*Tenodesis is a tendon problem. It is included in the joint assessment section because it can influence joint ROM evaluation and is easily assessed at the time of joint measurement.

motion refers to aberrant motion in the digit joints due to tightness or tethering of a tendon at a proximal location. The excursion of the tendon can become limited secondary to several conditions, including: the proximal end of a ruptured tendon becoming adherent to an adjacent tendon; swelling and tenosynovitis in the carpal tunnel, blocking flexor tendon motion; and adherence of the long finger extensors or flexors at the wrist. (In cases of hand trauma, the tendon can become limited because of scarring at any point along its course.)

For a tight tendon to create tenodesis action, it must cross over two or more joints. Consequently, this results in the motion of the distal joint(s) varying, depending on the position of the proximal joint. This process is also referred to as **extrinsic tightness,** a preferable term since it connotes an abnormal process and avoids confusion with normal tenodesis (full wrist extension elicits finger flexion and full flexion elicits finger extension) and with desirable tenodesis created by positioning or surgery.

The following are examples of extrinsic tendon tightness:

1. Binding of the flexor tendons in the carpal tunnel can result in lack of PIP joint extension when the wrist is in neutral but full PIP joint extension when the wrist is flexed. (If the condition is severe, MCP joint motion will also be altered.) Upon cursory evaluation, it may appear as if the patient has PIP joint flexion contractures. If the PIP joints straighten with the wrist or MCP joints in different positions, the problem is in the tendons, not in the PIP joints. (Evaluation and treatment for flexor tenosynovitis are discussed under a separate section in this chapter.)

2. The distal ends of a ruptured extensor tendon can become adherent to an adjacent tendon or structure on the dorsum of the hand in a manner that reduces tendon excursion. In this case, PIP and DIP joint motion can vary depending on the position of the MCP joint. When the MCP joint is flexed, the PIP joint will lack full active or passive flexion; when the PIP joint is fully flexed, the MCP joint will lack flexion.[37] In other words, the new length of the tendon is only long enough to go around one bend or corner at a time.

3. Tendons can also become limited because of adhesions following surgery.

Evaluation

The test for extrinsic tightness refers to assessing distal joint motion with the proximal joint in different positions. It is positive if the position of the proximal joint influences the ROM of the distal joint.[38]

Measuring ROM when tenodesis is present: To determine the effectiveness of treatment for this type of tendon problem it is necessary to document ROM of the joints distal to the tendon fixation both pre-treatment and post-treatment. There are two methods for doing this. Method 1: (This is the most accurate method for patients with polyarthritis.) Stabilize the proximal joints in neutral (0 degrees), for example, the wrist and MCP joints; then measure the maximal motion possible at the PIP joint. (The DIP joint should be measured if it is affected.) Method 2: Position the proximal joint, for example, the wrist, in full flexion or extension and measure the maximal motion of the distal joint, for example, MCP and PIP joints. The motion measured depends on which tendon is tight. This method can be reliable in patients with normal proximal joints, for example, in hand trauma patients.

Subluxation and Dislocation

Subluxation describes any degree of malalignment between normal and dislocated. Dislocation occurs when the articular surfaces are no longer in functional contact (Figs. 19–9 and 19–10).

In the MCP joint, the proximal phalanx slips volar or ulnar and volar on the metacarpal head. This is evaluated by palpating over the dorsum of the joint. When the joint is in neutral, an abnormal "step" can

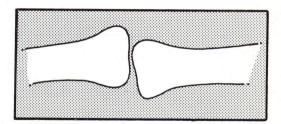

Figure 19–9. Subluxation of two digit bones includes any degree of malalignment between normal and dislocated.

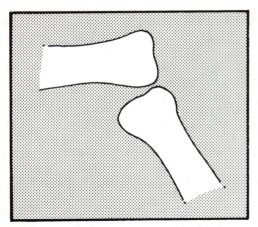

Figure 19–10. Dislocation occurs when the bones are no longer in functional contact.

be felt between the two bones if it is subluxed[1] (Fig. 19–11).

In the presence of chronic synovitis, subluxation is common in the radiocarpal joint (Fig. 19–12), the radioulnar joint, and the MCP joints. In the PIP and DIP joints, volar subluxation is rare because flexion contractures predominate and help keep the joint stable. Typically, the joint is described in terms of the contracture or deformity pattern, such as swan-neck. Occasionally, bone erosions or osteophytes cause lateral deviation of the PIP or DIP joints. In the thumb, volar subluxation of the distal phalanx and CMC joint is more common than the MCP joint.[38]

Subluxation can be described in the following manner: **mild:** palpable subluxation, no interference with function, full extension possible; **moderate:** visible subluxation limits range slightly, may or may not interfere with function; **severe:** gross malalignment of articulating bones; there is definite interference with ROM but articulating surfaces are still in functional contact.

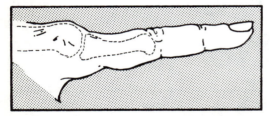

Figure 19–11. Metacarpophalangeal volar subluxation is illustrated here.

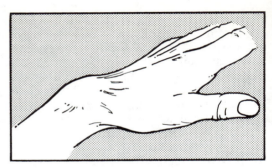

Figure 19–12. Volar wrist subluxation is shown here.

Ligamentous Instability (Laxity)

In the digits, the **collateral ligaments** are the structures that prevent excessive lateral motion (see Fig. 19–1). The digital collateral ligaments reinforce the joint capsule on either side of the joint. Each is composed of two sections: the cord portion that extends from the dorsal lateral side of the proximal bone to the volar lateral side of the distal bone, and the accessory section that attaches into the volar plate (Fig. 19–13). Chronic synovitis can result in stretching or lengthening of the collateral ligaments and abnormal lateral motion.[39,40]

Evaluation

The evaluation procedures are different for the MCP joint, compared with the PIP and DIP joints, because the shape of the metacarpal head alters the length of the ligaments. In the MCP joints, the cord portion predominates in determining mobility and stability of the joint. In the PIP and DIP joints, the cord and accessory portions appear to play a more equal role.

In the MCP joint, the collateral ligaments have a variable length, depending on the position of the joint. When the joint is flexed, the full length of the collateral ligament is required to accommodate the wide volar aspect of the lateral condyles of the metacarpal head.[39,41] When the joint is in extension, the full length is not required, and this section of the ligament is slack. This allows greater lateral mobility in extension. Consequently, *to evaluate the integrity of the collateral ligament in the MCP joint, it is necessary to position the joint in full passive flexion,* so the ligament is at full length and there is minimal lateral

Figure 19–13. This lateral view of the proximal interphalangeal joint shows the collateral ligament (CL), cord portion, and the accessory collateral ligament (ACL) attaching the middle phalanx and volar plate (VP). The flexor tendon sheath containing the superficialis tendon (ST) and the profundus tendon (PT) is closely attached to the periosteum of the phalanges and volar plate. The asterisk notes the recess between the volar plate and phalanx. The collateral ligaments are similar in the DIP joints. (From Wilson and Carter,[43] with permission.)

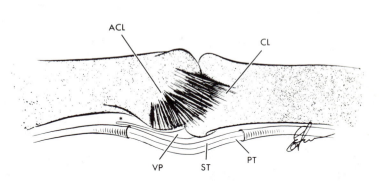

motion (Fig. 19–14). The metacarpal bone should be stabilized and the proximal bone moved from side to side. This positioning also applies to the thumb MCP joint. The PIP and DIP joints receive equal support from both sections of the ligament. When the joint is in extension, the cord portion of the collateral ligament is slack and the accessory ligament is taut. When the joint is flexed, the reverse occurs—the collateral ligament becomes taut and the accessory ligament is slack.[42]

This dual ligament structure ensures stability in any position, but unfortunately it also makes the PIP joints very prone to stiffness during immobilization. When the joint is splinted in extension, the cord portion of the collateral ligament tends to become fibrosed in a shortened position; and when the joint is splinted in flexion, the accessory collateral ligament can become contracted in a shortened position. Either ligament can prevent mobility.[43]

In arthritis, laxity tends to occur simultaneously in both ligaments, and testing the PIP and DIP joints in extension is sufficient. In cases of traumatic injury, only one ligament may be torn, and it is necessary to test the integrity of the cord portion of the collateral ligament with the joint in flexion and the accessory portion with the joint in nearly full extension. Nearly full extension centers the middle phalanx over the proximal phalanx, creating maximal tension on the accessory ligament.[43]

Normal joint stability is highly variable.

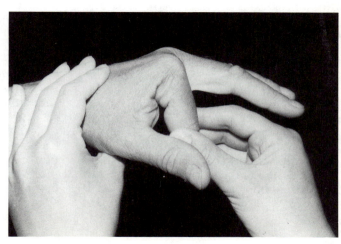

Figure 19–14. The collateral ligaments of the MCP joint are lax in extension and stretched their full length in flexion. To test the integrity of the collateral ligaments of the MCP joint, position the joint in full flexion and move the phalanx from side to side. Excessive lateral motion in this position is indicative of damage to the collateral ligaments.

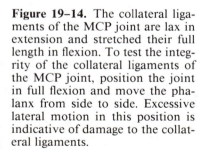

Normal for a specific person can be determined by comparing the digit being evaluated with an unaffected contralateral joint, when possible.

Excessive anteroposterior motion without lateral excess indicates laxity of the capsule and volar plate, rather than the collateral ligaments.

Ligamentous laxity can be described as **slight,** approximately 5 to 10 degrees in excess of normal; **moderate,** approximately 10 to 20 degrees in excess; and **severe,** approximately 20 degrees in excess.

Mutilans Deformity (Opera Glass Hand, La Main Lorgnette)

Mutilans deformity (opera glass hand, la main lorgnette) refers to severe resorption of the bone ends; that is, the bone ends are removed by being absorbed into the body, shortening the bone and leaving the joint completely unstable. This process most commonly occurs at the MCP and PIP joints and the radiocarpal and radioulnar joints. The cause is unknown. In severe cases, the entire carpus can be resorbed. (It can also occur in the toes.) It is associated with one subtype of psoriatic arthritis and is an uncommon sequela of severe RA. Mutilans is a devastating deformity and severely limits functional ability.[45]

The fingers appear shortened because of loss of phalangeal and/or metacarpal bone. In the early stages this condition may be mistaken for a ruptured collateral ligament. In this instance, an x-ray would confirm whether the joint instability is due to resorption or ligamentous laxity. As the condition progresses, loose overlying skin and tissue become folded, producing a telescoping appearance. The fingers tend to feel soft or fleshy. Joints are unstable and floppy as a result of resorption.[44] *Severity is described in terms of instability, resorption, and degree of shortening.*

The only treatment for mutilans is surgery. Arthrodesis *arrests* the resorption process and preserves the length of the digit, but this can be done only in the early stages of mutilans (Fig. 19–15).[44] This procedure is preferable to reconstructive surgery, using bone grafts to restore length. If a patient with early to moderate mutilans in the digits is not a candidate for surgery

because of concomitant problems or because he or she does not want a fusion, a tripoint orthosis such as the Silver-Ring Splint[45] may prove helpful in stabilizing the joint and improving function. However, it will not retard the resorption process (see Chapter 23).

Joint Contractures

Contracture is a term used to describe a fixed or more permanent limitation in joint motion, rather than a temporary limitation caused by pain, edema, or inflammation. A **flexion contracture** limits or prevents full extension. (The term assumes that the limitation is on the flexor surface.) Consequently, an **extension contracture** limits or prevents full flexion.

In the presence of rheumatic disease, contractures can result from any of the following:

1. Synovial hypertrophy can block motion and lead to secondary fibrosis. Also, dry synovitis without swelling (dry form) can result in fibrosis of the capsule and supporting structures (see Chapter 14).

2. Ineffective tendon motion (ROM lag). If a patient does not actively (or passively) utilize full available joint motion daily, permanent contractures of the capsule and ligaments can develop.

3. Shortening of the collateral ligaments due to chronic positioning or inappropriate orthotic treatment (see section on ligamentous instability).

4. Periarticular edema causes compression of the joint structures, leading to adhesions in a tight or shortened position.

5. Subluxation can block motion creating a fixed limitation; for example, radioulnar subluxation can prevent supination.

6. Osteophyte formation can block motion and eventually lead to ankylosis.

7. Muscle weakness. When muscle strength is 3.5/5 (fair plus) or less, the muscle is no longer able to balance antagonistic forces, resulting in chronic positioning that leads to contractures; for example, adduction contractures of the thumb are common sequelae if the abductor pollicis brevis becomes weak due to carpal tunnel syndrome.

8. Skin tightness occasionally appears to

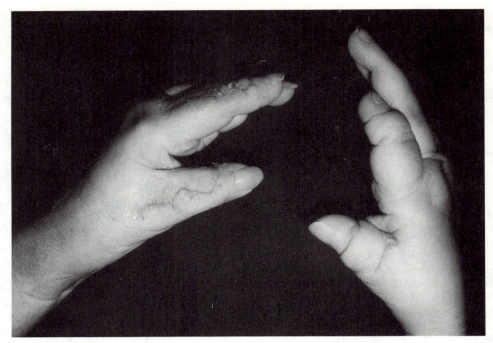

Figure 19–15. This woman has severe bilateral mutilans deformity of the thumb and index fingers. Resorption of the bone ends results in shortening of the digits and instability of the joints, impairing prehension skills. In the left hand the length and stability of the thumb and index finger have been restored by means of a bone graft and arthrodesis. Surgical fusion can prevent progress of bone resorption if performed early. Note the loss of length of the right index finger compared with the middle finger and the telescoping appearance of the shortened digits created by redundant skin.

be a causal factor, but it is usually secondary to joint or muscle limitations. In scleroderma (systemic sclerosis) limitations are due to fibrosis of all the soft tissues.

The importance of chronic or habitual positioning cannot be emphasized enough. In the treatment of hand trauma, a condition called **extensor habitus** is frequently seen. Classically, it involves complete stiffness of the entire index finger, secondary to minor trauma. This condition occurs when a patient keeps the index finger in an extended position to avoid pain or allow healing. The patient begins to use the middle finger habitually for prehension. The index finger gradually becomes stiff and immobile, solely as a result of this unconscious positioning process. Interestingly, upon taking the initial history, these patients often report that their finger became stiff overnight. Later, when the process is explained, the patient recalls gradual changes. Fortunately, this form of contracture can be readily resolved if treated early. This same physiological process can occur in patients with rheumatic diseases in a more subtle form. Patients with an unstable or painful DIP joint or isolated synovitis of a PIP joint may avoid using that finger. Patients with advanced carpal tunnel syndrome and a diminished 2-point discrimination (7 mm or more) often start using their ulnar fingers instead of the median fingers for prehension. *Altered patterns of functional use should be considered as a possible causal factor in digits with inordinate stiffness.*

Contractures are usually described by the degree of limitation; for example, left elbow has a 40-degree flexion contracture; patient cannot straighten elbow to neutral.

Ankylosis

When a joint becomes immobile, it is referred to as **ankylosed.** The fixation can be

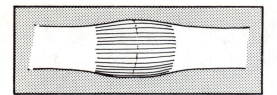

Figure 19–16. Fibrous ankylosis is illustrated here.

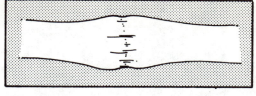

Figure 19–17. Bony ankylosis is illustrated here.

fibrous, that is, due to growth of fibrous tissue around the joint; or it can be **bony,** resulting from ossification within or around the joint (Figs. 19–16 and 19–17).[47] (The term **arthrodesis** described a surgical fusion.)

Fibrous ankylosis is the most common in rheumatoid arthritis. Since the limitation is due to changes in the soft tissue, there may or may not be slight motion present in this type of ankylosis. In bony ankylosis, there is no motion. This form is more common in psoriatic arthritis and JRA.[46,47]

Complete fibrous ankylosis can only be distinguished from bony ankylosis by x-ray study.[46] Therefore, for documentation purposes, it is best to describe the joint as ankylosed or describe the amount of motion available and the angle of fixation; for example, left middle finger PIP joint is essentially ankylosed (has a jog of motion) in 45 degrees of flexion; or right wrist is ankylosed in 20 degrees of flexion; left wrist has a jog of motion in neutral.

Tuft Resorption

This is a condition in which the tuft of the distal phalanx becomes resorbed. Seen in systemic sclerosis, it causes distinct shortening of the distal phalanx and nail.[48]

Evaluate by comparing length of finger with contralateral digit, if unaffected. Describe severity in terms of loss of digit length; for example, distal shortening of index and ring fingers. The length of loss, for example, 1 cm, can be measured and compared with a normal contralateral digit.

COMMON HAND AND WRIST DEFORMITIES

Radiocarpal Joint Subluxation

The carpal bones may slide volarward or ulnarward on the distal radius, or they may sublux in both planes simultaneously.[38]

Volar Subluxation and Dislocation

Chronic synovitis of the wrist joint weakens the supporting ligaments about the wrist. Loss of ligamentous support combined with the normal 10 to 15 degrees of volar inclination of the distal radius results in volar slippage of the carpal bones on the radius (Fig. 19–18). This volar subluxation may be further enhanced by volar displace-

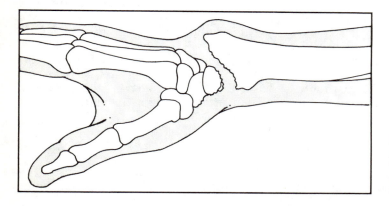

Figure 19–18. This illustration depicts volar subluxation of the carpus on the radius as a result of erosive synovitis of the radiocarpal joint.

ment of the extensor carpi ulnaris tendon. Once displaced volarly the extensor carpi ulnaris loses its effectiveness as an extensor and creates an additional flexor force on the carpus. The carpus may dislocate completely beneath the radius if erosion of the volar lip of the distal radius occurs.

Ulnar Subluxation and Dislocation (Radial Deviation Deformity)

Chronic synovitis of the wrist leads to loss of radial ligamentous support and destruction of the triangular fibrocartilage on the ulnar side of the wrist. Loss of radial and ulnar support allows the carpus to slide down the distal radius, which has a normal incline toward the ulna. It is most common for the proximal carpal bones to *sublux ulnarward* and for the distal carpal bones to rotate in a radial direction, resulting in the hand being *radially deviated on the forearm*. This condition often contributes to ulnar drift of the MCP joints (Fig. 19–19). Less frequently, the distal carpal bones do not rotate, and the hand may appear ulnarly deviated on the forearm.[49] This is a favorable consequence, since it creates less stress on the MCP joints.

If erosive synovitis continues, the carpus may eventually slide completely off the radius and dislocate on the ulnar side of the forearm, at a marked 90-degree angle, resulting in a right angle wrist deformity.

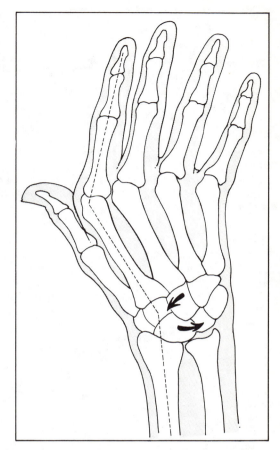

Figure 19–19. Shown here is the relationship between wrist and metacarpophalangeal joint deformity. In this drawing, the proximal end of the carpus has subluxed in an ulnar direction, rotating the hand radially on the forearm. This requires ulnar deviation of metacarpophalangeal joints to bring the index finger in line with the radius. The resulting articular alignment indicated by the dotted line produced the term zigzag effect.

Distal Radioulnar Joint Subluxation

In RA, the distal radioulnar joint is often one of the first sites of wrist disease. Weakening of the supporting ligaments results in subluxation between the ulna and radius, which creates a prominence on the dorsal aspect of the wrist (Fig. 19–20). If subluxation is severe, it can limit supination and wrist extension.[49,50] The literature describes this as "dorsal subluxation of the ulna on the radius." Dr. Adrian Flatt was the first to point out to me (1978) that this is highly unlikely—since the ulna is stabilized proximally to the humerus it is more probable that the floating radius (with attached carpal bones) has subluxed volarly on the ulna. Over the past 10 years, several leading hand surgeons have concurred on this

point, but the literature and clinical teaching have yet to catch up. Probably the dorsal prominence of the ulna makes it so easy to call this dorsal subluxation, even if this is not the case.

Evaluation

To evaluate subluxation between the ulna and the radius: Face the patient and stabilize the head of the radius with a lateral pinch grip. With the opposite hand, move the ulna head in a dorsovolar plane. Exces-

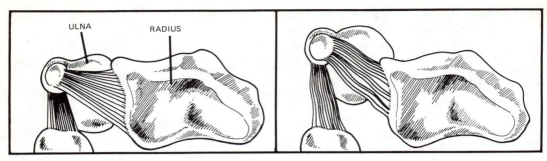

Figure 19–20. The distal radioulnar joint is illustrated here: *(left)* normal alignment, showing intact ligaments between the ulna, radius, and carpal bones; *(right)* laxity of the supporting ligaments allows volar subluxation of the radius, creating a dorsal prominence of the ulna.

sive motion indicates subluxation—referred to as a positive "piano key" sign.[38] Caution is needed in documentation since the normal degree of laxity is highly variable; compare with the other wrist if normal.

Metacarpophalangeal Ulnar Drift and Volar Subluxation

The term **drift** refers to an abnormal amount of deviation. Ulnar drift is most common in adult RA. Radial drift rarely occurs in adults but is frequently seen in children with JRA.[51]

MCP ulnar drift (Fig. 19–21) occurs because of the interrelationship of several fac-

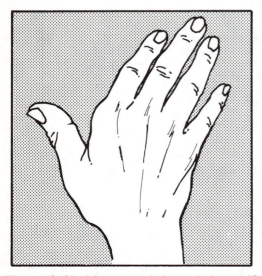

Figure 19–21. Metacarpophalangeal ulnar drift is depicted here.

tors, including: anatomical structure of the hand, which favors ulnar deviation; functional patterns of use and the influence of the flexor tendons during prehension; presence of chronic synovitis; and the position of the wrist, which is the keystone of the hand.

Anatomical Structure of the Hand

In the normal hand, both at rest and during motion, the phalanges are on an ulnar incline in relation to the metacarpals. This incline occurs because all the structural components favor the ulnar direction: the shape of the bones, placement and length of the collateral ligaments, and insertion of the intrinsic muscles. In addition, the flexor tendons cross the MCP joint from an ulnar angle. This in itself does not appear to produce ulnar motion at the joint because of the restraining power of the proximal annular ligaments (fibrous portion of the flexor sheath). However, when this ligament is weakened by synovitis, it loses its restraining power and the anatomical alignment of the flexor tendons creates a strong ulnar component for drift deformity, particularly for the index and middle fingers (Fig. 19–22).[52,53]

Functional Use of the Hand

All functional activities that involve MCP flexion, especially power pinch and grasp, increase the ulnar forces across the MCP joint (see Fig. 19–22). (See section later in this chapter regarding functional components of the hand.)[53,54]

When the flexor tendon sheath is dam-

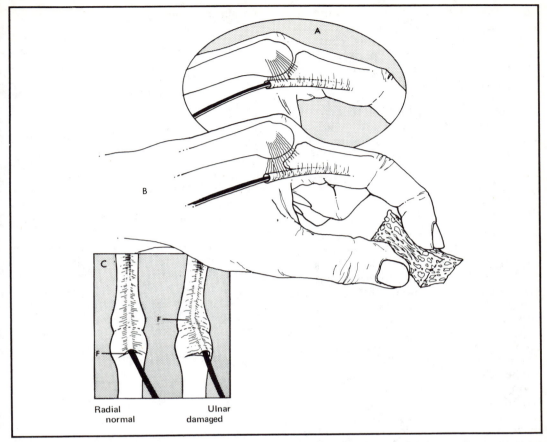

Figure 19–22. Influence of the long flexors in metacarpophalangeal drift deformity is illustrated. (*A*) This is the MCP joint with normal ligamentous stability. (*B*) The flexor tendons bowstring across the joint and elongate the supporting fibers during power pinch (or grasp), resulting in volar subluxation of the proximal phalanx. This can occur only when the fibers are weakened by chronic synovitis. (*C*) Volar view of the MCP joint shows that, with damage to the supporting fibers, the fulcrum of force (F) from the flexor tendon changes, placing the ulnar pull on the proximal phalanx.

aged by chronic synovitis, the flexor tendon is allowed to pull across the MCP joint in an exaggerated volar-ulnar direction during power pinch and grasp. In addition, the ulnar interossei demonstrate a power dominance over the radial interossei during functional use.[54]

The forces imposed on the MCP joint during prehension have been analyzed by Smith and his colleagues.[54] They determined that for every unit of force exerted during 2-point pad pinch, six units of force are required by the long finger flexors and three units of force are displaced over the MCP joint. Thus, if a person uses a 5-pound pinch to open a container, 15 pounds of force are exerted on the MCP

joint. If the MCP joint ligaments are damaged, this creates 15 pounds of volar force on the proximal phalanx. It is Smith's[54] work and this understanding of flexor forces that forms the theoretical basis for joint-protection instruction for the MCP joints (see Chapter 24).

Chronic Synovitis

The main cause of ulnar drift deformity is *chronic* MCP joint synovitis. Single limited acute bouts of MCP synovitis for the most part do not cause permanent deformity. Early synovitis appears to affect the joint in three ways. **First,** the inflammatory process, often referred to as *inflammatory* *infiltration,* damages and weakens the capsule and supporting ligaments.[55] **Second,** chronic intra-articular swelling, caused by synovial effusion and hypertrophy, distends the supporting joint structures and reduces their restraining power against ulnar forces, thus allowing the tendons to pull across the joint in a manner that enhances ulnar drift and volar subluxation. **Third,** pain and stretch of the joint capsule are hypothesized to cause **reflex muscle spasm (muscular splinting)** of the lumbricals and interossei.[56]

Position of the Wrist

In functional positions the index finger is in line with the radius. This requires the wrist to be in about 5 to 10 degrees of ulnar deviation. If the wrist becomes radially deviated with loss of ulnar ROM (the most common early wrist deformity in RA), the fingers deviate ulnarly to bring the index finger back into line with the radius. This theory or process is commonly referred to as the **zigzag effect** (see Fig. 19–19).[49]

The position of the wrist can have such a strong influence that some patients (with RA of the wrist and MCP synovitis) who develop an ulnar deviation deformity of the wrist can go on to develop a mild radial drift (instead of ulnar drift) of the MCP joints. In clinical practice patients with a natural ulnar deviation deformity *of the wrist* seem to have less MCP ulnar drift than patients with a radial deviation deformity of the wrist (the most common form). Occasionally, a patient will position his or her wrist radially to make ulnar deviated fingers appear straighter. These patients may appear to have wrist deformity, but a detailed assessment reveals an absence of wrist pain and radiographic changes.

Ulnar Drift in Late Stages

In advanced stages of ulnar drift, synovium may herniate through the radial transverse fibers of the extensor hood and the extensor communis tendons may slip ulnarward between metacarpal heads, giving the extensor tendon a mechanical advantage in an ulnar direction; however, these conditions usually occur after ulnar drift is established.[57]

Evaluation

Severity is determined by the degrees of drift present. Methods for measuring ulnar drift vary across the country. One of the most effective methods is to measure the angle between the phalanx and metacarpal joint *during active extension, without active correction.* For some patients, it is also helpful to know the amount of drift they have in flexion when the hand is relaxed. (The measurement method is described in detail in Chapter 20, Evaluation of Range of Motion.) When evaluating ulnar drift, it is important to keep in mind that the index finger normally has about 10 to 20 degrees of ulnar deviation during active extension.[19] Asking the patient actively to correct the drift provides additional information regarding the integrity of the joint structures.

Severity can be described as follows: *for the index finger,* slight (20 to 30 degrees); moderate (30 to 50 degrees); severe (50 degrees or more); and *for the other digits:* slight (0 to 10 degrees); moderate (10 to 30 degrees); severe (30 degrees or more).[58]

Swan-Neck Deformity

The crooked shape of this deformity may or may not remind you of a swan's neck; however, it impressed someone in this manner, and the name has been retained ever since. The complete swan-neck deformity consists of three components: PIP joint hyperextension, DIP joint flexion, and MCP joint flexion. Many people have natural hyperextensibility of the PIP joint, but this is referred to as such, and not as a deformity.

Most deformities result from damage to a single joint. The swan-neck deformity can occur secondary to synovitis at either the MCP, PIP, or DIP joint. It is a common deformity resulting from trauma in the nonarthritic patient. It has also been shown to occur because of intrinsic musculotendon imbalance secondary to carpal collapse. This etiology is based on the premise that carpal collapse alters the functional relationship between the length of the extrinsic tendons and skeletal length of the wrist–hand unit. Fortunately in many cases the musculotendon unit will contract or fibrose if it is not fully mobilized, recreating a bal-

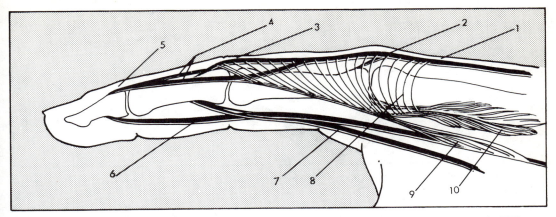

Figure 19–23. Normal finger extensor mechanism is depicted here: (*1*) extensor communis (EC) tendon; (*2*) EC insertion to proximal phalanx; (*3*) EC insertion to middle phalanx (forms the central slip); (*4*) fibers from the EC separate to form the lateral bands; (*5*) EC insertion to distal phalanx; (*6*) profundus tendon: (*7*) superficialis tendon; (*8*) extensor hood fibers; (*9*) lumbrical muscle originates from the profundus tendon; (*10*) interosseous muscle with dual insertion, one part into the hood fibers and one part into the proximal phalanx.

ance between tendon length and the hand bones. If this does not occur, the tendons become too long and slack, making it difficult to initiate PIP flexion. Shapiro reports on two cases of RA with carpal collapse and swan-neck deformities in which carpal distraction reversed the swan-neck deformities by facilitating PIP flexion.[59] This theory creates a fourth etiology for swan-neck deformity.

The normal extensor mechanism is shown in Figure 19–23 for comparison with Figures 19–24 to 19–26, which demonstrate the imbalance that can result from synovitis at each of the digit joints.

Initial Involvement at MCP Joint (Fig. 19–24)

This is the most frequent etiology for swan-neck deformity in RA. Chronic synovitis in the MCP joints is hypothesized to cause reflex intrinsic muscle spasm and eventual muscle contracture.[56] The arrows in Figure 19–24 indicate the direction of pull that the intrinsic muscles produce on the extensor mechanism.

Contracture of the intrinsic muscles in association with natural hypermobility of the PIP joint (or PIP synovitis stretching the volar capsule) can lead to flexion of the

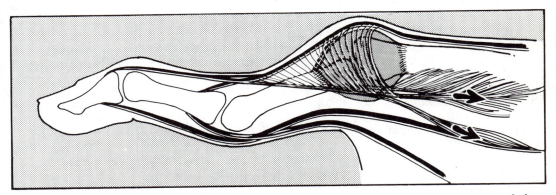

Figure 19–24. Shown here is swan-neck deformity with the initial synovitis at the metacarpophalangeal joint. This is the most common cause of the swan-neck deformity in RA.

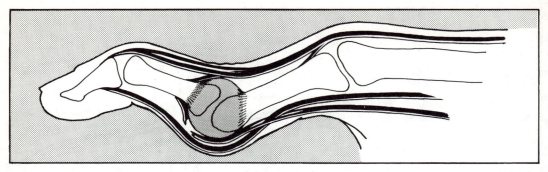

Figure 19–25. Shown here is swan-neck deformity with initial synovitis at the proximal interphalangeal joint.

MCP joints and hyperextension of the PIP joints.[60]

Initial Involvement at PIP Joint (Fig. 19–25)

This is the *least* likely cause of a swan-neck deformity because synovitis of the PIP joint most frequently results in a flexion contracture or a boutonnière deformity. It is possible but rare that chronic synovitis of the PIP joint can cause stretching of the volar capsule and the dorsal migration of lateral bands. Hyperextension of the PIP joint creates tension on the profundus tendon, flexing the DIP joint.[60]

Synovitis of the PIP joint may also lead to rupture of the flexor digitorum sublimis insertion, which predisposes the PIP joint to swan-neck deformity.[60]

Initial Involvement at DIP Joint (Fig. 19–26)

Chronic synovitis of the DIP joint (most commonly seen in psoriatic arthritis and JRA) can cause stretching or rupture of the insertion of the extensor tendon into the base of the distal phalanx.

As the DIP joint is pulled into flexion by the flexor digitorum profundus tendon, the PIP joint hyperextends because of the resultant imbalance.[60]

It is also possible for patients with OA to develop a mallet deformity when osteophyte formation ruptures the distal attachment of the extensor communis, consequently leading to a swan-neck deformity.

Late Stages

In the late stages, intrinsic contracture, stretching of the volar PIP capsule, collateral ligament shortening, tight skin, and tension on the profundus tendon become an integral part of most swan-neck deformities regardless of the initiating source.[60]

Other Etiologies

Approximately 10 percent of the general population has natural hyperextensibility of the PIP joint that creates a swan-neck appearance upon active extension. Occasionally, a patient with arthritis will have a swan-neck deformity from a prior traumatic injury. Traumatic swan-neck injuries primarily result from rupture of the extensor attachment at the DIP joint, rupture of the volar plate of the PIP joint and dorsal dislocation of the PIP joint, or an imbalance created by laceration, excision, or transfer of a flexor superficialis tendon.[43]

Evaluation

The swan-neck deformity involves a pattern of MCP joint flexion, PIP joint hyperextension, and DIP joint flexion. *Severity is determined by loss of PIP joint flexion.*[58] It can be described as (approximate guidelines): **mild,** 15 degrees hyperextension to 90 degrees flexion or more; **moderate,** 25 degrees hyperextension to 70 degrees flexion; and **severe,** 30 degrees hyperextension to 40 degrees flexion or less.[58] (Measure PIP flexion with the MCP joint flexed to rule out the effects of intrinsic tightness.) It is

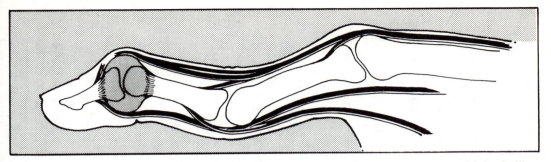

Figure 19–26. Swan-neck deformity with initial synovitis at the distal interphalangeal joint is illustrated here.

the loss of PIP joint flexion that reduces functional ability.

For surgical correction, the swan-neck deformity can be divided into four categories. These categories are described in detail in Chapter 29, Hand, Wrist, and Forearm Surgery.

Boutonnière Deformity (Fig. 19–27)

Boutonnière is a French word for buttonhole. The term is used to describe this deformity because the lateral bands separate, like a buttonhole, allowing the joint to protrude between them.

Initially, the deformity involves a flexion deformity of the PIP joint and hyperextension of the DIP joint. However, with chron-

icity, the PIP joint becomes a fixed contracture necessitating hyperextension of the MCP joint to achieve grasp.[61]

The boutonnière is the most difficult deformity to treat conservatively. Part of the reason is that by the time the lateral bands have displaced sufficiently to create a boutonnière, significant stretching of the supporting fibers has already taken place. Occupational therapists at the University of Michigan, Ann Arbor, have conducted a study evaluating the effectiveness of a 6-week extension orthotic immobilization program for reducible early (less than 20-degree loss of extension) boutonnière deformities. They found the program effective in reducing the deformity, but prolonged intermittent splinting was necessary to prevent its return.[62]

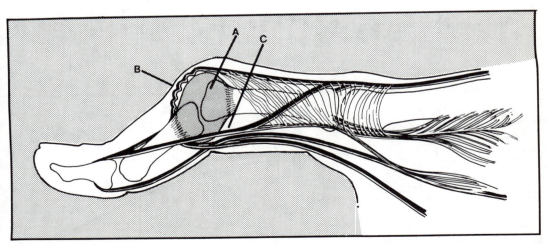

Figure 19–27. Depicted here is boutonnière deformity: (*A*) chronic synovitis; (*B*) lengthening of the central slip; (*C*) volar displacement of the lateral bands.

Chronic Synovitis (Fig. 19–27, A)

The boutonnière deformity differs from the swan-neck deformity in that the primary etiology is in the PIP joint. The inflammatory process damages the extensor structures to the PIP joint and weakens their attachments. Synovial hypertrophy distends the dorsal capsule mechanically, thus stretching or displacing the extensor structures.[61]

Lengthening of the Central Slip (Fig. 19–27, B)

Rupture or lengthening of the central slip attachment of the extensor communis tendon limits its effectiveness as an extensor for the middle phalanx.[61]

Volar Displacement of the Lateral Bands (Fig. 19–27, C)

Weakening and synovial distention of the transverse fibers that connect the lateral bands to the central slip allow the lateral bands to displace in a lateral-volar direction. This limits the ability of the interossei and lumbricals to extend the PIP joint. In addition, this process increases the mechanical advantage of the extensor mechanism for extending the DIP joint, thereby creating a hyperextension deformity of the DIP joint. With severe deformity, the lateral bands can be displaced volarward to the axis of the PIP joint and thus become an active flexor mechanism to the joint.[61] Compare alignment of structures in Figure 19–27 with normal alignment in Figure 19–23.

The deformity involves a pattern of PIP flexion, DIP hyperextension, and in the late stages, MCP hyperextension. *Severity is determined by loss of active PIP joint extension.*[58] It can be described as mild, loss of 5 to 10 degrees; moderate, loss of 10 to 30 degrees; and severe, loss of approximately 30 degrees or more.

Mallet Finger Deformity (Fig. 19–28)

This deformity involves flexion only of the DIP joint due to partial or complete rupture of the distal attachment of the EC tendon. In degenerative joint disease, osteophyte formation can stretch the extensor tendon, reducing its effectiveness for DIP joint extension, or cartilage loss can result in a collapse of the distal phalanx into flexion. In inflammatory joint disease, particularly psoriatic arthritis, synovitis causes lengthening or rupture of the distal EC tendon, removing the extension force to the DIP joint and thus allowing the profundus insertion to pull the joint into flexion.[58] Mallet finger deformity can also be caused by trauma to the distal extensor mechanism that is unrelated to arthritis.[43]

Since this deformity involves flexion only of the DIP joint, *severity is determined by loss of DIP extension.* Involvement can be described as mild, partial active extension; moderate, no active extension, but joint is mobile; and severe, fixed DIP contracture in flexion.[58]

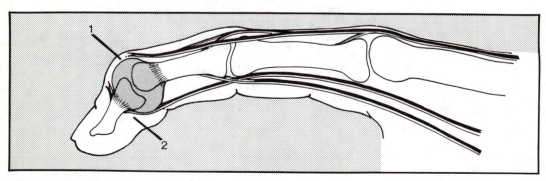

Figure 19–28. Mallet finger deformity secondary to synovitis is depicted: (*1*) rupture of the extensor tendon to the distal joint; (*2*) attachment of the profundus tendon.

Thumb Deformities—Rheumatoid

Thumb deformities are frequently referred to by their appearance, for example, "boutonnière" or "swan-neck." This type of label creates confusion about the dynamics of the deformity because these labels imply that the deforming force at the thumb MCP joint is similar to that of a finger PIP joint, which is not the case.

Nalebuff developed a classification for rheumatoid thumb deformities in 1968.[63] This was the classification presented in previous editions of this text. In 1984, he revised the classification to address critical dynamic factors and to reorder the types according to frequency of occurrence.[64] This classification includes only the most common deformity patterns. More patterns are possible, and thumbs that defy classification are documented by description. This classification system is more helpful to surgeons than to therapists.

However, it does provide a structure for understanding and thinking about the pathodynamics of the thumb, whereas labels such as boutonnière are not helpful at all. In a rheumatology program where all members of the team understand the classification, the use of "types" can provide for succinct documentation.

In the following descriptions a deformity in one joint results in the opposite deformity in adjacent joints. This is often described as a collapse or zigzag deformity. This is the typical sequela as long as the tendons are intact. If a patient has two adjacent joints deformed in the same direction, the most likely cause is tendon impairment either from rupture, tenosynovitis, or a nodule blocking excursion.[64] (Fig. 19–29 illustrates the normal extensor mechanism of the thumb for comparison with the deformity patterns in Figures 19–30 and 19–31.) Table 19–1, at the end of this chapter, provides a summary of the

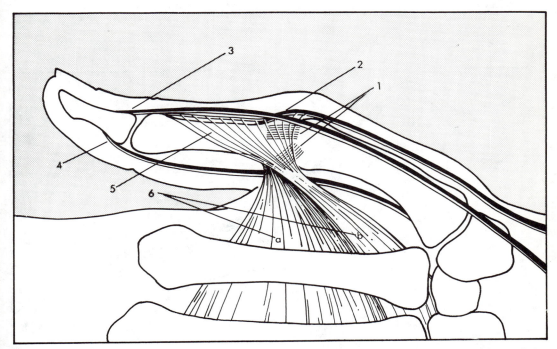

Figure 19–29. This figure presents the dorsal-ulnar view of normal extensor mechanism of the thumb: (*1*) collateral ligaments; (*2*) extensor pollicis brevis tendon (inserts into the extensor hood fibers and the base of the proximal phalanx); (*3*) extensor pollicis longus (inserts into the base of the distal phalanx and is attached to the hood mechanism); (*4*) flexor pollicis longus tendon; (*5*) extensor hood fibers; (*6*) adductor pollicis in which the transverse fibers (*a*) attach to the proximal phalanx and the oblique fibers (*b*) attach into the hood mechanism and assist in interphalangeal extension (on the radial side, the abductor brevis inserts into the radial hood fibers).

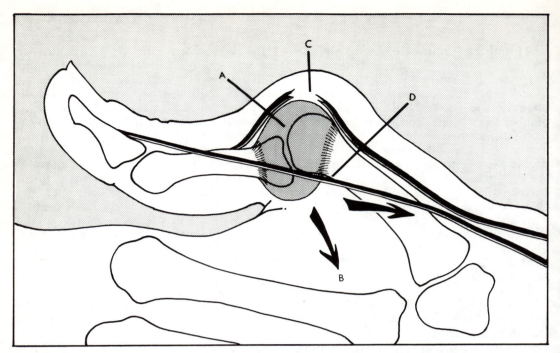

Figure 19–30. This figure shows the most common thumb deformity, Nalebuff classification type 1, extrinsic minus thumb: (*A*) chronic synovitis of the metacarpophalangeal joint; (*B*) intrinsic muscle tightness; (*C*) weakening or attenuation of the extensor pollicis brevis tendon; (*D*) ulnovolar displacement of the extensor pollicis longus. Pull of muscles is shown by arrows.

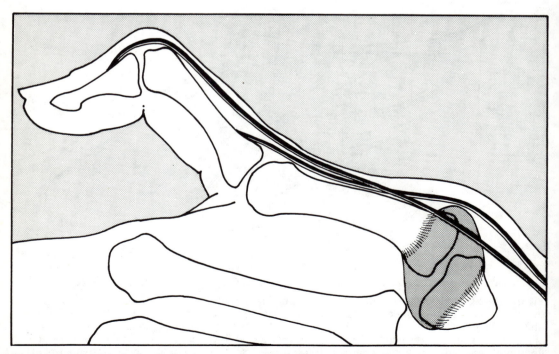

Figure 19–31. This figure shows the second most common thumb deformity, Nalebuff classification type II. This is the most frequent deformity resulting from OA.

pathomechanics of the most common deformity patterns defined by the Nalebuff classification.

Type I—Flexion of MCP Joint with Hyperextension of IP Joint and Compensatory CMC Abduction ("Extrinsic Minus Thumb"; Fig. 19–30)

This is the most frequently seen deformity in RA. This deformity starts with chronic synovitis of the MCP joint, resulting in the following events:

1. Stretching of the joint capsule and collateral ligaments.[63]
2. Stretching of the dorsal hood mechanism, thus reducing the effectiveness of the extensor pollicis brevis and creating an extrinsic minus condition.[63]
3. The extensor pollicis longus tendon, which normally passes directly over the MCP joint, may be displaced ulnarward, creating a flexor force for the MCP joint and a hyperextension force for the IP joint.[63]

It is also theorized that pain and distention of the joint capsule can elicit a reflex spasm of the intrinsic muscles of the thumb, resulting in an intrinsic plus posture of MCP flexion and IP hyperextension.[57] However, in many hands it appears that an extrinsic minus condition such as weakness or rupture of the extensor pollicis brevis (EPB), extensor pollicis longus (EPL), or flexor pollicis longus (FPL) can initiate this deformity and that the thumb intrinsic muscles become shortened secondary to the chronic flexion posture.[63]

The dynamics of Type I deformities result in flexion of the MCP joint and hyperextension of the IP joint. Pinch during functional activities adds another strong dynamic force to this process that further increases deformity. In order to approximate the pad of the thumb in pinch and grasp activities the patient needs to abduct the thumb and consequently develops an abduction posture of the CMC joint. This is only a compensatory alteration and there is no disease or damage to the CMC joint.

In its most severe form, the deformity consists of fixed contractures of both the PMCP and IP joints with subluxation resulting in as much as 90 degrees of IP hyperextension and 90 degrees of MCP joint flexion.[63] *Severity* is determined by the loss of active MCP joint extension and the degree of IP joint instability. It may be described as mild, loss of 5 to 20 degrees of active MCP joint extension; moderate, loss of 20 to 40 degrees; and severe, loss of 40 degrees or more.

Type II—CMC Joint Subluxation (Adduction) with MCP Joint Hyperextension and IP Joint Flexion (Fig. 19–31)

This is the second most common deformity pattern in RA and also the most common sequela to osteoarthritis (OA) of the CMC joint. In fact, one reason this deformity is so common in RA is because of the high incidence of OA of CMC joint, which affects people (especially women) with RA as well as the general population.

The initial site of involvement is the CMC joint. Synovitis of the CMC joint stretches the joint capsule, allowing the joint to sublux or dislocate in adduction. This adducted posture results in shortening of the adductor pollicis muscles and web space.[63] MCP joint hyperextension develops as the patient attempts to abduct the contracted first metacarpal bone.[63]

Severity is determined by the loss of active MCP flexion and the degree of CMC limitation present.

It is possible for a person with CMC subluxation and metacarpal adduction to develop MCP flexion and IP hyperextension, giving the appearance of a Type I deformity. (This was designated Type II in the previous classification but it is so uncommon it was dropped from the new classification altogether.)

Type III—MCP Lateral Deviation with CMC Joint Adduction

This deformity is the third most common type. Initially, it involves synovitis of the MCP joints with attenuation of the capsule and ulnar collateral ligaments. The MCP joint develops lateral instability and the first metacarpal drifts into adduction secondary to MCP involvement.[19] The first dorsal interosseous and adductor muscles

	Type I	Type II	Type III	Type IV	Type V
Initial Event	MCP Synovitis ↓	CMC Subluxation (due to synovitis or OA) ↓	MCP Synovitis ↓	MCP Synovitis ↓	MCP or IP Restoration (Mutilans) ↓
Sequela	MCP Flexion ↓ IP Hyperextension ↓ CMC Abduction (no CMC limitation)	CMC (Metacarpal) Adduction ↓ MCP Hyperextension ↓ IP Flexion	MCP Lateral Deviation (ulnar ligament instability) ↓ CMC Adduction Posture (no CMC limitation)	MCP Hyperextension (volar instability) ↓ IP Flexion CMC Adduction Posture (no CMC limitation)	MCP or IP Shortening and Instability
Prior Classification	Type I	Type III	Type IV	—	—

Figure 19–32. This is a summary of thumb deformities (Nalebuff classification, 1984).[64]

then become shortened and the web space becomes contracted. Although the first metacarpal is adducted, there is no associated CMC synovitis or subluxation of the CMC joint as seen in the Type II deformity.

Severity is determined by the degree of lateral deviation present and the extent of the adduction contracture. (See Fig. 29–5 for an example of this type of deformity.)

Type IV—MCP Hyperextension and IP Flexion (Normal CMC Joint)

This thumb looks similar to a Type II deformity, with MCP hyperextension and IP flexion. However, there is no CMC adduction or in fact any CMC involvement. This deformity originates in the MCP joint, where synovitis results in stretching of the volar capsule and MCP hyperextension. This ultimately leads to IP flexion.

Type V—Mutilans Thumb

Collapse or loss of bone substance, as seen in mutilans arthritis, results in shortening of the phalanges or metacarpal bone and total instability of the affected joints. This may occur solely in the thumb or in association with other affected joints. Surgical fusion with bone grafts to restore

length is the only effective treatment for this condition.

Figure 19–32 presents a summary of thumb deformities.

MUSCLE INVOLVEMENT

Intrinsic Muscle Atrophy

Assessment of intrinsic muscle atrophy (or the loss of muscle mass) is done to determine median and ulnar nerve involvement and to help define the extent of the disease on the peripheral structures.

When there is neurological impairment, the degree of atrophy correlates with muscle weakness, that is, the greater the atrophy, the weaker the muscle. Atrophy of thenar muscles is indicative of median nerve entrapment (carpal tunnel syndrome).[65] Atrophy of the hypothenar muscles may possibly be due to ulnar nerve entrapment.[8]

Atrophy can also occur secondary to disuse and systemic rheumatic disease. In the absence of neurological impairment the degree of atrophy does not necessarily correlate with weakness. It is possible to have severe atrophy and muscle strength at the grade 4 or 5 level. When atrophy is present, it is important first to evaluate for neurological involvement and second to assess for functional strength.

Evaluation

Diffuse atrophy of the intrinsic muscles (interossei and lumbricals), as indicative of the chronicity and severity of the disease, is determined by *visual assessment* of the first dorsal interosseous muscle. If there is atrophy of this muscle, it can be assumed that the other interossei have diminished in size also. Atrophy of the thenar and hypothenar muscles is also determined by visual assessment and comparison to a normal contralateral hand when possible.

Severity is generally described as slight or marked.

Intrinsic Muscle Weakness

Muscle weakness can occur due to peripheral nerve entrapment, cervical radiculopathy, and disuse.[8] All of the muscle can be affected. If there is a neurological deficit, an individual muscle examination should be performed.

In a routine arthritis hand assessment, it is generally sufficient to test selected muscles in order to screen for neurological impairment or disuse weakness. Testing the abductor pollicis brevis is critical for screening for carpal tunnel syndrome, median nerve entrapment. Testing the first dorsal and palmar interossei provides sufficient screening for ulnar nerve entrapment. The first dorsal interosseous is the last to be innervated by the ulnar nerve so it is the first to become weak. However, weakness in the third palmar interosseous or little finger adductor demonstrated by inability to adduct the little finger to the ring finger may be the first visual sign of ulnar nerve impairment. As a screening assessment it is easiest to apply resistance to the first dorsal interossei and abductor digiti quinti at the same time, and then to do the **snap test** (see below) for the first and third palmar interossei. (See Chapter 21 on muscle strength evaluation and the section on nerve entrapment in this chapter.)

Abductor Pollicis Brevis

This muscle should be checked in all arthritis hand assessments since weakness is often indicative of carpal tunnel syndrome. It is an important muscle and provides abduction for grasping objects. Patients with chronic weakness of this muscle often develop thumb adduction contractures.

Evaluation

Support the patient's hand in supination and stabilize the ulnar metacarpals and wrist. Have the patient abduct the thumb volar to the index finger and perpendicular to the palm. Apply resistance to the radial side of the thumb proximal phalanx. Grade according to a standard muscle strength evaluation.[66-68]

Dorsal and Volar Interossei

The interossei are prime MCP joint flexors. In some patients strengthening of the interossei can help compensate for extrinsic finger flexors that are not working effectively owing to tenosynovitis, attenuation, or contractures.

Evaluation

Dorsal interossei. Have the patient place his or her hand (palm down) on the table, and abduct the fingers. Stabilize the MCP joints. For the first and third muscles, apply resistance (to the proximal phalanx) to the radial side of the index and the ulnar side of the middle finger. For the second and fourth muscles, apply resistance to the ulnar side of the ring finger and the radial side of the middle finger.

Volar interossei: Snap test. Have the patient tightly adduct the fingers, with MCP and PIP joints in extension, and the hand supported in mid air, not on the table (to minimize flexor muscle substitution). During active adduction, attempt to abduct the patient's little finger and then the index finger. The resistance or abduction should be applied in a manner that allows the digit to snap. The muscles are graded on the following scale: 5/5 if the digit snaps back strongly, 4/5 if it snaps weakly, 3/5 if it adducts but cannot resist abduction, 2/5 if it partially adducts, and 1/5 for trace motion.

Abductor Digiti Quinti

Have the patient place his or her hand on the table and actively abduct the little finger. Apply resistance to the ulnar border of the proximal phalanx.[67] This can be done during the testing of the volar interossei.

Intrinsic Muscle Tightness

For patients with beginning swan-neck deformities, intrinsic muscle tightness can be a major deforming force.[19,39]

Shortening or tightness of the intrinsic muscles contributes to hand limitations in the following ways: (1) it can be a deforming causal factor for swan-neck deformity; (2) by itself, it can reduce dexterity; (3) it can contribute to flexion deformity of the MCP joints; and (4) if severe, it can limit the patient's ability to grasp large objects by prohibiting PIP and DIP flexion while the MCP joints are in extension.[69]

It is recommended that intrinsic muscle length be evaluated on all patients with inflammatory arthritis of the hands. It is theorized that pain and swelling in the MCP joints elicit a reflex spasm of the associated interossei muscles.[56] If this spasm is prolonged, the muscles can become contracted in a shortened position.[19] It is also possible for the intrinsic muscles to become contracted secondary to chronic flexion positioning of the MCP joints. Only a position of zero MCP extension and complete PIP flexion requires full excursion of the interossei muscles. Patients with painful MCP joints may not experience this position for months or even years.

Rationale for the test for intrinsic muscle tightness. The function of the interossei muscles is flexion of the MCP joints and extension of the PIP joints (Fig. 19–33).[39] When a person actively maintains a position of MCP joint flexion and PIP extension, the interossei muscles are contracting and are in their shortest position. Consequently, the opposite position (Fig. 19–34), MCP extension and PIP joint flexion, places the interossei muscles on stretch, and they have to extend their full length to allow this positioning. If a person's intrinsic muscles are tight or shortened they will not be able to fully flex the PIP joint while the MCP joint is in full extension (Fig. 19–35).[19] In fact, they will have greater PIP flexion with the MCP joint flexed than with the MCP joint extended. A patient has to have nearly full PIP flexion to be able to test the full length of the muscles.

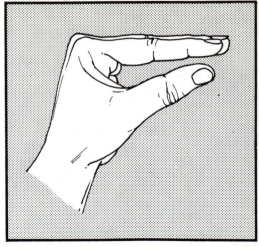

Figure 19–33. Shown here is the intrinsic plus position. The interossei and lumbricals act together to provide PIP extension when the MCP joints are flexed. In this position they are actively contracted and at their shortest length. This position should be avoided in swan-neck deformity. The opposite position (see Fig. 19–35) puts the muscles on stretch.

If a patient has MCP ulnar drift the standard test may not demonstrate tightness in the ulnar intrinsics. For these patients the test should be done with the digit radially deviated so the MCP joint is in neutral deviation during testing (except for the index finger, which should be in 20 degrees of

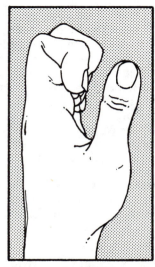

Figure 19–34. Shown here are normal intrinsic muscles stretched full length.

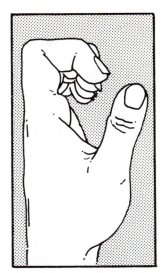

Figure 19–35. Tight intrinsic muscles do not allow full proximal interphalangeal flexion with the MCP joints in zero extension.

ulnar deviation). This is referred to in the hand surgery literature as the **test for "winged intrinsic tightness."**

Evaluation

1. This test must be done with *passive* motion. The patient has to be able to relax and not actively move the hand during the procedure.
2. Place the MCP joint in comfortable mid range. (Each finger must be done separately.)
3. Passively and gently flex the PIP joint as fully as possible. (Note ROM.)
4. Passively extend the MCP joint to neutral (zero extension).
5. Repeat passive PIP flexion. (Note ROM.) A loss of PIP flexion when the MCP joint is extended is indicative of intrinsic tightness.

The objective of this procedure is to determine if there is a difference in PIP joint ROM when the MCP joint is flexed, compared with when it is extended.[39]

Intrinsic tightness can be described in the following manner: *zero* or *absent,* PIP joint flexion is the same with MCP flexion or MCP extension; *minimal shortening,* tightness is palpable or there is less than 10 degrees change in PIP joint ROM; *marked shortening,* there is greater than 10 degrees difference in PIP joint ROM. Intrinsic tightness is documented in the degrees of difference of PIP joint motion; for example, 15 degrees tightness. (The criteria for goniometric measurement of the PIP joint in patients with arthritis are described in Chapter 20, Evaluation of Range of Motion.)

TENDON INVOLVEMENT

Tenosynovitis

In the hand, the tendons pass through a synovial-lined sheath at four locations: the volar aspect of the wrist; the volar aspect of the fingers; the volar aspect of the thumb; and the dorsum of the wrist (Fig. 19–36).[20] The purpose of the sheath is to facilitate lubrication and gliding of the tendons, particularly where the tendons slide over several bones. The sheaths have a double wall construction, and inflammation of the synovial lining results in excessive fluid being trapped within the walls of the sheath. If the inflammation becomes chronic, synovial tissue will proliferate and granulation tissue can form. Tenosynovitis impedes the gliding of tendons and, through an enzymatic process, directly attacks the tendons, reducing their integrity.[19]

Tenosynovitis differs from joint synovitis in two ways. First, in most cases, there is no warmth present; and second, there may not be any pain associated with it. The only indicative signs may be swelling and possibly impaired tendon function.[70]

Volar Wrist Tenosynovitis

The signs and symptoms of volar wrist tenosynovitis can include one or all of the following:

1. Swelling over the volar aspect of the wrist.
2. Carpal tunnel syndrome (median nerve entrapment).
3. Decreased excursion of the profundus and/or superficialis tendons affecting all four digits. This can result in decreased active finger flexion or decreased passive finger extension and tenodesis motion in the fingers.[72]
4. Pain and warmth may or may not be present.

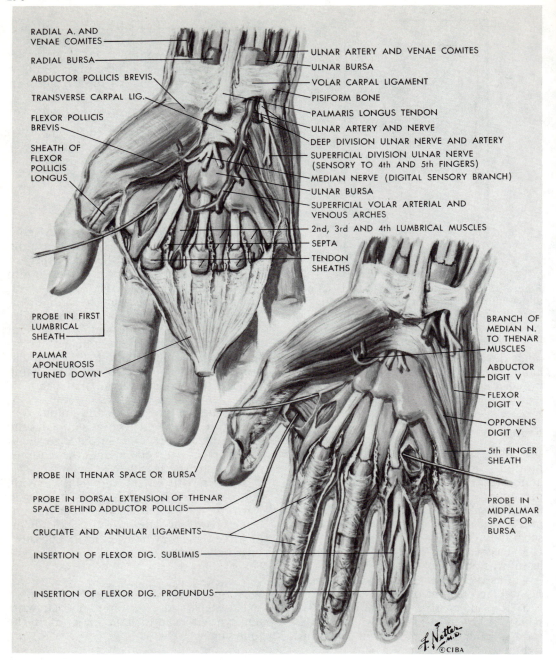

RADIAL A. AND VENAE COMITES

RADIAL BURSA

ABDUCTOR POLLICIS BREVIS

TRANSVERSE CARPAL LIG.

FLEXOR POLLICIS BREVIS

SHEATH OF FLEXOR POLLICIS LONGUS

ULNAR ARTERY AND VENAE COMITES

ULNAR BURSA

VOLAR CARPAL LIGAMENT

PISIFORM BONE

PALMARIS LONGUS TENDON

ULNAR ARTERY AND NERVE

DEEP DIVISION ULNAR NERVE AND ARTERY

SUPERFICIAL DIVISION ULNAR NERVE (SENSORY TO 4th AND 5th FINGERS)

MEDIAN NERVE (DIGITAL SENSORY BRANCH)

ULNAR BURSA

SUPERFICIAL VOLAR ARTERIAL AND VENOUS ARCHES

2nd, 3rd AND 4th LUMBRICAL MUSCLES

SEPTA

TENDON SHEATHS

PROBE IN FIRST LUMBRICAL SHEATH

PALMAR APONEUROSIS TURNED DOWN

BRANCH OF MEDIAN N. TO THENAR MUSCLES

ABDUCTOR DIGIT V

FLEXOR DIGIT V

OPPONENS DIGIT V

5th FINGER SHEATH

PROBE IN THENAR SPACE OR BURSA

PROBE IN DORSAL EXTENSION OF THENAR SPACE BEHIND ADDUCTOR POLLICIS

CRUCIATE AND ANNULAR LIGAMENTS

INSERTION OF FLEXOR DIG. SUBLIMIS

INSERTION OF FLEXOR DIG. PROFUNDUS

PROBE IN MIDPALMAR SPACE OR BURSA

Figure 19–36. Illustrated here are flexor sheaths at four levels: wrist, thumb, palm, and digits. In the digits the annular ligaments (pulleys) are the transverse fibers that encircle the flexor sheath and maintain the alignment of the flexor tendons. These fibers are strong and close fitting; nodules or thickened areas on the tendon can catch on these annular fibers, producing a trigger finger. In this illustration the flexor sheaths are filled with air to demonstrate that they are a closed space. This emphasizes how the sheaths would expand if they were filled with synovial fluid during flexor tenosynovitis. Normally the sheaths are close-fitting to the tendons. Palpation for digital flexor tenosynovitis is most effective over the cruciate (criss-cross) fibers, because they are weaker than the annular fibers and allow swelling to protrude. (Copyright 1969 CIBA Pharmaceutical Co, Division of CIBA-Geigy Corp. Reprinted with permission from Clinical Symposia, illustrated by Frank H. Netter, M.D. All rights reserved.)

Evaluation

1. Support the patient's wrist in neutral and palpate the volar aspect of the wrist just proximal to the palm. In patients with early disease, distention or visible swelling of this area is indicative of volar wrist tenosynovitis.

2. Evaluate for carpal tunnel syndrome (see section on median nerve entrapment later in this chapter).

3. To determine the excursion capability of flexor tendons, gently and passively extend the patient's fingers and wrist (Fig. 19–37). If the flexor tendons are not extending fully, there will be a difference in PIP or MCP joint extension when the wrist is extended compared with when the wrist is flexed, that is, tenodesis motion.

4. It is often difficult to determine if a patient has pain associated with the tenosynovitis, since most patients with RA also have painful radiocarpal or radioulnar synovitis.[72]

When tendon excursion is reduced, generally all four digits are affected. However, it is possible for only three or two digits to be involved. If the limitation is only in a single digit, it is probably due to digital rather than wrist tenosynovitis.[71]

If there is a decrease in active finger flexion, it is important to rule out extensor tendon tightness as a cause.

Severity can be related either to the degree of swelling or to the interference with tendon functioning. Some patients have a minimal amount of swelling but severe loss of tendon excursion, while others can have severe swelling but full tendon excursion.

If tendon excursion is limited and left untreated, permanent contractures can develop (Fig. 19–38). This condition should be treated as early as possible. The most effective conservative measures are ice compresses and intrasynovial steroid injections (not at the same time). If neither of these measures is successful, surgery is indicated.

To document tendon limitations, particularly before and after conservative treatment, the following methods are recommended. Measure MCP, PIP, and DIP joint ROM with the wrist in neutral; or record the maximal degree of wrist extension at which full MCP, DIP, and PIP joint extension is possible. Either method will rule out the influence of tenodesis motion.

Palmar Tenosynovitis

Severe hypertrophy of the tenosynovium can distend the sheath into the palm as well as fill the entire length of the sheath of the fifth digit tendons, which is often continuous between the wrist and digit level. Early tenosynovitis in the palmar region is difficult to detect because of overlying muscle

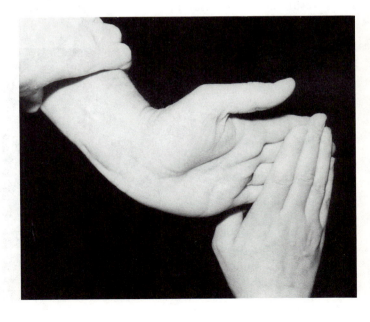

Figure 19–37. Flexor tenosynovitis at the wrist can cause limitations of the flexor tendons. Here the therapist is gently, passively extending the patient's wrist and fingers to determine if the flexor tendons can complete full excursion. If the tendons were blocked, the patient would not be able to fully extend the wrist and digits at the same time. This patient has normal excursion.

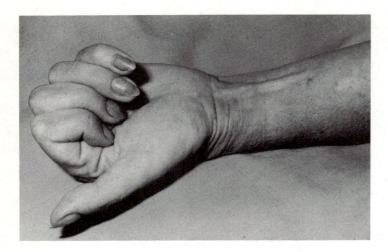

Figure 19–38. This young woman presented with a carpal tunnel syndrome. The hand evaluation revealed a flexion lag in the middle, ring, and little fingers, indicating that the profundus tendons were not gliding freely through the carpal tunnel. This suggested flexor tenosynovitis in the wrist, despite the absence of wrist pain or warmth. Her symptoms were alleviated and ROM restored following a tenosynovial steroid injection and orthotic immobilization of the wrist for 2 weeks.

and fascia. It is only palpable after marked hypertrophy has occurred.

When palmar tenosynovitis is associated with hand use, marked reduction of hypertrophied tissue can occur if the stressful activity is eliminated.

Digital Flexor Tenosynovitis

The signs and symptoms of digital flexor tenosynovitis can include any of the following.[71]

1. Swelling along the volar aspect of the digit (Fig. 19–39).
2. Decreased excursion of the flexor tendons, resulting in decreased active flexion or decreased passive extension (in a single digit).
3. Trigger finger due to tenosynovium (or nodule) catching on the pulleys (annular ligaments: see Fig. 19–37).
4. Pain or warmth may or may not be present.

Evaluation

1. Tendon sheath effusions are first evident over the volar aspect of the proximal phalanx.[1] Palpate this area with the digit in extension. Swelling, fullness, or tension in this area is indicative of tenosynovitis. When possible, compare swelling with uninvolved contralateral digits. Moderate or

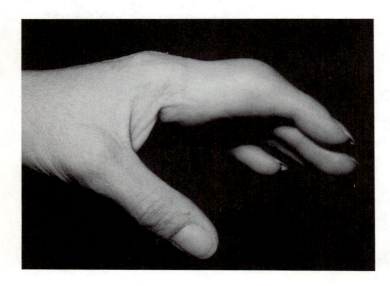

Figure 19–39. This is an example of severe digital flexor tenosynovitis and hypertrophy. Digital swelling secondary to flexor tenosynovitis is most evident when viewed from the lateral aspect.

severe tenosynovitis can also be palpated over the volar aspect of the middle phalanx.

2. If tenosynovitis is not readily palpable, stabilize the patient's MCP joints in extension and have him or her actively flex the PIP and DIP joints. Palpate over the volar aspect of the proximal phalanx. This procedure may allow a minimal effusion to be detected.

Tenosynovitis is considered slight if it is palpable but does not limit finger flexion or tendon excursion; moderate if there is some joint or tendon limitation; and severe if there is marked limitation in motion.

Treatment is similar to that for wrist tenosynovitis. Ice compresses and steroid injections are the recommended conservative measures. From personal experience, orthotic immobilization can be very effective in those cases in which there is a great deal of warmth and pain. Orthotic immobilization has not proven effective in cases without these two symptoms, and in most of these cases has increased stiffness.[70]

The flexor pollicis longus tendon has its own synovial sheath that is continuous from the IP joint to approximately 3 cm proximal of the wrist (see Fig. 19–37).[20] Tenosynovitis of this tendon can be nonpainful, with the effusion easily detected over the volar aspect of the proximal phalanx, or it can be painful and difficult to detect if inflammation is in the region beneath the thenar muscles.[70] Sometimes resistance applied to IP joint flexion can elicit pain along the tendon, distinguishing tendon involvement from CMC joint pain, which can also radiate into the thenar eminence. During palpation of this tendon, keep in mind that there are two small sesamoid bones over the volar aspect of the MCP joint. These can often be misinterpreted as nodules.

Dorsal Wrist Tenosynovitis

Each extensor tendon passes through a separate tendon sheath over the dorsal aspect of the wrist. As the tendons pass beneath the dorsal retinacular ligament, they are divided into six compartments (Fig. 19–40). Tenosynovitis can occur in a single compartment or in all six compartments at one time (Fig. 19–41).[20] Since the skin over the dorsum of the wrist is thin, effusions tend to feel puffy and are readily detectable; they often clearly delineate the length of the sheath. Synovitis of the radiocarpal and intercarpal joints can also cause swelling in this area. Joint synovitis is firm to the touch and is usually warm and painful.

Inflammation of the first compartment, which contains the abductor pollicis longus and the extensor pollicis brevis, is referred to as **de Quervain's disease.**[72] Unlike other areas of tenosynovitis, inflammation of the first compartment is almost always painful. Since this is a common condition, which frequently is primary and unrelated to arthritis, it is discussed in a separate section following the discussion of trigger finger.

The incidence of pain in dorsal tenosynovitis varies. The first compartment is usually painful; the sixth compartment, containing the extensor carpi ulnaris, is frequently painful; and compartments two through five are rarely painful.[70] It is theorized that the first and sixth compartments have more pain because of their close approximation to the superficial branch of the radial nerve and dorsal cutaneous branch of the ulnar nerve, respectively. When the tenosynovitis is painful, splinting can be very effective for reducing pain and inflammation. When there is no pain, it is very difficult to get patients to wear wrist orthoses. A full hand orthosis would be required to provide rest for the tendons in compartments three, four, and five. This would be impractical, particularly for patients without any symptoms. The value of orthotic immobilization for painless tenosynovitis needs much more investigation. For some patients immobilization can increase stiffness and swelling by eliminating muscle action as a mechanism for venous and lymphatic return. For conservative management, ice is more effective than heat in reducing swelling and pain.

Tenosynovitis of the extensor carpi ulnaris (ECU) tendon in the sixth compartment is of special concern. If the supporting ligaments that maintain the alignment of the insertion of the ECU are stretched, the tendon can displace volarward to become a major flexor force causing volar subluxation of the wrist (see discussion under common rheumatoid deformities). All conservative measures should be employed early to protect this tendon, before displacement occurs.

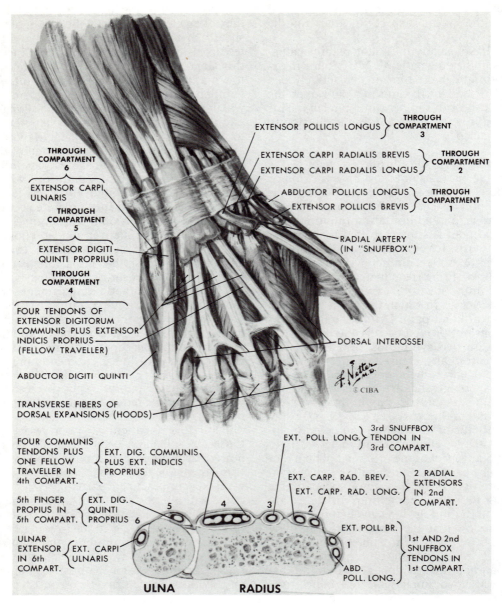

Figure 19–40. This illustration defines the extensor tendon sheaths and the compartments they pass through. In this drawing, the sheaths are filled with air to demonstrate that they are a closed structure and their expansiveness if filled with tenosynovial fluid. Tenosynovitis may afflict a single compartment or all compartments. Because the dorsal covering is thin, swelling is readily detected and conforms to the length of the sheath. (Copyright 1969 CIBA Pharmaceutical Co, Division CIBA-Geigy Corp. Reprinted with permission from Clinical Symposia, illustrated by Frank H. Netter, M.D. All rights reserved.)

The major consequence of dorsal tenosynovitis is ruptured extensor tendons at the wrist.[73] Chronic tenosynovitis compromises the integrity of the tendons, rendering them vulnerable to rupture as they slide over sharp or subluxed wrist bones.[73] (Evaluation of tendon ruptures is discussed in a separate section.)

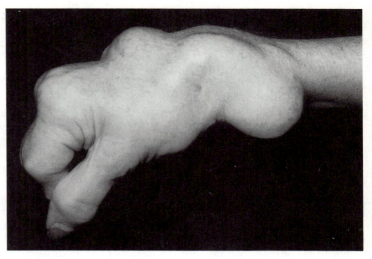

Figure 19–41. This woman demonstrates the extreme of dorsal tenosynovitis with involvement of multiple tendon compartments. The apparent enlargement of the MCP joints is created by volar subluxation of the proximal phalanges, which also gives the digits a shortened appearance. There is also marked synovitis of the thumb IP joint and a mild type III thumb deformity.

Trigger Finger

Trigger finger refers to a snapping or catching of a finger during active flexion or extension resulting from a nodule, tenosynovium, or a thickened flexor tendon becoming trapped at either the proximal, middle, or distal flexor pulley (Fig. 19–42).[72]

A network of fibrous bands (annular and cruciate ligaments) covers the flexor tendon sheath. These bands are thickest directly over the volar aspect of the MCP, PIP, and DIP joints (annular ligaments).[20] This strong thickened portion or band is referred to as a **pulley.** (This pulley functions similarly to a mechanical pulley, which maintains the position of a rope but allows it to slide.) The pulley hugs the tendon to the joint during flexion. If a pulley were cut, the flexor tendons would bowstring across the joint.[74]

A nodule or tenosynovial build-up on a tendon can get caught on any one of the three pulleys during either flexion or extension. Clinically this presents in one of the following ways: a slight catch or snap during motion; inconsistency in the degree of active motion; and inability actively to extend or flex a digit completely.

In the early stages, it is usually annoying but not painful. As the lump becomes larger the catching can be quite painful. Triggering can occur in one or more digits. It occurs most frequently at the MCP joints of the fingers and thumb, followed by the PIP joints and thumb IP joint; rarely does it occur at the DIP joints.[72]

Evaluation

1. First, ask the patient if his or her fingers ever catch or stay closed when opening or closing the hand. Most patients are aware of this problem if it is present.

2. Determine if it occurs rarely, occasionally, or consistently; if there is any pain associated with it; and if it interferes with function.

3. Palpate for a nodule over the flexor pulleys.

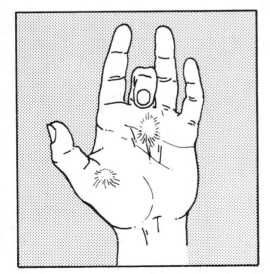

Figure 19–42. Common palpation sites for trigger finger are indicated in this drawing.

Severity can be described as *minimal,* inconsistent, painless triggering during active ROM; *moderate,* constant triggering during active ROM or intermittent but painful triggering; *severe,* prevents full active flexion or extension or is severely painful.

If the condition interferes with function or is painful, the patient should be advised to see a physician. Many patients do not mention the problem to their doctor because they believe the only solution is surgery. It is often encouraging for them to find out that the initial treatment of choice is an intrasynovial steroid injection.[72,74] In some cases, surgeons have found a regimen of orthotic immobilization following corticosteroid injection to be more effective than injection alone.[75] In my practice, I have had some (approximately 10) patients in whom the triggering was moderate and occurred near the end of maximal PIP flexion that responded favorably to wearing an elastic sleeve made of 2-inch wide, medium-strength, wristband elastic. The sleeve allowed them motion but prevented the end of range that created triggering; after 3 to 4 months the triggering stopped. Apparently elimination of an irritating force (catching on the pulley) was therapeutic in reducing the nodules or thickening.

de Quervain's Tenosynovitis

This is tenosynovitis of the first dorsal wrist compartment, which encloses the **abductor pollicis longus and the extensor pollicis brevis tendons.** This condition is common and frequently occurs in people without arthritis secondary to trauma or occupational stress.[72] The most common cause is repetitive lateral pinch (or prehension) with the wrist in ulnar deviation. In the past few years there has been an increased incidence of de Quervain's tenosynovitis in new mothers. Bilateral lifting and placing of the baby creates the classic aggravating force. As the baby gets heavier, the stress on the first compartment gets stronger. If the mother is nursing she may not be inclined to take anti-inflammatory medications, leaving orthotic immobilization and adapted lifting techniques as the sole treatment.[76] (See Chapter 23 on wrist–thumb orthoses and Chapter 25 on assistive devices.)

Signs and symptoms include pain over the first compartment and thumb with active or passive motion; swelling; and decreased thumb ROM secondary to pain. Warmth may or may not be present.

Evaluation

The Finkelstein Test.[1] The original version of this test is to have the patient make a fist, with the fingers holding the thumb in flexion, then to deviate the wrist ulnarward. *This method is too painful for patients with arthritis.* Therefore, the following adapted version is recommended. Passively and gently fully flex the patient's thumb and have the patient identify pain areas; then gently deviate the wrist ulnarward, keeping the thumb flexed (Fig. 19–43).

The test is positive if the maneuver elicits pain over the first compartment, possibly radiating to the first metacarpal bone. The test may elicit pain localized to the thumb IP or MCP joints or to the wrist joints, but this is usually indicative of joint involvement, not tenosynovitis.

When de Quervain's tenosynovitis is secondary to trauma or functional use, it is generally responsive to orthotic immobilization or a combination of steroid injection and immobilization. The ideal orthotic design is a radial wrist splint with an extension to immobilize the thumb MCP joint. This type of orthosis allows patients to make a fist and use their thumb IP for prehension. This design prevents excursion of the extensor pollicis brevis and abductor pollicis longus tendons, yet allows the patient to continue working (see Chapter 23). If de Quervain's syndrome becomes chronic and is nonresponsive to splinting, injections, and activity modification, then surgical tenosynovectomy may be indicated.

Tendon Ruptures

The most frequent cause of tendon rupture is a combination of tenosynovitis diminishing the strength and integrity of the tendons (attenuation) and attrition over rough subluxed bones or bone spurs. Occasionally the tenosynovium can cause sufficient pressure to compromise the blood supply to the tendon, creating ischemic areas.[73]

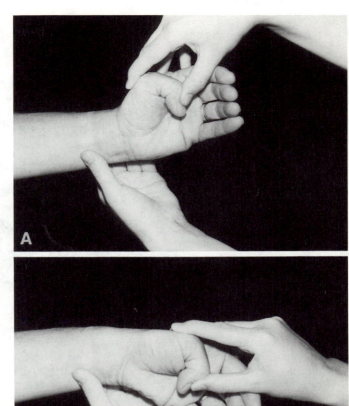

Figure 19–43. Demonstrated here is the Finkelstein test (adapted for patients with arthritis) for de Quervain's tenosynovitis. (*A*) Support the patient's wrist in neutral, gently passively flex the thumb, and note any pain. (*B*) Then deviate the wrist ulnarward, while maintaining thumb flexion. This maneuver places the tendons in the first wrist compartment, that is, the extensor pollicis brevis and the abductor pollicis longus on stretch. The test is considered positive if the maneuver elicits pain directly over the first compartment (see Fig. 19–40). Joint pain is not characteristic of tenosynovitis and may indicate arthritis. *Caution:* Try this procedure on several normal hands before trying it on a patient. The mechanics of the maneuver can create discomfort in normal hands.

Ruptures of the finger extensors are usually found over the distal end of the ulna (Fig. 19–44). The extensor pollicis longus tendon commonly ruptures at Lister's tubercle, where it turns radially to the thumb. The flexor tendons most frequently rupture over the scaphoid carpal bone. However, they can rupture at the palm or digit level.[73,74]

Because of the manner in which the extensor tendons slide over the carpal bones, rupture of the dorsal tendons is more common than rupture of the flexor tendons. The extensor digiti quinti (EDQ) is generally the first tendon to rupture. Interestingly, this muscle, which is of little functional importance, is the key tendon to evaluate in an arthritis hand assessment.[73] If this tendon is ruptured, the extensor communis tendons are in danger of attri-

tion also. Patients with partial or complete rupture of the EDQ are candidates for a dorsal tenosynovectomy to protect the other extensor tendons from attrition. In many cases, it is necessary to use a wrist orthosis to protect the remaining tendons until surgery can be scheduled. Rupture of the EDQ does not impair function, and since it is rarely noticed by patients, it requires a specific testing procedure.

The following tendons have the highest incidence of rupture. They are listed in order of greatest frequency.[73]

Extensor Digiti Quinti (EDQ)

Test procedure: Hold the MCP joints of the ring, middle, and index fingers in flexion to prevent function of the extensor communis tendon. Have the patient ac-

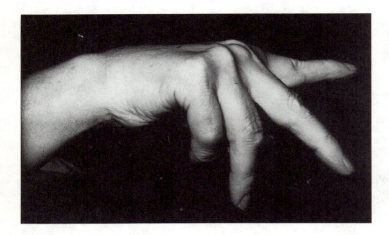

Figure 19–44. Extensor tendons are typically ruptured at the wrist level as a result of attrition by the eroded and roughened end of the ulna. This woman has complete rupture of the extensor digitorum quinti tendon and the extensor communis tendons to the little, ring, and middle fingers, as evidenced by the inability to fully extend the MCP joints of these fingers and the inability to palpate tendon function during active extension. Partial extension of the middle finger is possible due to intertendinous connections to the index finger. The extensor communis tendon to the index finger and the indicis proprius tendon are intact.

tively extend the little finger. Inability to actively extend the little finger MCP joint in this position indicates damage to the EDQ tendon (Fig. 19–44).

Considerations: It is necessary to rule out displacement of the extensor tendons as a cause for loss of MCP extension. PIP joint extension is accomplished by the intrinsic muscles.[73]

Extensor Digitorum Communis (EDC)

Rupture of this tendon occurs most frequently to the little and ring fingers. If there is a rupture, the patient will be unable actively to extend the associated MCP joint.

The indicis proprius provides extension to the index finger (see Fig. 19–44).

Considerations: The EDC tendons may displace into the ulnar MCP valleys and lose their mechanical advantage for extension. Rule out tendon displacement by positioning the MCP joints in extension. If the patient can maintain extension, once positioned, the tendons are intact. Palpate for tendon function over the dorsum of the hand during active extension. Inability actively to extend the little finger MCP joint indicates possible rupture of the fifth EDC as well as the EDQ (see Fig. 19–45).[73] Although rare, it is possible to have paralysis of the digit extensors due to entrapment of the posterior interosseous branch of the radial nerve.[10]

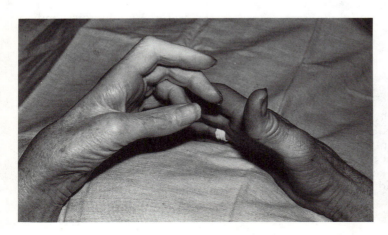

Figure 19–45. The extensor pollicis longus tendon is ruptured in this woman's left hand. To evaluate for EPL rupture it is advisable to palpate for tendon function. Observation of IP joint motion alone is not sufficient, inasmuch as the thumb intrinsic muscles are also capable of extending the IP joint.

Extensor Pollicis Longus (EPL)

Rupture of this tendon results in decreased active thumb IP joint extension (when the MP joint is extended) and possible decreased active MCP extension (Fig. 19–45).[73]

Considerations: The abductor pollicis brevis, adductor pollicis, and the flexor pollicis brevis (superficial head) also extend the IP joint of the thumb through their attachment to the dorsal expansion. Their pull on the IP joint is strongest when the MCP joint is flexed. To determine an EPL rupture, evaluate active thumb IP extension with the thumb MCP stabilized in extension. Have the patient put his or her hand flat on the table and raise the thumb up. This is retropulsion and can only be accomplished by the EPL. If joint limitations prevent this test, palpate for EPL function during active IP extension.

Flexor Pollicis Longus (FPL)

Rupture of this tendon results in loss of active thumb IP flexion and decreased ability for pinch. To determine if there is a partial rupture, test IP flexion with the thumb MCP and CMC joints stabilized in extension. This places the tendon on tension and allows slight motion to be detected.[73]

Considerations: A tendon nodule catching on the IP and MCP flexor pulley can also prevent thumb IP flexion. A rare condition that can impair FPL function is entrapment of the anterior interosseous nerve in the forearm. (See section on nerve entrapment and Fig. 19–47.)

Flexor Digitorum Profundus

Rupture of this tendon occurs primarily in the index finger. Rupture results in absent or diminished active DIP joint flexion, and the patient may lose the ability for tip-to-tip pinch.[73] Entrapment of the anterior interosseous nerve (AIN) in the forearm can result in weakness or loss of DIP flexion in the index finger and appears as an FDP rupture. See Figure 19–48 and the section on nerve entrapments.

Evaluation

Elicit active DIP joint flexion while stabilizing the PIP and MCP joints in extension.

Considerations: The ruptured distal tendon end may become adhered to other flexor tendons, resulting in partial flexion with the digit in extension. If this occurs there would be an absence of active flexion with the digit flexed.[73] A flexor tendon nodule can block profundus tendon excursion and imitate a rupture. This phenomenon can be ruled out by palpating for a nodule and observing the resting digital posture. If the tendon is ruptured, the finger will assume a more extended position than the other digits.[73]

Flexor Digitorum Superficialis (FDS)

Fortunately, rupture of the FDS is uncommon.[73] However, when it occurs, it is often in conjunction with rupture of the FDP tendon, to the index finger.

Evaluation

Stabilize all of the digits in full extension (to rule out profundus function), except the digit to be assessed. Have the patient actively flex the PIP joint.

Considerations: Rupture of the FDS usually does not interfere or reduce the patient's functional ability. However, the proximal end of the ruptured tendon may retract and become adherent to the profundus tendon and consequently limit profundus excursion. In the presence of severe digital flexor tenosynovitis, hand function may be improved by surgical removal of the FDS (or one slip of the FDS) to provide more room for the profundus tendon to slide effectively. To evaluate the superficialis tendon in the little finger it may be necessary to apply additional stabilization of the proximal phalanx in extension and adduction, while having the patient attempt active flexion, since many patients do not have independent function of the superficialis tendon in the little finger.

SKIN AND VASCULAR INVOLVEMENT

Skin Changes

There are characteristic skin lesions associated with systemic sclerosis (and mixed connective tissue disease), psoriatic arthritis, systemic lupus, dermatomyositis, and juvenile rheumatoid arthritis.[77] These are discussed in detail in the chapters on each disease in Parts II and III.

The following terms are often used to describe skin rashes in medical documentation.[77]

Macule: A circumscribed area of alternation of normal skin color. It is neither raised nor depressed compared with surrounding skin. It can be of any size and is the result of pigmentary or vascular abnormality.

Papule: A solid lesion, most of which is elevated above the skin.

Plaque: A lesion that is elevated above the skin with a relatively large surface area. It is formed by a confluence of papules.

Evanescent: This is used to describe a rash that appears and disappears over a short period of time, that is, within hours or a day. This is characteristic of the rash seen with juvenile rheumatoid arthritis.

Skin Ulcerations

Skin breakdown typically can occur in three ways.

1. In systemic sclerosis, fingertip ulcerations due to ischemia are common and extremely painful. Also, the skin may break down over the dorsum of the PIP joints or over calcium deposits.[48]

2. In RA, the skin may break down over bony prominences created by joint subluxation, such as over the dorsum of a severely flexed PIP joint. Nodules over the dorsum of the PIP joints are particularly vulnerable to trauma.

3. In hands with severe deformity or contractures, the skin can become macerated between the digits resulting from the difficulty in washing and drying the hands thoroughly in these areas.

Drug Reactions

Skin rashes are a common consequence of gold therapy, antimalarials (Plaquenil), penicillamine, or less commonly any of the NSAIDs.[77] In all cases, the rash is highly variable and can have any appearance; there is no characteristic pattern. All rashes that cannot be explained should be reported to the physician.

Chronic use of systemic steroids can re-sult in atrophic skin changes. The skin feels dry and smooth; there is decreased height in the dorsal folds over the digit joints and atrophy of the fingertip pulp. The skin appears thin and delicate and is sometimes referred to as *tissue paper skin.*[77] Multiple intradermal hemorrhages, which occur particularly on the arms after minor abrasion, are common.

Skin Tightness

This occurs primarily with systemic sclerosis or diabetes. If the skin is tight in the hands, it is usually difficult to pinch the skin over the dorsum of the middle and proximal phalanges.[48]

Vasculitis

Patients with RA can develop an arteritis of the small digital arteries. This can result in a peripheral neuropathy, nailfold infarcts, ulcers, and digital gangrene.[77] When it develops, vasculitis usually becomes the primary diagnosis. Therapy is generally minimal. Custom orthoses are often helpful for protecting ulcerated areas.

Telangiectasia

These are small reddish spots in the skin that result from a chronic dilatation of the capillaries.[77] They are indicative of the vascular changes that are taking place internally as well as cutaneously. They are most common in systemic sclerosis but occasionally can occur in rheumatoid arthritis.

Palmar Erythema

In patients with systemic diseases, the thenar and hypothenar eminences appear red, with discrete small red irregular-shaped blotches. The erythema is evidence of the vascular systemic involvement of the disease.[1]

Purpura

This refers to a spontaneous hemorrhage into the skin. The appearance varies with the type of purpura, and the color of the lesion varies from red to purple to brownish-yellow, as it dissipates.[77]

Purpura can occur in several disorders, including Henoch-Schönlein (anaphylactoid) purpura, erythema nodosum, severe RA, thrombocytopenia (low platelets), and in certain drug reactions. Patients on disease-modifying or immunoregulatory drugs should immediately report unusual or unexplained bruising to their physician.

Purpura can be purely cutaneous, or it can be indicative of hemorrhage in the internal organs. The term **ecchymosis** has the same definition as purpura but is generally used to describe a singular bruise or skin hemorrhages resulting from trauma.

Keratoderma Blennorrhagica

This is the characteristic skin lesion that occurs with Reiter's syndrome. The skin changes most frequently involve the acral (peripheral) regions, especially the soles, toes, and fingers, but can occur anywhere on the body. The lesions begin as vesicles (small blisters) on an erythematous base, progress to sterile pustules, and evolve to manifest keratotic scale. Psoriasis-like lesions can also appear in Reiter's syndrome.[77]

Temperature Changes and Sweating

Systemic diseases can alter vasomotor and sudomotor stability, resulting in hands that feel cold and clammy with increased sweating. As a result of these changes, the hand may feel very soft to the touch.[77]

Raynaud's Phenomenon

In this disorder, vasoconstriction causes blanching or cyanosis of the skin, with subsequent erythema upon vasodilation. The vasoconstriction can be in response to exposure to cold, emotional stress, or to dependent positioning of the arm to the side; or it can appear spontaneously. The color changes may be limited to the tip of a finger or encompass the entire hand.[78]

Raynaud's phenomenon most commonly occurs with systemic sclerosis, mixed connective tissue disease, and systemic lupus erythematosus. It is *not* associated with RA, but occasionally a person with RA can also have Raynaud's phenomenon as an unrelated but concomitant condition. The incidence in people with rheumatic diseases other than systemic lupus erythematosus, PSS, and MCTD is probably the same as for the general population. However, in 40 to 50 percent of patients, Raynaud's phenomenon may exist without underlying rheumatic disease.

The only clinical sign of Raynaud's phenomenon may be the white, blue, or red color changes in the skin, or there may be symptoms of pain and paresthesias.[78]

Evaluation

First ask the patient if he or she has noticed color changes in the hand, that is, turning red, white, or blue. Most patients are aware of these changes when they occur. Second, determine the extent of the changes—whether or not it is painful and how the symptoms interfere with functional ability. Also, can the patient identify any causal factors or measures that relieve the symptoms? Smoking habits should also be addressed. Patients with Raynaud's phenomenon should not smoke or use nicotine, a vasoconstrictor.[78] (See Chapter 10 for treatment).

Severity may be described in the following manner: *mild,* patient is aware of skin changes but does not experience any discomfort or functional loss; *moderate,* changes are uncomfortable but are of short duration and do not interfere with functional use; *severe,* skin changes are painful and may last 10 minutes or longer and functional ability of the hand is limited during attacks.

Documentation should include a description of the skin changes, their severity, and location.

NEUROLOGICAL INVOLVEMENT

The most common or widely recognized neurological conditions that can occur secondary to arthritis will be reviewed in this section. All of these conditions can result from other causes such as trauma or occupational use and are covered in detail in the neurological and orthopedic surgery literature. Practical guidelines for sensory evaluation are discussed at the end of this section.

Cervical Radiculopathy or Nerve Root Compression Syndrome

This condition can result from osteophyte formation or from cervical subluxation. Initial symptoms typically include pain, paresthesias, and sensory loss in the upper extremity and hand along dermatome patterns, followed by motor weakness of the affected associated muscles. Cervical nerve root compression should be the first differential diagnosis considered when sensory deficits in the hand are not consistent with typical median or ulnar nerve loss. For example, sensory loss isolated to the thumb can be due to C-6 compression.[5,6,79]

Entrapment Neuropathies

These conditions refer to direct compression of peripheral nerves from edema, synovitis, synovial hypertrophy, or trauma. In association with arthritis, the median nerve is the most commonly affected, the ulnar nerve is next in frequency, and radial nerve entrapment is uncommon but not rare.[8] Entrapment can occur at various sites, resulting in both sensory and motor impairment distal to the lesion.

Median Nerve Entrapment

The median nerve can be compressed at the wrist or in the forearm.

Carpal Tunnel Syndrome (CTS) Wrist Level (Fig. 19–46)

This is the most common entrapment syndrome seen in association with arthritis in adults.[8] Evaluation for CTS should be a part of every arthritis hand evaluation. Symptoms of CTS are rare in children with juvenile rheumatoid arthritis.

The carpal tunnel is bordered on three sides by the carpal bones. The volar side or roof is formed by the strong transverse carpal ligament. This narrow, rigid passageway contains nine flexor tendons and their

sheaths, blood vessels, and the median nerve. (See Fig. 19–37.) Any swelling in the tendon sheaths or thickening of the tendons or bones can cause compression of the nerve.[65]

The position of the wrist can expand or decrease the space of the carpal tunnel, thereby diminishing or increasing symptoms accordingly. The space in the tunnel is maximized when the radius and the scaphoid are in neutral alignment. When these two bones are in neutral, the second metacarpal is in approximately 10 degrees of extension, using standard goniometric placement. (When the second metacarpal is at zero degrees extension, the scaphoid is in 10 degrees of flexion.) Any position other than 10 to 15 degrees of wrist extension reduces the carpal tunnel space.[69]

All patients with RA or wrist synovitis are at high risk for developing CTS. Therefore, it is recommended that all wrist or hand orthoses made for patients with RA be in 10 degrees wrist extension. The main exception to this would be patients who are rapidly losing wrist extension and developing wrist flexion contractures. For these patients, the treatment of choice may be to maintain wrist extension by positioning in their maximal extension (which may be very limited).

The classic early *symptoms* of CTS include wrist pain or paresthesias in the fingers occurring only at night.[65] This pattern is attributed to prolonged positioning in either flexion or extension at night and nocturnal hand swelling that occurs in everyone when not actively using the hand. Occasionally patients report the symptoms occur only during certain functional activities such as driving, using a telephone, and so forth. The earliest *sign* of CTS is skin dryness or decreased sudomotor (sweat) function of the volar aspect of the affected digits.

Orthotic positioning of the wrist in 10 degrees of extension can be a very effective treatment for early CTS or for patients who have symptoms only at night. Once motor loss occurs, orthotic treatment may reduce discomfort but generally it will not alleviate or reverse symptoms. Surgery is indicated to release the transverse carpal ligament if motor loss is evident.[8]

There are two specific test procedures commonly used to diagnose CTS: (1) a per-

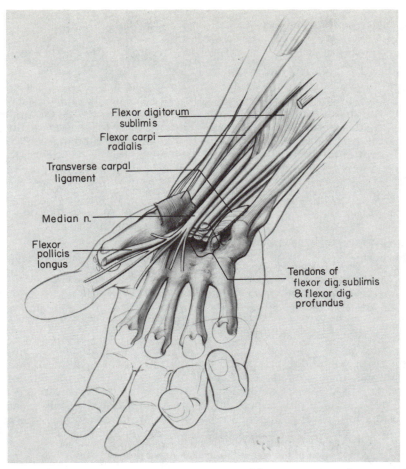

Figure 19–46. This shows reflection of the transverse carpal ligament to reveal passage of the median nerve and nine flexor tendons through the narrow carpal tunnel. Note the rigid bony floor and sides of the tunnel formed by the carpal bones. (From Liveson, JA, and Spielholz, NI: Peripheral Neurology. FA Davis, Philadelphia, 1979, with permission. Illustration by Hugh Thomas.)

cussion test (incorrectly referred to as the Tinel test) involves percussion over the median nerve at the wrist, which lies just lateral to the palmaris longus tendon. The test is positive if the maneuver elicits paresthesias along the median distribution. (2) The Phalen test: passive flexion of the wrist for 1 minute. The test is positive if the maneuver reproduces the symptoms.[65] If flexion is painful, a reverse Phalen test, holding the wrist in extension, can be done. These assessments are helpful in locating the site of the compression. If the patient has negative Phalen and percussion tests and no obvious wrist pathology, such as tenosynovitis, it is likely that the entrapment

is more proximal in the forearm or neck. The most reliable clinical assessment is a clear accurate history, identification of altered sudomotor function, a sensory evaluation for two-point discrimination, and an individual muscle test if motor loss is suspected.

Muscles affected: Abductor pollicis brevis, opponens pollicis, flexor pollicis brevis (superficial head) and the first and second lumbricals.[8]

Sensation and sudomotor function affected: Palmar surface of the thumb, index, and middle fingers, and the lateral half of the ring finger.[8]

Muscles to monitor: The abductor pollicis brevis is the key muscle to evaluate, since it can be easily isolated and is the first to be affected.

Symptoms: The sole symptom may be wrist pain at night. The pain may radiate into the palm or occasionally up the forearm. Paresthesias or numbness along the median distribution (with or without pain) may be presented. These symptoms may also occur with cervical nerve root and proximal forearm entrapment; thus, these conditions need to be ruled out before a diagnosis of CTS can be made. Numbness in all digits may mean the ulnar nerve is also involved.[65]

Median Nerve Entrapment in the Proximal Forearm

Although uncommon, it is possible for the median nerve to be compressed by fibrous bands at several levels as the nerve passes through the pronator teres and under the flexor superficialis arch (Fig. 19–47).[80]

Symptoms of proximal compression include paresthesias in the median innervated fingers; pain in the proximal forearm, increased by resistance to pronation, with occasional radiation to the upper arm; clumsy use of the hand with decreased grip or prehension skill; and tenderness over the pronator teres muscle.[80]

Johnson, Spinner, and Shrewsbury[80] in a report of 71 cases of proximal entrapment identified the following clinical pattern: (1) tenderness, firmness, or enlargement of the pronator teres muscles; (2) a positive Tinel's sign on percussion of the pronator teres muscle; (3) no weakness of the median innervated muscles (no significant conduction defect); (4) marked increase in paresthesias in the affected fingers during resistance to pronation with the elbow flexed and an increase in paresthesias when the elbow is gradually extended localizes the lesion to the pronator teres; (5) paresthesias or pain following resistance to elbow flexion and forearm supination identifies entrapment by the lacertus fibrosus of the biceps tendon; (6) a reproduction of paresthesias in the median innervated fingers upon independent flexion of the flexor superficialis of the middle finger localizes the entrapment to the fibrous arcade of the flexor superficialis; and (7) reproduction of

symptomatology with a tourniquet above diastolic pressure on the upper arm. Additionally, these patients may have a negative Phalen test and their symptoms are generally *not responsive to orthotic immobilization of the wrist.*[80]

In RA, the high incidence of flexor tenosynovitis makes wrist entrapment the most likely source for sensory disturbances in the median innervated digits. Proximal entrapment should be considered in patients with no apparent wrist involvement; early or mild symptoms that do not increase at night (due to positioning); a negative Phalen's test; or in cases that do not respond to conservative measures.

Anterior Interosseous Nerve (AIN) Syndrome

The anterior interosseous nerve is a motor branch of the median nerve (see Fig. 19–47). Entrapment of this nerve can occur in adults in the forearm; however, it is rare. Typically patients present with nonspecific pain in the forearm or elbow and weakness of the flexor pollicis longus muscle, resulting in a characteristic pinch (Fig. 19–48). Testing further reveals weakness of the flexor profundus to the index and occasionally the middle fingers.

In addition to the AIN syndrome several other conditions can cause weakness or inability to flex the thumb IP joint and index DIP joint. These conditions include partial or complete rupture of the FPL or flexor digitorum profundus (FDP) at the wrist; flexor tenosynovitis; tendon nodules in the digital or palm sheath; and proximal median nerve compression above the AIN. The presence of tenodesis motion can help rule out the possibility of tendon rupture.

Muscles affected: Flexor pollicis longus, pronator quadratus, and the flexor digitorum profundus to the index and middle fingers.[81]

Sensation affected: None

Muscles to monitor: This condition is so rare that it is usually not part of a routine assessment. However, evaluation of the flexor pollicis longus can help distinguish between a high (forearm) and a low (wrist) entrapment of the median nerve. Patients with a complete lesion (usually traumatic) demonstrate a characteristic 2-point pinch in which the thumb IP joint and the index

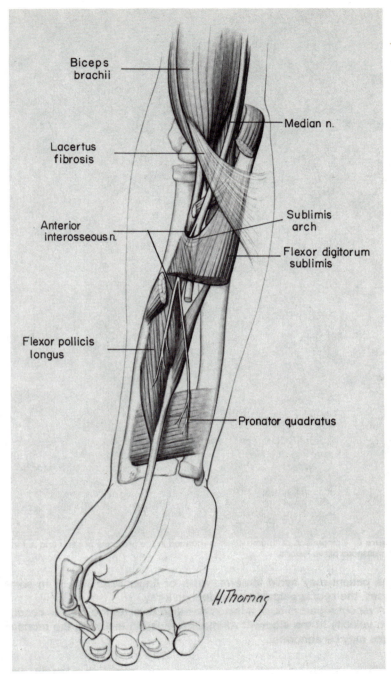

Figure 19–47. This shows the course of the median nerve and its anterior interosseous branch. Entrapment of the median nerve in the forearm is uncommon but should be considered in patients with median nerve paresthesias, a negative Phalen's test, and no apparent wrist involvement. (From Liveson, JA, and Spielholz, NI: Peripheral Neurology. FA Davis, Philadelphia, 1979, with permission.)

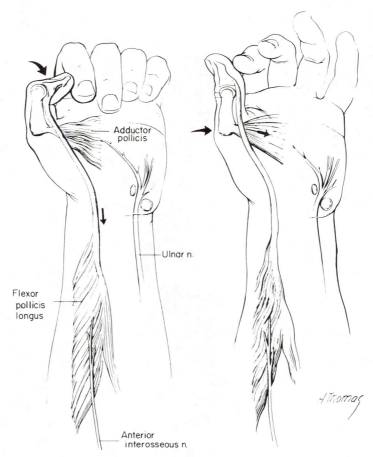

Figure 19–48. Comparison of characteristic thumb pinch between an ulnar nerve lesion *(left)* and an anterior interosseous nerve lesion *(right)* is illustrated. In an ulnar nerve lesion the flexor pollicis longus substitutes for the weakened adductor pollicis, resulting in marked flexion of the IP joint during pinch (Froment's sign). In the uncommon AIN paralysis, the patient loses the ability to flex the IP joint actively and achieves pinch force by using the adductor pollicis. (From Liveson, JA, and Spielholz, NI: Peripheral Neurology. FA Davis, Philadelphia, 1979, with permission.)

DIP joint are in neutral extension during prehension. This pattern may not be as easily recognized in a partial lesion.

Double Crush Syndrome

Occasionally a patient with cervical spine arthritis develops nerve root compression and median nerve compression at the same time, a condition referred to as the **double crush syndrome.**[82] It is theorized that the cervical lesion causes primary damage to the nerve fibers, which renders them more vulnerable to a superimposed entrapment.[82] This condition can also affect the ulnar nerve.

Physicians do not recognize this syndrome when there are no clear or obvious symptoms of cervical nerve root compression. Clinically, there are a large number of patients with CTS, *without* wrist inflammation or other signs of wrist pathology that have cervical muscle tightness or spasm or pain. The coexistence of these two problems is so great that it cannot be ignored. It is quite possible that there is a range of subclinical cervical compression (i.e., compression that does not produce classic symptoms) that can alter the physiology of the distal nerves, rendering them more vulnerable to compression. Because of this experience *we evaluate cervical func-*

tion in all patients with CTS (or ulnar nerve entrapment). Resolution of the cervical involvement is essential for preserving or improving the integrity of the peripheral nerves. (See the section on treatment of the cervical spine in Chapters 4, 6, 14, and 32.)

Ulnar Nerve Entrapment

Ulnar Nerve Entrapment at the Elbow

Compression of the ulnar nerve at this location (ulnar groove, posterior to medial epicondyle) is quite common in the presence of severe elbow synovitis. It occurs only occasionally in *early* RA. There is considerable variability in the depth of the ulnar groove. When a patient has a shallow groove, there is less space to accommodate any synovitis and higher risk of traumatizing or subluxing the ulnar nerve. The nerve is most vulnerable to pressure when the elbow is flexed.[79] So the patient with elbow synovitis and a flexion contracture is particularly at risk. Ulnar nerve compression can also result from improper positioning following upper extremity surgery.

Typically, conservative management includes a steroid injection to reduce synovitis and ice compresses for acute episodes. Occasionally splinting (with the elbow in extension) is helpful on a temporary basis to reduce inflammation or alleviate pressure on the nerve.

Muscles affected: Flexor carpi ulnaris, flexor digitorum profundus to the ring and little fingers, all hypothenar muscles (palmaris brevis, abductor digiti quinti, opponens digiti quinti, flexor digiti quinti), lumbricals to the ring and little fingers, all interossei, flexor pollicis brevis (deep head), and the adductor pollicis.[8]

Sensation affected: Palmar and *dorsal surface of the little finger,* the medial half of the ring finger, and ulnar side of the hand.[8] Sensation to the dorsum of the little finger is a key area to test to distinguish between elbow and wrist compression syndromes, because the dorsal cutaneous branch is proximal to the wrist. Thus, if the dorsal sensation is diminished, the lesion is above the wrist. If only the volar sensation is altered, the lesion is at Guyon's canal or lower.

Muscles to monitor: The first dorsal interosseous and the adductor pollicis. Patients with an ulnar nerve lesion demonstrate a characteristic pinch, in which there is marked flexion of the thumb IP joint and extension or hyperextension of the thumb MCP joint during active prehension due to substitution of the FPL for the weak adductor pollicis (see Fig. 19–49). This prehension pattern is referred to as **Froment's sign for ulnar nerve palsy.** It is also important to observe for clawing of the ring and little fingers, which is characteristic of ulnar nerve compression.[8]

Symptoms: Paresthesias along both the dorsal and volar ulnar distribution and

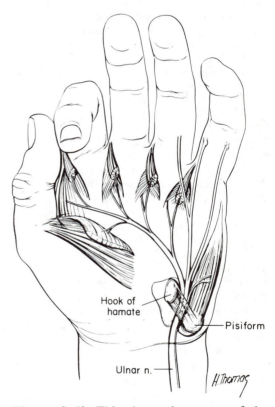

Figure 19–49. This shows the course of the ulnar nerve through Guyon's canal. Within the canal, the ulnar nerve is both motor and sensory; but beyond the hook of the hamate, the nerve divides into a separate deep motor branch and sensory fibers to the ring and little fingers. Therefore, lesions distal to the hamate may cause pure motor or sensory loss. (From Liveson, JA, and Spielholz, NI: Peripheral Neurology. FA Davis, Philadelphia, 1979, with permission.)

pain radiating down the forearm or occasionally upward to the arm.[8]

Ulnar Nerve Entrapment at the Wrist (at Guyon's Canal)

Guyon's canal is between the pisiform bone and the hook of the hamate bone. It is covered by the pisohamate ligament, thus forming a fibro-osseous tunnel (Fig. 19–49). Compression can be in the canal or just distal to it. The most common sources of compression are carpal synovitis, trauma, deep ganglions, and occupational stress.[8,79] Motor branches arise within the canal to the hypothenar muscles. Innervation of other intrinsic muscles occurs distal to the canal; therefore, different patterns of involvement can result, depending on the specific side of the compression.

Entrapment of the ulnar nerve at the wrist is less common than at the elbow, but comprehensive hand assessments often reveal ulnar sensory loss that is apparently overshadowed by coexistent carpal tunnel syndrome. This is easy to understand when you consider that sensory skills in the ulnar fingers are not as critical as those in the median fingers, and atrophy and weakness of the intrinsic muscles may be masked by chronic rheumatoid disease and joint contractures. Undetected ulnar nerve entrapment in RA may be a source of diminished grip since the interossei and lumbricals are prime flexors of the MCP joints.[9]

Muscles affected: Palmaris brevis, abductor digiti quinti, opponens digiti quinti, flexor digiti quinti, lumbricals to the ring and little fingers, all interossei, flexor pollicis brevis (deep head), and the adductor pollicis. (The FDP and FCU are unaffected.)[8]

Sensation affected: Only the palmar surface of the little finger and medial side of the ring finger. Dorsal sensation is normal, since the dorsal cutaneous branch is proximal to the wrist.[8] If dorsal sensation is diminished the lesion is above the wrist. Compare sensation with the contralateral hand.

Muscles to monitor: Little finger abductor and adductor.

Symptoms: There can be either motor loss *or* sensory impairment, *or* both, depending on the location of the compression. Sensory impairment is more common

and early symptoms can include decreased sensation and paresthesias along the ulnar half of the hand. There may also be marked tenderness over Guyon's canal, compared with the contralateral hand.[8]

Radial Nerve Entrapment

Impingement of this nerve occurs in the elbow and forearm.

Posterior Interosseous Nerve (PIN) Syndrome

The PIN is a motor branch of the radial nerve (Fig. 19–50). Elbow synovitis can impinge on this nerve as it passes through the supinator muscle in the forearm. This condition is considered uncommon in association with trauma, tumors, ganglions, or bursitis and rare in association with rheumatoid arthritis[10]

Muscles affected: The PIN has two branches: the first is usually compressed; the second branch may be involved or spared. First branch: extensor carpi ulnaris, extensor digiti quinti, extensor communis. Second branch: extensor pollicis longus, extensor pollicis brevis, abductor pollicis longus, and extensor indicis proprius.[10]

Sensation affected: None.

Symptoms: Typically, there is a history of elbow synovitis with pain anterior to the elbow, which can radiate both proximally and distally along the radial distribution. Over a period of days, the patient develops weakness in the fingers and partial or complete inability to extend one or more of the MCP joints, and possibly the thumb. Wrist extension may be in a radial direction as a result of compression of the first branch and loss of the extensor carpi ulnaris. This condition can mimic extensor tendon rupture; however, the presence of tenodesis motion can confirm tendon integrity.[10] Weakness of the finger extensors may also be confused with dislocation of the EC tendons. This can be demonstrated by the ability to maintain MCP extension once positioned.

Radial Tunnel Syndrome (RTS)

The **radial tunnel** refers to a 5-cm area where the radial nerve crosses anterior to

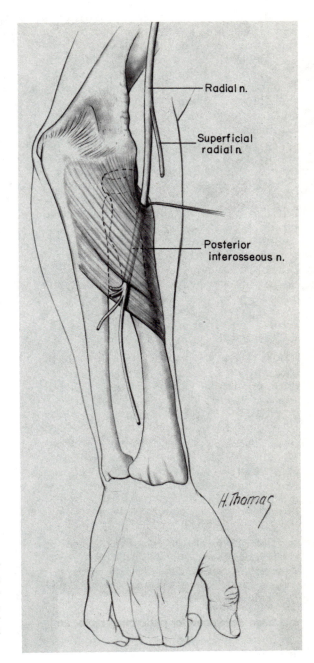

Figure 19–50. The course of the posterior interosseous branch of the radial nerve through the radial tunnel deep to the supinator muscle is shown here. (From Liveson, JA, and Spielholz, NI: Peripheral Neurology. FA Davis, Philadelphia, 1979, with permission.)

the radiohumeral joint and courses between the supinator and the arcade of Frohse (see Fig. 19–50). As the nerve travels through this area, one or all of the following structures can impinge on the nerve.[83,84] The fibrous origin of the extensor carpi radialis brevis (ECRB) can create a flat rigid medial edge to the tunnel and may be densely adherent to the underlying fibrous origin of the supinator. The transverse fibrous bands that cross the nerve anterior to the head of the radius can become thickened. A fan of radial recurrent vessels crosses over and is often interwoven into the structure of the posterior interosseous nerve. The arcade of Frohse can become thickened and fibrous with age.

Patients with radial tunnel syndrome complain primarily of aching pain localized to the extensor muscle mass just below the elbow. The pain is initiated and intensified by repetitive motion involving forearm pronation or pronation and wrist flexion. Grip strength may be diminished secondary to pain. Generally these patients do not have any sensory or motor loss.[83,84]

Initially, these patients may appear to have tennis elbow (lateral epicondylitis), but they do not respond to conservative treatment (i.e., steroid injections, wrist orthoses, or exercise) because they have a structural compression not a tendinitis. Since 1972 when this syndrome was first described, many cases of resistant tennis elbow have been identified as RTS.[84]

Lister, Belsole, and Kleinert have described four diagnostic procedures for distinguishing RTS from tennis elbow.[83]

1. The point of maximum pain as indicated by history and by indirect testing is over the radial tunnel, not the lateral epicondyle.

2. The point of maximum tenderness is over the radial tunnel.

3. Resistance applied to the proximal phalanx of the middle finger, with the elbow and wrist extended, produces more pain in the radial tunnel than does resistance to the ulnar fingers or passive stretching of all the extensors. Resistance to the middle finger (occasionally the index finger) transmits the force directly to the insertion of the ECRB, which forms the lateral edge of the tunnel.[83]

4. Pain is elicited over the radial tunnel when supination is resisted, with the elbow in extension.[83] Lister, Belsole, and Kleinert also note that it is not uncommon for patients to have multiple compression syndromes and that it is possible for a patient to have both RTS and tennis elbow.[83]

Thoracic Outlet Syndrome

Entrapment of the neurovascular supply to the upper extremity as it passes through the thoracic outlet can be due to bony, fascial, or muscular impingement.[85,86] This condition is not specifically related to arthritis, but it is included here because its presence may first be detected during a hand assessment.

One of the first symptoms that patients often complain of is numbness only when they elevate the arm overhead. More severe symptoms include pain throughout the upper extremity and numbness and paresthesias, often perceived in the C-8-T-1 dermatome.

Compression of the subclavian artery can result in numbness, coldness, and weakness in the upper extremity.[85,86] There are several specific maneuvers that help locate the area of compression.[86,87] If this condition is suspected by the therapist, patients should be advised to bring the symptoms to the attention of the physician. The symptoms of TOS can be confused with those of fibromyalgia (see Chapter 5).

EVALUATION OF SENSATION FOR PERIPHERAL NERVE ENTRAPMENT

For all practical purposes in rheumatological rehabilitation of the hand, sensation is evaluated to determine if median or ulnar nerve entrapment has affected sensory nerves. It provides a guidepost for appreciating the severity of the compression and in the early stages provides a guide for determining the effectiveness of conservative measures. Damaged sensation should return to normal if conservative measures are effective. If it does not, the patient is a candidate for surgery. For these purposes the most efficient quantitative sensory assessments are the Weber 2-point discrimination (2PD) test and the moving 2-point discrimination (M2PD) test. These tests are the most valuable to use because the results of these tests correlate highly with function in nerve entrapment syndromes.[88,89]

There is a wide range of other sensory assessments. Each is effective for determining a certain aspect of sensibility. No single test provides a complete assessment. The sensory nerve conduction study is considered the most sensitive means of determining the integrity of median and ulnar sensory nerves. It can be a valuable diagnostic tool, but it is expensive and must be administered by a physician. It is not indicated in all cases and is not feasible as an initial screening tool. The Weinstein-Semmes monofilament provides a precise means for mapping light touch and point localization for the documentation of injury, anomalous innervation, and nerve regeneration. However, this assessment is time consuming and thus costly. It should be reserved for cases in which the outcome of the sensory evaluation will alter or determine the treatment to be administered.[90] Testing sharp-dull discrimination provides information about protective sensibility but does not provide quantitative measures that correlate with function.[88] The Weber 2PD and the M2PD tests are efficient and inexpensive as screening measures and can be administered in all clinical settings.

Weber Two-Point Discrimination Test

The static 2-point discrimination test (Fig. 19–51) developed by Weber in 1835 is a measure of the shortest distance at which a person perceives two distinct points touching the skin.[88] At a lesser distance the person perceives two points as one. This test has long been considered to have a direct positive correlation with hand function, that is, as the 2PD distance increases (becomes less sensitive), patients have increasing difficulty performing tasks. It is currently considered to have a strong positive correlation with the ability to perform various grips, but it *does not* always correlate with tactile gnosis as a key to hand function. Many patients have demonstrated higher tactile gnosis skills than would normally be expected considering their 2PD. Because of this, the test is no longer used for monitoring progress following nerve repair.

Currently, the main value of this test is screening for differences of sensation between the digits to detect sensory loss from nerve compression. If a therapist develops a precise, consistent technique for applying this test, it may also serve to monitor progress in a patient. Unfortunately, the amount of applied pressure is critical to the outcome, and it is difficult to control the pressure. Therefore, test-retest and inter-tester reliability is poor.

From personal experience in working with hundreds of patients with nerve entrapment associated with rheumatic diseases, the Weber 2PD test performed cor-

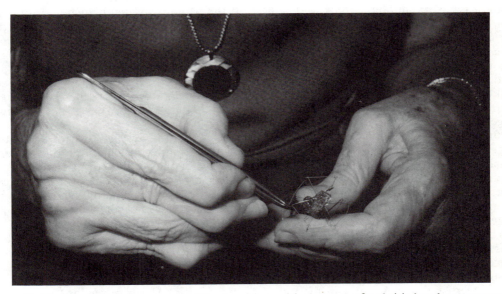

Figure 19–51. Functional assessment of the hand is a critical aspect of arthritis hand management. Rarely is it possible to predict functional skills simply from the appearance of the hand alone. This woman clearly illustrates this point. Despite severe fixed deformities, she is able to perform the dexterous skills required in her work as an electronics parts assembler. (Photo courtesy of Edward Nalebuff, M.D.)

rectly and consistently has proven to be an excellent screening measure that correlates strongly with the patient's subjective report of functional skills. For example, if a patient's 2PD is 3 mm on all digit finger pads, except the median innervated fingers on the right hand, which are 4 to 5 mm, the patient will report slight difficulty with dexterity and often avoid using the affected fingers for certain tasks such as gripping things with his or her ulnar fingers and palm for better control. At 10 mm of 2PD, patients have great difficulty and avoid using the median fingers if at all possible. This test is not recommended for mapping regeneration or measuring tactile gnosis but is very effective for quantitating sensory loss resulting from peripheral nerve entrapments, particularly if the patient's normal 2PD is used for a comparison with the affected area.

The measures cited in the above examples refer to the finger pad area. There are different norms for 2PD in various areas of the hand; the finger pad area is the most sensitive area. The norms in this area are 3 to 5 mm.[88] However, each person has his or her own normal distance. The majority of adults have 3 to 3.5 mm 2PD; some have 2 mm 2PD; and a few have 4 to 5 mm. Generally people with a distance of 5 mm perform heavy work and have thickened skin. *When the evaluation is performed, it is important that the patient's own normal 2PD be determined.* This is done by comparing the ulnar and median fingers bilaterally. Gellis and Pool tested 105 normal subjects and found all subjects had less sensation in their thumb and index finger; the middle finger had the same 2PD as the ring and little fingers.[91] (This may be because the ulnar fingers are used less and are therefore more sensitive.) This finding indicates that the median nerve compression may be most clearly detected by comparing the 2PD of the middle finger with the 2PD of the little finger. They also found that sensitivity varied between age groups. Subjects 10 to 19 years of age had an average 2PD of 2 mm. Subjects 70 to 79 years of age had an average of 3 to 3.5 mm in the middle, ring, and little fingers and 4 to 5.5 mm in the index finger and thumb.

Method: First, all therapists should experience this test before they administer it to a patient.

Equipment: a 2- or 3-point anesthesiometer (available from Fred Sammons, Inc.) or a Boley gauge or dull-pointed eye calipers. The instrument used should not have sharp points that elicit a pain response. (Some professionals use a reshaped paper clip, but with this device it is difficult to keep the points even or to ensure consistency among different evaluators.)

1. Explain the test and demonstrate the procedure while the patient is observing. It is often helpful to demonstrate how 2PD sensitivity increases from the palm to the fingertip.
2. Have the patient close his or her eyes or occlude vision in some manner.
3. Alternate touching the skin with 1 point or 2 points simultaneously. Ask the patient to identify if he or she feels 1 or 2 points. (The pressure from the instrument should not blanch the skin, and the 2 points need to touch with even pressure.) The recommendations for a correct response vary. Some surgeons recommend that 2 out of 3 correct responses are needed; others say 7 out of 10 correct answers are needed.[88,90,91] Basically you need sufficient applications to ensure that the patient is perceiving the points and not guessing at the answer.
4. Generally it is easiest to start at 3 mm. If the patient can distinguish at 3 mm easily, test at 2 mm. If the patient cannot discern 2 points at 3 mm, gradually increase the testing 1 mm at a time, attempting at least three tries at each distance. If the person does not have 10 mm it is usually sufficient to indicate his or her sensation at greater than 10 mm and not continue testing.
5. When this test is done for evaluation of hand trauma in which the digital nerve may be damaged, the points should be applied in a longitudinal axis of the finger.[88] For nerve entrapment syndromes the placement does not alter the response.
6. Explain the results of the test to the patient.

Moving Two-Point Discrimination

This test was developed by Dellon as a means for quantitating a person's ability to discern moving touch.[90] The test, which was introduced in 1978, is based on the theory that the sensation of touch is mediated by two types of nerve fibers: quickly adapting fibers (which innervate Meissner's and Pacini's corpuscles) that are detectors of transient touch, that is, movement and vibration; and slowly adapting fibers that mediate the sensation of pressure by responding to increasing frequency of indentation of the skin.[89]

The test is performed in a manner similar to the Weber 2PD test, only the finger is stroked instead of touched (see method below). Dellon has reported a limited study, using the test on 39 normal hands and 63 patients with nerve injuries. Only the finger pad areas were tested, using a reshaped paper clip. Dellon found that in this population the average or normal M2PD was 2 mm in the thumb pad. Some of the normal subjects had a M2PD of 3 mm. The response was equal bilaterally, except in one person. In 25 hands ipsilateral digits were compared. In 17 of these hands, the thumb and little finger were equal; in 7 of the hands the thumb had a M2PD of 2 mm and the little finger had 3 mm. In one hand the little finger was more sensitive than the thumb. Static 2PD and M2PD were equal in 30 hands, and in the remaining 9 hands the M2PD was 2 mm and the static 2PD was 3 mm. (In this study Dellon found the average Weber 2PD to be 2 mm, which differs from the averages in other studies.) In the patient population studied, there was a much wider variation in the distances between 2PD and M2PD. It was also found that following nerve repair, M2PD returned faster than static 2PD. This variability between these two sensory functions (perceiving static versus moving 2PD) appears to account for the discrepancy between tactile gnosis and static 2PD seen in the clinic.[89]

The M2PD test appears to be more sensitive than the static 2PD test for evaluating sensory regeneration and tactile gnosis. It also adds additional information regarding functional sensibility.[89] However, only one limited survey has been reported and the data conflict with previously reported larger studies on the Weber 2PD test. This may be due to different testing instruments or procedures. *The M2PD is easier to perceive because considerably more skin is touched than with the static 2PD.* This factor has not been integrated into the theory proposed by Dellon.

For purposes of evaluating sensory involvement in nerve entrapment syndromes, both the static 2PD and M2PD tests can be used effectively. More experience is needed in using the M2PD in this area. Future studies and experience may reveal that the M2PD is more sensitive for this function also. Therapists are encouraged to use both tests to determine the more effective test for their clinical needs.

Evaluation:

Described by Dellon

1. A paper clip is rearranged so the points are even and any sharp barbs are not touching the patient.
2. The hand to be tested is supported on a table.
3. The patient is oriented to the test. The technique is demonstrated.
4. The patient is stroked along the length of the finger pad with the points 5 to 8 mm apart and then proceeding in stages down to 2 mm apart. Vision is occluded. Stroking is parallel to the long axis of the finger at an angle to the majority of the fingerprint ridges.
5. The testing stimulus is alternated between 1 and 2 points. If the patient perceives the changes correctly, the next lower value is tested. Seven out of 10 correct responses are required before going to the next level.

Dellon does not describe the amount of pressure used, that is, whether the skin is blanched or not; nor is the exact length of the stroke described. Both of these variables could certainly affect the outcome. It is recommended that the technique used be as similar as possible to the method used for static 2PD.

ASSESSMENT OF HAND FUNCTION

Measurement of Range of Motion and Muscle Strength

Methods of assessing ROM and strength of the hand are discussed in detail in Chapter 20, Evaluation of Range of Motion, and Chapter 21, Evaluation of Muscle Strength.

Descriptive and Quantitative Assessment of Functional Hand Ability

A functional hand assessment determines **functional ability;** that is, how does a patient use his or her hand in spite of limitation; and **functional disability.** Knowing this information will allow you to more effectively plan and assess treatment. The ROM and strength assessments provide some of this information, but they do not demonstrate how the patient can use muscular substitutions and adaptive methods to perform a functional task. In fact, there is often very little direct correlation between hand ROM and the patient's ability to perform functional activities (see Fig. 19–51).

There are many types of functional hand assessments currently in use, ranging from simple to complex, quantitative to nonquantitative, and standardized to nonstandardized. The type best suited to a clinic depends on the patient population and the specific reasons for assessment.

Since no single assessment method can be recommended for all clinics, this section reviews the basic functional components of the hand, the relationship to treatment for arthritis, and a description of published functional hand assessments. The assessment summary at the end of this chapter is included primarily as a reference source for therapists interested in designing their own evaluations or adopting an established test.

Functional Components of the Hand

Often hand function is defined only in terms of grip and pinch.[92,93] I believe it is critical to take a much broader approach in assessing and treating the hand to include nonprehension and bilateral prehension function.[69]

It is true that grip and pinch represent function unique to the hand; that is, it is difficult to substitute for them if the hand is damaged. It is reasonable that they constitute an area of prime concern in conservative and surgical management. The nonprehension and bilateral prehension skills are not basic to hand function; most of them could be performed even if the fingers were amputated. However, they plan an important role in activities of daily living and in rehabilitation for arthritis. Patients with various hand problems, such as MCP synovitis, wrist limitations, ruptured extensor tendons, MCP subluxation, and boutonnière deformities, frequently report difficulty or inability in performing nonprehension tasks.

One of the major goals in preventive treatment for the arthritic hand is to substitute nonstressful hand use for that which is stress producing. For the rheumatoid hand with active synovitis all of the prehensile patterns carry a potential for deformity when used with significant pressure. However, the nonprehension and bilateral prehension patterns do not present the same potential for deformity and therefore play a key role in joint-protection strategies. Additional instruction in compensatory adaptive methods or assistive equipment is indicated for patients with difficulty in performing nonprehension tasks. (See Chapter 24 on joint protection and Chapter 25 on assistive devices.)

Defining and assessing prehension by the following four-part classification provide the broad structure necessary for working with the hand with rheumatic disease.

Finger–Thumb Prehension. The holding of objects between the thumb and fingers of a single hand (Figs. 19–52 to 19–54). This includes all forms of pinch: lateral, 2-point and 3-point tip, and 2-point and 3-point pad. The object can be any size, that is, the fingertips do not have to be approximated. The pinch terminology used here reflects the recommendations of Smith and Benge.[95]

Full Hand Prehension. The holding of an object so that the palm forms one of the gripping surfaces (Figs. 19–55 and 19–56). This includes all of the typical grasps: gross (palmar), power, and cylinder.

Nonprehension. The following are nonprehensive uses of the hand:

1. Use of the hand as a base for the application of upper extremity strength. This includes hookgrip (when the fingers literally form a hook at the end of the forearm) and use of the extended hand to push large objects (Fig. 19–57).
2. Use of the fingers to apply pressure such as in patting soil around a plant (Fig. 19–58), smoothing cloth while ironing, tucking in a shirt at the waist, or tucking in sheets.
3. Use of the fingertip, usually the index

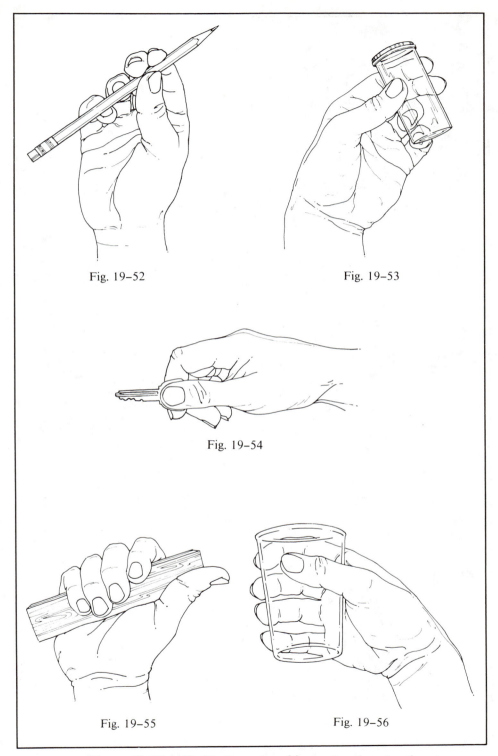

Fig. 19–52

Fig. 19–53

Fig. 19–54

Fig. 19–55

Fig. 19–56

Figures 19–52 to 19–56. Examples of finger–thumb prehensions.

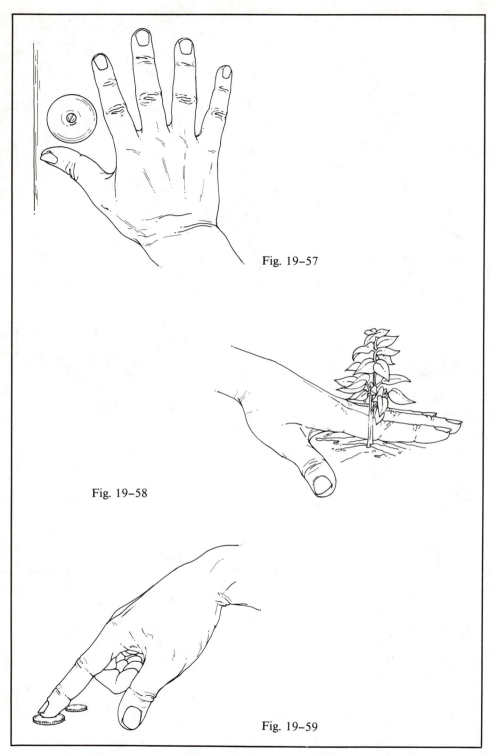

Fig. 19–57

Fig. 19–58

Fig. 19–59

Figures 19–57 to 19–59. Examples of nonprehensive function.

or middle finger, for precision sorting motions such as sorting coins on a counter (Fig. 19–59), dialing a telephone, or pushing buttons.

4. Use of the heel of the hand or the ulnar edge of the palm to apply pressure.

Bilateral Prehension. This is the holding of objects between the palmar surfaces of both hands as in unilateral nonprehension. The hand functions as a static extension of the upper extremity. Prehension is performed because both hands are used. It is essentially used to hold objects too large or too heavy to hold with a single hand.

DOCUMENTATION OF HAND INVOLVEMENT

Purpose of Documentation

The primary purpose of documenting hand involvement is communication. It assists in the following:

1. Documentation is effective if another therapist or physician, re-evaluating the patient's condition several months later, can determine the alterations from the documentation. Phrasing or recording should be directed toward facilitating the re-evaluator's assessment.

2. The written description is an effective method for learning and teaching how to do hand assessments simply because it requires a full qualitative evaluation.

Methods of Documentation

There are two principal ways of documenting hand involvement:

1. Photograph the hands and add a written description of aspects that cannot be pictorially displayed such as instability, triggering, or ankylosis. This is the most efficient method, but it is time consuming and requires photographic skills.

2. Write a systematic description of involvement, itemized by joints or anatomical areas in paragraph form, or create a form to document measurements and a summary of the assessment.

I developed the hand evaluation form at the end of this chapter with the Occupa-

tional Therapy staff at the Robert B. Brigham Hospital to provide an organized method for recording and documenting hand status. The form allows for flexibility in recording methods and was designed to meet the therapists' documentation needs. A brief summary of the patient's hand status accompanied the form in the medical chart to facilitate physician and team communication. The use of this form was designated for patients with active *complex* hand involvement who could benefit from a systematic review and documentation process. It was not indicated for patients with minimal involvement, for example, carpal tunnel syndrome or monoarticular arthritis, or patients with severe burned out, end-stage deformity who were not candidates for hand therapy.

Documentation Procedures

Photographic Documentation

Procedure

When using photographic documentation of hand involvement it is helpful to have a standard protocol for positioning the hands. *All members of the team involved with the photography must be aware of the positioning procedure.*

For some deformities, positioning is crucial in order to obtain a reliable interpretation of the photograph. For example, it is impossible to evaluate the degree of MCP ulnar drift present in a photograph unless it is known whether the fingers are in active or passive extension. (See Chapter 20, Evaluation of Range of Motion, for discussion on how to assess ulnar drift.) Medical photographers commonly use the same positioning procedures used in radiology for taking x-ray pictures. This method involves placing the hands on a table, which means passive pressure from the table can distort the degree of ulnar deviation and the degree of finger flexion deformities. This method does not allow for accurate assessment of ulnar drift. *The fingers should be off the table and in active extension to assess MCP involvement.*

Photographic Views

The six standard photographic views are

Posteroanterior (PA), dorsal
(Fig. 19–60, left)

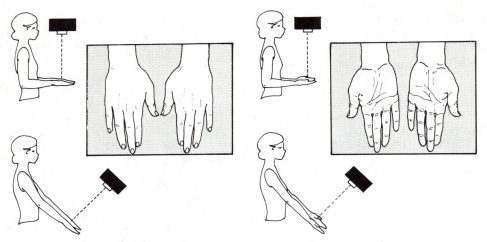

Figure 19–60. Illustrated here are photographic fields: *(left)* posteroanterior (PA) view, *(right)* antero-posterior (AP) view.

Anteroposterior (AP), ventral
  (Fig. 19–60, right)
Ulnar, medial (Fig. 19–61, left)
Radial, lateral (Fig. 19–61, right)
Ulnar oblique (Fig. 19–62, left)
Radial oblique (Fig. 19–62, right)

Note the proper positioning of the camera for each view. The view recommended depends on the type of problem demonstrated and the number of photographs to be taken. Adrian Flatt describes the 16 standardized views that he uses for surgical documentation in his book, *Care of the Rheumatoid Hand.*[19]

Joint structures are more readily visible from the dorsum of the hand; therefore, the dorsal (PA) approach is usually the view used for most common joint deformities such as boutonnière, swan neck, ulnar drift, wrist deviation, and synovitis or when only

one photograph is to be taken to document multiple joint problems.

A radial, ulnar, or oblique view may be more effective for documenting decreased finger extension resulting from triggering, Dupuytren's contracture, ruptured extensor tendons, and MCP subluxation.

In addition to the standard views, photographs of the hand during functional use such as in pinch or grip may be a helpful adjunct for certain treatment situations.

Patient Consent Form

Every hospital has a patient release or consent form that should be signed by any patient even if only the hands are photographed. Make sure it includes patient permission to use the photos in professional publications. Many publishers will not use a photo unless there is a written consent form. Sometimes a publisher will use the

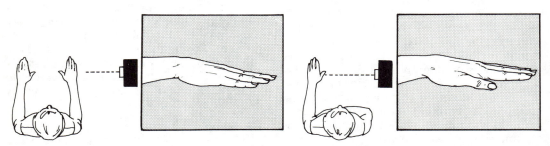

Figure 19–61. Photographic fields are illustrated: *(left)* ulnar (lateral) view, *(right)* radial (medial) view.

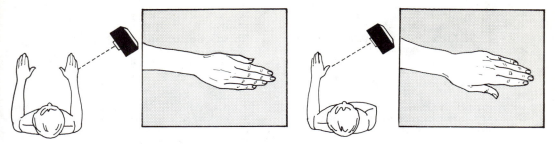

Figure 19–62. Photographic fields are illustrated: *(left)* ulnar (oblique) view, *(right)* radial (oblique) view.

photo without consent but will block out the eyes, but this should be avoided.

Background

Background color is an important consideration in photography and can significantly influence the appearance of the skin color. Red tones tend to reflect off the hand and increase any redness present. Very pale colors and white tend to reflect light; this results in diminished skin tone. Warm tones such as brown and gold usually do not provide sufficient contrast.

Moderate intensity shades of blue or green (e.g., surgery green, sky blue) or *flat black* (for light skin) provide the overall best results. A black background provides optimal contrast for black and white photographs for publication. When doing re-evaluations of the same hand it is helpful to use the same background color with each documentation.

Lighting

Usually regular clinic lighting with flashbulbs or a strobe light is sufficient; if extra lighting is used, it should be kept consistent in re-evaluations. For close-up hand photography a weak flash is needed. If the strobe or bulb is too bright it will reflect off the hand, leaving a light or washed-out area in the center of the hand. The strobe light can be muted by putting white paper tape directly on the strobe light or covering it with any thin white opaque material (e.g., tissue paper).

Film

The selection of film depends on the type of camera used. Top-quality film should be used for color slides and prints.

Kodachrome (ASA 25 or 64) is often recommended for close-up photography because it offers the highest resolution. Ectachrome can also be used. It offers the advantage of a faster speed but has less resolution. If you need the slides in a hurry, keep in mind that Kodachrome may take up to a week to be developed because it has to be sent to an authorized center for processing. Only high-speed films can be processed in one day at most photo centers.

There are two excellent inexpensive publications available for therapists interested in pursuing clinical photography: *Clinical Photography*, No. N-3, 1972, 117 pages; and *Planning and Producing Slide Programs*, 1975, 68 pages. Both books are available from Eastman Kodak Co., Department 454, Rochester, NY 14650.

REFERENCES

1. Polley, HF, and Hunder, GG: Rheumatological Interviewing and Physical Examination of the Joints, 2nd ed. WB Saunders, Philadelphia, 1978.
2. D'Ambrosia, RD: Musculoskeletal Disorders: Regional Examination and Differential Diagnosis. JB Lippincott, Philadelphia, 1977.
3. Hoppenfeld, S: Physical Examination of the Spine and Extremities. Appleton-Century-Crofts, New York, 1976.
4. Kapandji, IA: The Physiology of the Joints. Vol 1. Upper Limb. Churchill-Livingstone, Edinburgh, 1968.
5. Jackson, R: The Cervical Syndrome, 4th ed. Charles C Thomas, Springfield, IL, 1978.
6. Cailliet, R: Neck and Arm Pain. FA Davis, Philadelphia. 1964.
7. Kozin, F: Painful shoulder and the reflex sympathetic dystrophy syndrome. In McCarty, DJ (ed):

Arthritis and Allied Conditions. Lea & Febiger, Philadelphia, 1978, pp 1091–1120.

8. Nakano, KK: Entrapment neuropathies. In Kelley, WM et al (eds): Textbook of Rheumatology. WB Saunders, Philadelphia, 1981.

9. Dawson, DM, Sallett, M, and Millender, LH: Entrapment Neuropathies. Little, Brown & Co, Boston, 1983.

10. Millender, LH, Nalebuff, EA, and Holdsworth, DE: Posterior interosseous nerve syndrome secondary to rheumatoid synovitis. J Bone Joint Surg 55A(4):753, 1973.

11. Coonrad, RW, and Hooper, WR: Tennis elbow: Its course, natural history, conservative and surgical management. J Bone Joint Surg 55A:1177, 1973.

12. Lehman, JL, and Kushner, S: Tennis elbow. Physiotherapy (Can) 31(5):251, 1979.

13. deAndrade, Jr, GC, and Dixon, AstJ: Joint distension and reflex muscle inhibition in the knee. J Bone Joint Surg 47A:313, 1965.

14. Vasey, JR, and Crozier, LW: A neuromuscular approach to knee joint problems. Physiotherapy 66(6):193, 1980.

15. Goldner, JL: Pain: General review and selected problems affecting the upper extremity. J Hand Surg 8(5):740–745, 1983.

16. Huskisson, EC: Measurement of pain. Lancet 2(7889):1127, 1974.

17. DeCeulaer, K, and Dick, WC: The clinical evaluation of antirheumatic drugs. In Kelley, WM et al (eds): Textbook of Rheumatology. WB Saunders, Philadelphia, 1981.

18. McCarty, DJ, and Gatter, A: A dolorimeter for quantification of articular tenderness. Arthritis Rheum 8:551, 1965.

19. Flatt, AE: Care of the Rheumatoid Hand, 3rd ed. CV Mosby, St Louis, 1974.

20. Lampe E: Surgical Anatomy of the Hand. CIBA Pharmaceutical Co, Summit, NJ, 1969. (Still available in 1988.)

21. Hunter, JM, and Mackin, EJ: Edema and bandaging. In Hunter, JM, Schneider, LH, Mackin, EJ, and Bell, JA: Rehabilitation of the Hand. CV Mosby, St Louis, 1978.

22. Wright, V: Psoriatic arthritis. In Kelley, WM et al (eds): Textbook of Rheumatology. WB Saunders, Philadelphia, 1981.

23. Harris, E: Rheumatoid arthritis: The clinical spectrum. In Kelley, WM et al (eds): Textbook of Rheumatology. WB Saunders, Philadelphia, 1981, p 951.

24. Ginsberg, MH, Genant, HK, Yu, TF, and McCarty, DJ: Rheumatoid nodulosis: An unusual variant of rheumatoid disease. Arthritis Rheum 18:49, 1975.

25. Ganda, OP, and Caplan, HI: Rheumatoid disease without joint involvement. JAMA 228:228, 1974.

26. Brower, AC, NaPombepra, C, Stechschulte, DJ et al: Rheumatoid nodulosis—Another cause of juxta-articular nodules. Diagn Radiol 118:669, 1977.

27. Simons, FER, and Schaller, JG: Benign rheumatoid nodules. Pediatrics 56:29, 1975.

28. Rush, PJ, Bernstein, BH, Smith, CR et al: Chronic arthritis following benign rheumatoid nodules of childhood. Arthritis Rheum 28:1175–1179, 1985.

29. Williams, HJ, Biddulph, EC, Coleman, SS, and Ward, JR: Isolated subcutaneous nodules (pseudo-rheumatoid). J Bone Joint Surg 59a:73–76, 1977.

30. Angelides, AC, and Wallace, PF: The dorsal ganglion of the wrist—Its pathogenesis, gross and microscopic anatomy and surgical treatment. J Hand Surg 1(3):228, 1976.

31. Fogel, GR, Younge, DA, and Dobyns, JH: Pitfalls in the diagnosis of the simple wrist ganglion. Ortho 6:990–992, 1983.

32. Calabro, J: Rheumatoid arthritis. Clinical Symposia, CIBA, Vol 23, No 1, 1971.

33. Swanson, AB, Goran-Hagert, C, and Swanson, GdG: Evaluation of impairment of hand function. In Hunter, JM, Schneider, LH, Mackin, EJ, and Bell, JA (eds): Rehabilitation of the Hand. CV Mosby, St Louis, 1978.

34. Brandt, KD: Pathogenesis of osteoarthritis. In Kelley, WM et al (eds): Textbook of Rheumatology. WB Saunders, Philadelphia, 1981, p 1463.

35. Dell, PC, Brushart, MD, and Smith, RJ: Treatment of trapeziometacarpal arthritis: Results of resection arthroplasty. J Hand Surg 3(3):243, 1978.

36. Lockie, LM: Examination of the arthritic patient. In Hollender, J, and McCarty, DJ (eds): Arthritis and Allied Conditions. Lea & Febiger, Philadelphia, 1972, p 87.

37. Rosenthal, EA: The extensor tendons. In Hunter, JM, Schneider, LH, Mackin, EJ, and Bell, JA (eds): Rehabilitation of the Hand. CV Mosby, St Louis, 1978, pp 206–210.

38. Kleinert, HE, and Frykman, G: The wrist and thumb in rheumatoid arthritis. Orthop Clin North Am 4:1085, 1973.

39. Boyes, JH: Bunnell's Surgery of the Hand, 5th ed. JB Lippincott, Philadelphia, 1970.

40. Eaton, RG: Joint Injuries of the Hand. Charles C Thomas, Springfield, IL, 1971.

41. Fess, EE, Gettle, KS, and Strickland, JW: Hand Splinting—Principles and Methods. CV Mosby, St Louis, 1981.

42. Palmer, AK, and Louis, DS: Assessing ulnar instability of the MCP joint of the thumb. J Hand Surg 3(6):542, 1978.

43. Wilson, RL, and Carter, MS: Joint injuries in the hand: Preservation of proximal interphalangeal joint function. In Hunter, JM, Schneider, LH, Mackin, EJ, and Bell, JA (eds): Rehabilitation of the Hand. CV Mosby, St Louis, 1978, p 172.

44. Nalebuff, EA, Garrett, J: Opera-glass hand in rheumatoid arthritis. J Hand Surg 1(3):210, 1976.

45. Silver-Ring Splint Company, PO Box 1063, Charlottesville, VA, 22902.

46. Forrester, D, Brown, JC, and Nesson, A: The Radiology of Joint Disease. WB Saunders, Philadelphia, 1979.

47. Adamson, JD: Treatment of the stiff hand. Orthop Clin North Am 1:467, 1970.

48. Entin, MA, and Wilkinson, RD: Scleroderma hand: A reappraisal. Orthop Clin North Am 4:1031, 1973.

49. Pahle, JA, and Raunio, P: The influence of wrist position on finger deviation in the rheumatoid hand. J Bone Joint Surg 51B:664, 1969.

50. Taleisnik, J: Rheumatoid synovitis of the volar

compartment of the wrist joint: Its radiological signs and its contribution to wrist and hand deformity. J Hand Surg 4(6):526, 1979.

51. Chaplin, D, Pulkki, T, Saarimaa, A, and Vainio, K: Wrist and finger deformities in juvenile rheumatoid arthritis. Acta Rheum Scand 15:206, 1969.

52. Backhouse, KM: The mechanics of normal digital control in the hand and an analysis of the ulnar drift of rheumatoid arthritis. Ann R Coll Surg Engl 43:154, 1968.

53. Hakstian, R, and Tubiana, R: Ulnar deviation of the fingers: The role of joint structure and function. J Bone Joint Surg 49A:299, 1967.

54. Smith, EM, Juvinall, RC, Bender, LF, and Pearson, JR: Flexor forces and rheumatoid metacarpophalangeal deformity. JAMA 198:130, 1966.

55. Laine, VAI, Sairanen, E, and Vainio, K: Finger deformities caused by rheumatoid arthritis. J Bone Joint Surg 39A(3):527, 1957.

56. Swezey, RL, and Fiegenberg, DS: Inappropriate intrinsic muscle action in the rheumatoid hand. Ann Rheum Dis 30(6):619, 1971.

57. Smith, RJ, and Kaplan, EB: Rheumatoid deformities at the MCP joints. J Bone Joint Surg 49A:31, 1967.

58. Swanson, AB: Flexible Implant Resection Arthroplasty in the Hand and Extremities. CV Mosby, St Louis, 1973, p 109.

59. Shapiro, JS: Wrist involvement in rheumatoid swan neck deformity. J Hand Surg 7(5):484–491, 1982.

60. Nalebuff, EA, and Millender, LH: Surgical treatment of swan neck deformities in rheumatoid arthritis. Orthop Clin North Am 6(3):733, 1975.

61. Souter, WA: The problem with boutonniere deformity. Clin Orthop 104:116, 1974.

62. Mitchell, DM, Palchik, NS, Gilbert, NL et al: Successful splinting for boutonniere deformities: Issues for arthritis health professionals. AHPH Annual Meeting Poster Session, Washington, DC, 1987. (Contact OT Department, University of Michigan, Ann Arbor, Michigan, for information about this approach.)

63. Nalebuff, EA: Diagnosis, classification and management of rheumatoid thumb deformities. Bull Hosp Joint Dis 24:119, 1968.

64. Nalebuff, EA: The rheumatoid thumb. Clin Rheum Dis 10:589–608, 1984.

65. Phalen, GS: The carpal tunnel syndrome: Seventeen years experience in diagnosis and treatment of 654 hands. J Bone Joint Surg 48A:211, 1966.

66. Guide for Muscle Testing of the Upper Extremity. Occupational Therapy Department, Rancho Los Amigos Hospital. Published by the Professional Staff Association of RCAH. Downey, California, 1976.

67. Kendall, HO, Kendall, FP, and Wadsworth, GE: Muscles—Testing and Function, 2nd ed. Williams & Wilkins, Baltimore, 1971.

68. Daniels, L, and Worthingham, C: Muscle Testing: Techniques of Manual Examination. WB Saunders, Philadelphia, 1972.

69. Melvin, JL: Rheumatoid Disease—Occupational Therapy and Rehabilitation. FA Davis, Philadelphia, 1977.

70. Melvin, JL: Rheumatoid Disease—Occupational

Therapy and Rehabilitation, 2nd ed. FA Davis, Philadelphia, 1983.

71. Millender, LH, and Nalebuff, EA: Preventive surgery—Tenosynovectomy and synovectomy. Orthop Clin North Am 6(3):765, 1975.

72. Medl, WT: Tendinitis, tenosynovitis, "trigger finger," and de Quervain's disease. Orthop Clin North Am 1:375, 1970.

73. Nalebuff, EA: The recognition and treatment of tendon ruptures in the rheumatoid hand. In American Academy of Orthopedic Surgeons, Symposium on Tendon Surgery in the Hand. CV Mosby, St Louis, 1975.

74. Gray, RG, Kiem, IM, and Gottlieb, NL: Intratendon sheath corticosteroid treatment of RA, associated and idiopathic hand flexor tenosynovitis. Arthritis Rheum 21(1):92, 1978.

75. Rhoades, CE, Gelberman, RH, and Manjarris, JF: Stenosing tenosynovitis of the fingers and thumb. Results of a prospective trial of steroid injection and splinting. Clin Orthop (190):236–238, 1984.

76. Schumacher, HR Jr, Dorwart, BB, and Korzeniowski, OM: Occurrence of De Quervain's tendinitis during pregnancy. Arch Intern Med 145(11):2083–2084, 1985.

77. Soter, NA: Cutaneous manifestations of rheumatic disorders. In Kelley, WM et al (eds): Textbook of Rheumatology. WB Saunders, Philadelphia, 1981.

78. Leroy, EC: Scleroderma (systemic sclerosis). In Kelley, WM et al (eds): Textbook of Rheumatology. WB Saunders, Philadelphia, 1981, p 1217.

79. Spinner, M: Injuries to the Major Branches of Peripheral Nerves of the Forearm. WB Saunders, Philadelphia, 1972.

80. Johnson, RK, Spinner, M, and Shrewsbury, MM: Median nerve entrapment syndrome in the proximal forearm. J Hand Surg 4(1):48, 1979.

81. Nakano, KK, Lundergan, C, and Okihiro, MM: Anterior interosseous nerve syndrome. Diagnostic methods and alternative therapies. Arch Neurol 34:477, 1977.

82. Upton, ARM, and McComas, AJ: The double crush in nerve entrapment. Lancet 2:359, 1973.

83. Lister, GD, Belsole, RB, and Kleinert, HE: The radial tunnel syndrome. J Hand Surg 4(1):52, 1979.

84. Roles, NC, and Maudsley, RH: Radial tunnel syndrome—Resistant tennis elbow as a nerve entrapment. J Bone Joint Surg 54:499, 1972.

85. Urschell, HC, and Razzuk, MA: Management of the thoracic outlet syndrome. N Engl J Med 286:1140, 1972.

86. CIBA Symposia: Thoracic Outlet Syndrome. CIBA Pharmaceutical Co, Summit, NJ, 1970.

87. Britt, LP: Nonoperative treatment of the thoracic outlet syndrome symptoms. Clin Orthop 51:45, March–April, 1967.

88. Omer, GE Jr, and Spinner, M: Peripheral nerve testing and suture techniques. American Academy of Orthopedic Surgeons Instructional Course Lectures, Vol XXIV. CV Mosby, St Louis, 1975.

89. Dellon, AL: The moving two-point discrimination test: Clinical evaluation of the quickly adapting fiber/receptor system. J Hand Surg 3(5):474, 1978.

90. Bell, JA: Sensibility evaluation. In Hunter, JM, Schneider, LH, Mackin, EJ, and Bell, JA (eds):

Rehabilitation of the Hand. CV Mosby, St Louis, 1978.

91. Gellis, M, and Pool, R: Two-point discrimination distances in the normal hand and forearm. Plast Reconstr Surg 59:57, 1977.
92. Landsmeer, JM: Power grip and precision handling. Ann Rheum Dis 21:164, 1962.
93. Napier, JR: The prehensile movements of the human hand. J Bone Joint Surg 38B:902, 1956.
95. Smith, RO, and Benge, MW: Pinch and grasp strength: Standardization of terminology and protocol. Am J Occup Ther 39(8):531–535, 1985.

ADDITIONAL SOURCES

Anatomy

Arkless, R: Cineradiography in normal and abnormal wrists. Am J Roentgenol 96:837–844, 1966.

Bachdahl, M, and Carlsoo, S: Distribution of activity in muscles acting on the wrist. Acta Morphol Nerrl Scand 4:136–144, 1961.

Backhouse, KM, and Catton, WT: An experimental study of the functions of the lumbrical muscles in the human hand. J Anat 88:133–141, 1954.

Bowers, WH, Wolf, JW, Nehil, JL, and Bittinger, S: Proximal interphalangeal joint volar plate I: Anatomical and biomechanical study. J Hand Surg 5:79, 1980.

Brand, PW: Clinical Mechanics of the Hand. Year Book Medical Publishers, Chicago, 1985.

Brumfield, RH Jr, Nickel, VL, and Nickel, E: Joint motion in wrist flexion and extension. South Med J 59:909–910, 1966.

Close, J, Kidd, R, and Kidd, CC: The functions of the muscles of the thumb, the index, and long fingers. J Bone Joint Surg 51a:1601–1620, 1969.

Cooney, WP, and Chao, EYS: Biomechanical analysis of static forces in the thumb during hand function. J Bone Joint Surg 59a:27–36, 1977.

Doyle, JR: Anatomy of the flexor tendon sheath and pulleys of the thumb. J Hand Surg 2(2):149, 1977.

Evans, DM: The PIP joint. Clin Rheum Dis 10(3):631–656, 1984.

Kaplan, EB: Functional and Surgical Anatomy of the Hand, 2nd ed. JB Lippincott, Philadelphia, 1965.

Napier, JR: The form and function of the CMC joint of the thumb. J Anat 89:363, 1955.

Shrewsbury, MM: A systematic study of the oblique retinacular ligament of the human finger: Its structure and function. J Hand Surg 2:194, 1977.

Smith, RL: Intrinsic muscles of the fingers: Function, dysfunction, and surgical reconstruction. American Academy of Orthopedic Surgeons, Instructional Course Lectures, XXIV. St Louis, CV Mosby, 1975.

Taleisnik, J: The ligaments of the wrist. J Hand Surg 1:110, 1976.

Tubiana, R (ed): The Hand—Vols I, II, III. WB Saunders, Philadelphia, 1981, 1985, 1986.

Wyke, B: The neurology of joints: A review of general principles. Clin Rheum Dis 7(1), April 1981. (Excellent description of joint pain mechanisms.)

Diabetic Hand Involvement

Borsey, DQ, Roger, EC, Fraser, DJ, et al: Small muscle wasting of the hands in diabetes mellitus. Diabetes Care 6(1):10–17, 1981.

Campbell, RR, Hawkins, SJ, Maddison, PJ, and Reckless, JPD.: Limited joint mobility in diabetes mellitus. Ann Rheum Dis 44:93–97, 1985.

Clark, CV, Pentland, B, Ewing, DJ, and Clarke, MB: Decreased skin wrinkling in diabetes mellitus. Diabetes Care 7(3):224–227, 1984.

Garza-Elizondo, MA, Diaz-Jouanen, E, Franco-Casique, JJ, and Alarcon-Segovia, D: Joint contractures and scleroderma-like skin changes in the hands of insulin-dependent juvenile diabetics. J Rheum 10(5):797–800, 1983.

Grgic, A, Rosenbloom, AL, Weber, T, et al: Joint contracture: Common manifestation of childhood diabetes mellitus. J Pediatrics 88(4):584–588, 1976.

Jung, Y, Hohmann, TC, Gerneth, JA, et al: Diabetic hand syndrome. Metabolism 20(11):1008–1015, 1971.

Lawson, PM, Maneschi, F, and Kohner, EM: The relationship of hand abnormalities to diabetes and diabetic retinopathy. Diabetes Care 6(2):140–143, 1983.

Rosenbloom, AL, Silverstein, JH, Lexotte, DC, et al: Limited joint mobility in childhood diabetes mellitus indicates increased risk for microvascular disease. N Engl J Med 305:191–194, 1981.

Seibold, JR: Digital sclerosis in children with insulin-dependent diabetes mellitus. Arth Rheum 25(11):1357–1361, 1982.

Sturfelt, G, Leden, I, and Nived, O: Hand symptoms associated with diabetes mellitus. Acta Med Scand 210:35–38, 1981.

Heat/Cold Modalities

Flinn-Wagner, S, and Rajan, H: The effect of dry heat on normal hands. J Hand Surg 9A( ):609, 1984.

Hawkes, J, Care, G, Dixon, JS, Bird, HA, and Wright, V: Comparison of three physiotherapy regimens for hands with rheumatoid arthritis. Br Med J (Clin Res) 12.291(6501):1016, 1985.

Pospisilova, J, Samohyl, J, Koprivova, M, and Jelinkova, A: Our experience with the use of ultrasound in rehabilitation of hand. Acta Chir Plast (Prague) 22(4):191–199, 1980.

General Philosophy and Rehabilitation Treatment

Arthritis Information Packet. American Occupational Therapy Association, 1383 Piccard Drive, Rockville, MD 20850.

Bear-Lehman, J: Factors affecting return to work after hand injury. Am J Occup Ther 37:189–194, 1983.

Bear-Lehman, J, and McCormick, E: The expanding role of occupational therapist in the treatment of industrial hand injuries. OT in Health Care 2(4), 1985/1986.

Blair, SJ: Rehabilitation of the hand. In Nickel, VL (ed): Orthopedic Rehabilitation. Churchill-Livingstone, New York, 1982, pp 193–208.

Callahan, AD: Occupational therapy and hand rehabilitation. Am J Occup Ther 37(3):166, 1983.

Hand Information Packet. American Occupational Therapy Association, Practice Division, 1383 Piccard Drive, Rockville, MD 20850.

Hunter, JM, Schneider, LH, Mackin, EJ, and Callahan, AD (eds): Rehabilitation of the Hand, 2nd ed. CV Mosby, St Louis, 1984.

Makuc, D, Utginger, PD, Yount, WJ, Slosser, D, and Moskowitz, N: Hand structure and function in an industrial setting. Arthritis Rheum 21(2):210, 1978.

McLaughlin, JE, and Reynolds, WJ: An evaluation of the therapeutic exercise on hand function in rheumatoid arthritis. Physiotherapy (Canada) 25(2):71, 1973.

Melvin, JL: Roles and functions of occupational therapy in hand rehabilitation. Am J Occup Ther 39(12):795–798, 1985.

Parry, W: Rehabilitation of the Hand. Butterworth, Boston, 1981.

Urbaniak, JR et al: Office diagnosis and treatment of hand pain. Orthop Clin North Am 13(3):477–495, 1982.

Hand Assessment

Baxter, PL, and Ballard, M: Evaluation of the hand by functional tests. In Hunter, JM, et al (eds): Rehabilitation of the Hand, 2nd ed. CV Mosby, St Louis, 1984.

Bendz, P: Systemization of the grip of the hand in relation to finger motor systems. Scand J Rehabil Med 6:158–165, 1974.

Chao, EY, Opgrande, JD, and Axmear, FE: Three dimensional analysis of finger joints in selected isometric hand function. J Biomechanics 9:387–396.

DeVore, GL, and Hamilton, GF: Volume measuring of the severely injured hand. Am J Occup Ther 22:16, 1968.

DeVore, GL, Meredith, KE, Jones, PB, and Parmenter, E: Development and validation of a self report hand functioning checklist. J Hand Surg 9A(4):611, 1984.

Drake, BL: Student speaks gross motor skills and hand grip in the elderly: A pilot study. Am J Occup Ther 34(4):274–276, 1980.

Evans, DM, and Lawton, DS: Assessment of hand function. Clin Rheum Dis 10(3):697–725, 1984.

Hohlstein, RR: The development of the prehension in normal infants. Am J Occup Ther 36(3):170–176, 1982.

Kamukura, N, Matsuo, M, Ishil, H, Mitsuboshi, F, and Miura, Y: Patterns of static prehensions in normal hands. Am J Occup Ther 34:437, 1980.

Louis, DS, Jacobsen, KE, Rasmussen, CJ, Green, TL, and Goldstein, SA: An evaluation of normal values for and variations between stationary moving 2 point discrimination. J Hand Surg 8:617, 1983.

Rudge, S, and Drury, PL: Finger joint size measurements and changes in body weight (letter). Lancet 17.2(8251):877–878, 1981.

Schwanholt, C, and Stern, PJ: Measuring cone for thumb abduction/extension. Am J Occup Ther 38(4):263, 1984.

Tubiana, R, Thomine, JM, and Mackin, E: Examination of the Hand and Upper Limb. WB Saunders, Philadelphia, 1984.

Nerve Entrapment Syndromes—Carpal Tunnel Syndrome

Armstrong, TJ, and Chaffin, DB: Carpal tunnel syndrome and selected personal attributes. J Occup Med 21:481–486, 1979.

Dorwart, BB: Carpal tunnel syndrome: A review. Semin Arthritis Rheum 14(2):134–140, 1984 (review).

Ditmars, DM Jr, and Houin, HP: Carpal tunnel syndrome. Hand Clin 2(3):525–532, 1986.

Gelberman, RH, Szabo, RM, and Mortensen, WW: Carpal tunnel pressures and wrist position in patients with Colles' fractures. J Trauma 24(8):747–749, 1984.

Groneman, L: Carpal tunnel syndrome can be lessened with early treatment. Occup Health Safety 54(10):39–46, 1985.

Hirsh, LF, and Thanki, A: Carpal tunnel syndrome. Avoiding poor treatment results. Postgrad Med 77(1):185–187, 190–192, 1985.

Inglis, A: The universal operative complications in the carpal tunnel syndrome. J Bone Joint Surg 62a:1208–1209, 1980.

Kasdan, ML, and Janes, C: Carpal tunnel syndrome and vitamin B6. Plast Reconstr Surg 79(3):456—462, 1987.

Kessler, FB: Complications of the management of carpal tunnel syndrome. Hand Clin 2(2):401–406, 1986 (review).

Parent, LH, and Bear-Lehman, J: Muscle Re-education in Median Nerve Injury. Illinois Center for Educational Development, Chicago, 1983.

Schlacter, LB, and Tindall, GT: Carpal tunnel syndrome—A disabling yet treatable condition. J Med Assoc Ga 70(12):861–865, 1981.

Szabo, RM, Gelberman, RH, and Dimick, MP: Sensibility testing in patients with carpal tunnel syndrome. J Bone Joint Surg 66a:60, 1984.

Nerve Entrapment Syndromes—Other

Bohannon, RW, and Gajdosik, RL: Spinal nerve root compression—Some clinical implications. A review of the literature. Phys Ther 67(3):376–382, 1987.

Chan, KM, and Lamb, DW: The anterior interosseous nerve syndrome. J R Coll Surg Edinb 29(6):350–354, 1984.

Chuman, MA: Risk factors associated with ulnar nerve compression in bedridden patients. J Neurosurg Nurs 17(6):338–342, 1985.

Coccia, MR, and Satiani, B: Thoracic outlet syndrome. Am Fam Physician 29(2):121–126, 1984.

Collins, DN, and Wever, ER: Anterior interosseous nerve syndrome. South Med J 76(12):1533–1537, 1983 (review).

Crawford, FA Jr: Thoracic outlet syndrome. Surg Clin North Am 60(4):947–956, 1980.

Daskalakis, MK: Thoracic outlet compression syndrome: Current concepts and surgical experience. Int Surg 68(4), 1983.

Dyck, PD et al: Peripheral Neuropathy. WB Saunders, Philadelphia, 1984.

Eversmann, WW Jr: Compression and entrapment neuropathies of the upper extremity. J Hand Surg 8(5,Pt 2):759–766, 1983.

Fahey, VA: Arm yourself against thoracic outlet syndrome. Nursing '84 14(12):42–45, 1984.

Gross, MS, and Gelberman, RH: The anatomy of the distal ulnar tunnel. Clin Orthop (196):238–247, 1985.

Hirsh, LF, and Thanki, A: The thoracic outlet syndrome. Meeting and diagnostic challenge. Postgrad Med 77(1):197–199, 202–203, 206, 1985.

Hogue, RE: Compression of the deep palmar branch of the ulnar nerve. A case report. Phys Ther 65(2):203–205, 1985.

Miller, RG: Acute vs. chronic compressive neuropathy. Muscle Nerve 7(6):427–430, 1984 (review).

Sallstrom, J, and Celegin, Z: Physiotherapy in patients with thoracic outlet syndrome. Vasa 12(3):257–261, 1983.

Szabo, RM, Gelberman, RH, Williamson, PV, Dellon, AL, et al: Vibratory sensory testing in acute peripheral nerve compression. J Hand Surg 9a:104, 1984.

Young, HA, and Hardy, DG: Thoracic outlet syndrome. Br J Hosp Med 29(5):457, 459, 461, 1983.

Rheumatic Disease Hand Involvement

Akeson, W, Amiel, D, and Woo, S: Immobility effects of synovial joints the pathomechanics of joint contractures. Biorheology 17:95–110.

Apfelberg, DB, Maser, MR, Lash, H et al: Rheumatoid hand deformities: Pathophysiology and treatment. West J Med 129:267–272, 1978.

Bennett, JB: Hand injuries and disorders. Principles of management for the family physician. Postgrad Med 73(4):171–185, 1983.

Blackhouse, KM: Extensor expansion of the rheumatoid hand. Ann Rheum Dis 31:112-117, 1972.

Bleifeld, CH, and Inglis, AE: The hand in systemic lupus erythematosus. J Bone Joint Surg 56A:1207–1215, 1974.

Colditz, JC: Arthritis. In Malick, MH, and Kasch, MC (eds): Manual on Management of Specific Hand Problems. AREN Publications, Pittsburgh, 1984.

DeFlaviis, L, Nessi, R, Del-Bo, P, Calori, G et al: High resolution ultrasonography of wrist ganglia. JCU 15(1):17–22, 1987.

DeSalamanca, FE: Swan-neck deformity: Mechanism and surgical treatment. Hand 8:215–221, 1976.

Flatt, A: Care of the Rheumatoid Hand, 3rd ed. CV Mosby, St Louis, 1974, pp 12–32.

Foster, RJ: Wrist pain. How to identify the cause and treat it. Postgrad Med 76(5):117–128, 1984.

Grundberg, AB, and Reagan, DS: Pathologic anatomy of the forearm: Intersection syndrome. J Hand Surg 10(2):299–302, 1985.

Gunther, SF: The carpometacarpal joints. Orthop Clin North Am 15(2):259–277, 1984.

Helal, BH: Extra articular causes of PIP joint stiffness in RH. Hand 7:37–40, 1975.

Helal, BH: Distal profundus entrapment in rheumatoid disease. Hand 2:48–51, 1970.

Hergenroeder, PT, et al: Bilateral scapholunate dissociation with degenerative arthritis. J Hand Surg 6(6):620–622, 1981.

Linscheid, RL, and Dobyns, JH: Rheumatoid arthritis of the wrist. Orthop Clin North Am 2:649, 1971.

Menon, J: The problem of trapeziometacarpal degenerative arthritis. Clin Orthop (175):155–165, 1983.

Miura, T, Nakamure, R, and Torii, S: Conservative treatment for a ruptured extensor tendon on the dorsum of the proximal phalanges of the thumb (mallet thumb). J Hand Surg 11(2):229–233, 1986.

Neviaser, JS: Musculoskeletal disorders of the shoulder region causing cervicobrachial pain: Differential diagnosis and treatment. Surg Clin North Am 43:1703, 1963.

Read, GO, Solomon, L, and Biddulph, S: Relationship between finger and wrist deformities in rheumatoid arthritis. Am Rheum Dis 42(6):619–625, 1983.

Serup, J: Ring size measurement of the digits in females suffering from generalized scleroderma (acrosclerosis). A simple method to quantify skin and soft tissue affection. Dermatology 171(1):41–44, 1985.

Sheon, RP, Moskowitz, RW, and Goldberg: Soft Tissue Rheumatic Pain—Recognition, Management, Prevention, 2nd ed. Lea & Febiger, Philadelphia, 1987.

Sturge, RA: The remote effects of rheumatic diseases on the hand, and their management. Clin Rheum Dis 10(3):449–477, 1984.

Tirlapur, VG et al: The hand in practice. Practitioner 226(1367):943–951, 1982.

Trumble, TE, and Watson, HK: Posttraumatic sesamoid arthritis of the metacarpal joint of the thumb. J Hand Surg (Am) 10(1):94–100, 1985.

Viikari-Juntura, E: Tenosynovitis, peritendinitis and the tennis elbow syndrome. Scand J Work Environ Health 10(6, Spec No):443–449, 1984.

Wilson, RL: Rheumatoid arthritis of the hand. Orthop Clin North Am 17(2):313–343, 1986.

Sport and Performing Arts Injuries

Aronen, JG: Problems of the upper extremity in gymnastics. Clin Sports Med 4(1):61–71, 1985.

Birrer, RB: Sports medicine rheumatology. Clin Rheum Prac 2(5):196, 1984.

Frykman, GK, Wood, VE, and Miller, EB: The psycho-flexed hand. Clin Orthop 174:153–157, 1983.

Hochberg, FH, Leffert, RD, Heller, MD et al: Hand difficulties among musicians. JAMA 249:1869–1872, 1983.

Kaplan, PE: Posterior interosseous neuropathies: Natural history. Arch Phys Med Rehabil 65(7):399–400, 1984.

Lederman, RJ: Nerve entrapment syndromes in instrumental musicians. Med Prob Perf Artists, June 1986.

Morgan, JV, and Davis, PH: Upper extremity injuries in skiing. Clin Sports Med 1(2):295–308, 1982.

Spiegel, D, and Chase, RA: The treatment of contractures of the hand using self-hypnosis. J Hand Surg 5(5):428–432, 1980.

Stulberg, SD: Sport injuries and arthritis. Compr Ther 6(9):8–11, 1980.

Understanding or Developing Functional Hand Assessments

Downie, W, Leatham, P, Rhind, V, Wright, V, Branco, J, and Anderson, J: Studies with pain rating scales. Ann Rheum Dis 37:378–381, 1978.

Hall, EA, and Long, CA: Intrinsic hand muscles in power grip. Electromyography 8:379–421, 1968.

Landsmeer, JM: Power grip and precision handling. Ann Rheum Dis 21:164, 1962.

Lansbury, J: Methods for evaluating rheumatoid arthritis. In Hollander, JL (ed): Arthritis and Allied Conditions, 7th ed. Lea & Febiger, Philadelphia, 1966, pp 269–291. (Also in 6th ed, 1960. The same chapter in 8th ed is abbreviated. Contains a review of evaluations of joint status.)

Napier, JR: The prehensile movements of the human hand. J Bone Joint Surg (Br) 38:902, 1956.

Robinson, HS et al: Functional results of excisional arthroplasty for the rheumatoid hand. Can Med Assoc J 108:1495, 1973. (Application of C.A.R.S. hand function assessment to document surgical treatment contains normative data on grip strength using a sphygmomanometer.)

Schultz, KS: The Schultz structured interview for assessing upper extremity pain. Occup Ther Health Care 1(3):69, Fall 1984.

Sherik, S, Weiss, AE, and Flatt, AE: Functional evaluation of the congenitally anomalous hand. Part I. Am J Occup Ther 25:98, 1971.

Swanson, AB: Flexible Implant Resection Arthroplasty in the Hand and Extremities. CV Mosby, St Louis, 1973.

Taylor, N, Sand, PL, and Jebson, R: Evaluation of hand function in children. Arch Phys Med 54:129, 1973.

Weiss, AE, and Flatt, AE: Functional evaluation of the congenitally anomalous hand. Part II. Am J Occup Ther 25:139, 1971.

Table 19–1 Summary of Published Functional Hand Evaluations (Listed in Chronological Order)

Author	Title	Where Published	Test Items	Grading System	Method Standardized	Normative Data
Agnew, P, and Masis, F	Hand Function Related to Age and Sex	Arch Phys Med Rehabil 63:269–271, 1982	Jebsen Hand Function Test (See Jebsen, below.)	Timed individual subtest scores	Yes	Yes for sex and age under 60 years (N = 318)
Carroll, D	A Quantitative Test of Upper Extremity Function	J Chronic Dis 18:479–491, 1965	*Timed Functional Tasks:* 1. Moving a series of items from a table to a shelf 14″ higher than the table. Items include graduated wooden blocks, metal pipe, spheres, a slate of wood, a washer, an iron. 2. Pouring water: pitcher to glass, glass to glass, using pronation and then supination. 3. Placing hand: behind head, top of head, and at mouth. 4. Writing name.	Thirty-three subtests, each item rated on a scale of 0–3; grade equals total score.	Yes	Yes
Carthum, CJ, Clawson, DK, and Decker, JL	Functional Assessment of the Rheumatoid Hand	Am J Occup Ther 23:122–125, 1969	*Hand Strength:* 1. Grip (sphygmomanometer). 2. Pinch (adapted sphygmomanometer). 3. Cylindrical (adpated dowel and weights). 4. Finger flexion (special measurement device). *Disease Status:* Presence of: pain, heat, tenderness and crepitation indicated by color-coded chart.	Based on percentage of normative time.	Yes	Yes

ROM: using a goniometer.

Jebsen, RH	An Objective and Standardized Test of Hand Function	Arch Phys Med Rehabil 50:311–319, 1969	*Timed Functional Tasks:* 1. One-handed activities: opening and closing a safety pin, unbuttoning and buttoning button boards, cutting out a square and straight line with scissors. 2. Two-handed activities: cutting plasticized clay with knife and fork, unlacing relacing, and tying a shoelace. *Timed Functional Tasks:* 1. Writing a short sentence. 2. Turning over 3 × 5 inch cards. 3. Picking up small objects and placing them in a container. 4. Stacking checkers. 5. Simulated eating. 6. Moving empty large cans on a table. 7. Moving weighted large cans.	Timed individual subtest scores	Yes	Yes (Extensive, N = 360)
MacBain, KP (Assessment used at C.A.R.S.— British Columbia)	Assessment of Function in the Rheumatoid Hand	Can Occup Ther J 37:95–102, 1970	*Hand Strength:* 1. Grip (sphygmomanometer). 2. Pinch (sphygmomanometer). 3. Hook grasp (weight-pulley system).	Based on percentage of normative time	Yes	Yes

Table 19–1 Summary of Published Functional Hand Evaluations (Listed in Chronological Order) (Continued)

Author	Title	Where Published	Test Items	Grading System	Method Standardized	Normative Data

			ROM:
			1. Fingertip inches to crease.
			2. Hand tracing.
			
			Timed or Weighted Functional Tasks:
			1. For applied strength:
			  a. Cutting play dough with a knife and fork.
			  b. Pouring a full kettle of water into a bowl.
			  c. Pouring from a large measuring cup into a teacup.
			2. For precision:
			  a. Buttoning and unbuttoning a Montessori board.
			  b. Pinning and unpinning a safety pin into cloth.
			  c. Threading and tying a shoelace.
			  d. Opening, closing, and locking a model door.
			  e. Picking up and retaining 3 coins.			

Kellor, M et al	Technical Manual Hand Strength and Dexterity Norms	1. Sister Kenny Institute Pub. # 721	*Hand Strength:* 1. Grip (dynamometer). 2. Pinch: palmar, lateral, 3-point (pinch meter).	Individual subtest scores	Yes	Yes (Extensive for age, sex, hand dominance)

Author	Title	Reference	Description	Score		
	2.	Am J Occup Ther 25:77–83, 1971	*Dexterity:* Placing and removing 9 pegs in a board.			
Treuhaft, PS, Lewis, MR, and McCarthy, DJ	A Rapid Method for Evaluating the Structure and Function*† of the Rheumatoid Hand	Arthritis Rheum 14:75–86, 1971	*ROM:* 1. Active ROM is measured on all joints. 2. Grades of range are assigned a numerical score. *Structure:* Common hand pathologies, e.g., ulnar deviation and instability, are assigned a numerical rating. *Scores:* Written on a hand outline (functional activities not included).	Sum of subtest ratings	Yes	Yes
Potvin, AR et al	Simulated Activities of Daily Living Examination	Arch Phys Med Rehab 53:476–486, 1972	*Timed Functional Tasks:* There are 7 subtests that involve walking, standing, or dressing. *Additional Hand Function Subtests Include:* 1. Unbuttoning and buttoning buttons on a cloth board. 2. Opening and closing a zipper on a cloth board. 3. Putting on garden gloves. 4. Tying a bow in shoelaces. 5. Opening and closing a safety pin.	Timed individual subtest scores	Yes	Yes

335

Table 19–1 Summary of Published Functional Hand Evaluations (Listed in Chronological Order) (*Continued*)

Author	Title	Where Published	Test Items	Grading System	Method Standardized	Normative Data
			6. Unwrapping a Bandaid. 7. Squeezing toothpaste. 8. Threading a needle. 9. Picking up coins. 10. Dialing a telephone. 11. Cutting soft plastic substance with a knife. 12. Using a fork.			

Smith, H	Smith Hand Function Evaluation	Am J Occup Ther 27:244–251, 1973	*Timed Functional Tasks:*
			1. Unilateral grasp-release tasks:
			  a. Placing and replacing 3 graduated blocks to a prescribed position on the table.
			  b. Placing 4 graduated nails in a glass.
			  c. Placing 4 coins in a glass.
			  d. Placing 16 pegs in a board (8 small, 8 large).
			2. Activities of daily living:
			  a. Opening and closing a safety pin.
			  b. Unbuckling and buckling a belt on a cloth board.
			  c. Unbuttoning and buttoning three buttons on a cloth board.
			  d. Opening and closing a zipper on a board.
				Separate timed scores for each subtest	Yes	Yes

e. Tying a double knot in shoelaces on a board.
f. Tying a bow with shoelaces on a board.
g. Simulated shoelacing on a cloth board.
3. Writing sample: Write name, trace rectangle and a curved line.

Hand Strength:
Grip (dynamometer).

Bell, E, Jurek, K, and Wilson, T	Physical Capacities Evaluation of Hand Function (PCE) (Article titled: Hand Skill Measurement.)	Am J Occup Ther 30(2):80–86, 1976	*Unilateral Tasks:* 1. Picking up straight pins 2. Peg, washer, sleeve assembly 3. Nut, bolt assembly 4. Card sorting 5. Turning blocks over *Bilateral Tasks:* 1. Erector set assembly 2. Removing coins from purse 3. Peg washer assembly 4. Nut, bolt assembly 5. Card sorting 6. Bennet Hand Tool Dexterity Test 7. Turning blocks over *Strength:* Dynamometer	Timed subtest scores. Averaged total. — Yes — Yes (N = 50)

*Method is described in adequate detail for reproduction.
†In this study, function is defined as active ROM.

337

OCCUPATIONAL THERAPY
ARTHRITIS HAND EVALUATION

☐ INPATIENT   ☐ OUTPATIENT

Dx:_____ Onset:_____ Age:_____ Date:_____ Time:_____

Referral:_____ Occupation:_____

Medications/Surgeries: _____

Prior OT/PT _____ ARA Class ___

JOINT INVOLVEMENT	Right	Left
Neck		
Shoulders		
Elbows		
Forearms		
Wrists		

RIGHT HAND

		Thumb		Index	Middle	Ring	Little
	CMC		MCP				
	MCP		PIP				
	IP		DIP				

Type _____ Fingertip to Palm Crease: T_____ I_____ M_____ R_____ L_____ cm
Comments:

LEFT HAND

		Thumb		Index	Middle	Ring	Little
	CMC		MCP				
	MCP		PIP				
	IP		DIP				

Type _____ Fingertip to Palm Crease: T_____ I_____ M_____ R_____ L_____ cm
Comments:

Circle Dominance

Note the following conditions in above section.

Pain	Crepitation (Crep)	Synovial Hyper. (Syn Hyp)	Synovitis (Syn)
Swelling	Osteophytes	Dislocation (Disloc)	Ankylosis (Anky)
Nodules	Boutonniere (Bout)	Bone Resorption (Resorp)	Mallet
Lag	Subluxation (Sublux)	Ulnar Drift (Ul-Dr)	Swan Neck (S-N)

MUSCLE INVOLVEMENT	RIGHT	LEFT
Intrinsic Muscle atrophy		
Intrinsic Muscle strength		
Abd. Pollicis Brevis Strength		
Intrinsic Tightness		

TENDON INVOLVEMENT

Flexor Tenosynovitis Wrist and Digits		
Trigger Finger		
Flexor Tendon Excursion		
Extensor Tenosynovitis		
DeQuervain's (APL, EPB) Finklestein Test		
Tendon Ruptures EDQ, EDC, EIP, EPL, FPL, FDP		

SKIN/NEUROVASCULAR INVOLVEMENT

Skin Integrity/ulcers		
Raynaud's Phenomenon		
Sensation med./ul. nerve		

PREHENSION	RIGHT		LEFT		Comments
	able	unable	able	unable	
Full Grip					
Palmar Grip					
Lateral Pinch					
2 Pt. Pinch					

Morning Stiffness _____

ADL STATUS _____

_____

_____

MAIN FUNCTIONAL HAND LIMITIATIONS: _____

_____

TREATMENT RECOMMENDATIONS/PLAN: _____

_____

_____

Therapist: _____

Chapter 20

Evaluation of Range of Motion

The range of motion (ROM) evaluation not only provides information on the degrees of motion present but also affords the therapist an opportunity to assess joint status in general, pain tolerance, and, in part, functional ability. A system of recording joints that (1) are painful with motion, (2) are painful without motion, and (3) manifest crepitation during the ROM evaluation is recommended as a simple means of charting disease activity as well as providing an easy reference for treatment planning. In addition, *the time of the assessment and the amount and type of anti-inflammatory or analgesic medication* *taken prior to the assessment should be noted, since these medications can significantly affect objective assessments.*

METHOD OF MEASUREMENT

The method for measuring joint ROM in this chapter is based on procedures for measuring and recording adopted by the American Academy of Orthopedic Surgery (AAOS) in 1965.[1] This method assumes the extended "anatomical position" of extremity joints as zero degrees rather than 180 degrees. All motions of a joint are measured from a starting position defined as zero degrees; the degrees of motion of a joint are added in the direction the joint moves from the zero starting position.

The AAOS manual published by the American Academy of Orthopedic Surgeons entitled "Joint Motion—Method of Measuring and Recording"[1] defines the direction, range, and axis of all joint motions. Although it *does not* show the actual positioning of the goniometer, lines depicting the axis of the joint suggest its appropriate placement. In addition to the procedures outlined in the manual for measuring normal joints, special considerations are needed to ensure consistent and accurate measurement of the arthritic joint.

JOINT MEASUREMENT USING A GONIOMETER

The procedures and rationales in this chapter supplement the content of the AAOS manual. However, only joint motions that need special consideration are included here.

Shoulder

The patient may not be able to perform pure abduction or flexion because of pain or joint changes. Frequently the patient will substitute flexion on an oblique plane. Therefore, motion in other than a standard plane should be noted. It is important to have the patient externally rotate the arm when performing abduction so there will be no interference from the greater tuberosity of the humerus jamming against the acromion process.

Elbow

When the elbow is in full extension, the radius and ulna do not extend in a straight line from the humerus but are at an angle. This is often referred to as the **carrying angle** or **cubitus valgus**[2] (Fig. 20–1). The angle is usually greater for females than for males. This angle can easily be confused with flexion or extension range, especially if forearm rotation is limited.

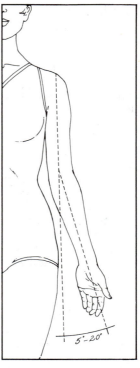

Figure 20–1. Normal "carrying angle" of the elbow is indicated in the illustration.

The standard procedure of measuring elbow range is with the forearm supinated (anatomical position), but frequently this is not possible with patients who have arthritis. When elbow range is being measured precisely for surgical or splinting treatment, accuracy can be enhanced by also noting the degree (or position) of forearm rotation.

Forearm

When evaluating forearm supination or pronation, it is essential that the elbow be at a 90-degree angle and next to the side of the body to prevent substitution of shoulder rotation.

Wrist

Flexion and Extension

Placement of the goniometer for evaluation of the wrist varies from clinic to clinic. The AAOS manual diagrams indicate placement for flexion over the dorsum of the wrist joint, but common arthritic wrist deformities (e.g., synovial hypertrophy or subluxation) often prohibit accurate measurement with this method. The following method is recommended for consistent measurement of both flexion and extension on patients with or without wrist involvement.

Alignment of the axis of the goniometer with the axis of the radiocarpal joint. The stable bar of the goniometer is placed along the shaft of the radius and the movable bar is placed along the shaft of the second metacarpal bone (Fig. 20–2). Alignment with the second metacarpal is preferred over the fifth metacarpal because (1) wrist motion takes place principally at the radiocarpal joint, and (2) rotational forces on the fifth metacarpal distort the measurement of wrist motion.

Although wrist flexion and extension ranges are determined by measuring the angle between the shaft of the second metacarpal and the shaft of the radius, orthopedic surgeons may refer to wrist flexion and extension as the angle between the scaphoid (or carpal navicular) and the shaft

of the radius rather than the second metacarpal. There is a difference of about 10 to 15 degrees between these two reference points. This is a minor point, but it will facilitate communication if the therapist is aware that the physician *may* have a different frame of reference in discussing joint range. For example, the surgeon may state that he fused the wrist at 15 degrees of flexion to facilitate perineal care but measurement along the axis of the radius and *second metacarpal* may read neutral or zero degrees. To understand this, palpate your radiocarpal joint in neutral and notice the angle of the second metacarpal—it is probably in 15 degrees of extension.

Ulnar and Radial Deviation

Align the stable bar along the median of the forearm and the movable bar with the shaft of the third metacarpal. The end of the bar should be directly over the third metacarpal joint (Fig. 20–3).

Caution: Make sure that you align with the shaft of the bones and not the extensor tendons.

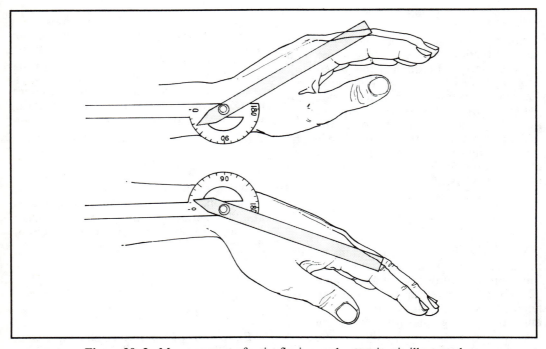

Figure 20–2. Measurement of wrist flexion and extension is illustrated.

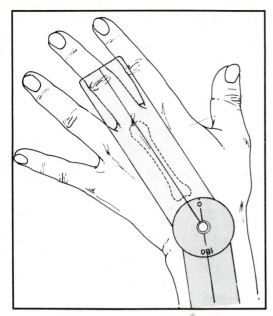

Figure 20–3. This figure depicts measurement of wrist deviation.

Fingers

It is important that a small 180-degree goniometer be used for the fingers so the arms can be aligned accurately and not be distorted by pressure distal to the joint. It is recommended that one cut off and round the ends of a small plastic goniometer so the arms are about 2½ inches from the axis. *The goal is to measure the angle between the shafts of the bones.* When subluxation is present, the true axis of the joint is lost and only approximate, not accurate, measurements can be obtained with a single-axis goniometer. To handle this problem, I have arrived at the following solution in my clinical practice.

Measurement of Subluxed Joints

1. Align the proximal arm over the stable (usually proximal) bone; then align the distal arm so it *parallels* the subluxed or distal bone. This usually means the distal arm does not touch the subluxed bone.
2. I try to use this technique every time I measure a subluxed joint, and I mark the resultant range with an **S** to indicate I used this technique.

3. If accuracy is particularly important for a specific treatment, I often measure the joint in the standard way and with the subluxed technique.

This is clearly a less than perfect solution but it has made my measurements more reliable than having no system at all.

Flexion and Extension

Flexion of all joints is most accurately measured by placing the goniometer over the dorsum of the joint; however, if deformities, swelling, or nodules make placement difficult, move the goniometer *slightly* lateral to the protuberance and align the arms of the goniometer with the shafts of the bones being measured.

Metacarpophalangeal Joints. (Metacarpophalangeal joints are commonly termed *proximal finger joints* by surgeons.) *Caution:* The directive, "make a fist," often is effective to elicit full proximal interphalangeal (PIP) flexion but *not effective* for eliciting full metacarpophalangeal (MCP) flexion, because full power grip ("fist") limits MCP flexion of the index and middle fingers. To measure MCP flexion, have the patient bend his knuckles as far as possible (with the PIP joints relaxed).

Proximal Interphalangeal Joints (Middle Finger Joints). *Caution:* The AAOS manual and other ROM texts[3] indicate that measurement of the distal interphalangeal (DIP) and PIP joints should be done with the MCP joints in extension. This method will give an inaccurate measurement if the patient has intrinsic muscle tightness. (See Chapter 19 for information on intrinsic tightness.) *Measurement of the PIP joint should be done with the hand in a comfortable position with MCP joints flexed (in about midrange).*

Distal Interphalangeal Joints (Distal Finger Joints). The DIP joints should be measured in the position that allows maximal DIP flexion. Often this is in the position of a full fist, which makes placement of the goniometer difficult. If this is the case, it is better to estimate the ROM in this position than to have the patient open his fist and lose range.

Hyperextension

Metacarpophalangeal Joints. The most accurate method that I have found for measuring hyperextension of the MCP joints is to align a finger goniometer with the axis of the index and little finger MCP joints, then estimate, or "eyeball," the range of the long and ring fingers. Measuring over the volar surface of the hand distorts the range. Measurement with a full-circle goniometer is advocated by some authors, but in my opinion it places the axis of the goniometer too far from the axis of the joint. When measuring the MCP joints, it is critical to use a short goniometer because otherwise the proximal end will hit the wrist and distort the range measurement. A standard small goniometer is also a clumsy tool to use on the small joints.

The Importance of Hyperextension. I consider the measurement of MCP hyperextension to be an important aspect of an arthritis hand evaluation; and I find exercise to maintain this motion, especially in the early hand, a critical treatment. When arthritis (or any problem) affects the MCP joints, the first motion that is lost is hyperextension. Therefore, maintaining hyperextension is essential to maintaining normal baseline function. If you normally have hyperextension mobility and you lose it due to arthritis or swelling, your hand will not "feel" normal to you; your hand will feel tight, less agile, and less dexterous.

The role of hyperextension has not been discussed in the rheumatology/hand rehabilitation literature. Several factors contribute to this. Some people (mostly men) do not have hyperextension range. It is not considered as essential to hand function as, for example, flexion or extension, because you can perform daily activities without it. There is a wide variability in normal range (0 to 50 degrees), which makes it harder to define abnormal range. The degree of normal hand hyperextension varies between joints and between hands in a given individual. Some major ROM reviews to establish norms have not even included hyperextension.

Another point to consider is that in most digital joints, active ROM and passive ROM are equal or vary by no more than 5 degrees. In the normal hand the difference between active and passive hyperextension can vary by as much as 20 degrees, and probably more in some people. (Test your own hand and see the difference.)

If a patient has MCP flexion contractures, hyperextension is going to be a moot point. But, for all of my patients with near-normal or minimal hyperextension, I document their ROM and give them simple exercises and awareness techniques to maintain or improve hyperextension, such as holding the hands together in a prayer position and then actively hyperextending the MCP joints while keeping the MCP heads in contact.

Proximal and Distal Interphalangeal Joints. Place the goniometer on the *lateral* edge of the joint, aligning the axis of the goniometer with the axis of the joint. Lateral placement is preferred over volar because volar fat pads and tenosynovitis can distort goniometer placement.

Ulnar Deviation of the Metacarpophalangeal Joints

The technique for measuring this motion is probably the most controversial of all joint motions. A variety of methods can be found throughout the country. Some therapists measure the MCP joint in active extension; others measure the MCP joint with the hand lying on a table; and still others measure it with the hand in a resting position.

In the past I have advocated measurement in active extension because it appeared to be the most accurate and consistent. If only one measurement can be taken this is probably the best one, but it does not give a complete picture of the relationship of ulnar drift to hand function. In order to evaluate and treat patients effectively, *I find it necessary to measure ulnar drift in active extension, to appreciate the influence of ulnar drift during extension activities, such as reaching for a glass, and in a position of rest, to appreciate the influence of drift during light flexion activities* (e.g., typing). Assessment of ulnar drift during strong grasp has not been an issue so far.

Another advantage to evaluating the hand in both active extension and at rest is that you can determine which position increases the ulnar drift. Some patients have more drift in extension whereas others have more in flexion.

I do not recommend measuring ulnar drift with the hand resting on a surface, because the surface can create variable degrees of distortion, making follow-up assessments unreliable.

Method of measurement using active extension: Have the patient hold his or her hand in pronation, in mid air, and raise his or her fingers toward the ceiling without trying to correct the drift. For some patients it may be necessary to stabilize the palm. The axis of the goniometer is placed over the dorsum of the MCP joint and the arms of the goniometer are aligned with the proximal phalanx and metacarpal bone (Fig. 20–4). Care should be taken *not* to align the goniometer with the extensor tendons. When measuring the MCP joints it is also important to keep in mind that the

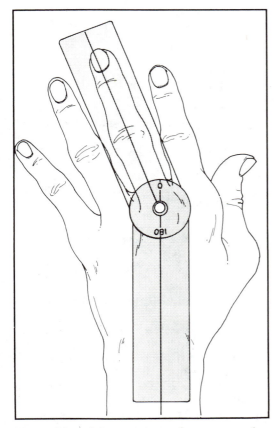

Figure 20–4. Measurement of metacarpophalangeal deviation during active extension is depicted.

index finger normally has about 20 degrees of ulnar deviation.[4] Thus, if a patient had 10 degrees of drift in the middle, ring, and little fingers and 30 degrees of drift in the index finger, only 10 degrees of the index measurement would be pathological, and it would be appropriate to report that the patient has 10 degrees of MCP ulnar drift. Most clinics record the 30 degrees because it is the goniometric reading, but this can be misleading to the patient, treating physician, or therapists following the patient.

Degrees of range are recorded as a single measurement and not as a range, for example, 40-degree ulnar deviation and not 0 to 40 degrees.

Additional information regarding the integrity of the joint and muscles can be obtained by measuring the degree of active drift correction. Have the patient actively extend his or her fingers, place the palm of the hand on the table, relax the fingers; then have the patient radially deviate each finger to neutral. Measure at the point of maximal correction.

A two-axis goniometer has been developed by Hasselkus and associates for measuring MCP joint subluxation.[5] There is seldom a need for this amount of precision, but in specific situations it could be helpful.

Thumb

Metacarpophalangeal and Interphalangeal Joint

Flexion, extension, and hyperextension are measured in the same manner as the finger PIP joints.

Carpometacarpal Joint

The unique structure of the carpometacarpal (CMC) saddle joint allows for more complex motion. In rheumatology and orthopedics the motions of the CMC joint are described using the following terminology.

Abduction (palmar)
Motion: The maximal span of the thumb perpendicular or at right angle to the palm.
Measurement: The angle between the first and second metacarpal bones, with the apex of the goniometer placed directly

over the CMC joint with the thumb perpendicular to the palm.

Significance: Palmer abduction is essential for allowing grasp around objects. Limitations can be due to joint disease or soft tissue (web space) contracture, or both.

Abduction in extension

Significance: This refers to a combined motion; it could also be referred to as *extension in abduction,* which would actually have more meaning because extension has more functional significance in this position; that is, extension allows the palm to be pressed against a flat surface. Abduction plays a somewhat lesser role of increasing the span of the hand during manipulation or handling of large objects.

Adduction

Motion: Approximation of the thumb to the radial side of the palm.

Measurement: Distance of the thumb to the second metacarpal indicates loss of adduction.

Significance: Loss of active adduction usually indicates weakness of the adductor pollicis muscles and ulnar nerve impairment.

Opposition

Motion: A combination of abduction, flexion, and rotation. Opposition represents the approximation in abduction of the first metacarpal to the fifth metacarpal.

Measurement: Determined by the ability to bring the center tip of the thumb in contact with the tip of the fifth digit. If the little finger is limited, observe for rotation of the thumb nail when the patient attempts opposition.

Significance: Opposition allows precision pinch to the other digits. In the rheumatic diseases, the loss of opposition occurs with the loss of abduction.

Flexion

Motion: Movement of the thumb metacarpal medially from neutral. Flexion is the ability to bring the first metacarpal volar to the second metacarpal.

Significance: This brings the thumb into the palm, out of harm's way, and allows a fist and power grasp. Flexion range is short, approximately 20 degrees. Loss of flexion due to joint disease is uncommon and overshadowed by the more serious and obvious loss of extension or abduction. Trauma could result in an extension contracture.

Extension

Motion: All movement that brings the distal head of the first metacarpal lateral to the distal head of the second metacarpal.

Extension is the return of flexion and the return of opposition. It can occur in any degree of abduction.

Measurement: Extension is determined by the ability to bring all five metacarpal heads in contact with a flat surface at the same time. Extension is an end point, and the goal is zero extension.

Significance: Extension allows the entire palm to be placed flat against a surface. Inability to achieve zero extension is referred to as an *adduction contracture* even though, in reality, it is probably a combination of an adduction-flexion-opposition contracture.

Retropulsion

Motion: Retroversion is the equivalent of hyperextension for the CMC joint. With the hand flat on the table (with all the metacarpals touching the surface), it is the ability to raise the distal metacarpal head off the table.

Measurement: If the patient has normal MCP and IP joint function, you can use the distance that the tip of the thumb raises off the table as a measure of retropulsion. If these joints have excessive hyperextension, it may be preferable to use the distance between the table and the volar aspect of the distal first metacarpal head.

Significance: This motion is accomplished by the extensor pollicis longus (EPL). If the CMC joint is normal or not limited, retropulsion is the test to determine EPL function and strength. Rupture of the EPL is one of the more common ruptures in rheumatoid arthritis. Also, retropulsion is the recommended motion or plane for applying resistance to strengthen the EPL following repair.

ALTERNATE METHODS OF ASSESSING RANGE OF MOTION

Functional Range of Motion

This type of assessment involves having the patient touch various body landmarks to determine if there is sufficient ROM to accomplish self-care tasks in each body region (Table 20–1). Consequently this method provides information about multiple joint range rather than a single specific joint.

Using the index MCP joint is recommended because it is more reflective of

Table 20–1 Landmarks for Assessing Functional Range of Motion[6] (Touching Landmarks with Index MCP Joint)

Common Body Landmarks	Range of Motion for
Top of head	Hair care, face hygiene, shoulder abduction, and flexion
Back of neck	Neck hygiene, managing clothes, shoulder abduction, and external rotation
Mouth	Feeding and facial and dental hygiene
Back of waist	Managing clothes and shoulder internal rotation
Toe of shoe (while sitting)	Lower extremity dressing (assess back, hip, and knee flexion and elbow extension)

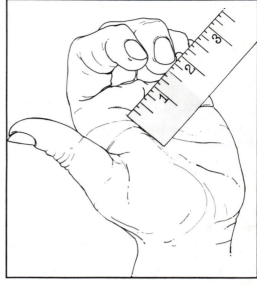

Figure 20–5. This drawing shows measurement of composite finger flexion using fingertip to palmar crease method.

function. For example, if a person is just able to touch his or her mouth with the fingertip, there is probably not sufficient range for facial hygiene, dental care, or feeding. If the person can touch the mouth with the index MCP, there is adequate ROM for function.

I developed this method to be used as a rapid clinical screening procedure.[6] It provides information concerning mobility for all self-care activities, except perineal care. This needs to be considered separately.

Composite Flexion Range of Motion of the Fingers

1. Measurement of distance between fingertip and the distal palmar (midpalmar) crease.
    a. Equipment
      (1) Ruler with a zero starting edge[1]
      (2) Digit-o-meter[7]
    b. Procedure: Have the patient flex his fingers and measure the distance between either the tip of the fingers (not the pad) or the fingernail edge and the distal palmar crease (Fig. 20–5). For greater ac-

curacy the distance of the tips proximal or distal to the crease should be noted; for example, 1 inch from crease *proximal* + ½ inch off of palm indicates greater MCP flexion, whereas 1 inch from crease *distal* + ½ inch off of palm indicates very little MCP flexion. The landmark (tip or fingernail) selected for measurement is arbitrary but should be used consistently throughout the clinic. Personally, I have found the fingernail edge less accurate, as many patients do not have fingernails that extend to the end of the finger.

2. Measurement of distance between fingertips and distal wrist crease. This method is recommended only for hands with severely limited finger flexion.

Finger Abduction and Web Space Excursion

1. Measurement of finger abduction span from tip of the little finger to tip of the index finger[1] and from tip of the little finger to the tip of the thumb.
    a. Procedure: Have the patient abduct fingers on a piece of paper. Place a dot above the tip of the little finger and above

the tip of the index or thumb. Remove the hand and measure the distance between the dots. *Note:* MCP ulnar drift may influence the accuracy of this form of measurement.

This method is particularly valuable for documenting abduction mobility for people with scleroderma. A copy of their hand outline and documented finger span can be given to them to use at home as a guide for maintaining mobility.

2. Measurement of web space. The position of maximal stretch of the web space is with the thumb abducted at about a 45-degree angle to the palm. If precise measurement is needed, it is best to measure the distance between the first and second metacarpal heads at the point where the web starts. Using a stacking cone with markings works very well for this. If a more general assessment is needed, paper tracings of digit span may be sufficient. It is important to keep in mind that if you use the tip of the thumb to the tip of the index finger as a measure of web space, you are also including lateral deviation of the MCP joint and hyperextension of the IP joint. Using the juncture of the web at the digit provides a more precise reference point even on paper tracings.

Wrist or Finger Deviation

A record can be kept of the degree of deviation by tracing an outline of the hand and forearm. With one color of ink, trace the position of greatest deviation, and with another color, trace the position of active correction.

REFERENCES

1. Joint Motion—Method of Measuring and Recording. American Academy of Orthopaedic Surgeons, Chicago, 1966.
2. Smith, FM: Surgery of the Elbow, 2nd ed. WB Saunders, Philadelphia, 1972, pp 19–20.
3. Norkin, CC, and White, DJ: Measurement of Joint Motion: A Guide to Goniometry. FA Davis, Philadelphia, 1985.
4. Flatt, A: Care of the Rheumatoid Hand, 3rd ed. CV Mosby, St Louis, 1974, p 250.
5. Hasselkus, BR, Kshepakaran, KK, Houge, JC, and Plautz, KA: Rheumatoid arthritis: A two-axis goniometer to measure metacarpophalangeal laxity. Arch Phys Med Rehabil 62:133–135, 1985.
6. Melvin, JL: Rheumatic Disease—Occupational Therapy and Rehabilitation. FA Davis, Philadelphia, 1977, p 138.
7. Brayman, S: Measuring device of joint motion of the hand. Am J Occup Ther 25:173, 1971.

ADDITIONAL SOURCES

Boone, DC, and Azen, SP: Normal range of motion of joints in male subjects. J Bone Joint Surg 61A:756, 1979.
Boone, DC et al: Reliability of goniometric measurements. Phys Ther 58:1355, 1978.
Brown, ME: Rheumatoid arthritic hands: Tactual-visual evaluation approaches. Am J Occup Ther 20(1):17, 1966.
Esch, D, and Lepley, M: Evaluation of Joint Motion: Method of Measurement and Recording. University of Minnesota Press, Minneapolis, 1974.
Gowitzke, BA, and Milner, M: Understanding the Scientific Basis for Human Movement, 2nd ed. Williams & Wilkins, Baltimore, 1980.
Hamilton, GF, and Lachenbruch, PA: Reliability of goniometers in assessing finger joint angle. Phys Ther 49:465–469, 1969.
Hellebrandt, FA, Duvall, EN, and Moore, ML: Measurement of joint motion: Part III: Reliability of goniometry. Phys Ther Rev 29:302–307, 1949.
Holland, GJ: Physiology of flexibility: Review of literature. Kinesiology Review 49–62, 1949.
Hoppenfeld, S: Physical Examination of the Spine and Extremities. Appleton-Century-Crofts, New York, 1976.
Kendall, HO, and McCreary, EK: Muscles: Testing and Function, 3rd ed. Williams & Wilkins, Baltimore, 1983.
Low, JL: The reliability of joint measurement. Physiotherapy 67:227, 1976.
McRae, R: Clinical-Orthopedic Examination. Churchill-Livingstone, New York.
Mitchell, WS, Millar, J, and Sturrock, RD: Evaluation of goniometry as objective parameter for measuring joint motion. Scott Med J 20:57–59, 1975.
Moore, ML: Clinical assessment of joint motion. In Licht, S: Therapeutic Exercise. Elizabeth Licht, New Haven, 1972.
Norkin, CC, and Levangie, PK: Joint Structure and Function. FA Davis, Philadelphia, 1983.
Rothstein, JM, Miller, PJ, and Roettger, F: Goniometric reliability in a clinical setting. Phys Ther 63:1611, 1983.
Spilman, HW, and Pinkston, D: Relation of test positions to radial and ulnar deviation. Phys Ther 49:837, 1969.
Tata, JA et al: A variable axis electrogoniometer for

measurement of single plane movement. J Biomech 11:421, 1978.

Thomas, DH, and Long, C: An electrogoniometer for the finger: A kinsiologic tracking device. Am J Med Elec April–June:96, 1964.

Trombley, CA, and Scott, AD: Occupational Therapy for Physical Dysfunction, 3rd ed. Williams & Wilkins, Baltimore, 1987.

Waugh, KL, Minkel, JL, Parker, R et al: Measurement of selected hip, knee, and ankle joint motions in newborns. Phys Ther 63:1616, 1983.

Chapter 21

Evaluation of Muscle Strength

MANUAL MUSCLE TEST FOR PATIENTS WITH ARTHRITIS
   Method
   Grading Terminology
   Recording
OBJECTIVE ASSESSMENTS OF HAND STRENGTH
Grip Strength
        Measuring Grip with the Jamar Dynamometer
        Standardized Procedures from Mathiowetz and Co-
        workers
        Measuring Grip with an Adapted Sphygmomanometer
Pinch Strength
        Standardized Procedures from Mathiowetz and Co-
        workers

This chapter discusses the specific elements to consider when measuring manual or objective strength of patients with joint involvement. Evaluation of individual muscle strength is not covered in this chapter because the procedure for patients with arthritis, which is the same as the one for patients with neurological disorders, is described in detail in other texts.[1,2]

Assessment of muscle strength in patients with rheumatic diseases commonly involves three forms of testing: (1) manual group muscle test, (2) manual individual muscle test, and (3) objective grip and pinch strength test. For most clinical needs, a group muscle test is sufficient. Measuring individual muscle strength is indicated when assessing specific neurological impairment (e.g., median nerve entrapment) or when there is a need to strengthen specific muscles (e.g., in a postoperative therapy program). There is a new system for measuring muscle strength (not grip) using a hand-held dynamometer. Procedures have been established but normative studies have not been done at this time.[3]

Because a manual test can determine only gross differences in muscle strength and is inadequate for determining increments of normal (grade 5) strength (e.g., both a 30-pound grip and a 70-pound grip would test as normal on a manual test), objective measures are employed for hand strength assessment. Over the past 5 years, a considerable amount of work has been done to standardize and improve the reliability and validity of grip and pinch assessment.

MANUAL MUSCLE TEST FOR PATIENTS WITH ARTHRITIS

Method

Basic information on specific positioning and grading procedures for both group and individual tests can be found in the major texts on muscle testing.[1,2] However, the procedures in these books are designed for patients with normal joints and, therefore, need to be adapted for evaluation of the patient with arthritis.

The important difference in assessing strength of patients with arthritis versus other disability groups is that *resistance should be applied within the patient's pain-free range and not at the end of his or her active range.*[4] (Standard muscle testing procedure involves application of resistance at the end of complete range.[1,2]) Patients with arthritic joints frequently have pain at the end of active range or have marked discomfort the last 30 to 40 degrees of active motion. Resistance should be applied when the joint is positioned within the pain-free range because this avoids pain-inhibition of muscle strength and is the range of the patient's functional strength.[4]

For example, Mr. S. has shoulder flexion range 0 to 120 degrees passively and 0 to 90 degrees actively (with pain at the end of range). If the shoulder flexor muscles are tested at the end of active range, they may be scored as a grade 3 (fair—unable to take resistance against gravity) due to pain inhibition, but if tested at 45 degrees of flexion (within the pain-free range) they may be scored as a grade 4 (good—able to take moderate resistance). The amount of resistance this patient can take within the pain-free range will be indicative of the kinds of functional tasks he can perform. For instance, Mr. S. could probably lift or transport moderate-weight items or lift pans when cooking. Reporting a grade 3 for this patient would not accurately portray his actual muscle strength.[4]

Grading Terminology

The most common system of grading utilizes descriptive terms such as *good* or *fair* to convey degrees of muscle strength. The inherent problem with this terminology is that the connotations of the terms are in conflict with the precise definition ascribed them. For example, a grade of good indicates a muscle is able to move the joint through complete range of motion against gravity and hold against some resistance.[1] But, a muscle graded as good is not *good;* it is a damaged or weakened muscle. The term *fair* implies okay; but a fair muscle is not *okay;* it is severely damaged. Likewise muscle strength with a grade of normal may not be *normal* for that particular in-

dividual. This descriptive terminology can be misleading and hinder communication with health professionals, especially with physicians or nurses who are not familiar with the precise clinical definitions ascribed by therapists.[4]

A solution to this semantic conflict is to substitute a numerical scale for the descriptive terms. The system that follows was first published in 1946 by the National Foundation for Infantile Paralysis.[1]

5 = Normal (able to take full resistance against gravity)
4 = Good (able to take moderate or some resistance against gravity)
3 = Fair (not able to take resistance against gravity)
2 = Poor (able to move part through complete range of motion with gravity eliminated)
1 = Trace (muscle contraction can be palpated)
0 = Zero (no palpable contraction)

When using a numerical system it is helpful to report the baseline score. This indicates the points achieved compared with the total possible; for example, elbow flexors: 4/5 (4 out of 5 points). Muscle strength that is between two scores can also be represented numerically instead of by a plus-minus system; for example, a score of 3.5 can be used instead of fair plus (F+) to indicate a muscle that can take *slight* resistance against gravity. The combination of numbers and math signs can also be effective, for example, 3+/5.

Recording

Documentation of strength of muscles surrounding painful joints should include a simple notation system (e.g., an asterisk) to indicate that the grade recorded represents *resistance applied within a (relatively) pain-free range* instead of the standard end-of-range position.[4] A special notation is also required when painful joints prohibit the standard testing procedure of applying full or moderate resistance. If this occurs, an accurate evaluation is not possible, although it is usually possible to determine, and valuable to know, whether the muscles can tolerate at least slight resistance. Grade 3.5 is the minimal amount of strength required to counteract opposing muscle groups (important in preventing contractures).

A sample notation is "Accurate evaluation not possible because of pain; elbow and shoulder muscles can tolerate at least slight resistance." The recording should also note the time of day and amount of anti-inflammatory or analgesic medication taken, prior to assessment, because these medications can significantly affect objective assessments.

OBJECTIVE ASSESSMENTS OF HAND STRENGTH

The current hydraulic adjustable dynamometer had been a standard assessment tool since 1954. Kellor and co-workers (1971) developed the first extensive normative data controlled only for age and sex. These norms are the most frequently used and cited. In her protocol, Kellor used the highest scores of two trials as the measure of grip and pinch strength.[5] This measure has since been proven to have low reliability (the average of three trials has proven to be most reliable[6]). The Kellor protocol also did not control for arm position or verbal instructions, nor were there any test-retest or inter-rater reliability measures of the protocol. Additionally, the pinch gauge used in the original study is no longer commercially available.

For all of these reasons, Mathiowetz and associates have developed new normative values for grips and pinch for adults and children using commonly available equipment.[6-8] These norms correct for the deficits described above and are in accord with the guidelines for assessment recommended by the American Society of Hand Therapists.[9]

To compare your client to new norms you must use the standardized protocol used for establishing the norms. If you use a different protocol, you should not compare your results to the norms.

Grip Strength

People with arthritis have a wide range of hand involvement, and two methods used to assess grip strength are recommended. The standard Jamar dynamometer is considered the most accurate of the commercially available instruments for measuring grip.[6,10] Although its accuracy is approximately within 5 percent (i.e., within a 5-percent error factor) a recent study has shown that the percentage of measurement error can vary between models of the Jamar dynamometer.[11] Another study demonstrated the dial model to be more accurate than the digital readout.[6] I recommend it for hands with minimal involvement or 60 pounds or more of grip strength, or both. In most instances, the Jamar dynamometer will work for patients with mild or even moderate osteoarthritis.

For people with active arthritis or significant hand deformity, the shape and rigidity of the Jamar dynamometer can cause pain that inhibits or prevents the application of grip force. In some situations, the coldness of the metal can also create discomfort. The Jamar dynamometer may be difficult for people with very weak hands to hold or maneuver, and it can be discouraging to use because there is no sense of impact; that is, there is no physical feedback to indicate that the hand is making an impact on the device. Also, verbal encouragement to grip hard on a rigid handle can damage inflamed PIP or MCP joints. For these reasons, an adapted sphygmomanometer is recommended for people with severe weakness, active inflammation, or significant deformity, or all three.[3]

One advantage of using the Jamar dynamometer is that standardized norms exist for adults and children.[6-8] However, the norms are not useful if the device itself diminishes grip strength.

Measuring Grip with the Jamar Dynamometer

To use the normative values established by Mathiowetz and co-workers,[6-8] you must use the standardized procedures, which include verbal commands. If you alter the procedure in any way, your data should not be compared to the norms.

Calibration accuracy of the dynamometer is certainly critical to using the normative data. There are currently three versions of the Jamar dynamometer: version A, the older gray, metal style with a dial readout; version B, one with a digital readout; and version C, a newer black model with a flat, rather than sloping, handle. Model A was used to establish the Mathiowetz norms.[6,8] The newer model (C) is considered to have greater accuracy than version A. A comparison study showed 6 to 12 percent higher scores with version C compared to version A.[11] This should be factored in when using normative data.

No simple clinical method exists for testing the accuracy of a dynamometer. One possible solution is to do a standardized trial on staff members when a new dynamometer is purchased or when one is recalibrated at the factory. Therapists could then retest themselves periodically. If scores begin to vary by more than 5 percent, the other staff members could be tested. If the scores are off for several staff members, the dynamometer probably needs recalibration.

If you are in a clinical situation where you *do not* want to use the norms—if, for example, your main interest in measuring grip is to evaluate progress by comparing the patient to himself or to compare one hand to the contralateral hand—you can develop your own protocol, as long as it is administered consistently on each retest. But again, you *should not* compare the results to the norms.

Standardized Procedures from Mathiowetz and Co-Workers[6-8]

Equipment. Standard Jamar dynamometer (not the digital type) with accurate calibration from the factory.

Procedure
1. Determine hand dominance; test the dominant hand first.
2. Test grip before pinch.
3. Seat the patient. Test with
   a. Shoulder adducted and in neutral rotation
   b. Elbow flexed at 90 degrees
   c. Forearm in neutral
   d. Wrist at 0 to 30-degree extension and 0 to 15-degree ulnar deviation
4. Three successive trials should be recorded.
5. The adjustable handle is set at the second notch from the dial for all patients.
6. The dynamometer is held lightly around the dial to prevent accidental dropping.
7. *Verbal instructions:* "I want you to hold the handle like this and squeeze as hard as you can." The examiner demon-

strates and then gives the dynamometer to the subject. After the subject is positioned appropriately, the examiner says, "Are you ready? Squeeze as hard as you can." As the subject begins to squeeze, say, "Harder! . . . Harder! . . . Relax." After the first trial score is recorded, the test is repeated with the same instructions for the second and third trial and for the other hand. (*Note:* This testing procedure with a hard dynamometer is not appropriate for people with inflamed MCP or PIP joints because they can be damaged by excessive force.)

8. *Scoring:* Use the average of three trials. (This measure has the highest reliability).[6] Normative data are available in references 6 and 7.

Measuring Grip with an Adapted Sphygmomanometer

A standard mercury sphygmomanometer can be used with all patients who have grip strength of less than 300 mm Hg (approximately 70 pounds). It is necessary to use a dynamometer with patients who have a grip of 70 pounds or more.

The sphygmomanometer is adapted by rolling up the cuff and securing it so that when inflated to a specific point the cuff attains a constant circumference. The point of inflation and the size of the circumference are arbitrary. The most common circumference sizes are 6, 7, and 8 inches, with starting points of 20, 30, and 40 mm Hg, respectively. However, the only normative data gathered to date have been on a cuff with an 8-inch circumference and a starting point of 40 mm Hg.[12]

Note: When ordering a sphygmomanometer for this purpose, request a *cloth* arm cuff. The new models come with a nylon cuff that is difficult to roll and to stabilize.

Procedure
The following are two methods for adapting a sphygmomanometer for grip strength (Fig. 21–1). An aneroid sphygmomanometer may be used; however, it is easier to maintain the starting point with a mercury sphygmomanometer.[4]

Method I (Fig. 21–1)

1. Make a bag to hold the cuff using a nonslippery, nonstretch, washable preshrunk material.
2. The size of the bag should allow the

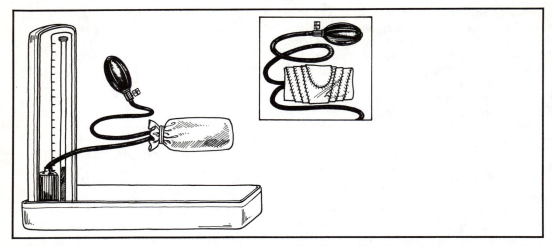

Figure 21–1. How to adapt a sphygmomanometer for grip strength is indicated: method I (*left*); method II (*inset*). (See text for explanation.)

cuff to expand to the desired circumference when inflated to the initial starting point (e.g., a 3½-inch wide bag will allow for a 7-inch circumference).

Method II (Fig. 21–1)

1. Roll up the cuff starting with the bladder end until it is about 6 inches in circumference when deflated. Tape with masking tape.

2. Inflate the cuff to the selected starting point, either 20, 30, or 40 mm Hg. Adjust the cuff until it has the desired circumference of 6, 7, or 8 inches.

3. Remove tape and pin, then whip stitch the edges, being careful not to puncture the rubber.

Have the patient seated for the procedure. Inflate the sphygmomanometer to the designated starting point (e.g., 30 mm Hg). (Be sure there is no pressure on the cuff when this is done.) Have the patient grip the cuff as hard as possible. Test each hand three times, alternating hands to minimize the fatigue factor. The forearm or hand *should not* rest on the table or lap and should be in midrotation to start with. After each recording, make sure the mercury returns to the designated starting point.[4]

Every method possible for recording results has been reported in the literature; however, the following method seems the most reliable and is the one I use.[4] How-

ever, it has not been tested for validity or reliability.

1. Record three readings and report an average of the three; this can significantly reduce the error factor. (In a study on grip strength in Scotland, investigators found the first reading had a significantly higher range of error over the second and third readings.[13]

2. Record the highest sustained pressure with each test. This can be difficult. If the patient grips slowly, there is no problem, but if he or she grips hard and fast, the mercury will show a high initial spurt because of the momentum of the mercury (not the muscle strength). Do no record spurts that appear as a result of momentum but record the sustained high point.

Caution: If the purpose of the test is to determine the patient's functional strength, the mercury column *should not* be in view of the patient nor should the therapist offer verbal encouragement. However, if the purpose is to determine absolute muscle function (e.g., in a drug study) encouragement or visual feedback may be desired. *Whatever is done must be consistent with each patient and each retest.*

Pinch Strength

Because the surface contact between the pinch-measuring device and the fingers is minimal, the design of the equipment is not as crucial as it is for measuring grip strength. Most standard pinch gauges are sensitive enough for low measurements. Mathiowetz and co-workers have found the pinch gauge manufactured by B & L Engineering to be the most accurate.[6,14] Normative data for three types of pinch have been established for adults and children using the following protocol.

Standardized Procedures from Mathiowetz and Co-Workers[6-8]

Equipment. B & L Engineering pinch gauge with accurate calibration (this can be determined by suspending a known weight from the finger grooves).

Procedure

1. Determine hand dominance; test the dominant hand first.
2. Test grip before pinch.
3. Seat the patient. Test with
    a. Shoulder adducted and in neutral rotation
    b. Elbow flexed at 90 degrees
    c. Forearm in neutral
    d. Wrist at 0 to 30-degree extension and 0 to 15-degree ulnar deviation
Note: To maintain the standard position during testing, present the gauge with the dial face up for lateral pinch and on its side for 2-point tip and 3-point pad (palmar) pinch.
4. Read gauge on needle side of red marker.
5. Three successive trials should be recorded.
6. The gauge is held by the examiner at the distal end to prevent dropping. (New gauges come with a cord loop to slip over the examiner's wrist as a safety measure against dropping.)

7. Give verbal instruction:
    a. 3-point pad (palmar) pinch: "I want you to place your thumb on this side and your first two fingers on this side as I'm doing and pinch as hard as you can." The examiner demonstrates the position and gives the pinch gauge to the subject. After the subject is positioned appropriately, the examiner says, "Are you ready? Pinch as hard as you can." As the subject begins to pinch, say, "Harder! ... Harder! ... Relax." After the first trial score is recorded, the test is repeated with the same instructions for the second and third trials and for the other hand.
    b. 2-point tip pinch: "I want you to place the tip of your thumb on this side and the tip of your index finger on this side as if to make an O. Curl your other finger into your palm as I'm doing." The examiner demonstrates the position and gives the pinch gauge to the subject. After the subject is positioned appropriately, the examiner repeats the series of questions and statements used for testing palmar pinch.
    c. Lateral (key) pinch: "I want you to place your thumb on top and your index finger below as I'm doing and pinch as hard as you can." The examiner demonstrates the position and gives the pinch gauge to the subject. After the subject is positioned appropriately, the examiner repeats the series of questions and statements used for testing palmar pinch.
8. *Scoring:* Use the average of three trials. (This measure has the highest reliability.) Normative data are available in references 7 and 8.
Note: Testing using verbal encouragement should not be used with patients who have acute synovitis of the thumb and finger joints.

REFERENCES

1. Daniels, L, and Worthington, C: Muscle Testing: Techniques of Manual Examination. WB Saunders, Philadelphia, 1972.
2. Kendall, HO, Kendall, FP, and Wadsworth, GE: Muscles: Testing and Function, 2nd ed. Williams & Wilkins, Baltimore, 1971.
3. Smidt, GL: Strength Testing—A System Based on Mechanics. Spark Instruments and Academics, Inc, PO Box 5123, Coralville, IA 52241.
4. Melvin, J: Rheumatic Disease: Occupational

Therapy and Rehabilitation. FA Davis, Philadelphia, 1977.
5. Kellor, M et al: Hand strength and dexterity: Norms for clinical usage: Age and sex comparisons. Am J Occup Ther 25:77, 1971.
6. Mathiowetz, V, Weber, K, Volland, G, and Kashman, N: Reliability and validity of grip pinch and strength evaluations. J Hand Surg 9A:222–226, 1984.
7. Mathiowetz, V, Kashman, N, Volland, G, Weber,

K, Dowe, M, and Rogers, S: Grip and pinch strength: Normative data for adults. Arch Phys Med Rehabil 66:69–74, 1985.

8. Mathiowetz, V, Wiemer, DM, and Federman, SM: Grip and pinch strength: Norms for 6- to 19-year-olds. Am J Occup Ther 40(10):705–711, 1986.

9. Fess, E, and Moran, C: Clinical Assessment Recommendations. American Society of Hand Therapists, 1981.

10. Kirkpatrick, JE: Evaluation of grip loss: Factor of permanent disability in California. Calif Med 85:314–320, 1956.

11. Flood-Joy, MM, and Mathiowetz, V: Grip strength measurement: A comparison of three Jamar dynamometers. Occup Ther J Res June–July, 1987.

12. Robinson, HS et al: Functional results of excisional arthroplasty for the rheumatoid hand. Can Med J 108:1495, 1973.

13. Lee, P et al: An assessment of grip strength measurement in rheumatoid arthritis. Scand J Rheum 3:17, 1974.

14. B & L Engineering, Santa Fe Springs, CA, 90670.

ADDITIONAL SOURCES

Measurement of Grip Strength for Both Sphygmomanometer and Dynamometer

Ager, CL, Olivett, BL, and Johnson, CL: Grasp and pinch strength in children 5–12 years old. Am J Occup Ther 38:107, 1984.

Anderson, WF, and Cowan, NR: Hand grip pressure in older people. Br J Prev Soc Med 20:141, 1966.

Bechtol, CO: The use of a dynamometer with adjustable handle spacings. J Bone Joint Surg 36:4, 1954.

Bower, LE: Investigation of the relationship of hand size and lower arm girth to hand grip strength as measured by hand dynamometers. Res Quart 32:308–314, 1961.

Bowie, W, and Cumming, GR: Sustained handgrip in boys and girls: Variation and correlation with performance and motivation to train. Res Quart 43:131–141, 1972.

Burke, WE, Tuttle, WW, Thompson, CW, Janney, CD, and Weber, RJ: The relation of grip strength and grip strength endurance to age. J Appl Physiol 5:628–630, 1953.

Caleb, B: Fluid squeeze dynamometer. Physiotherapy 48:3, 1968.

Carthum, C, Clawson, D, and Decker, J: Functional assessment of the rheumatoid hand. Am J Occup Ther 23:122–125, 1969.

Cousins, GF: Effects of trained and untrained testers upon the administration of grip strength tests. Res Quart 26:273, 1955.

Drake, BL: Gross motor skills and hand grip in the elderly: A pilot study. Am J Occup Ther 34:274, 1980.

Fike, ML, Laurita, M, and Rousseau, E: Measurement of adult hand strength: A comparison of two instruments. Occup Ther J Res 2:43, 1982.

Fisher, MB, and Birren, JB: Standardization of a test of hand strength. J Appl Psychol 380–387, 1946.

Kai-nan, A, Chao, EYS, and Asker, LJ: Hand strength measurements (using special designed strain-gauge instruments). Arch Phys Med Rehabil 61:366, 1980.

Lee, P, Baxter, A, Dick, WC, and Webb, J: An assessment of grip strength measurement in rheumatoid arthritis. Scand J Rheumatol 3:17, 1974. (Uses a sphygmomanometer.)

MacBain, KP: Assessment of function in the rheumatoid hand. Can J Occup Ther 37:95, 1970. (Describes use of a sphygmomanometer.)

Montoye, HJ, and Faulkner, JA: Determination of optimum setting of an adjustable grip strength. Res Quart 35:29–36, 1964.

Myers, DB, Grenna, DM, and Palmer, DG: Hand grip function in patients with rheumatoid arthritis (using an electric dynamometer). Arch Phys Med Rehabil 61:369, 1980.

Pearson, R, MacKinnon, MJ, Mark AP et al: Diurnal and sequential grip functions in normal subjects and effects of temperature change and exercise of the forearm on grip function in patients with RA and normal controls. Scand J Rheum 11:113, 1982.

Pryce, J: The wrist position between neutral and ulnar deviation that facilitates maximum power grip strength. J Biomech 13:505, 1980.

Rose, GA et al: A sphygomomanometer for epidemiologists. Lancet 1:296, 1964.

Schmidt, RI, and Toews, JV: Grip strength as measured for the Jamar dynamometer. Arch Phys Med Rehabil 5:321, 1970.

Scott, JT: Morning stiffness in rheumatoid arthritis. Ann Rheum Dis 19:361, 1960. (Describes use of an adapted sphygmomanometer that records up to 600 mm Hg.)

Smith, RO, and Benge, MW: Pinch and grasp strength: Standardization of terminology and protocol. Am J Occup Ther 39(8):531, 1985.

Sollerman, C, and Sperling, L: Grip function of the healthy hand in a standardized hand function test. Scand J Rehab Med 9:123–129, 1977.

Teraoka, T: Studies on the peculiarity of grip strength in relation to body positions and age. Kobe J Medical Science 25:1–17, 1979.

Tuttle, WW, Janney, CD, and Thompson, CW: Relation to maximum grip strength to grip strength endurance. J Appl Physiol 2:663–670, 1950.

Wainerdi, HR: Simple ergometers for measuring strength of hand grip. JAMA 144:8, 1950.

Weiss, MW, and Flatt, A: Pinch strength and hand size in the growing child: A pilot study of 198 normal children. Am J Occup Ther 25:10, 1971.

Wilson-MacDonald, J, Caughey, MA, and Myers, DB: Diurnal variation in nerve conduction, hand volume, and grip strength in the carpal tunnel syndrome. Br Med J [Clin Res] 289(6451):1042, 1984.

Chapter 22

Evaluation of Activities of Daily Living at Home, Work, and Leisure

The concept of activities of daily living (ADL) was introduced in rehabilitation at a time when most patients requiring rehabilitation had a severe disability that prevented return to work or were housewives who did not work outside the home. Consequently, most ADL assessments focused on self-care and household activities. Now, with the majority of women in the work force and the majority of patients with rheumatic disease treated on an outpatient basis, assessing only self-care and housework is no longer adequate. For the employed person, the ADL assessment should include daily activities in the workplace. Treatment such as joint protection, energy conservation, and assistive devices should include the workplace and leisure activities.

The assessment of self-care and school activities for children is included in Chapter 15.

PURPOSE OF THE ADL EVALUATION

The primary goal of the evaluation is to provide a database necessary for effective treatment planning that will (1) reduce pain from needless stress, (2) increase functional independence, and (3) prevent unnecessary deformity (through patient education). Secondarily the assessment can serve as a measure of change following treatment. The ADL assessment should answer the following questions:

1. Is the patient performing any daily tasks that are causing pain or potentially deforming stresses to his or her involved joints?

and

Are there adaptive methods, instructions, or equipment that could minimize or eliminate the pain or joint stress in these activities?

2. Is the patient limited in performing daily tasks as a result of a physical limitation?

and

Are there adaptive methods or equipment that could increase the patient's independence or ability in these tasks?

(The need for physical treatment is determined by the musculoskeletal evaluation.)

METHOD OF ASSESSMENT

The evaluation procedure can take several forms: interview, observation of patient performance (timed or untimed), or patient self-report. Usually a full evaluation is a combination of all three. The choice depends on the following:

1. The nature of the patient's disability
2. The patient's reliability in reporting
3. The clinical setting in which the evaluation is taking place
4. The reason for the assessment
5. The level of disease activity: acute, subacute, chronic

For example, interview and patient self-report may be sufficient for an ADL assessment on an employed man with chronic degenerative joint disease of the knees in an outpatient clinic; however, interview, self-report, and demonstration of tub/

shower transfer ability may be indicated for a severely disabled inpatient. *Interview and self-report are not sufficient and patient demonstration is essential for accurate assessment of functional ability in patients with (1) severe multiple joint involvement, (2) recent onset of disease or an increase in debility (when they may not be aware of their limitations), or (3) psychological overlay.*

The nursing assessment can provide a valuable resource for understanding the hospitalized patient's actual, rather than reported, functional ability. The nurse's observations and chart report should be considered before finalizing the ADL treatment plan.

SPECIAL FACTORS TO CONSIDER

Factors that are typical of rheumatic disease patients and that need special consideration in the ADL evaluation are

1. Morning stiffness (duration, location, severity)
2. Percent of good days versus bad days
3. Fatigue (time of onset, duration) and endurance
4. Pain during activities
5. Medication (amount, type, when taken, if taken)
6. ARA functional classification

These factors are discussed in detail in Chapter 18, Evaluation of Medical History and Symptoms. In addition to these medical conditions, seven activity areas need special attention.

1. Positioning at night and during leisure activities such as watching television or reading
2. Use and height of seats for lower extremity problems (bed, chairs, toilet) in the home or at work
3. Amount of stair climbing for patients with lower extremity involvement
4. Use and height of work surfaces and materials for neck and back involvement
5. Ability of the patient to use private or public transportation
6. Taking medication (ability to open bottles, swallowing, or problems with remembering)[1,2]

7. Quality of sleeping mattress and pillow—appropriateness for medical condition

WHEN THE SELF-CARE EVALUATION SHOULD BE DONE

The time of the day that the evaluation is done is an important factor. It also needs to be taken into account when doing re-evaluations and longitudinal comparisons. This is especially true for the patient with morning stiffness or poor endurance. An ADL evaluation (with demonstration) done on a patient with rheumatoid arthritis at 2:00 PM only provides information about how the patient performs in the afternoon, and this can be quite different from the person's performance in the morning when stiffness is at a maximum.

In assessing outpatients it is important to determine their early morning functional status as well as their ability during the clinic evaluation. In assessing inpatients, an early morning (before breakfast) evaluation has the advantage of providing information about the patient's most dysfunctional state, but this may not be representative of his or her average level throughout the day. A more representative assessment is possible for both inpatients and outpatients, when it occurs at midday and precedes physical therapy, especially hydrotherapy.

EMOTIONAL FACTORS TO CONSIDER DURING THE ASSESSMENT

Regardless of whether an interview or demonstration is done, the ADL evaluation is a very personal procedure. It is as personal as going into the doctor's office and undressing for an examination. Not only is the patient going through a literal or figurative undressing, but also, as the procedure takes place, the patient has to discuss his or her worst attributes, that is, list inabilities.

No matter how empathetic the therapist is, there is no way of completing an ADL assessment by stressing only the positive aspects. One avenue open for positive counteraction is in giving the patient feedback about the positive things that can be done to increase his or her independence. But in order for the therapist to be able to give this kind of feedback, the therapist needs to know the patient's physical status before starting the ADL evaluation.

ACTIVITIES IN THE WORKPLACE— VOCATIONAL ASSESSMENT

In rheumatology, assessment of a person's vocational activities is needed in two distinct situations:

1. When the arthritis *does not* interfere with his or her ability to continue employment. The patient is working and "employability" is not an issue. In this case, the purpose of the assessment is to plan strategies to reduce physical and emotional stress and pain, and improve endurance and function. This is basically an extension of the ADL assessment to the workplace.

2. When the arthritis *does* interfere with a person's ability to continue employment. In this case, the purpose of the assessment is to determine appropriate referral options. If the disease is severe and the person cannot find suitable work, then he or she may have to collect disability insurance. For some manual laborers or blue-collar workers, mild to moderate disease can prohibit continued employment. People in these situations should be referred to a counselor at the state department of rehabilitation. The work-capacity evaluation and work hardening play a limited role in the face of progressive active disease.

This section will focus on what to do when the person is still working, because this situation is by far the most common and holds the greatest potential for prevention and to influence the patient's health. The nature of a person's vocation, the physical requirements of the work, the amount of control a person has to vary the job to accommodate symptoms, the support given by co-workers and employer, and the amount of enjoyment that a person derives from the work are all factors that play a powerful role in a person's health and illness. Consequently, reducing physical and emotional stress in the workplace can reduce fatigue and influence the immune system and reduce symptomatology.

Assessment

The tasks and environmental factors in the workplace are much more varied than in the home, so no single assessment questionnaire is adequate for use in all work situations. The following questions provide a loose structure to assess the major areas of physical and emotional stress and functioning in the workplace.

Preparing for Work

1. What are the effects of morning stiffness when preparing for work and at the beginning of the work day?

2. How hectic or stressful is the morning preparation time? Is there anything that could make the morning time more manageable? For example, morning time can be hectic if a young child or more than one child must be readied for school.

3. What are the person's scheduled work hours?

Transportation

4. How does the person get to work? Commuting will be made easier or more difficult depending on the level of stiffness at the beginning of the day and fatigue at the end of the day.

5. What is the person's commute time and distance?

Work Setting

6. What are the physical working conditions? If a desk or work station is used, what type are they? What type of seating is available?

7. Where is this work area in relation to other facilities, for example, the cafeteria, restrooms, meeting rooms, parking?

8. What are the walking, standing, and sitting requirements of the job? Does the person walk to other floors or buildings or sit in one place all day? Are there elevators or escalators?

9. What are the writing or hand skill requirements?

10. What level of strength is needed to do the job? What is the weight of material that must be lifted, carried, lowered, pulled, or pushed? Is this work done in a standing, sitting, or walking posture? Levels of strength needed in work are described as sedentary, light, medium, heavy, and very heavy work.

11. What are the stooping, kneeling, crawling, and crouching requirements, in terms of frequency and duration?

12. What are the climbing and balancing requirements, in terms of frequency and type, e.g., are ladders, stairs, or scaffolds used?

13. If the person works in a confined space, does this create excessive strain on the joints?

14. What are the environmental risk factors of the workplace? Consider the exposure to toxic chemicals and fumes, heat or cold, sun, dangerous mechanical processes, radiation, air pollution, excessive noise, and inadequate lighting. These factors can create additional physical and psychological stress at work.

Lunch and Rest Breaks

15. What are the nature, quality, and length of breaks?

16. Does the person hurriedly eat junk food from a machine for lunch at his or her desk in a busy office while working? Or is there a pleasant, relaxed area in which to eat and take a 45- to 60-minute lunch break?

17. Is a pleasant, smoke-free rest area available? (Even smokers hate smoke-filled rooms.)

18. Is there a quiet place where the person could practice a relaxation exercise?

19. If the person eats in a cafeteria, can he or she handle the tray, dishes, cups, and so forth?

20. Does the person take advantage of available rest breaks, and if so, how?

21. Nutrition and eating patterns can have a major influence on fatigue. For example, sugar and caffeine create a temporary energy high that a few hours later depletes energy and causes fatigue. Mild dehydration, associated with not drinking

water or liquids for long periods of time, can also bring on fatigue. Eating foods high in fat can slow one's metabolism, which also increases the feeling of tiredness. (If you would like to do counseling on this subject, ask a nutritionist familiar with these concepts to give an inservice presentation to your occupational therapy department.)

Work Activities

22. What activities at work aggravate joints or symptoms the most? How does the person handle these activities? What adaptive methods are used?

23. What power or control does the person have to alter the work to reduce joint stress or accommodate symptoms?

Interpersonal Relationships

24. Are the person's supervisor and co-workers supportive and pleasant to work with, or is there interpersonal strife?

25. Do the person's supervisor and co-workers know that the person has arthritis or back pain? If yes, what is their reaction? If no, how does this affect the person at work?

26. What are the sources of psychological stress on the job? For example, what is the nature of the person's relationship with the boss and co-workers? What is the amount of work to be done? What is the schedule? Is the person bored at work?

27. Does the person avoid taking actions at work that would reduce his or her pain, such as stretching during breaks, using orthoses, using ice packs, or using a cane, because others would react negatively?

If a person has mild arthritis or pain that does not require any special consideration, there may be no need to tell co-workers about it. But if a supervisor and co-workers do not know about a serious involvement, then this suggests that the person has significant feelings of denial or lack of self-acceptance. These feelings and the "keeping a secret" process can be sources of emotional stress. A person may also avoid telling an employer if there is fear of discriminatory reprisal—unfortunately, a very real situation in many jobs.

HOME ASSESSMENT

The ideal method for a home assessment is an on-site home visit. Such a visit affords a unique opportunity to

1. Assess architectural barriers in the home that limit the patient's functional independence.

2. Give the patient specific instructions on how to adapt his or her furniture or home to minimize joint stress and improve function.

3. Assess the quality of home life in terms of family attitudes, interpersonal relationships, cooperation, and stress factors that significantly influence patient compliance.

4. Assess the ease or difficulty of maintaining the house and yard. (Homes that are cluttered or have poorly divided work areas require more energy to maintain than homes with adequate space.)

The procedure for the home assessment depends primarily on the patient's ambulation status. When ambulation aids or wheelchairs are involved, the assessment is essentially the same as for patients with ambulation aids in nonarthritic disorders. There are a few exceptions. The height of chairs or seats is an important consideration for joint protection of the knees for people using crutches, canes, or walkers. The type and height of chairs can also influence neck positioning during reading or leisure activities.

The type of handrim is a special consideration for people using wheelchairs. Regular wheelchair handrims increase ulnar drift deformity. For clients with beginning ulnar drift (or the potential for it), handrims with projections or knobs are preferred since they can be used in a non-deforming manner. However, these projections increase the width of the wheelchair and may limit accessibility through inside passageways and doorways.

In general the home assessment should include the following:

1. Evaluation of the safety and accessibility of entrances and passageways

2. Types of floor coverings, especially if ambulation aides or a wheelchair is used

3. Patient's ability to open, close, and lock windows and doors (If a person is disabled, methods of escape in event of fire should be explored.)

4. Accessibility of light switches, outlets, and heat controls

5. Height of counters, tables, tub, bed, and chairs

6. Consideration of work areas in regard to work-simplification and energy-conservation measures

7. Ease of use of faucets, locks, controls

The slide/tape program developed by Tillman and Haviland is an excellent resource for reviewing these criteria. (See resource list at the end of the chapter.)

SAMPLE ADL AND HOME ASSESSMENT FORMS

Two ADL and home assessment forms are included here as samples to stimulate thinking and to provide a starting point for therapists to develop their own forms. Each occupational therapy clinic serves a unique population and each therapist has a different assessment bias or technique. Forms developed in a clinic should reflect these differences.

The first sample form is a screening form I developed for use in an arthritis medical clinic. This screening interview takes approximately 10 to 15 minutes and was designed as a case-finding tool—to determine if patients could benefit from a complete evaluation and treatment. A copy of the form was kept in the patient's clinic chart for a medical record and to orient resident physicians as to some of the activities of daily living that need consideration. Notations on status were spelled out for physicians not familiar with occupational therapy jargon.

The second form is a complete ADL assessment developed for patients with rheumatic diseases. Parts 1 and 3 were designed at the Los Angeles County-University of Southern California (LAC-USC) Medical Center. Part 2 was developed by the Canadian Arthritis and Rheumatism Society (C.A.R.S.) of British Columbia. The sequence of the C.A.R.S. form has been reordered and items on female hygiene, child care, endurance, and housework assistance added. Part 3, Occupational Therapy Recommendations, has proven extremely valuable for emphasizing or summarizing the many joint-protection or safety suggestions made to patients during the ADL assessment or treatment sessions. For example, a patient may consider a recommendation to put safety strips or a safety mat in the tub to be a casual, common-sense suggestion. Formally writing it out as a professional recommendation often makes the patient appreciate the structure and purpose of the ADL assessment.

LITERATURE ON ADL ASSESSMENTS

Most of the research and development of ADL assessments in occupational therapy has been done on an individual clinic basis. Each clinic has either adapted an established assessment or developed its own evaluation forms and procedures.

Most assessments involve an ADL analysis checklist with or without a scoring procedure. Two reports that utilize a standardized ADL assessment procedure with rheumatic disease patients have been published and are mentioned here for therapists who wish to develop or incorporate a quantitative ADL assessment procedure in their program. Dr. Edward Lowman used an itemized ADL assessment (106 items) scored on the basis of "percentage of functional deficiency" (percentage of items the patient was not capable of performing).[3] Dr. H. Robinson and Ms. D. Bashall, O.T.Reg., at the Canadian Arthritis and Rheumatism Society (C.A.R.S.) in British Columbia developed a timed "self-care assessment" that quantitates the patient's performance as a percentage of normal time range for all basic dressing tasks; for example, putting on a blouse: normal time 15 to 25 seconds.[4]

K. P. MacBain, O.T.Reg., has published the only functional assessment specially related to children with arthritis.[5] I. L. Coley, O.T.Reg., has published a text addressing evaluation of self-care skills in children.[6] (See Chapter 15 for ADL assessment of children.)

FUNCTIONAL ASSESSMENTS VERSUS ADL ASSESSMENTS

A major area of concern in the treatment of chronic disease is the determination of patient progress or outcome as a result of medical, surgical, or rehabilitative intervention. A wide range of instruments described as functional assessments has been developed for this purpose. These functional assessments differ from ADL assessments in that they tend to be more general and are designed to be administered by physicians or research assistants with the overall objective of measuring change in the patient. ADL assessments are primarily designed for treatment planning and therefore are very detailed in format. For example, most functional assessments do not include specific questions about the patient's ability to write or to open food packages. (See Additional Sources at the end of this chapter.)

REFERENCES

1. Lisberg, RB, Higham, C, and Jayson, MI: Problems for rheumatic patients in opening dispensed drug containers. Br J Rheumatol 22(2):95–98, 1983.
2. Lambert, JR, Hopkins, R, Wright, V, and Cardoe, N: Child-resistant containers: An appraisal in arthritic patients. Rheumatol Rehabil 17:89–90, 1978.
3. Lowman, EW: Rehabilitation of the rheumatoid cripple: A five-year study. Arthritis Rheum 1:38, 1958.
4. Robinson, H, and Bashall, D: Functional assessment in rheumatoid arthritis. Can J Occup Ther 29:123–138, 1962. (Reprinted in Ehrilich, G (ed): Total Management of the Arthritic Patient. JB Lippincott, Philadelphia, 1973.)
5. Coley, IL: Pediatric Self-Care Evaluation. CV Mosby, St Louis, 1978.
6. MacBain, KP, and Hill, RH: A functional assessment for juvenile rheumatoid arthritis. Am J Occup Ther 27(6):326, 1973.

ADDITIONAL SOURCES

Architectural and Accessibility Barrier Assessment

American National Standard for Making Buildings and Facilities Accessible and Usable for Physically Handicapped People. American National Standards Association, New York, 1980.
Bingham, B: Cooking with Fragile Hands. Creative Cuisine, Inc, PO Box 578, Naples, FL 3339.
Dickson, TL: Adaptations for independent infant care by mothers who are disabled. In Cromwell, FS (ed): Occupational Therapy Strategies and Adaptations for Independent Daily Living. Haworth Press, New York, 1984, pp 69–77.
Kliment, SA: Into the Mainstream: A Syllabus for a Barrier-Free Environment. RSA, HEW, Washington, DC, 1975.
Resource Guide to Literature and Barrier Free Environments. Architectural and Transportation Compliance Board, Washington, DC, 1981.
Sorensen, RJ: Design for Accessibility. McGraw-Hill, New York.

Taira, ED: An occupational therapist's perspective on environmental adaptations for the disabled elderly. In Cromwell, FS (ed): Occupational Therapy Strategies and Adaptations for Independent Daily Living. Haworth Press, New York, 1984, pp 25–33.
Tica, P: Barrier-Free: Accessibility for the Handicapped. Institute for Research and Development in Occupational Education, 1411 Broadway, New York, NY 10018.

Community Assessment

Boblitz, MH: Transportation evaluation, counseling, and training. In Ehrlich, GE (ed): Rehabilitation Management of Rheumatic Conditions. Williams & Wilkins, Baltimore, 1980.
Chamberlain, MA, Buchanan, JM, and Hands, H: The arthritic in an urban environment. Ann Rheum Dis 38:51, 1979.
Rosenthal, D, Boblitz, MH, and Rao, VR: Bus use by disabled arthritics: Functional requirements. Arch Phys Med Rehabil 58:220, May 1977.

General Functional Assessments

Berendsin, EMJ, and Heijne-van der Kleij, MF: Rehabilitation aspects of rheumatoid arthritis. Part III. Activities of daily living. Analysis and treatment of patients with rheumatoid arthritis. EULAR Bulletin (Basel) 12(3):88–92, 1983.
Chambers, LW, MacDonald, LA, Tugwell, P, Buchanan, WW, and Kraag, G: The McMaster Health Index Questionnaire as a measure of quality of life for patients with rheumatoid disease. J Rheumatol 9:780–784, 1982.
Conaty, JP, and Nickel, VL: Functional incapacitation in rheumatoid arthritis: Rehabilitation challenge. J Bone Joint Surg 58:624, 1971. (A correlative study of function before and after hospital treatment.)
Convery, FR, Minteer, MA, Amiel, D, and Connett, KL: Polyarticular disability: A functional assessment. Arch Phys Med Rehabil 58:494, November 1977.

Cristarella, MC: Visual functions in the elderly. Am J Occup Ther 31(7):432–440, 1977.

Donaldson, SW, Wagner, CC, and Gresham, GE: Unified ADL evaluation form. Arch Phys Med Rehabil 54:175–179, 185, 1973.

Feigenson, J, Polkow, L, Meikle, R, and Ferguson, W: Burke Stroke Time-Oriented Profile (BUSTOP): Overview of patient function. Arch Phys Med Rehabil 60:508–511, 1979.

Granger, CV: Health accounting—Functional assessment of the Long-Term Patient. In Kottke, FJ, Stillwell, GK, and Lehmann, JF: Krusen's Handbook of Physical Medicine and Rehabilitation, 3rd ed. WB Saunders, Philadelphia, 1982, pp 253–274.

Granger, CY, Albrecht, GL, and Hamilton, BB: Outcome of comprehensive medical rehabilitation: Measurement by PULSES Profile and Barthel Index. Arch Phys Med Rehabil 60:145–154, 1979.

Halsted, L, and Hartley, RB: Time care profile: Evaluation of new method of assessing ADL independence. Arch Phys Med Rehabil 56:110–115, 1975.

Jette, AM: Functional status instrument: Reliability of a chronic disease evaluation instrument. Arch Phys Med Rehabil 61:395–401, 1980.

Katz, S, Ford, AB, Moskowitz, RW, Jackson, BA, and Jaffe, MW: Studies of illness in aged: Index of ADL: Standardized measure of biological and psychological function. JAMA 185:914–919, 1963.

Liang, MH, and Jette, AM: Measuring functional ability in chronic arthritis. Arthritis Rheum 24:80–86, 1981.

Liang, MH, Cullen, KE, and Larson, MG: Measuring function and health status in rheumatic disease clinical trials. Clin Rheum Dis 9:531–539, 1983.

Mahoney, FI, and Barthel, DW: Functional evaluation. Barthel Index. MD State Med J 14:61–65, 1965.

Meenan, RF, Gertman, PM, and Mason, JH: Measuring health status in arthritis. Arthritis Rheum 23:146–152, 1980.

Meenan, RF, Gertman, PM, Mason, JH, and Dunaif, R: The arthritis impact measurement scales. Arthritis Rheum 25(9):1048–1053, 1982.

Potts, MK, and Brandt, KD: Evidence of the validity of the Arthritis Impact Measurement Scales. Arthritis Rheum 30(1):93–96, 1987.

Potvin, AR, Tourtellotte, WW, Dailey, JS, Albers, JW, Walker, JE, Pew, RW, Henderson, WG, and Snyder, DN: Simulated activities of daily living examination. Arch Phys Med Rehabil 53:476–486, 1972.

Sarno, JE, Sarno, MT, and Levita, E: Functional life scale. Arch Phys Med Rehabil 54:214–220, 1973.

Schoening, HA, and Iverson, IA: Numerical scoring of self-care status: Study of Kenney self-care evaluation. Arch Phys Med Rehabil 49:221–229, 1986.

Sheikh, K, Smith, DS, Meade, TW, Goldenberg, E, Brennan, PJ, and Kinsella, G: Repeatability and validity of a modified activites of daily living index in studies of chronic disability. Int Rehabil Med 1:51–58, 1979.

Home Assessment

Buchwald, E: ADL for Physical Rehabilitation. McGraw-Hill, New York, 1963. (Primary transfer training, functional assessment carried out by physical therapy.)

Cooper, S: Accidents and older adults. Geriatric Nursing 2(4):287–290, 1981.

Duurland, E: Rehabilitation aspects of rheumatoid arthritis. Part V. Home adaptation. EULAR Bulletin (Basel) 13(1):4–7, 1984.

Immink, J: Rehabilitation aspects of rheumatoid arthritis. Part IV. Domestic activities. EULAR Bulletin (Basel) 12(4):128–132, 1983.

Loomis, B: The home visit: An integral part of OT for patients with rheumatic diseases. Am J Occup Ther 19:264, 1965. (Only source on home visits for people with arthritis.)

Notelovitz, M, and Ware, M: The monetary cost. In Stand Tall: The Informed Woman's Guide to Preventing Osteoporosis. Triad Publishing, Gainesville, FL, 1982, p 40.

Peszczynski, M, and Fowles, B: Home Evaluations. Highland View Cuyahoga County Hospital, Highland View, IN, 1957.

Price, J: Unintentional injury among the aged. J Gerontol Nurs 4(3):36–41, 1978.

Rusk, HA et al: A Manual for Training the Disabled Homemaker, 2nd ed. Rehabilitation Monograph VIII. Institute of Physical Medicine and Rehabilitation, Bellevue Medical Center, 400 E 34th Street, New York, NY 11216, 1961. (Excellent resource.)

Tillman, R, and Haviland, N: 603 Elm Street: Overcoming Barriers to Independence, #P116. University of Michigan Media Library, G1302 Towsley Center, University of Michigan Medical Center, Ann Arbor, MI 48109. (This is an excellent slide/tape program designed for health professionals: includes evaluation of home-safety factors.)

Vocational Assessment

Allen, VR: Health Promotion in the office. Am J Occup Ther 40(11):764–770, 1986.

Arthritis and Industry, Annotated Bibliography. Arthritis Information Clearinghouse, Box 9782, Arlington, VA 22209.

Bettencourt, CM, Carlstrom, P, Brown, SH, Lindau, K, and Long, CM: Using work simulation to treat adults with back injuries. Am J Occup Ther 40(1):12–18, 1986.

Budic, C: Arthritis and employment on-site job intervention. Physical Disabilities Specialty Section Newsletter AOTA 3(1), 1980.

Cooper, CL, and Payne, RE (eds): Stress at Work. John Wiley & Sons, New York, 1978.

Coulton, C: Person-environment fit and rehabilitation. In Krueger, DW: Rehabilitation Psychology: A Comprehensive Textbook. Aspen, Rockville, MD, 1984.

Cromwell, FS: Work-related programs in occupational therapy. Haworth Press, New York, 1985. (Previously published as Occupational Therapy in Health Care, vol 2, no 4, 1985–1986.)

Fike, ML: The role of occupational therapy in psychological rehabilitation of the physically disabled. In Krueger, DW: Rehabilitation Psychology: A Comprehensive Textbook. Aspen, Rockville, MD, 1984.

A Guide to Job Analysis. Materials Development Center: Stout Vocational Rehabilitation, University of Wisconsin–Stout, Menomonie, WI, 1982.

Hadler, N: Medical ramifications of the Federal regulation of the Social Security Disability Insurance Program. Ann Int Med 96(5):665–669, 1982.

Hadler, NM, and Gillings, DB (eds): Arthritis and Society. Butterworth, Boston, 1985.

Holmes, D: The role of the occupational therapist-work evaluator. Am J Occup Ther 39(5):308–313, 1985.

Lytel, RB, and Botterbusch, KF: Physical Demands Job Analysis: A New Approach. Stout Vocational Rehabilitation Institute, University of Wisconsin–Stout, Menonomie, WI, 1981.

Mathesen, LN: Work Capacity Evaluation. Employment and Rehabilitation Institute of California, Anaheim, CA, 1984.

Matheson, L, Ogden, LD, Violette, K, and Schults, K: Work hardening: Occupational therapy in industrial rehabilitation. Am J Occup Ther 39(5):314–321, 1985.

Meenan, RF, Liang, MH, and Hadler, NM: Social Security disability and the arthritis patient. Bull Rheum Dis 33(1):1–8, 1983.

Moos, R: The Human Context: Coping with Social and Physical Environments. John Wiley & Sons, New York, 1975.

Partridge, AG: Determination of Social Security disability in rheumatic diseases. Clin Rheum Prac 275–280, 1984.

Pell, KL (Committee Chairperson): Vocational Evaluation and Work Adjustment Glossary. Stout Vocational Rehabilitation Institute, University of Wisconsin–Stout, Menomonie, WI, 1977.

Pitzele, SK: We Are Not Alone—Learning to Live with Chronic Illness. Thompson & Co, Minneapolis, 1985, p 208. (See the section on modifications at work.)

Rule, WR: Lifestyle Counseling for Adjustment to Disability. Aspen, Rockville, MD, 1984.

United States Department of Labor, Employment and Training Administration: Dictionary of Occupational Titles, 4th ed. US Government Printing Office, Washington, DC, 1977.

Yelin, E, Meenan, R, Nevitt, MA, and Epstein, W: Work disability in rheumatoid arthritis: Effects of disease, social, and work factors. Ann Int Med 93(4):551–556, 1980.

Zimmer, AB: Employing the handicapped. A Practical Compliance Manual. Amacon, New York, 1981.

Vocational Assessment: Sources for Regulations, Funding, and Opportunities

American Society of Handicapped Physicians (ASHP), 137 Main Street, Grambling, LA 91245

Department of Health and Human Services, Social Rehabilitation Services, Rehabilitation Services Administration, Washington, DC 20014.

Handicapped Organization of Women (HOW), Box 35481, Charlotte, NC 28235.

President's Commission on Employment of the Handicapped, 1111 20th Street, NW, Suite 636, Washington, DC 20036.

National Rehabilitation Association, 1522 K Street, NW, Washington, DC 20005.

Vocational Guidance and Rehabilitation Services, 2289 E 55th Street, Cleveland, OH 44103.

Sample #1

ACTIVITIES OF DAILY LIVING (ADL)

SCREENING

Name: *Jane Doe*   Age: *40* Hosp. #: *123456*

DX *R.A.*   Dominance *R*

A.D.L.		Date 9/4/81	Date	Date
Dressing:	UE & torso	indep.		
	LE & torso	indep		
	fasteners	assist needed with sm. buttons		
Grooming		indep.		
Hygiene:	toilet	indep		
	bath	unable to wash back		
Transfer:	chair	low seat causes pain		
	bed	indep.		
	toilet	causes pain		
	tub	needs a bench		
	car	needs assist.		
	public trans.	unable		
Kitchen work		husband helps		
Housework		husband helps		
Marketing		husband		
Yard work		husband		
Vocational skills		NA		
Hand skills (keys, writing, jars, etc.)		indep. except for strength tasks		
Assistive Equipment				
splints		none		
ambulation aids		cane		
adaptive devices		none		
Endurance		fair		
ROM		mod. limitations		

COMMENTS: 9/4/81 *patient needs a full ADL assessment*

Sample #2

ADL ASSESSMENT (PART 1)

Name _____ File No.: _____
Address _____ Age: _____
_____ ARA Functional Class:* _____
Phone _____

Diagnosis: (*onset joint involved*)†_____
Ambulation Status: (*household, community, etc. + gait*)_____
Posture: _____
Handedness: Dominant Hand _____ Preferred Hand _____
Morning Stiffness: From _____ to about _____; Average _____ hours.
Percent of good days vs. bad days: _____
Energy Pattern:
    Hours of sleep/night? _____ hrs. from _____ to _____.
    Rest breaks during day? _____
    Rest time of day? _____
    Amount of fatigue? (*onset, duration*)_____
Medications: (*type + quantity*)_____

Home Assessment

Home and Family Situation: (*type of home; people in home, their age & health*)_____
_____
_____
Entrances: (*steps, rails, inclines?*)_____
Inside Passageways: (*width, loose rugs, electrical cords?*)_____
Types of Floor Covering: Kitchen_____
    Living Room _____ Hall_____
    Bedrooms _____ Bathroom _____
Door & Windows: (*ability to open, close, lock*)_____
Height of:
    Tub: Inside: _____ outside _____ Toilet bowl (excluding seat)_____
    Bed_____ Sofa_____
    Dining room chair_____ Living room chair_____
    Kitchen counter_____
Wheelchair Measurements
    Height of seat _____ Width_____
    Type _____ Type of handrim (*regular or with projections?*)_____
Transportation: (*method, transfer ability?*)_____

Vocation Assessment

Type of Work Setting: _____
Physical Layout‡ (*problems or hindrances*)_____

Use of Entrances _____
Use of Lavatories _____
Amount of:
    Lifting _____
    Bending _____
    Walking _____
    Sitting _____
Height of work surface _____
Height and type of chair used: _____

SPECIAL OR ADAPTIVE EQUIPMENT (currently used by patient at home or work):_____
_____
_____

_____

*This is discussed in Medical History, Chapter 13.
†Notations in parentheses are not included on the original form but are included here to indicate some of the factors considered in each section.
‡When indicated have patient draw a house plan or work layout and furniture arrangement on back of paper.

ADL ASSESSMENT (PART 2*): ACTIVITY ANALYSIS

Name: _____

Date: _____

The purpose of this questionnaire is to discover any difficulties you might have in the stated area which the therapist may be able to help you with.

Please complete the following questionnaire putting a check in the appropriate column or drawing a line through the question if it is not applicable.

I. *SELF CARE SECTION*

BEDROOM: Can you ... ?	Easily	With diff.	Not at all	Solution
move from place to place in bed				
roll to right and then to left side				
turn and lie on abdomen				
sit up in bed				
get into bed				
get out of bed				

DRESSING: Are you able to put on and take off the following articles?

Women

	Easily	With diff.	Not at all	Solution
brassiere				
girdle				
garter belt				
panties				
slip				
stockings				
socks				
shoes				
dress with front opening				
dress with side opening				
dress with back opening				
blouse				
skirt				
sweater				
coat				
hat				
gloves				
slacks				

*Adapted from material from the Canadian Arthritis and Rheumatism Society (C.A.R.S.), British Columbia.

	Easily	With diff.	Not at all	Solution
Men				
vest or undershirt				
shorts				
trousers				
shirt				
sweater				
socks				
shoes				
suit jacket				
tie				
coat				
hat				
gloves				
Men and women: Can you manage...?				
zippers				
buttons: large				
small				
hooks and eyes				
snap dome fasteners				
buckles				
safety pins				
belts				
putting hand in: back pocket				
side pocket				
brushing clothes				
hanging up or putting away clothes				
putting on working or resting splints				
TOILET: Can you manage ... ?				
getting on and off toilet				
adjusting clothing for toilet needs				
using toilet paper				
flushing toilet				
maneuvering bedpan				
getting to toilet at night				
BATH: Can you manage ... ?				
getting into a bath				
out of a bath				
into a shower				
out of a shower				
turning taps (tub & sink)				

	Easily	With diff.	Not at all	Solution
BATHING: Can you manage ... ?				
washing: feet				
hands				
back				
chest				
neck				
face				
hair				
drying self				
drying between toes				
PERSONAL CARE: Can you manage ... ?				
Men and Women				
brushing teeth				
using dental floss				
using electric razor				
safety razor				
cutting: fingernails				
toenails				
brushing and combing hair				
Women				
applying makeup				
setting hair				
shaving legs				
shaving underarms				
using sanitary napkins or tampons				
douching				
grooming eyebrows				
application of contraceptives				
AMBULATION: Can you ... ?				
walk unaided or with cane				
with crutches				
walk: up steps (if applicable)				
down steps				
up a slope				
down a slope				
turn around				
walk on rough ground				
get up and down a curb				
cross a street in 30 seconds on green light				
get down to the floor and up again				

	Easily	With diff.	Not at all	Solution
stand for more than half hour while working				
get on and off living room chair				
get on and off kitchen chair				
EATING: Can you ... ?				
use a fork				
use a spoon				
cut meat				
butter bread				
drink from a cup				
from a glass				
stir coffee, tea, etc.				
open a bottle				
pour from a bottle				
pour a cup of tea or coffee				
II. *HOUSEHOLD ACTIVITY SECTION*				
FOOD PREPARATION: Can you ... ?				
do grocery shopping				
open: tin cans				
jars				
packaged goods				
reach shelves: above countertop				
below countertop				
prepare vegetables: peel				
slice				
bake a cake or cookies:				
measure dry ingredients				
measure liquids				
break an egg				
use an eggbeater				
stir batter				
knead dough				
pour batter into pan				
open oven door				
place pan in oven				
roll dough				
use a saucepan				
fill a saucepan				
carry pan to stove				
remove hot dish from oven				
drain vegetables				
pour hot water from kettle				
pour tea and/or coffee into cups				

	Easily	With diff.	Not at all	Solution
DINING: Can you ... ?				
set table				
carry to table: full glass				
full cup & saucer				
full plate				
hot casserole				
(other)				
CLEAN UP: Can you ... ?				
scrape and stack dishes				
wash dishes				
scrub pots and pans				
pick up object from floor				
wipe up spills on floor				
sweep floor				
use dustpan				
mop floor				
shake mop				
wash floor				
clean refrigerator				
clean oven				
dispose of garbage				
(other)				
OTHER HOUSEHOLD ACTIVITIES: Can you manage ... ?				
laundry: handwashing				
wringing				
machine washing				
machine drying (open dryer door?)				
hanging on line				
ironing blouse or shirt				
folding sheets				
hanging dress on hanger				
dusting/cleaning—high and low surfaces				
vacuuming/carpet sweeper				
making beds				
changing beds				
cleaning bathtub				
picking up a pin				
threading a needle and sewing				
using scissors				
handling coins				

	Easily	With diff.	Not at all	Solution
feeding pets				
(other)				
TRANSPORTATION: Can you ... ?				
get onto a bus				
stand on bus holding overhead bar				
descend from bus				
get into a car (open car door)				
out of a car				
drive a car				
MISCELLANEOUS: Can you ... ?				
manage medicine bottles				
take own medicine				
use a telephone				
open an envelope				
write for 15 minutes				
hold a book				
turn the pages				
shuffle and hold a hand of cards				
strike a match (use cigarette lighter)				
smoke a cigarette or pipe				
wind a clock				
a watch				
type				
care for garden				
mow lawn				
sweep porch				
open and close: a door				
window				
drawer				
reach shelves at head level				
open milk cartons				
turn taps on and off				
use pull-chain light				
use light switches				
manage wall-plugs				
push buzzer, doorbell				
use spray cans				
open doors with knobs				
with keys				
pour milk from bottle to glass				
operate stove burners and oven				
operate sink taps				

	Easily	With diff.	Not at all	Solution
open and close refrigerator				
use wall plug				
(other):				

CHILD CARE OR GRANDCHILD CARE: Can you ... ?

	Easily	With diff.	Not at all	
lift a small child (e.g. under age two)				
bathe a child				
fix child's hair				
dress small child				
change diapers				
do personal hygiene for small children				

ENDURANCE:

	Easily	With diff.	Not at all	
Does an average day's housework make you:				
extremely tired				
quite tired				
only slightly tired				

What activity during the week is the most strenuous for you?

_____

ASSISTANCE:

Who will do heavy cleaning duties, e.g. waxing floor, washing windows?

_____

How often is he/she available?

_____

DAILY ROUTINE:

Briefly describe your average daily routine or schedule:

_____
_____
_____
_____
_____

RECREATIONAL OR LEISURE INTERESTS: Difficulties with these activities due to the arthritis? Please list:

_____
_____
_____
_____
_____

OCCUPATIONAL THERAPY (PART 3)

RECOMMENDATIONS BASED ON ACTIVITY OF DAILY LIVING ASSESSMENT*

For: _____ File No.: _____

Rest/Sleep:

Morning Stiffness:

Ambulation:

Entrances, steps:

Inside Passageways:

Floor Coverings:

Doors and Windows:

Seating Heights:

Wheelchair:

Bedroom:

Toilet:

Bathing:

Washing:

Personal Care:

Dressing:

Eating:

Meal Preparation:

HOUSEHOLD ACTIVITIES

Best height for:
      toilet
      dining chair
      kitchen stool
      living room chairs or sofa
      bed

EQUIPMENT RECOMMENDATIONS:

_____ O.T.R.

_____ Date

*Complete this form in duplicate, one copy for patient.

PART V

OCCUPATIONAL THERAPY MODALITIES

This section reviews both treatments that are unique to arthritis, such as orthoses and joint protection, and general treatments, such as assistive devices, crafts, and exercise, that require special considerations before being applied to people with arthritis.

Chapter 24 on joint protection has been expanded to include assessment of joint protection needs in the workplace as well as protection measures for back and neck pain caused by muscular pain or joint or disc involvement.

Chapter 25 on assistive equipment has been extensively revised. The selection of equipment has been organized around the site of involvement (e.g., hand impairment) as well as around the type of activity (e.g., dressing) to accommodate the two problem-solving modes necessary when treating people with isolated involvement compared to total joint involvement.

Chapter 23

Orthotic Treatment for Arthritis of the Hand

Precautions
Patient Instruction
Wrist Orthosis
Design and Treatment Considerations
Impact of Wrist Orthoses on MCP Joints
Precautions
Patient Instruction
Wrist–MCP Orthosis and MCP Orthosis
Design and Treatment Considerations
Precautions
Patient Instruction
Wrist–MCP Orthosis: Dynamic Postsurgical Type
Design and Treatment Considerations
Precautions
Patient Instruction
Postoperative Procedure
Wrist–Thumb Orthoses
Type I: For de Quervain's Tenosynovitis
Design and Treatment Considerations
Type II: For Combined Wrist and Thumb CMC Joint
Dysfunction
Thumb Orthosis: CMC-MCP Stabilization Type
Design and Treatment Considerations
Precautions
Patient Instruction
Finger Orthoses: Tripoint Type
Design and Treatment Considerations
Precautions
Patient Instruction
Finger Orthosis: Cylinder Design
Design and Treatment Considerations
Precautions

While modifying a custom thermoplastic wrist orthosis for a 16-year-old girl with intercarpal instability, I asked if she minded wearing an orthosis to high school. She replied "No, it's no problem. Everyone is wearing them."

Orthotic hand treatment appears to be coming of age with rapid growth of application in sports and industry. The increased demand and use are helping reduce the stigma of wearing an "orthopedic looking device." This is especially true for people with traumatic injuries, like my patient above. But it is also helping reduce the stigma for people with polyarthritis—trickle-down stigma reduction. Societal acceptance of hand orthoses has a strong influence on patient acceptance and cooperation with wearing schedules. Patient cooperation and follow-through are essential for treatment to be effective. The most beautiful creative orthosis is wasted effort if it sits in a drawer. Throughout this chapter the emphasis is on using the lightest, thinnest, least obtrusive and most functional and aesthetically appealing orthoses possible. All these factors can influence patient acceptance and effective treatment.

Orthotic treatment is important to occupational therapy (OT) because in current practice it is a treatment that is often prescribed early in the course of a disease or condition and frequently provides the first point of access into occupational therapy. Thus it provides the therapist an opportunity to assess the patient and to determine if further OT or rehabilitation would benefit the patient, and to make appropriate recommendations to the referring physician.

RATIONALE FOR ORTHOTIC TREATMENT

The objectives of orthotic treatment for arthritis and tenosynovitis include (1) reducing pain and inflammation by restricting motion, (2) preventing dysfunctional contractures by maintaining the joint in optimal alignment, (3) providing stability for a joint to improve function, (4) preventing stress to a joint during activities, and (5) correcting or reducing contractures.

Reducing Pain and Inflammation

Pain and inflammation are effectively reduced by restricting or preventing joint/tendon motion.[1-3] **Immobilization** has a multifactorial impact on the joint. First, it reduces the functional demand on the capsule and synovial lining by providing "localized rest," thus allowing the immunological resources of the capsule to concentrate on erradicating the inflammation. The process is similar to that of bedrest, which helps one recover from the flu; that is, bedrest supports the embattled immune system, allowing it to concentrate on healing. Second, pain and swelling are a stimulus to **muscle contraction and spasm,**[4,5] which are natural internal mechanisms to restrict or "splint" the joint and thus reduce pain caused by motion. However, muscle contraction compresses the joint (and stresses tendons), increasing intra-articular pressure and consequently pain. Rigid orthoses can break this pain–spasm cycle by stopping pain with motion and providing joint support so the muscles can relax. For this outcome to occur, the patient needs to relax consciously into the orthosis and let the orthosis do the work. Muscular guarding is stimulated by conscious and subconscious fear of pain with motion or use. If a patient has had wrist pain, for example, for a prolonged period, **subconscious "guarding"** may become automatic and habitual. The patient may be totally unaware of it. All patients should be taught conscious relaxation for the treated extremity and be instructed to "relax into the orthosis and let it support the wrist." Often it is only after this type of training that the patient becomes aware of how much guarding was taking place. One vivid clinical example illustrating this point is that of a patient with acute lateral epicondylitis, treated with a circumferential wrist orthosis. I explained the purpose of the orthosis and simply instructed the patient to let the orthosis "do the work." A week later there had been no progress. Re-examination of the patient's arm revealed excessive muscular guarding with the orthosis on as well as off. The patient was instructed in tension awareness techniques and conscious forearm–wrist relaxation during hand activities. Within a few days the patient started making excellent progress.

When pain is associated with inflammation, which is typical of joint synovitis but not necessarily of tenosynovitis, a decrease in pain is an indicator of a decrease in inflammation. The pain is the result, in part, of increased intra-articular pressure. **Pain as a criterion of joint synovitis** includes the following classification: *severe*, pain at rest; *moderate*, pain with motion; and *minimal*, pain with palpation or compression. (See Chapter 19 on hand assessment for further discussion.)

When the wrist is inflamed the most likely cause of pain is the synovitis, as described above. When a wrist with chronic rheumatoid arthritis (RA) is in remission with no apparent inflammation, pain can result from a variety of conditions such as impingement of pannus, ligamentous damage, intracarpal instability, impingement of osteophytes, or eroded carpal bones and limitations from fibrosis (creating abnormal mechanics).[5] **Pain from any source can cause a reflex inhibition of the wrist muscles,**[4,6] often described by patients as "My wrist just gave away" or "I'm always dropping things, feels like my wrist just stops working." This loss of wrist strength may or may not be preceded by the perception of pain. When there is no perception of pain it is theorized that the wrist stimulus generated a spinal rather than a cortical muscle inhibition reflex. The wrist stimulus will generate "pain" if it completes the cortical pathway; this in turn will elicit muscle inhibition. The wrist stimulus will not generate pain if it elicits muscle inhibition at the spinal level. If this phenomenon is occurring frequently in a patient with minimal or no inflammation, a flexible wrist orthosis (with or without the volar support) can help resolve the problem and improve function.

Preventing Dysfunctional Contractures

Orthoses are extremely effective for positioning the hand and preventing dysfunctional deformities that can result from improper positioning. The most common deformities of the hand that can be prevented are wrist flexion and thumb adduction contractures. In some cases a full hand–wrist orthosis can prevent dysfunctional proximal interphalangeal (PIP) and metacarpophalangeal (MCP) contractures. Another conditon that is preventable is fixed ulna bayonet wrist deformities with the hand fixed at a 90-degree ulnar angle to the wrist. This results from radiocarpal instability occurring after surgical removal or erosion of the ulnar styloid. Patients without an ulnar styloid should be monitored for excessive ulnar mobility. When this is present, a high conforming thin circumferential wrist orthosis is an option to preventing ulnar dislocation. Preventing a fixed deformity reduces the amount of surgery necessary to stabilize the wrist.

An issue of major concern is the role of orthotic treatment in the prevention of deformities caused by musculotendon imbalance and dynamic forces, such as MCP ulnar drift, wrist subluxation, and swanneck deformities. There are several points at which preventive intervention is possible and can affect the final outcome. But the key to success is truly prevention, because corrective intervention is limited. These specific prevention strategies are discussed under the treatment for each condition.

Providing Stability for a Joint

Joint instability can result from direct damage to the ligament, which weakens and lengthens it; or from cartilage and bone erosions, which reduce the joint length or bone-to-ligament ratio. Both processes can result in the ligaments being slack and consequently excessively mobile. In severe inflammatory joint disease, usually a combination of both processes occurs. An orthosis can provide sufficient external support to an unstable joint to allow sufficient stability and function of the distal joints. The joints most commonly requiring this type of treatment include the wrist, thumb MCP, thumb IP, and finger PIP. The finger orthoses, tripoint type, described in this chapter can be very effective in stabilizing the thumb IP and finger PIP and distal interphalangeal (DIP) joints. When joint instability interferes with function, the ideal solution is usually surgical reconstruction or fusion. Orthotic treatment plays a primary role when the patient is not a candidate for surgery because of concomitant health problems or when there is going to be a prolonged delay before surgery can be scheduled.

Orthoses that provide rigid stability for a single joint also provide patients an opportunity to experience how an immobile, stable joint can influence hand function. In effect, this simulates a surgical fusion and generally makes the operation more acceptable to the patient. This is particularly helpful for people with monoarticular joint trauma or arthritis.

Preventing Stress to a Joint

When hand orthoses are used to treat inflammation, preventing stress to the joint or tendon is a key part of that function. After the inflammation has resolved or healed the orthosis can be used during specific activities to prevent recurrence of pain and inflammation. This is a common approach for treating osteoarthritis (OA) of the thumb carpometacarpal (CMC) joint and wrist tenosynovitis.

The commercial flexible wrist orthoses (e.g., the Freedom Splint) can play an invaluable role for joint protection of the wrist by preventing rotational torque forces. These orthoses allow up to 50 degrees of flexion and extension to accommodate function, but they effectively prevent circumduction. If a person has active wrist synovitis (and MCP synovitis), in my opinion it makes more sense to have "joint protection" for the wrist accomplished through use of a wrist orthosis rather than asking the patient to try and remember to "hold the wrist in straight alignment" during scores of functional tasks during the day.

Correcting or Reducing Contractures

The use of orthoses to correct or reduce contractures due to arthritis must be accomplished after the inflammation is resolved. Common treatments in this area include the application of serial orthoses to correct PIP flexion, thumb adduction, and wrist flexion contractures. Dynamic finger orthoses may also be used to correct MCP and PIP extension contractures. **Dynamic forces should never be applied to an inflamed joint.** The instructions for serial casting the wrist for children with juvenile rheumatoid arthritis (JRA) are included in Appendix 5, and the indications for use of cylinder orthoses for the digits are reviewed in this chapter. The protocol for use of dynamic orthoses to correct contractures is not unique to arthritis management and is covered in the hand rehabilitation and orthotic literature.[7-10]

ORTHOTIC TREATMENT FOR SPECIFIC CONDITIONS

The Referral

It is the role of the occupational therapist to *determine the specific orthosis that a patient needs,* to instruct the patient in the wearing and care protocol, and to determine the need for appropriate follow-up sessions.

When there is coordination among team members, the orthosis recommendations should be the same between the referring physician and the occupational therapist. A range of factors can result in a discrepancy in the orthosis determination between the physician and therapist. For example, the symptoms may change between the medical and OT examinations; the patient may present the symptoms or history differently to each practitioner; either the therapist or the physician may ask more specific questions about function or work, thus influencing the orthosis selection; or the physician may not be familiar with all the design nuances, especially of less common orthoses. Many physicians routinely write a specific order, for example, "wrist orthosis," to indicate their concern or focus for the patient, expecting that if the therapist has a better

idea he or she will implement it and then call the physician. Most physicians want the best orthotic program available for their patients. When a therapist determines that a patient should have a different orthosis from that ordered by the physician, it is the therapist's responsibility to convey his or her findings to the referring physician and to secure at least a verbal order for any changes on the referral.

Whenever *professionals* apply a treatment, they should be capable of instructing the patient in the application of the treatment, in this case the wearing protocol and follow-up. Orthotic *technicians* apply orthoses without responsibility for wearing instruction or for follow-up evaluation. In a facility with a coordinated team approach all other members of the team—physician, nurse, and physical therapist—should be knowledgeable in the general philosophy and indications for hand orthoses. For example, they should know the indications for a referral to OT. It is the role of the occupational therapist to determine effective protocols and to teach them to the other team members, including the rheumatologist. When a therapist fabricates and fits orthoses without evaluating the patient, understanding the reason for an orthosis, or knowing the wearing protocol, he or she is functioning as an orthotic technician.

When I lecture, the most frequent questions I am asked are related to orthosis wearing protocols for specific problems. First, it is very difficult to provide a single answer because each treatment should be individually tailored for the patient's unique situation and pattern of involvement. Second, I can only describe my personal experience, since research on protocol effectiveness is not very feasible considering the range of severity and joint/tendon involvement.

Treatment Protocols

In this section, I describe my personal approach to orthotic management, based on my training, the medical philosophy of the physicians I work with, the particular clinic populations I have worked with, and my philosophy and biases about orthoses. I am *not* presenting it as dogma, only as one example. If you are new to this area of treatment or do not have a protocol, those presented here can provide at least a starting point for effective treatment. Every experienced therapist has his or her own philosphy and approach. This is as it should be because each clinical population is different. The most important bottomline is effective *results.* Whenever orthotic treatment does not achieve the expected results, the therapist should re-evaluate the design, wearing protocol, and patient's response to the orthosis. If a problem or an answer cannot be found, a second opinion from another experienced therapist should be sought. An orthosis may not totally resolve inflammation but it should reduce it. *The patient should be able to report back that the orthosis is helping and that he or she is pleased with it and using it.*

If this is not happening, the following factors should be re-evaluated: patient selection, orthosis selection, evaluation techniques, patient education (patient expectations regarding the problem and treatment), patient instruction regarding use, orthosis design (Are joints unnecessarily restricted?), materials (thickness and comfort), patient use (Is he or she strapping it too tightly or "guarding" with the orthoses on?), and patient acceptance. Any one of these factors can prevent effective treatment.

If you do not have follow-up sessions with your patients you will never know if your approach is effective. Dissatisfied patients often don't come back. When an actual follow-up session is not indicated, I have patients call me in 1 to 2 weeks to report on their progress. (Patients really appreciate this.) Also, I do not charge for adjustments (they are factored into the cost) to encourage patients to come back, because if the orthosis is uncomfortable they won't wear it.

Personal Philosophy. These treatment protocols have been developed over the last 20 years. Although purely empirical, they represent the most effective treatment strategies I have found. As mentioned above, these protocols are based on the following orthotic and human considerations: *First,* that orthoses are unnatural things to wear; they are typically hard, cold or hot, and often sweaty; they are visual reminders of disability; and they are unsexy. Because

of these factors, I try to use the smallest, thinnest, least obtrusive, most aesthetically pleasing orthoses possible. *Second,* except for a couple of digit orthoses, most orthoses reduce overall dexterity and function in some fashion, despite some specific gains. Because of this, I try to use the most functional orthoses applicable. *Third,* immobilization of one joint alters the biomechanical forces to adjacent joints, causing stress that can increase inflammation in these joints. Thus, the impact of an orthosis on adjacent joints is a critical consideration.[11] I try to treat patients the way I would like to be treated and design orthoses that I would not mind wearing.

Orthotic treatment as described in this section is organized according to specific common clinical problems. The details on using each orthosis are covered later in this chapter. The symptoms and sequelae of each of the following conditions are described in detail and referenced in Chapter 4 on OA, Chapter 6 on RA, and Chapter 19 on hand assessment. Treatment for JRA is reviewed in Chapter 14.

Acute Wrist Synovitis without Digital Involvement

Orthosis. Wrist orthosis: rigid circumferential design, without restriction to thumb or MCP joints.

Wearing Time. Day and night. The orthosis is removed for bathing, handwashing, and gentle active range of motion (AROM) 3 to 5 times a day.

Duration. Until acute inflammation subsides, typically 1 to 4 weeks. (It can subside in as short a time as 2 to 3 days.) Then the options are (1) to continue wearing the above orthosis as long as there is any inflammation; (2) to reduce wearing to use during daytime activities and use a flexible wrist orthosis with a volar support at night (often preferable for people who do a lot of strenuous activities); or (3) to reduce to daytime flexible wrist orthosis when possible (preferable for long-term treatment or for sedentary people, as long as inflammation does not increase with reduction to a more flexible orthosis).

If there is synovial hypertrophy, the orthosis can be continued as long as there is progress in decreasing the circumference of the wrist. It may take up to 6 months or longer to allow the hypertrophied tissue to atrophy.

Comments. Gentle isometric exercises to the wrist extensors and flexors (in the orthosis) should be initiated as soon as they can be done without pain. When prolonged immobilization is indicated, referral to a physical therapist for portable home electrical stimulation *may* be indicated to maintain wrist flexor and extensor strength.

Some type of wrist orthosis should be used during activities as long as there is inflammation. Most patients find that if they stop using an orthosis, the wrist inflammation increases. In my experience treatment with a rigid circumferential orthosis is effective in reducing inflammation 100 percent of the time. If the patient does not improve within a week, the problem may be (1) excessive subconscious guarding (see previous section on reducing pain and inflammation); or (2) the patient may not be wearing the orthosis or may be doing strenuous activities, such as carrying luggage or shopping bags. If inflammation resolves and pain persists, noninflammatory causes such as ligamentous laxity, subluxation, and so forth should be considered.

Acute Wrist Synovitis with Minimal MCP Synovitis

Orthosis. Flexible wrist orthosis with volar support during daytime and rigid wrist orthosis during nighttime.

Comments. A rigid wrist orthosis worn during activities creates compensatory stress on the adjacent MCP joints.[11] In a person with active MCP synovitis, this stress can exacerbate MCP disease. This occurs in most but not all cases. If a patient came to me with the above problem, I would fit the person with the above two orthoses. Then I would have the patient do a 1-week trial of wearing the rigid wrist orthosis during the day, explaining the risk of exacerbating the MCP synovitis and teaching the patient how to determine if this is occurring. If the patient can tolerate the rigid wrist orthosis, I would have him or her wear the rigid orthosis both day and night. If the rigid orthosis aggravates the MCP joints, I would use the protocol first

designated above. This orthotic program is indicated as long as synovitis is present.

Acute Wrist Synovitis with Moderate MCP Synovitis

Orthosis. Flexible wrist orthosis during daytime and rigid wrist orthosis during nighttime.

Comments. When there is this much inflammation in the MCP joints, the joints are extremely sensitive to compensatory stress from wrist immobilization. In such cases I use this protocol without a trial of rigid orthosis. Although this does not provide the ultimate in immobilization for the wrist, it is better to sacrifice the wrist and preserve the MCP joints than to save the wrist and damage the MCP joints, because there are better surgical options for the wrist than for the MCP joints. This orthotic program is indicated as long as synovitis is present.

Why not use a full wrist–hand orthosis at night? From personal experience I have found the results of using a full wrist–hand orthosis to be equivocal with that of using simply a wrist orthosis at night. It appears that a full wrist–hand orthosis is most effective when there is severe inflammation present. The results I have encountered from using a wrist–hand orthosis at night in these cases have not warranted the restriction to function they cause. However, a trial of each type may be warranted to determine the best orthosis to use.

Acute Wrist Synovitis with Severe MCP Synovitis

Orthosis. Flexible wrist orthosis with or *without* a volar support during daytime and rigid wrist–hand orthosis during nighttime.

Comments. The more inflamed the MCP joints, the more flexible a wrist orthosis I use. In severe cases I remove the volar support, based on the philosophy stated in the above two comment sections.

If the patient has only wrist and MCP involvement and the PIPs are normal (no pain with palpation) I would use a wrist–MCP orthosis during the day. However, this is an extremely rare situation, since most patients with this involvement also have PIP inflammation. I would still use the wrist–hand orthosis at night because pressure on the fingertips can create pain in inflamed MCP joints.

Fortunately patients with this degree of inflammation are fairly uncommon, because current drug therapy regimens are able to control inflammation. Severe inflammation, as in this clinical scenario, tends to occur when a patient is not on an appropriate medical protocol or is unable to take anti-inflammatory medications.

MCP Synovitis

The occurrence of MCP synovitis without any wrist or PIP involvement is rare, but it can occur. I have seen it in more patients with psoriatic arthritis than in those with RA.

Orthosis. MCP orthosis: dorsal type.

Wearing Time. Day and night. It is removed for bathing and range of motion (ROM) exercises.

Duration. As long as acute inflammation persists, usually 1 to 4 weeks. If synovial hypertrophy exists, continue this schedule as long as swelling continues to diminish.

Comments. If the inflammation subsides to a minimal level, the orthosis can be worn during stressful activities during the day and discontinued at night for as long as some inflammation remains. See the section on MCP orthoses in this chapter for details on using this type of orthosis.

MCP Ulnar Drift

This is one of the most controversial and discussed clinical problems in orthotic treatment for arthritis. The big questions are: can you prevent it and can you correct or reduce established drift with orthoses?

Prevention. I believe it is possible to prevent MCP ulnar drift in *some* patients with RA, but not all. However, this has not been studied or proven. Prevention rests on two factors: (1) maintaining ulnar deviation at the wrist, and (2) avoiding strong grasp during MCP inflammation. At present there is no evidence at all that passive positioning with orthoses has any impact on reducing MCP drift.

The most important thing a therapist or patient can do to prevent MCP ulnar drift is to maintain ulnar deviation of the wrist. Radial drift or deviation of the wrist is the most powerful causal force for MCP ulnar drift. Patients who for some unknown reason develop fixed ulnar deviation of the wrist essentially *do not* develop MCP ulnar drift. (In fact, in some cases they develop MCP radial drift, similar to that seen in JRA.)

Maintaining ulnar deviation of the wrist can be achieved in a couple of ways. First, you can use orthotic positioning. All wrist orthoses for people with RA should hold the wrist in at least 10 degrees of ulnar deviation, if possible. For patients at high risk of losing ulnar deviation, 15 to 20 degrees may be appropriate. (See the section on wrist orthoses for more details on this point.) Second, you can use patient education to encourage ulnar positioning at rest by teaching the importance of this concept. Patients have a lot of misconceptions about their hands. If they have beginning MCP drift, they volitionally or subconsciously position their wrists in radial deviation to make their fingers look straighter. This only makes the problem worse.

Avoiding strong grip during periods of MCP inflammation by using joint-protection techniques (e.g., using the palm and bilateral prehension) can be very effective in reducing both inflammation and the deforming forces of the flexor tendons.

Correction. There is only one published study that seriously addresses the issue of passive orthotic correction for MCP ulnar drift. In 1967, orthopedists at Rancho Los Amigos Hospital had patients with RA and ulnar drift fitted with dynamic metal MCP orthoses that maintained the digits in neutral alignment (day and night) for 6 months. At the end of the study there was no significant change in MCP deviation.[12] Since this was a comprehensive trial, there has been no impetus to do further studies along this line. It is possible that orthoses will play a role in correcting drift in the future, but it is not likely to be through simply passive correction of the MCP joints.

Although it is frequently said that the capsule and ligaments have "stretched out," they do not have true stretch capacity. In fact, they actually lengthen as a result of damage. A rubberband provides an example of the difference between stretch and lengthening. When a rubberband becomes longer we say it has "stretched out" when in fact it has developed micro-tears resulting in greater length. In a capsule, micro-tears from chronic distention and synovitis would be filled in with fibrous tissue. Consequently, passive positioning in a shortened length is no more effective with a joint capsule than it is with an elongated rubberband—it is the damage, not the length, that is the problem.

Passive alignment of the digits with finger separators in wrist–hand orthoses does nothing to correct or prevent MCP ulnar drift. This procedure should only be used if it makes the orthosis more comfortable for the patient. With the hand, a static orthosis should never be used to achieve passive correction, because this creates focal pressure points. (This is a basic tenet of orthotic treatment.) For RA, finger separators can be used, but only for comfortable correction. That is, trying to achieve ideal alignment at the risk of creating pressure sores serves no purpose.

Intrinsic Muscle Tightness

Orthosis.   MCP orthosis: dorsal design.

Wearing Time.   At night and progressive daytime tolerance.

Comments.   The treatment protocol for this problem is highly variable. It depends on how well the patient can tolerate the orthosis and how restrictive it is to function during the day. I start patients with night use and begin daytime use with 2 to 3 hours progressing to tolerance. For some patients 2 to 3 hours is the limit; others are able to wear the orthosis 24 hours a day without a problem. The more hours they are able to wear it, the faster they progress toward the desired results.

The orthosis should maintain the MCP joints in 0 degrees of extension or as close to it as possible. Sometimes it is necessary to allow greater index flexion for function. Most of the results can be achieved by this approach in 1 to 2 weeks. For some it may take up to 4 to 6 weeks.

Swan-Neck Deformities

Orthotic treatment for this problem includes the reduction of intrinsic tightness, as above, if present and the use of tripoint design finger orthoses. The finger orthoses are indicated primarily if PIP hyperextension interferes with function. The Silver Ring custom-fitted orthoses provide an aesthetic option for long-term treatment of swan-neck deformities. (See the section on finger orthoses.)

PIP Synovitis

Orthosis.   Finger orthosis: cylinder design.

Wearing Time.   Day and night. It is removed during periods of day rest, hygiene, and for frequent gentle ROM.

Comments.   Orthotic immobilization for this problem is extremely difficult: first, because the orthosis keeps the digit extended and interferes with function; second, because prolonged immobilization in *any* position puts the collateral ligaments at risk for contracture; and third, the outcome of this treatment is unpredictable. I have had great success with rapid reduction of inflammation and swelling in some patients, and zero results in others. I start with an initial trial of 1 week. If there is progress, I continue until progress plateaus. Then I have the patient wear the orthosis only during very stressful activities. If there is no significant progress within 2 weeks I discontinue the orthosis or suggest the patient use it at his or her discretion to protect the joint.

DIP Joint: Acute Osteoarthritis

Orthosis.   Finger orthosis: cylinder design (for the IP joint only, with tip free for prehension).

Wearing Time.   As much and as long as it helps relieve pain.

Comments.   Generally orthotic treatment is not indicated for the DIP joints. But occasionally severe pain and inflammation can significantly impair function. Small cylinder-type orthoses made out of $\frac{1}{16}$-inch material can prevent painful motion. I present this treatment as an option and let the patient decide if he or she wants to try it. As an extra benefit the orthosis also creates some comforting warmth.

The orthosis should hold the joint in extension and be removed for hygiene and gentle ROM.

Thumb CMC Osteoarthritis

Orthosis. Thumb CMC-MP orthosis. (Wrist and IP joint should have full mobility.)

Wearing Time. For moderate or severe inflammation/pain, 2 to 4 weeks. For minimal inflammation/pain, 1 to 3 weeks.

Comments. The response to this orthotic treatment is highly variable. Some people get complete pain relief in 3 to 5 days; others need 4 to 6 weeks. I recommend patients wear the orthosis day and night (removed for hygiene and gentle ROM) for 1 week if pain/inflammation is minimal, and for 2 weeks if pain is moderate to severe or until they can go without the orthosis all day without pain. When this day arrives (determined by a trial test) I have them reduce wearing time to use during stressful activities as a preventive measure for 2 to 3 months.

When the orthosis is fitted I explain the wearing protocol and request that during a quiet time they carefully review their daily activities and identify those that elicit thumb pain. The most common offending activities typically are writing, child care, shopping, gardening, and driving.

The minimum goal is to have the patient become pain-free and, ideally, nontender. The rationale for using this specific design is described in detail in the section on thumb orthoses, later in this chapter.

Thumb MCP Synovitis

Orthosis. Thumb–MCP orthosis.

Wearing Time. Day and night until inflammation is brought under control and swelling is reduced, then during stressful activities as a preventive measure as needed.

Comments. If there is synovial hypertrophy, it can take 4 to 6 months to reduce the capsular tissue. When the treatment is for a traumatic collateral ligament sprain, the orthosis is worn until pain and tenderness are gone. Gentle ROM should be done daily to prevent stiffness.

Thumb IP Synovitis or Instability

Orthosis. Finger orthosis: tripoint type.

Wearing Time. For synovitis: as long as there is progress in the reduction of pain and swelling. For instability: during the daytime as long as it helps.

Comments. Thumb IP synovitis as a specific problem needing treatment is uncommon. Instability due to joint erosion is far more common. Occasionally severe OA may necessitate an orthosis. The design of the orthosis should prevent flexion/extension, as needed, as well as lateral motion, and it should leave the distal portion of the thumb pad free for prehension. Surgical fusion is the best treatment for IP instability, but for patients who are not surgical candidates a tripoint orthosis is very effective.

PATIENT EVALUATION

A thorough physical and functional hand assessment is essential both before and after fitting an orthosis. The initial assessment is necessary to determine the type/design of orthosis to use and the second assessment is necessary to determine if the orthosis fits properly and is of value. The therapist may elect to use a standardized assessment, such as the Jebsen Hand Function Test, or to create his or her own informal but systematic assessment. (See Chapter 19 for description of standard assessment.) The assessment should include pain, active and passive ROM, strength, sensation, joint stability, muscular guarding on spasm, contractures, dominance, prehension patterns and skills, use of assistive devices or work equipment, function for activities of daily living (ADL), effect of the orthosis' restrictions on adjacent joints and upper extremity function, ability for applying and removing the orthosis, and psychological acceptance.[7,13]

After both the pre- and postorthotic assessment the therapist should be able to answer the following questions:

1. What hand functions can the person perform? This includes lateral pinch, hook and power grasp, opposition, object manipulation, ADL, and strength.

2. What is the quality of performance? Are the skills done easily, with effort, slowly, with or without pain? This is important, because frequently an orthosis will not increase the skills possible but will improve the quality of function by reducing pain.

3. When there is a functional limitation, what is the cause? Is it pain, muscle tightness, fibrosis, triggering, weakness, instability, limited ROM, or malalignment?

4. How does the orthosis improve or restrict function? Most orthoses do both, and it is important for both the patient and the therapist to understand the functional trade-offs in order to have realistic expectations.

5. How does the orthosis affect other joints in the extremity? A heavy wrist–hand orthosis can aggravate elbow involvement. A rigid wrist orthosis can require different shoulder and elbow motions to accommodate restricted wrist ROM, especially for self-care tasks close to the body. These can result in increased shoulder or elbow pain. *Whenever you immobilize one joint, stress to the adjacent joints is increased.*

When the therapist is ready to recommend orthotic treatment to the physician or patient, the therapist should be able to specify the patient's need for the orthosis, the purpose of the orthosis, and wearing time protocol (e.g., at night, during activities, 24 hours a day, and so forth).

DESIGN AND FABRICATION OF THE ORTHOSIS

Since each orthosis is designed to accomplish a particular function, the design and materials used can vary as long as the desired function is achieved, the principles of orthosis application are adhered to, and the orthosis is well tolerated and aesthetically acceptable. Specific design requirements for each type of orthosis commonly used for treatment of arthritis in the hand are reviewed later in this chapter. The basics of orthotic design and fabrication are covered in several current publications.[7–9,14,15] Polyethylene is the only material used in the treatment of arthritis not covered in the basic texts. Therefore, fabrication procedures are provided in Appendix 3 at the end of this book.

SPECIAL PRECAUTIONS AND CONSIDERATIONS DURING FABRICATION OF THE ORTHOSIS

1. Fitting the Orthosis. There may be discomfort to the patient during fitting of the orthosis because of temperature, compression over synovitis, or sudden passive movement. People in pain are often very apprehensive about "being handled," so it is important to be gentle, to keep the patient's elbow or forearm supported, and to explain in advance what you are planning to do.

2. Effects of the Orthosis on Other Joints. The orthosis may affect the other joints in the extremity. For example, immobilization of a joint causes increased compensatory stress to adjacent joints, and a heavy wrist orthosis can aggravate an involved elbow or shoulder joint.

3. The Patient's Ability to Put on and Remove the Orthosis. This is especially important when bilateral orthoses are required. Strap closures should be adapted to allow independence in application.

4. The Weight of the Orthosis. In addition to affecting the proximal joints, the weight of the orthosis can influence patient compliance. A thumb (CMC–MCP) orthosis made of ⅛-inch thermoplastic material can feel "heavy" especially to someone with a small hand, making it less desirable to wear. Material ¹⁄₁₆-inch thick is recommended for small hand orthoses.

5. The Degree and Fluctuation of Joint and Periarticular Swelling. This is an important consideration for circumferential orthoses. Orthoses fabricated during the day need to allow room for diurnal or nocturnal swelling; and orthoses made for severely swollen joints often have to be adjusted as the swelling or inflammation decreases. It is important to ask patients about their swelling patterns. Also, many anti-inflammatory medications cause fluid retention.

6. Perspiration. Sweating is a problem with all thermoplastic materials, including perforated forms. For small hand orthoses, dusting the inside with athletic-type or foot talcum powder that contains antiperspirants and deodorant is generally sufficient for comfort and minimizes perspiration. For larger wrist or full hand orthoses, cotton (not nylon) stockinette liners are generally necessary to provide adequate wearing comfort and prevent skin irritation from perspiration. Moleskin lining is *not recommended* because it is difficult to clean and becomes unhygienic. It is helpful to show patients how to cut their own stockinette liners and to provide sufficient replacements with the orthosis.

7. Accommodating the Ulnar Styloid. If an orthosis covers the ulnar styloid it is essential to "bubble" the orthosis over the styloid to allow room for the styloid to move during forearm rotation. This is best done by padding the styloid with a circle of ⅛-inch adhesive foam (approximately 2.5 cm in diameter). To avoid adherence of the foam to the thermoplastic, put a thin layer of petroleum jelly on top of the foam.

ANATOMICAL LANDMARKS FOR ORTHOSIS FABRICATION

Dermal and skeletal landmarks are shown in Figures 23–1 and 23–2 to provide easy reference relevant to the discussions of

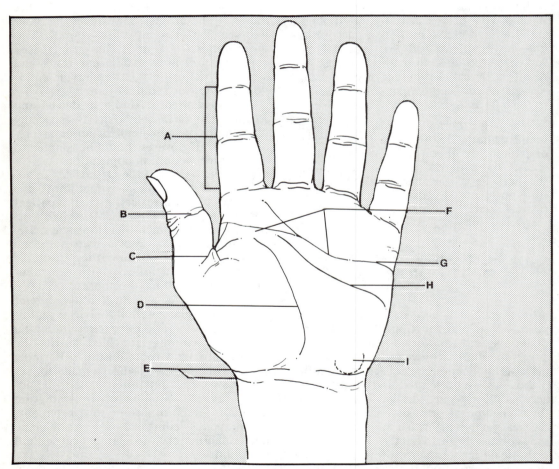

Figure 23–1. Palmar hand creases are shown here: (*A*) digital creases: distal, middle, proximal; (*B*) distal thumb crease; (*C*) proximal thumb creases; (*D*) thenar crease; (*E*) wrist creases; (*F*) composite (midpalmar crease); (*G*) distal palmar crease; (*H*) proximal palmar crease; (*I*) pisiform bone. The palmar hand creases are important because they delineate where joint motion takes place. The thenar crease (*D*) defines the area of thumb motion. The composite or midpalmar crease (*F*) delineates MCP joint flexion. The proximal palmar crease (*H*) indicates motion of the carpometacarpal joints of the fourth and fifth digits. The proximal palmar crease is frequently absent.

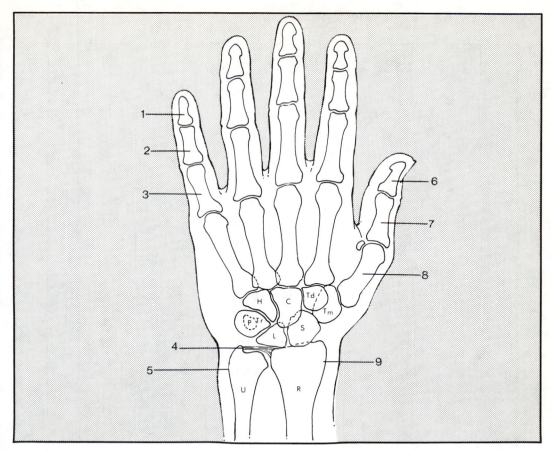

Figure 23–2. Bones of the hand and wrist are shown here: (*1*) distal phalanx; (*2*) middle phalanx; (*3*) proximal phalanx; (*4*) triangular fibrocartilage; (*5*) ulnar styloid; (*6*) distal phalanx; (*7*) proximal phalanx; (*8*) metacarpal; (*9*) radial styloid; (*H*) hamate; (*C*) capitate; (*Td*) trapezoid; (*Tm*) trapezium; (*S*) scaphoid (navicular); (*L*) lunate; (*Tr*) triquetrum; (*P*) pisiform; (*U*) ulna; (*R*) radius.

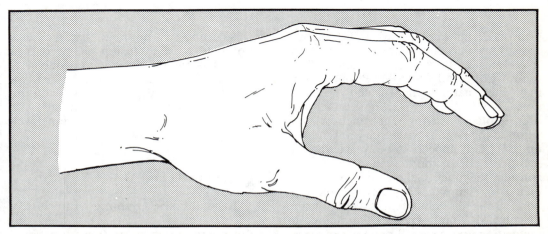

Figure 23–3. This drawing indicates the functional position of the hand, lateral view: 20 to 30 degrees wrist extension, thumb in opposition, finger joints slightly flexed. (MCP joints in 30 to 45 degrees of flexion.)

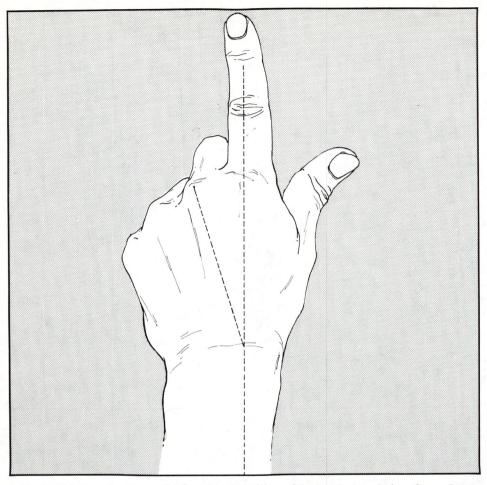

Figure 23–4. This drawing shows the functional position of the hand, dorsal view. Second metacarpal is in a straight line with the radius; wrist is in 5 to 10 degrees of ulnar deviation. Orthoses should maintain this functional position whenever possible.

orthosis design in this chapter. The palmar creases are particularly important because they designate the range of mobility of the thumb CMC and finger MCP joints. Normal functional alignment is shown in Figures 23–3 and 23–4. Sterling Bunnell has been quoted as saying "the functional position of the hand is with each joint in midrange."[10] This appears to be an accurate assessment. In orthotic management we consider the functional position to be as depicted in Figure 23–3. This position supports Bunnell's statement except for the thumb CMC joint, which is maintained in opposition and near full palmar abduction to protect against dysfunctional adduction and extension (abduction) contractures. It

is also important to note that the ideal amount of wrist extension, 30 degrees as depicted, is not appropriate for people with RA, wrist flexor tenosynovitis, or wrist synovitis because 30-degree extension diminishes the carpal tunnel and patients with these diagnoses are at high risk for developing carpal tunnel syndrome.

ORTHOTIC MATERIALS

Thermoplastic Orthotic Materials

Information on various low temperature thermoplastic orthotic materials is presented in Table 23–1. Materials with iso-

Table 23–1 Low Temperature Thermoplastic Orthotic Materials*

Low-Temperature Thermoplastic Orthotic Materials

Similarities
- Requires hot water bath to soften
- Applied directly to the skin
- Retains shape when cool
- Can be reshaped with heat
- Sheets are 18 × 24 inches unless otherwise specified

Differences
- Vary in ability to conform to hand contours
- Some self-bond, others require use of a solvent
- Vary in hardness and thickness
- Considerable variation in cost
- Vary in resistance to fingerprint and surface pressure

Product Name	Description	Properties				Use Indicies 3 = High 1 = Low 2 = Moderate			Manufacturer/Principal Source
		Temp to Heat	Thickness (inches)	Self-Bond	Non-Bond	Rigidity Index	Shrinkage Index	Conformity Index	
Aquaplast original or coated	Opaque, solid, or perforated sheet material, clear when fully heated, controlled stretch, excellent conformability. Original self-bonds.	160–180°	⅛ or 3⁄32 or 1⁄16	X	or X	2	2	3	WFR Aquaplast Corp. PO Box 635 Wyckoff, NJ 07481 1-800-526-5247
Aquaplast green stripe	Limited stretch and conformability.	160–180°	⅛ or 1⁄16	X	or X	2	2	2	
Aquaplast blue stripe	Extra pliable, maximal conformability.	160–180°	⅛ or 1⁄16	X		2	2	3+	

393

Table 23–1 Low Temperature Thermoplastic Orthotic Materials* *Continued*

Product Name	Description	Temp to Heat	Thickness (inches)	Self-Bond	Non-Bond	Rigidity Index	Shrinkage Index	Conformity Index	Manufacturer/Principal Source
				Properties		Use Indicies 3 = High 1 = Low 2 = Moderate			
Ezeform	Rubber-based sheet material, matt finish, fingerprint resistant, most rigid of the group when cooled.	170°	⅛	X		3	2	1	Smith & Nephew/Rolyan Corp. N93 W14475 Whittaker Way Menomones Falls, WI 53051 1-800-558-8633
Kay Splint Series I	Highly conforming sheet material, will stretch if unsupported, requires care to avoid fingerprint marks.	150°	⅛		X	2	2	3	Fred Sammons, Inc. Box 32 Brookfield, IL 60513 1-800-323-5547
Isoprene	Flexible material with less stretch, good for large orthoses and fracture bracing.	160°			X	2	2	1	
Series III	Rubber-based sheet material, mark resistant, very rigid when cool.	160°	⅛	X		3	2	2	

Product	Description	Temperature	Thickness						Manufacturer
Multiform I	Highly conforming sheet material, fingerprint resistant, controlled stretch, bonds strongly without use of solvent.	150–180°	$\frac{1}{8}$ or $\frac{1}{16}$	X		2	2	3	AliMed, Inc. 297 High Street Dedham, MA 02026 1-800-329-2900
Multiform II	Same as above, but will not bond unless surface coating is dissolved.	150–180°	$\frac{1}{8}$		X	2	2	3	
Multiform Soft	Thin thermoplastic bonded to closed-cell Aliplast for softness against the skin and rigid outer shell.	150°	$\frac{1}{8}$		X	1	2	1	
Orthoplast	Solid or perforated sheet material, self-adhesive, very rigid when cooled, good for fracture bracing.	160°	$\frac{1}{8}$	X		3	2	2	Johnson & Johnson Products, Inc. PO Box 4000 New Brunswick, NJ 08903 1-800-255-2500
Polyform	Highly conforming sheet material, drape for precision detail, bonds with solvent.	160°	$\frac{1}{8}$ or $\frac{1}{16}$		X	2	2	3	Smith & Nephew/Rolyan Corp. (as above)
Polyflex	Flexible sheet material, controlled stretch, isoprene rubber base.	160°	$\frac{1}{8}$		X	2	2	2	Smith & Nephew/Rolyan Corp. (as above)
Ultraform	Highly conforming sheet material, bonds with solvent.	160°	$\frac{1}{8}$ or $\frac{1}{16}$		X	2	2	3	Fred Sammons, Inc. (as above)
Ultraform 294	Rubber-based material, fingerprint resistant, bonds with solvent.	160°	$\frac{1}{8}$		X	2	2	2	

*Created by Alice Shafer, MS, OTR, FAOTA.

prene rubber content such as Orthoplast and Polyflex have a softer feel and appear to be better tolerated by people with arthritis and tender bony prominences, compared to Polyform, which has no rubber and feels rigid. Aquaplast ($\frac{1}{16}$- or $\frac{3}{32}$-inch thick) is rigid but its high contourability allows a close fit and an even distribution of pressure.

Aquaplast is available in the original uncoated self-adherent form or in a coated form that requires a solvent to permit self-adherence.

When marking patterns, it is best to use a pencil or awl so markings will not be visible on the finished orthosis.

Orthotic materials other than low temperature materials are presented in Table 23–2.

ORTHOTIC EVALUATION INDEX

Design Index

If the orthosis is well designed and of optimal value to the client, the following questions *should be answered yes.*

1. Does the orthosis conform to and maintain the normal transverse and longitudinal arches of the hand and wrist?[14]

2. Does the orthosis position the wrist in 10 degrees ulnar deviation?[13] (This only applies if the client can tolerate the position.)

3. When the orthosis is worn for a half hour and used in functional tasks, is the client's hand free of persistent redness or

Table 23–2 Orthotic Materials Other Than Low Temperature Thermoplastics

Materials	Advantages	Disadvantages
Plastazote	Soft, comfortable, lightweight, and has high skin tolerance. Porous and therefore causes less sweating.	Poor wearing properties (wearing ability about 3 months). Recommended only for splints involving low stress. Requires plastic reinforcement to provide stability or correction. Bulky.
Leather	High cosmetic and skin tolerance; greater male acceptance. Available in a variety of colors and thicknesses. Flexibility and nonslip surface helpful for some vocational demands.	Poor hygienic properties. Requires metal, elastic, or plastic reinforcement to provide stability. Circumferential splints create warmth and swelling.
Polyethylene (low density) (See Appendix)	Long wearing, cleans easily, maintains shape, and has cosmetic appearance. Inexpensive Can be worn in hot water tasks. Thickness determines rigidity.	Requires oven heating and positive mold. May shrink with heating. Slippery palmar surface may hinder gripping.
Plaster of Paris bandage	Fast curing, easy to use, requires no heat. Optimal contour property. Inexpensive. Recommended for short-term splints on patients who can tolerate weight or as an immediate temporary splint. It can be lightweight, attractive, and comfortable if skillfully constructed.	Breaks down with stress and exposure to water. Cannot be cleaned or remolded. It is heavy, bulky, and unattractive if constructed using a standard cast technique.

tenderness caused by splint or strap pressure? Red areas caused by the edge of an orthosis, similar to those made by a wristwatch or elastic waist band, are not a problem. Tender red focal areas indicate a pressure point that can lead to skin breakdown.

4. If MCP flexion is desired, does the palmar end extend *only to* the distal or mid-palmar crease?[14] If fourth and fifth metacarpal rotation is desired for power grasp, the orthosis should extend ½ inch proximal to the distal palmar crease or to the proximal palmar crease.[8]

5. If MCP joint protection is desired, does the palmar end extend to the middle of the proximal phalanx?

6. When thumb motion is desired, does the thenar clearance allow for full opposition?

7. Is the orthosis sturdy enough to provide the desired stability for the wrist when the client is using his hands?

8. Does the fit of the orthosis allow for distribution of pressure over the widest area possible?

9. When fitted, is the client free of pain caused by the orthosis? (It should not push the wrist into too much dorsiflexion or cause pressure over the ulnar styloid.)

10. Can the client put on and take off the orthosis without causing stress to the opposite hand?

11. If the patient has RA carpal tunnel syndrome or wrist flexor tenosynovitis, is his or her wrist maintained in 10 degrees of extension? (This is the angle that maximizes the carpal tunnel space.)

12. Are only the essential joints restricted by the orthosis?

13. Is there full mobility of all joints not encased by the orthosis?

14. Is the orthosis closely contoured to the body?

15. Are all edges and corners rounded and smooth?

16. On wrist orthoses does the forearm strap avoid pressure on the ulnar styloid?

Functional Index

When the orthosis is designed to increase hand function, an objective assessment of hand function should be made with and without the orthosis to determine if the orthosis is effective. Determining grip and pinch strength with and without the orthosis provides a rapid and objective means of assessing a wide range of functional factors. However, the more subtle motions of hand function are often hampered by an orthosis; therefore, manipulation tasks are equally important. Many of the subtests in standard functional hand evaluations can be adapted to provide effective assessments for specific orthoses. (A review of the published assessments appears at the end of Chapter 19, Hand Pathodynamics and Assessment.)

If a person has severe polyarticular limitations it is critical to evaluate functional ability for self-care tasks with the orthosis on and not limit the assessment to desk-top activities typically represented by "hand function tests." For example, a person with neck, shoulder, and elbow limitations may need wrist flexion in order to feed independently. An orthosis that maintains the wrist in the "ideal" 10-degree extension may not be ideal for this patient.

PATIENT EDUCATION

An orthosis is of value only if it is worn correctly. Because of the problems that may occur secondary to incorrect use of a splint, effective education regarding splint instruction is essential. To facilitate assessment of patient instruction and learning, information regarding orthosis usage has been delineated into behavioral objectives.

Therapist's Instructional Objectives

The objective is to teach the patient the following information in such a manner that the patient can achieve his or her objectives:

1. The purpose of the orthosis, including the advantages and disadvantages

2. When and for how long the orthosis should be worn

3. How to determine if the orthosis is effective and guidelines for discontinuing it

4. What exercises to do in conjunction with the orthosis

5. How to put on and take off the orthosis

6. How to determine if the orthosis is positioned correctly

7. How to care for and clean the orthosis and straps

8. How to check the skin for pressure areas

9. Who to call or see if problems with the orthosis should arise

Patient Objectives

Instructions for use, precautions, and orthosis care should be put in writing. Patients have so much on their minds during a clinic visit even simple instructions can be forgotten or become unclear once the patient tries to implement them.

Before the orthosis is issued or the patient is discharged, the patient should be able to

1. Tell the therapist the purpose of the orthosis, when it should be worn, and when it should be discontinued

2. Demonstrate prescribed exercises

3. Put the orthosis on and take it off independently, without any verbal or nonverbal cues from the therapist

4. Identify the landmarks to look for in order to determine if the orthosis is positioned correctly

5. Explain to the therapist what has to be done to the orthosis to care for it properly

6. Describe what to look for when checking the skin for pressure areas

HAND ORTHOSES FOR ARTHRITIS AND TENOSYNOVITIS

Wrist–Hand Orthosis: Resting Type

The wrist–hand orthosis (Fig. 23–5) is a static volar orthosis that restricts motion by preventing flexion of the wrist, thumb, and fingers and maintains the joints in the functional position. The indications and goals for the wrist–hand orthosis are listed in Table 23–3.

Design and Treatment Considerations

The orthosis should include the fingertips and the proximal two thirds of the forearm. Inclusion of the fingertips is important even if the PIP and DIP joints are not involved, because pressure on exposed fingertips can cause pain in the MCP joints. It is best to have the hand totally protected so the patient can relax and not have to "guard" the hand against external pressure.

If the patient does not have thumb involvement it is advisable to eliminate the C-bar so the patient can manage bed clothes more easily.

It is critical that the orthosis and strapping be sufficient to hold the hand in position. If the hand should slide proximal in the orthosis (a common problem) the MCP joints rest in extension where they can de-

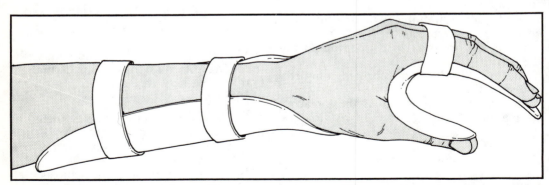

Figure 23–5. This figure shows wrist–hand orthosis (resting type) with C-bar. In this figure, the wrist is in 30 degrees of extension. Patients with RA, wrist synovitis, flexor tenosynovitis, or carpal tunnel syndrome should be positioned in 10 degrees of extension to maximize the carpal space. Thirty degrees of extension is appropriate for patients who are losing extension and appear to be developing wrist-drop or wrist flexion contractures. The MCP joint should be in 35 to 45 degrees of flexion.

Table 23–3 Indications and Goals for the Wrist–Hand Orthosis

Indications	Goals
Acute synovitis of the wrist, fingers, and thumb.	To provide localized rest to the involved joints, thereby decreasing inflammation and pain.
Wrist and finger extensor and/or thumb abductor muscles are less than grade 3.5 (not able to take slight resistance against gravity due to weakness).	To maintain optimal range until extensors are strong enough to counterbalance flexors (orthoses should be used in conjunction with a strengthening program).
Beginning multiple joint contractures.	To ensure proper positioning and maintain optimal range of motion during sleep.
Patients with acute systemic illness, severe disability, or peripheral nerve damage, who are not actively using their hands.	To obtain proper position and maintain optimal joint range and web space.

velop contractures of the collateral ligaments. Thermoplastic materials with high conformability can help secure the hand in position. Commercial orthoses with general shaping and excessive degree of extension (3 to 45 degrees) frequently result in slippage.

Positioning

Wrist. Adult and adolescent patients with acute (or chronic) wrist synovitis or tenosynovitis are at high risk for developing carpal tunnel syndrome; therefore, it is prudent to position their wrists in 10 degrees extension, which maximizes the carpal tunnel, compared to the classic functional resting position of 30 degrees, which diminishes the tunnel. The main exceptions to this rule are patients who appear to be rapidly losing extension and only have 20 to 40 degrees left (e.g., patients with acute PA or JRA) or when weakness, not pain, is the primary indication for the orthosis. In these cases it is more important to maintain extension mobility and position in 20 to 30 degrees (pain-free) extension. *Note:* Children with JRA do not appear to develop carpal tunnel syndrome. (See Chapter 14 for a discussion of JRA.)

The concept of positioning in extension is based on the principle that 30 degrees is a position that allows the greatest function in grip and desk activities. It is not the best position of function for self-care activities such as buttoning and toileting. If the pa-

tient's illness is so severe that bilateral wrist ankylosis appears imminent, the orthoses should hold the wrists in the position that allows the greatest function for that individual, taking into consideration upper extremity and trunk and neck function. For some patients this may mean one wrist in neutral and the other in slight extension or even flexion. Bilateral surgical wrist fusions are often done in neutral or with one wrist in slight flexion.

For all patients the orthosis should maintain the wrist in 10 degrees of ulnar deviation when possible, because this is the normal functional alignment of the wrist.

Thumb. In opposition and palmar abduction; that is, volar, not lateral, to the second metacarpal.

Fingers. Third MCP joint in zero deviation with the second, fourth, and fifth digits approximated to the third but not crowded. Spacers between the fingers may be needed to maintain optimal position, or an ulnar ridge may be indicated to keep the fifth digit in alignment. Spacers are used to increase comfort and keep the fingers from slipping in the orthosis. *They should not be used to passively correct a deformity.* Passive correction creates pressure areas and there is no evidence that it alters the deformity once the orthosis is removed. *Note:* From a dorsal view of the normal hand in the functional position, the index MCP joint should appear in slight ulnar deviation and the fourth and fifth MCP joints should appear in slight radial deviation.[16]

The MCP joints should be in 35 to 45 degrees of flexion—the greater the extension, the more likely the possibility that the collateral ligaments can become tight in a shortened position. The PIP joints should also be in about 45 degrees of flexion and the DIP joints in slight flexion. Children are positioned in greater extension because of the high risk of flexion contractures (see Chapter 14).

Precautions

1. Pressure against bony prominences should be avoided.
2. To accommodate nocturnal swelling, the sides of the forearm trough should not be higher than the midline of the forearm. The curve of the trough should be less than 180 degrees and all the edges of the forearm portion should be flared slightly.
3. Daily gentle ROM should be done to prevent contractures. If there is any ROM lag, passive ROM should be done.

Patient Instruction

Wearing Time
1. For acute inflammation of the full hand, wear during bedrest and sleeping. When swelling and pain in the fingers subside or become minimal, the patient can begin to use a wrist orthosis at night.
2. For weakness, a wrist–hand orthosis is used during sleep or bedrest and a wrist orthosis is used during the day.

Note: These orthoses are very incapacitating, damaging to one's self-image, and unsexy. For some people they can be very helpful, but patients should be progressed to a less restrictive orthosis as soon as possible. (Every therapist prescribing these orthoses should wear one to bed for one night to get a feel for their restrictiveness.)

Instructions, in addition to the general instructions given earlier in this chapter, are as follows:

1. If the orthosis is to be worn at night only, patients may remove it to accomplish self-care tasks.
2. If the patient has bilateral orthoses, the straps on the dominant hand should be such that they can be opened independently (e.g., with teeth) in order to get out of bed in a hurry or in an emergency.

3. If the patient needs bilateral orthoses and cannot manage both orthoses at the same time, it is sometimes effective to have the patient alternate with a wrist orthosis every other night. Thus, on any given night only one hand is in a full orthosis.

Wrist Orthosis

The functional wrist orthosis is one that restricts or immobilizes the wrist but allows for full MCP joint and thumb mobility. The indications and goals for a wrist orthosis are listed in Table 23–4.

Design and Treatment Considerations

There are four different types of orthoses in this classification.

Rigid Thermoplastic Volar Wrist Orthosis (Fig. 23–6). This orthosis was historically referred to as a volar cock-up splint. It stabilizes the wrist by preventing flexion and circumduction but allows some extension during activities. It does *not* im-

Table 23–4 Indications and Goals for Wrist Orthosis

Indications	Goals
Hand function limited by wrist pain (patient may report dropping things or wrist giving way).	To improve hand function and grip strength (immobilization of the wrist relieves pain with motion and consequently muscle inhibition secondary to pain[1,5]).
Inflammation.	To provide localized rest to the joint, decrease inflammation and pain, and protect extensor tendons from attrition and rupture. (See discussion on extensor tendon rupture in Chapters 19 and 29.)
Some cases of persistent carpal tunnel syndrome.	To reduce pressure on the median nerve.

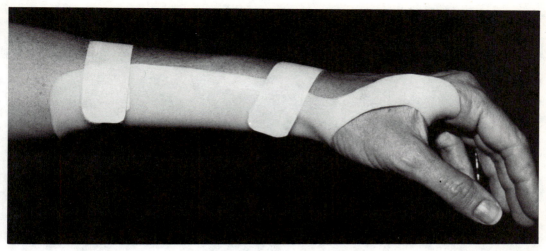

Figure 23–6. Wrist orthosis, volar type. For daytime use a third strap is needed over the dorsum of the hand to restrict wrist extension. The distal edge should not restrict the MCP joints. Wrist is 10 degrees of extension, appropriate for RA.

mobilize the wrist. It can be effective for positioning during bedrest and is preferred by many patients for this purpose because of the open design. For more stability a third strap can be added over the dorsum of the hand.

Rigid Thermoplastic Circumferential Wrist Orthosis (Fig. 23–7). This orthosis provides rigid support on all sides and immobilizes the wrist to approximately 5 degrees of motion. It is very effective for reducing inflammation or providing stability. The MCP joints must be pain free to use this orthosis.

Flexible Gauntlet-Style Wrist Orthosis with a Rigid Volar Reinforcement Bar (Fig. 23–8). This orthosis allows considerable flexion and extension, approximately 50 degrees, but prevents circumduction and flexed wrist positioning. The degree of flexion and extension reduces compensatory stress to the MCP joints, and limited circumduction reduces considerable rotational stress to the wrist. These are made of elastic, leather, canvas, or vinyl. The reinforcement bar is either aluminum or plastic.

Flexible Gauntlet-Style Wrist Orthosis with Rigid Dorsal or Dorsal and Volar Reinforcement. There are now numerous commercial gauntlet-type orthoses on the market. Generally these are more suited to industrial or traumatic wrist problems, because they tend to be bulky and dorsal pres-

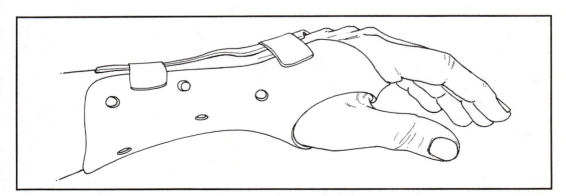

Figure 23–7. Rigid thermoplastic circumferential wrist orthosis is illustrated here (see Appendix 3).

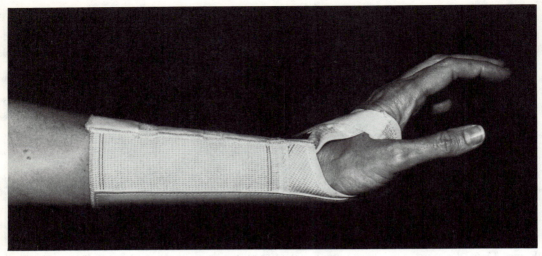

Figure 23–8. Flexible gauntlet-style wrist orthosis (Freedom Splint). In this photo the volar support is at a 10-degree angle. The patient is in active extension to demonstrate how much extension is possible in this orthosis. Some active flexion is also possible.

sure is not well tolerated by people with painful dorsal tenosynovitis or swelling and tender bony prominences.

Impact of Wrist Orthoses on MCP Joints

In some clients with active wrist and MCP joint synovitis a wrist orthosis can create or accentuate stress on the MCP joints and exacerbate the synovitis in these joints. The more severe or acute the MCP joint involvement is, the more vulnerable the MCP joints seem to be to any additional stress. Two factors seem to contribute to this process. First, immobilization of the wrist and carpal bones requires that all motion take place in the finger and elbow joints. The importance of this particular factor seems to depend on the type of work or hand skills a person does with the orthosis on. The heavier the work is, the more stress is involved. (I refer to this as **compensatory stress.**[11]) Second, in a plastic orthosis the palmar piece prevents sensation in that area. The only palmar area with sensation is over the MCP joints. This *may* require a person to apply more pressure to ensure a tight grip when picking up an object.

Those factors are described in conditional terms because the theory about this process is based on personal observation.[10] Studies are needed on how wrist orthoses affect digital joints. The hand is a complex mechanism. Immobilization of a major component is bound to have some effect on the adjacent structures. A review of the literature has not revealed any research on this topic.

In the early 1970s the rigid polyethylene wrist orthosis became a popular treatment for RA, based on the premise that complete immobilization of the wrist would eliminate wrist pain with motion and allow the patient to have greater hand strength and function. Essentially all of our patients with wrist synovitis were treated with this orthosis. At that time, I had an opportunity to work with a woman from the second day of her sudden onset RA with total joint involvement. Two weeks following onset she was discharged with bilateral rigid wrist circumferential orthoses. At the 1-month follow-up visit, she had severe (almost dislocated) MCP subluxation. With the orthoses on, her fingers literally "fell off" the end. This experience prompted me to re-examine the impact of this type of orthosis on MCP involvement in all of my patients and I found that in a majority of the patients the orthosis appeared to exacerbate the MCP synovitis. Neither the patient nor the treating physician had related the MCP exacerbation to the orthosis, and they both assumed the increased inflammation was the natural course of the disease. However, a change in wrist orthosis resulted in a decrease in MCP inflammation. The impact of a rigid wrist orthosis on MCP inflammation is variable. I have had patients with minimal MCP synovitis who did not *appear* to have any increase in MCP inflammation wearing a rigid wrist orthosis during the day. However, it is clear that the greater the MCP inflammation, the more vulnerable the joint is to compensatory stress generated by a rigid wrist orthosis. As a result of this experience I am very cautious about recommending rigid orthoses for daytime use. I have found the program for orthotic treatment outlined below to be the most effective for treating wrist synovitis in patients with coexistent MCP synovitis.

The primary guideline is the following: *the more active or acute the MCP joint involvement, the less restrictive the wrist orthosis for daytime use.* (This daytime protocol is in conjunction with a thermoplastic wrist or full hand orthosis at night.)

1. *Severe, acute wrist synovitis and minimal MCP joint involvement.* The patient with this condition may benefit the most from a thermoplastic orthosis with instruction to monitor the MCP joints carefully. If the orthosis appears to be making the MCP joints worse, a change to a more flexible orthosis is advised.

2. *Moderate wrist synovitis and moderate MCP synovitis.* The optimal orthosis is a flexible elastic-vinyl gauntlet (commercial) orthosis with the metal reinforcement included. These orthoses allow approximately 50 degrees of wrist flexion-extension but prevent circumduction; thus, they reduce considerable rotation forces to the wrist but do not alter flexion and extension dynamics as much as a rigid orthosis does.

3. *Moderate wrist synovitis and acute MCP synovitis.* If the PIP joints are not involved, a thermoplastic wrist–MCP stabilization orthosis may be ideal. If the PIP joints are inflamed, this type of orthosis may cause compensatory stress to the PIP joints. For these patients it may be necessary to use a flexible commercial orthosis with the metal bar removed.

These examples of orthotic treatment apply to patients with early active disease. For patients with damaged unstable wrist joints and essentially inactive MCP joint disease, thermoplastic wrist gauntlet orthoses are often ideal for daytime use.

Precautions

1. Orthoses may increase deforming stresses to the MCP joints.
2. To allow full MCP flexion, the distal end of the orthosis should extend about 1 cm proximal to the distal palmar crease.
3. Full thumb opposition should be possible.
4. The thumb web space section can irritate or cut the skin. (The edges should be smoothed or rolled; moleskin padding should be avoided if possible.) It is usually most comfortable if it does not impinge against the index MCP joint.
5. There should not be any pressure over the ulnar styloid.

Patient Instruction

Wearing Protocol

The following instructions are in addition to the general instructions given earlier in this chapter.

1. If the purpose of the orthosis is to decrease pain and increase hand function, the orthosis should be worn during hand activities.
2. The patient should remove the orthosis several times during the day or when needed; the wrist should be ranged and the skin should be checked for pressure areas.
3. When this orthosis is prescribed to increase hand function and is to be worn during activities, it is important that the patient has realistic expectations of the orthosis. The orthosis may relieve wrist pain, but the palmar piece and restricted mobility reduce dexterity, making many activities more difficult. Unrealistic expectations can lead to disappointment and discarding of the splint.
4. For circumferential orthoses, cotton stockinette liners are the most effective and hygienic. For the thermoplastic volar orthosis the liner is optimal but many patients prefer it for warmth and comfort.

Wrist–MCP Orthosis and MCP Orthosis

There are two basic types of orthoses that can immobilize the MCP joints to reduce inflammation and the deforming pull of the flexor tendons, yet allow hand function—the wrist–MCP orthosis (Figs. 23–9 and 23–10) and the MCP orthoses (Fig. 23–11). However, the use of these orthoses on patients with RA is very limited because these orthoses can cause severe compensatory stress to the PIP joints, and most RA patients with active MCP synovitis have PIP involvement also. *These orthoses can exacerbate the PIP synovitis.* These orthoses can be used effectively on people with active MCP synovitis with normal or inactive PIP involvement. Synovitis solely in the MCP joints is more common in psoriatic arthritis, systemic lupus erythematosus, and occasionally ankylosing spondylitis. Indications and goals for these orthoses are listed in Table 23–5.

Design and Treatment Considerations

Variable basic designs include

1. A static volar wrist cock-up splint with an extended palmar piece and individual finger separators. It may have an optional thumb post and ulnar ridge (see Fig. 23–9).
2. A dorsal design with volar digit loops as described by Quest and Cordery[17] (see Fig. 23–11).
3. Static short orthosis that fits entirely on the hand with a palmar piece over the MCP heads, individual finger separators, and dorsal strap closure (Fig. 23–12).
4. Circumferential wrist stabilization orthosis that extends to the middle of the proximal phalanges. This is used when there is both wrist and MCP joint involvement but no active PIP synovitis (see Fig. 23–10).

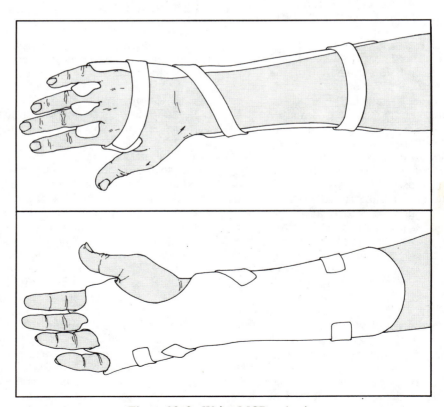

Figure 23–9. Wrist–MCP orthosis.

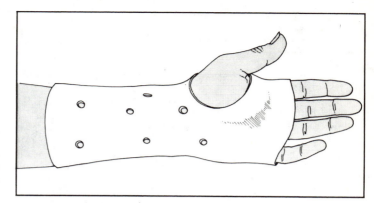

Figure 23–10. Wrist-MCP orthosis, made of high-temperature polyethylene (see Appendix 3).

The most important treatment consideration has already been stated; that is, immobilization of one joint can cause increased stress to the adjacent joints. In this case the PIP joints are the most vulnerable. I have used the MCP orthosis much more frequently than the wrist–MCP orthosis. Somehow patients with active MCP and wrist synovitis severe enough to warrant a rigid orthosis usually have PIP synovitis as well. I have used the MCP orthosis on a number of people with psoriatic arthritis whose PIPs were normal and wrist synovitis was minimal but had persistent active MCP synovitis. I find the dorsal MCP orthosis (see Fig. 23–10) made of ³⁄₃₂-inch Aquaplast (volar digit loops of ¹⁄₁₆-inch thickness) extremely effective in reducing MCP synovitis and stretching the intrinsic musculature.

For MCP synovitis without intrinsic tightness

1. The MCPs should be positioned in approximately 30 degrees of flexion.
2. The index digit should be in a position that allows lateral pinch and writing with the dominant hand.
3. For acute synovitis the orthosis immediately reduces pain and is well tolerated. For prolonged use patients often report they prefer the MCP joints in extension because they can't place their hand flat or stretch it out.

For MCP synovitis and intrinsic tightness

1. The MCP joints should be in zero extension except the index finger may have to

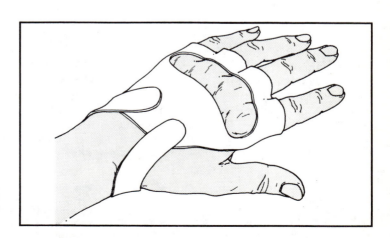

Figure 23–11. MCP orthosis: dorsal type (Quest-Cordery splint).[15]

Table 23–5 Indications and Goals for the Wrist–MCP and MCP Orthoses

Indications	Goals
MCP synovitis without active PIP synovitis, or MCP and wrist synovitis.	To prevent overstretching of the capsule during phases of inflammation and swelling. The capsular and articular ligaments are distended by joint effusions and are extremely vulnerable to overstretching during these phases. These orthoses minimize the three most damaging forces on the MCP joint: 1. Pull of the flexor tendons in strong grasp and pinch[18] 2. Passive pressure toward ulnar deviation 3. Reflex spasms of the intrinsic muscles
Beginning MCP volar subluxation, beginning swan-neck deformities, or intrinsic tightness (without active PIP synovitis).	To stretch tight intrinsic muscles by keeping the MCP joints in extension and allowing PIP flexion,[10] thereby producing gentle repetitive stretch to the intrinsic muscles. The orthosis can be used solely as a positioning device during stretching exercises or during activities.

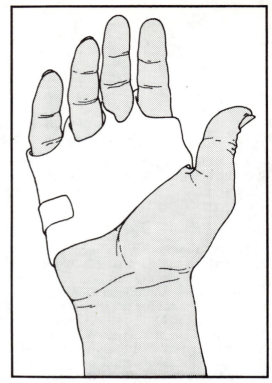

Figure 23–12. Palmar MCP orthosis (Johnson-Johnson pattern).

be in slight flexion to allow writing and pinch prehension.

2. Any orthosis that maintains the MCP joints in extension *must be carefully monitored because prolonged use can result in contracture of the collateral ligaments.* Treating the acute synovitis takes priority over the intrinsic tightness and should be done first.

Precautions

1. Careful, frequent skin inspection must be carried out for orthoses with finger separators. Patients with dry, atrophied, tissue-paper skin resulting from long-term steroid use may be prone to skin breakdown with these splints.

2. For volar designs, maximal allowance for the thenar eminence is necessary for hand function.

3. *Positioning of the MCP joints in extension can cause shortening of the collateral ligaments, especially in diagnoses other than MCP synovitis.* In the presence of chronic MCP synovitis, the radial collateral ligaments become overstretched. It is possible that splinting in extension may cause a desirable shortening of these ligaments, but further experimentation is needed in this area.

Patient Instruction

These instructions are in addition to the general instructions given earlier in this chapter.

1. For MCP synovitis, the orthosis is preferably worn both day and night with removal for ROM exercises and brief periods throughout the day when the patient is at leisure. If the patient cannot tolerate day and night wear, then the daytime hours, when hand function is greatest, are recommended for orthosis use.

2. If the orthosis is used for protection, its purpose is to counteract the ulnar deviating and subluxating forces that are created by the long finger flexors on the MCP joint capsule during grasp and pinch activities. (See Chapter 19, Hand Pathodynamics and Assessment, for pathodynamics of ulnar drift.) This is a difficult concept for patients to understand, but they need to have an awareness of the process in order to know how to protect their joints. They also must receive instruction in how to manage tasks in a protective manner when they are not wearing the orthosis, for example, during bathing and while handling sheets and blankets in bed. (See Chapter 24, Joint-Protection and Energy-Conservation Instruction.)

3. Treatment of intrinsic tightness is still experimental. It may be necessary to wear the orthosis for as little as 1 hour twice a day or as long as all day, or even during the night, depending upon severity of the tightness and the treatment objective.

4. Patients must be told that this orthosis, like most hand orthoses, decreases hand dexterity.

Wrist–MCP Orthosis: Dynamic Postsurgical Type

The wrist–MCP orthosis (Fig. 23–13) is used in the postoperative treatment of MCP joint implant arthroplasty. The orthosis positions and supports the wrist, controls position and alignment of the fingers while allowing active flexion, and allows for the application of dynamic flexion force. The goal of treatment is to apply controlled low-amplitude force over a prolonged period to influence the organization and synthesis of new scar tissue forming in and around the joint capsule—the **encapsulation process**[19] (Table 23–6). (See Chapter 29 on hand surgery for an explanation of the encapsulation process, specific surgical procedures, and timing of orthotic treatment.)

Design and Treatment Considerations

The low-profile dynamic outrigger (see Fig. 23–13) has gained in popularity over the last several years and has replaced the high-profile outrigger (Fig. 23–14) in the management of post MCP arthroplasty in most hand therapy clinics. The low-profile outrigger requires a dorsal design with a *rigid transverse palmar bar* to prevent wrist flexion. It is preferable to fabricate the orthosis from a thermoplastic material with high contourability and ease in bonding such as the polycaprolactone group (Aquaplast, Polyform, K-splint). A close-conforming orthosis prevents slippage when flexion assist force is applied. The orthosis should also have a transverse outrigger that allows individual alignment of the fingers. The outrigger can be a commercial design (see Fig. 23–13) or hand fabricated of wire. (See the article by Judy Colditz.[20]) The specific design of the orthosis can vary as long as the principles of dynamic application of force are adhered to, the goals can be achieved, and the orthosis is aesthetically acceptable.

Design Considerations for the Orthosis

1. The wrist should be positioned in 5 to 10 degrees of ulnar deviation (if possible) and in neutral or 10 degrees of extension. More than 10 degrees of wrist extension places the long extensors on slack and makes it difficult to maintain MCP joint extension.

2. The palmar surface should not extend beyond the proximal palmar crease in order to allow full MCP joint flexion.

3. The orthosis should allow full thumb opposition and extension.

4. The orthosis should cover the distal two thirds of the forearm.

5. The distal end should cover the MCP joints (over the incision). If it is too short, the incision area will be pinched by the end of the orthosis during MCP extension.

6. The orthotic design must allow for stable attachment of the extensor and, if necessary, flexor outrigger.

7. The orthosis should not create pressure on the ulnar styloid. It is best to di-

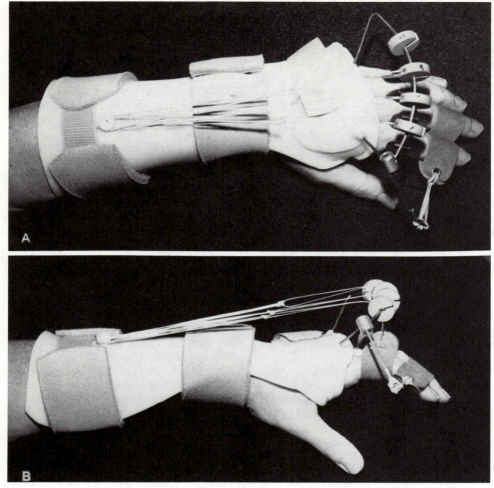

Figure 23–13. Dorsal wrist–MCP orthosis with dynamic low-profile Phoenix outrigger. This orthosis has a rigid palmar support to prevent wrist flexion.

rectly pad the styloid before forming the orthosis. (A thin layer of petroleum jelly over the foam will prevent it from sticking to the thermoplastic.)

Principles of Dynamic Application of Force for Postoperative Management of MCP Arthroplasty

1. *Providing force perpendicular (90 degrees) to the long axis of the proximal phalanx.* This allows the most efficient application of force and prevents compression or distraction of the phalanx. It also helps prevent the slings from cutting into the web space.[9]

2. *Providing constant application of force.* This is done by using long rubber-bands and stretching them twice their resting length. This provides a more constant tension than a shorter band stretched twice its resting length.[20] A long rubberband maintains more tension if the MCP joint increases in extension.

The distance of the outrigger to the point of force application and the length of plastic (fishing) line can often be adjusted to allow maximal rubberband length.

3. *The appropriate amount of applied force is the minimal amount that will support the phalanges in neutral extension at rest and allow full available active flexion.* Some surgeons recommend maintaining the ring finger in 10 degrees of flexion and the little finger in 10 to 20 degrees so their

Table 23–6 Indications and Goals for the Wrist–MCP Orthosis: Dynamic Postsurgical Type

Indications	Goals
Post-MCP joint implant arthroplasty.	To position the wrist optimally.
	To position the fingers in optimal dorsovolar, radioulnar, and rotational alignment (at rest and in motion) to facilitate optimal encapsulation.
	To minimize ulnar deviating forces.
	To reduce extensor lag, thereby increasing the mechanical advantages and functional strength of the extensor communis tendons.
	To increase MCP flexion range.
	To prevent or minimize postsurgical adhesion.

post-treatment range will have greater flexion than the radial fingers, so essential for grip.

4. *The assists should pull the fingers just radial of their normal deviation.* For the index finger, this would mean 10 degrees ulnar deviation since normal deviation for this digit is approximately 20 degrees ulnarly. This is to allow tightening of the radial capsule.[19]

5. *If the fingers pronate abnormally, additional lateral supination assists may be necessary to correct rotation.*[19]

6. *Flexion force should be applied by a method that allows individual adjustment for each digit.* This can be done with individual digit slings. In some instances flexion and rotational forces can best be applied to a dress hook fastener attached to the fingernail with cyanoacrylate adhesive. A single flexion cuff does not allow for individualization of applied force.

7. *The pull of the flexor force should be toward the scaphoid (navicular) and not toward the center of the wrist.*[8]

8. *The appropriate amount of flexion force is the minimal amount necessary to pull or maintain the digit at the end of available flexion range.* The flexion force should be light, not heavy. The goal is to gently maintain the joint in flexion for a prolonged period, and not to use force to increase range.

9. *Adequate stabilization of the orthosis so it does not migrate distal during the application of flexor assists.* The purpose of the assists is to increase flexion. If the orthosis slides distal because of the rubberbands pulling the orthosis to the fingers instead of the fingers to the orthosis, the palmar bar or edge slides over the MCP heads, preventing flexion. If the orthosis conforms closely to the contours of the hand, the orthosis should not slide. In this case, sliding is often due to excessive force. If a commercial orthosis is used, with low conformability a figure-eight elbow strap may be necessary to provide proximal stabilization of the orthosis during application of the flexion assists.[19,20]

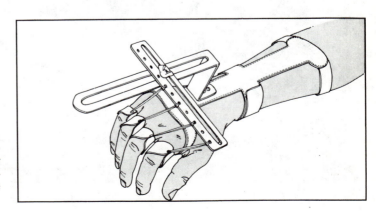

Figure 23–14. High-profile dynamic, wrist–MCP orthosis for post-MCP-arthroplasty treatment (Swanson design Pope brace).

Precautions

1. If finger slings are too tight or of a hard, nonporous material such as plastic, skin breakdown or irritation may occur. Recommended materials include ultra-suede and moleskin with the adhesive backing left on. Commercial slings frequently need to be trimmed.

2. Finger slings should be narrow enough to allow full PIP flexion.

3. Too much extensor band tension may cause undue joint stress; therefore, adjust the tension to patient's tolerance.

4. Flexion assists that pull the fingers toward the center of the wrist rather than to the scaphoid may cause rotational stress to the MCP joints.

5. If swelling occurs distal to the orthosis or distal to the assist slings, the orthosis is too tight and needs adjusting.

6. The design of the orthosis needs to allow easy application and adjustment so that the assists remain in adjustment during patient application at home.

Patient Instruction

These instructions are in addition to the general instructions given earlier in this chapter.

1. The patient should be *given written instructions* explaining when to wear the orthosis and how to position it and the assist bands. It is helpful to identify visual landmarks that he or she can use to spot check that the orthosis is positioned correctly. Usually the patient should be able to change from flexion to extension assists independently.

2. The patient should have a clear understanding of the postoperative goals and treatment procedures and the importance of positioning the orthosis correctly.

Postoperative Procedure

See Chapter 29 on hand surgery. Therapists treating MCP arthroplasties should be familiar with Dr. Alfred Swanson's postoperative guides and the article by Madden, DeVore, and Arem on postoperative management.[21,22]

Wrist–Thumb Orthoses

Type I: For de Quervain's Tenosynovitis

The type I orthosis (Fig. 23–15) is ideal for treatment of de Quervain's (first compartment) tenosynovitis because it provides a radial post to prevent motion of the abductor pollicis longus (APL) and the extensor pollicis brevis (EPB), the two tendons in the first wrist compartment, yet it allows wrist and IP motion. Thus, this design complies with one of the basic principles of orthotic management; that is, restricting the minimal number of joints possible to achieve the therapeutic goal.

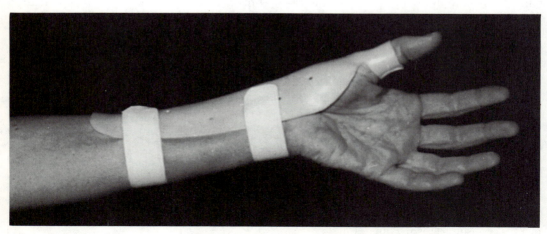

Figure 23–15. Wrist–thumb orthosis for de Quervain's tenosynovitis.

Design and Treatment Considerations

To treat de Quervain's tenosynovitis it is essential to restrict or block wrist deviation but *not* flexion and extension. The radial design (i.e., the forearm sides do not extend beyond the midline of the forearm) allows midrange flexion and extension but not deviation.

Thumb flexion and ulnar wrist deviation put the greatest stress on the tendons in the first compartment. It is *not* necessary to restrict thumb IP motion or thumb abduction (with a C-bar). The type I design allows CMC motion by stabilizing the thumb and allowing the hand to approximate to the thumb.

The distal end of the thumb post should allow full IP flexion wide enough to prevent pinching of the flexor surface during full IP flexion. If the patient has inflammation of the IP joint, this orthosis could aggravate the IP arthritis by restricting proximal joint motion. In this case it may be necessary to extend the distal portion to cover the IP joint but leave the thumb tip exposed for pinch.

Patients with de Quervain's tenosynovitis can return directly to work or activities after being fitted with this orthosis without fear of stressing the affected tendons.

The orthosis should be fitted with the wrist in 10 degrees of ulnar deviation and approximately 35 degrees of extension, so the patient can accomplish desk-top, writing, and grip activities easily. This design is appropriate only for people who do not have wrist involvement; therefore, there are no restrictions against extension positioning. After fitting the orthosis, it is critical that the edge over the dorsum of the hand does not cut in or restrict the hand during writing or other functional activities.

On occasion people with chronic carpal tunnel syndrome or wrist synovitis will develop acute de Quervain's tenosynovitis or inflammatory OA of the CMC joint and it is necessary to restrict both the wrist and the thumb. If the patient has de Quervain's tenosynovitis it is *not* necessary to have a C-bar. If the patient has CMC arthritis it is essential to prevent CMC motion with a C-bar. The wrist should be positioned in 10 degrees of extension and 10 degrees of ulnar deviation. The distal palmar edge should not restrict MCP flexion. If the patient also has MCP inflammation, this type of orthosis can create compensatory stress on the MCP joints. In this case it would be preferable to treat the De Quervain's tenosynovitis with the type I design, even though it is not ideal for the wrist, and to treat CMC arthritis with a thumb (CMC-MCP) orthosis and a flexible wrist orthosis (e.g., the Freedom Splint).

Type II: For Combined Wrist and Thumb CMC Joint Dysfunction (see Fig. 23–16)

There are a number of wrist disorders that are treated with complete prolonged immobilization. For example, intercarpal instability, acute or chronic wrist synovitis, intercarpal arthritis, and wrist instability (when surgery is not feasible). For most patients, a circumferential wrist orthosis is sufficient. However, when the CMC joint is directly involved, has concomitant OA, or when CMC motion aggravates wrist pain, it is necessary to enclose the CMC joint. (Unfortunately this requires inclusion of the MCP joint even if it is not involved.)

Design and Treatment Considerations

1. In order to immobilize the wrist there has to be rigid volar and dorsal support; dorsal straps are not sufficient.

2. To achieve a close fit, the orthotic material has to have high conformability and be thinner than ⅛-inch thick. Material ⅛-inch thick is too bulky and heavy for this design. The orthosis in Fig. 23–16 is made out of ³⁄₃₂-inch thick Aquaplast.

3. The circumferential design requires that the material be "bubbled" over the ulnar styloid and flared away from the radial styloid.

4. The edges along the forearm opening need to be slightly flared to prevent pinching of the skin.

5. The distal palmar end should not limit MCP flexion.

6. The thumb portion should allow full IP flexion and position the thumb in a manner that maintains maximal CMC abduction but allows writing with the dominant hand.

Wearing Protocols. Immobilization for intercarpal instability or trauma related in-

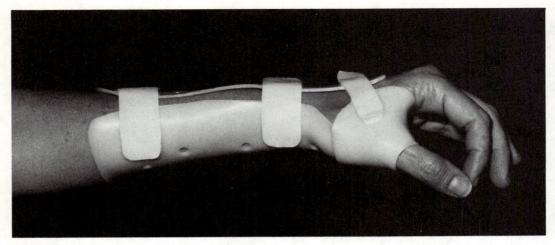

Figure 23–16. Wrist–thumb orthosis, circumferential type, immobilizes the wrist and thumb CMC-MCP joints (can be made without the thumb section). Wrist is in 10 degrees of ulnar deviation.

juries can vary from 2 to 12 months. The treatment for wrist synovitis and concomitant thumb involvement is the same as outlined for "acute wrist synovitis without digital involvement" in the section on orthotic treatment for specific conditions in the beginning of this chapter.

Thumb Orthosis: CMC-MCP Stabilization Type

The thumb orthosis for CMC stabilization restricts motion of the thumb CMC and MCP joints but allows full function of the wrist, thumb IP, and index MCP joints (Fig. 23–17). It maintains the thumb in palmar abduction. It is not necessary to immobilize the wrist to treat the thumb CMC

joint effectively. The indications and goals for this orthosis are listed in Table 23–7.

Design and Treatment Considerations

It is critical to fabricate small hand orthoses of this type out of a thermoplastic material with high contourability. The lighter and thinner the material, the less the orthosis interferes with hand function and the greater the patient acceptance. Thermoplastic in ⅟₁₆-inch thickness (e.g., Aquaplast) is ideal.

The design of the orthosis must include the MCP joint because the structure of the thumb makes it impossible to immobilize the CMC joint and simultaneously allow full MCP joint motion. Treatment of a

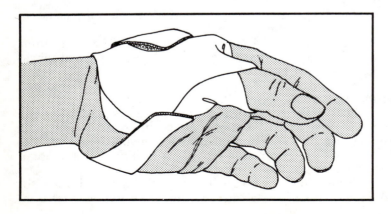

Figure 23–17. Thumb orthosis for CMC stabilization.

Table 23–7 Indications and Goals for the Thumb Orthosis: CMC Stabilization Type

Indications	Goals
Thumb CMC pain with motion.	To relieve pain, reduce inflammation, and increase hand function. This orthosis is most effective for isolated joint involvement typically seen with osteoarthritis.
To maintain CMC web space (e.g., for systemic sclerosis).	

CMC fracture requires immobilization of the wrist to total restriction of movement. However, total elimination of motion is not necessary to treat CMC arthritis effectively. I created the design shown in Figure 23–15 in 1976, and since that time it has been used by more than a thousand patients with a very high success rate. A follow-up mail survey of my patients regarding compliance with this orthosis revealed that 82 percent found the orthosis effective in reducing pain and inflammation and wore it as prescribed.[23]

When the orthosis is not effective, the problem is usually that compression force applied to the tip of the thumb is the aggravating factor; this cannot be avoided and function permitted at the same time. The small amount of motion that would be eliminated by a wrist–thumb orthosis is rarely if ever the source of pain. Treating CMC arthritis with a wrist–thumb orthosis violates one of the primary principles of orthotic management: *An orthosis should encompass the minimal number of joints required to achieve the therapeutic goal.*

The only part of the orthosis that is therapeutic is the abduction C-bar, which creates a wedge that restricts CMC joint motion. The rest of the orthosis simply holds it in place. Theoretically the C-bar should be made as wide as possible for maximal restriction of motion, with the thumb positioned in palmar abduction. However, I have found that if positioning the thumb in

maximal abduction limits writing or pinch prehension, patients will not wear the orthosis. After the fitting, I therefore make sure patients can perform pinch prehension and writing (if it is the dominant hand) comfortably. If not, I sacrifice some restriction and narrow the C-bar. The degree of MCP flexion is also critical for comfortable writing. When treating the dominant hand, I advise observing the patient write before fitting the orthosis and noting the degree of thumb MCP joint flexion he or she uses (everyone is different). The orthosis should be fabricated with the same degree of MCP flexion.

Precautions

1. A careful functional performance checkout is necessary to determine if the orthosis binds, rubs, or limits IP joint flexion or index MCP joint flexion.
2. This orthosis should *not* be used on patients with active thumb IP joint inflammation, because immobilization of the MCP joint will create compensatory stress to the joint, exacerbating the synovitis. In some cases the orthosis can be made longer to include the IP joint, but leaving the tip or pad free.
3. The inside seam should be smoothed flat, because it crosses over the delicate dorsal skin.
4. If a person has an enlarged thumb IP joint and a narrow phalanx shaft, be sure to slide the orthosis distal so the neck of the opening is over the widest part of the IP joint, just before the material is cool or full set. This prevents the orthosis from getting stuck on the thumb. The thumb opening must be wide enough to slide over the IP joint and to accommodate the volar tissue during IP flexion as well as diurnal swelling.

Patient Instruction

These instructions are in addition to the general instructions given earlier in this chapter.

Wearing Protocol for CMC Joint Inflammation. I have the patient wear the orthosis day and night for 2 to 3 weeks to give the joint maximal rest. At the end of the second week I have the patient "test the waters," that is, go without the orthosis for

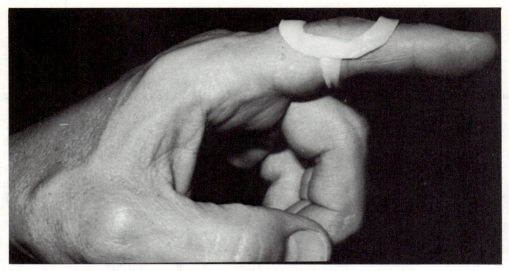

Figure 23–18. Finger orthosis, tripoint design (Aquaplast pattern).

the morning or day. If the patient has pain after a couple of hours, he or she should wear the orthosis for another few days or a week and then again "test the waters." When the patient gets to the point that he or she can get through the day without any pain, I recommend that the patient begin wearing the orthosis during stressful activities for another month or two to keep the inflammation out of the joint for a prolonged period. The more complete the elimination of inflammation, the more re-sistant the joint appears to be to the stress of physical activity.

Finger Orthoses: Tripoint Type

The tripoint design applies pressure at three points and can be used to restrict either joint flexion or extension (Figs. 23–18 and 23–19). Indications and goals for its use are listed in Table 23–8.

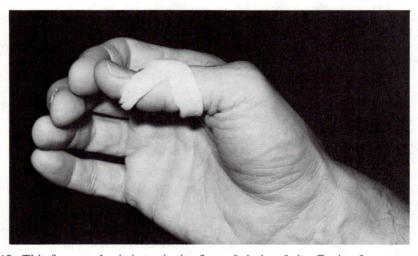

Figure 23–19. This finger orthosis is a tripoint-figure 8 design. It is effective for preventing flexion and for stabilizing the thumb IP joint.

Table 23–8 Indications and Goals for the Tripoint Design Orthosis

Indications	Goals
Swan-neck deformities.	To improve hand function and relieve stress to the volar aspect of the PIP joint resulting from severe hyperextension. To improve cosmesis (occasionally).
Postsurgical swan-neck repair (Littler procedure).	To prevent overstretching of ligaments and expansion of fibers during postoperative healing phase.[24]
Thumb hyperextension.	To improve function, especially pinch prehension.
Boutonnière deformity.	To decrease or prevent PIP contractures usually requiring the Bunnell safety pin splint.
Mutilans or PIP/IP instability.	To improve stability for function.

Design and Treatment Considerations

The tripoint finger orthosis is a small, lightweight orthosis that applies pressure at three points: proximal and distal to the dorsal surface of the joint and centrally to the opposing surface (Fig. 23–18). These orthoses are most frequently made from thermoplastic material but can be made out of metal.[25] Aquaplast (⅟₁₆-inch) can be quickly shaped to a highly cosmetic, lightweight slip-on orthosis. The Silver Ring Company will custom create an orthosis to your specifications (Fig. 23–16). The designs can vary. I currently use the Aquaplast design (see Fig. 23–18), a figure-eight design (see Fig. 23–19), and the Silver Ring splints (see Fig. 23–20).

Aquaplast and Silver Ring orthoses appear to have the highest patient acceptance. Plastic orthoses are suitable for one to three fingers with swan-neck deformities, but they are not practical for all of the digits except for short-term postsurgical treatment. The Silver Ring orthoses can be worn on all

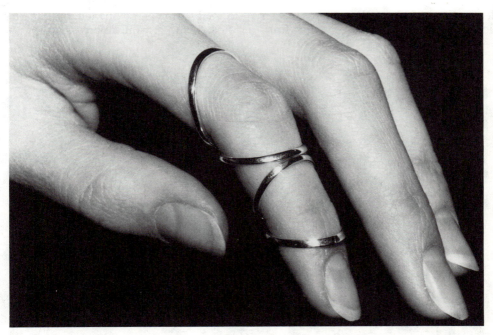

Figure 23–20. Two Silver Ring Splints are demonstrated on a normal hand. The one on the PIP joint prevents hyperextension associated with swan-neck deformities and provides lateral stability. The splint on the DIP joint prevents hyperextension associated with a boutonnière deformity.

digits. (See Chapter 19, Hand Pathodynamics and Assessment, for dynamics of swan-neck deformities.) They also have the advantage of being adjustable.

Orthoses for the thumb usually need to be custom contoured because they are the most difficult to fit. They can also be used to reduce lateral forces to the thumb as a protective or preventive measure during functional activities such as needlework.

The PIP joint following swan-neck surgery should not extend to neutral and be restricted to −10 degrees of extension or 10 degrees of flexion in order to encourage shortening of the volar structures and, it is hoped, to inhibit recurrence.[24]

Precautions

In swan-neck deformities the skin over the volar surface of the PIP joint may be especially tender or vulnerable as a result of the constant stretch from PIP subluxation (hyperextension). Frequently the desired close fit may become constrictive with diurnal or nocturnal swelling.

Patient Instruction

See earlier section in this chapter for instructions pertaining to patient education.

Finger Orthosis: Cylinder Design

A cylinder orthosis (Fig. 23–21) can be designed to prevent motion in either a PIP or a DIP joint.

Design and Treatment Considerations

This orthosis needs to be made out of a thin thermoplastic (e.g., $\frac{1}{16}$-inch thick) so it will not rub against the adjacent fingers. It is also important that it be lightweight to avoid stress and fatigue to the proximal adjacent joint(s). This orthosis can also be made out of plaster of Paris bandage, but since this material is bulkier and cannot be cleaned, there is no advantage to using it for people with arthritis.

Cylinder orthoses for the PIP joint should not interfere with MCP or IP joint flexion. Those for the DIP joint should not restrict the PIP joint and should expose as much of the finger pad as possible for prehension.

Fabrication of the cylinder with a dorsal seam is recommended. If variations in swelling require an adjustable orthosis, the dorsal seam can be opened and the orthosis closed with a mini Velcro strap.

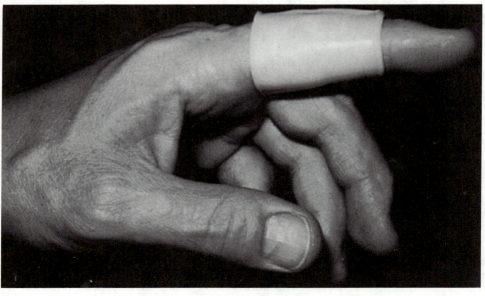

Figure 23–21. Finger orthosis, cylinder design. This orthosis allows full MCP and DIP mobility.

When the orthosis is being used for serial treatment to increase PIP joint extension (serial casting), the dorsal portion distal to the PIP joint can be removed (leaving a half cylinder distal to the joint). This adaptation allows easy donning and removal over a PIP joint flexion contracture.

Solid Aquaplast with punched airholes seems easier to work with because the edges are smooth and it adheres more easily to strapping material. The perforated material leaves rough edges.

For the protocol for treatment of PIP synovitis and osteoarthritis of the DIP joint see the section on orthotic treatment for specific conditions at the beginning of this chapter.

Precautions

During fabrication it is important to *avoid stretching* the material. If the material is stretched the finished orthosis tends to be too tight. The orthosis should slide on and off easily.

If the finger swells and the orthosis is hard to remove (i.e., stuck) the patient should hold the finger under *cold* water.

The indications and goals for the cylinder design finger orthosis are given in Table 23–9.

Table 23–9 Indications and Goals for a Cylinder Design Finger Orthosis

Indications	Goals
PIP synovitis.	To reduce stress and inflammation.
Inflammatory osteoarthritis of the DIP joint.	To decrease pain and inflammation.
To block PIP motion during exercise Anti-boutonnière exercises.	To encourage DIP flexion during PIP extension.
Post-MCP arthroplasty	To encourage MCP flexion.
Serial extension treatment of the PIP joint.	To increase PIP extension (in a noninflamed joint).

REFERENCES

1. Partridge, REH, and Duthie, JJR: Controlled trial of the effect of complete immobilization of the joints in rheumatoid arthritis. Ann Rheum Dis 22:91, 1963.
2. Gault, SS, and Spyker, JM: Beneficial effect of immobilization of joints in rheumatoid arthritis and related arthritides: A splint study using sequential analysis. Arthritis Rheum 12:34, 1969.
3. Ehrlich, GE (ed): Total Management of the Arthritic Patient. JB Lippincott, Philadelphia, 1973, p 52.
4. d'Andrade, JR et al: Joint distension and reflex muscle inhibition in the knee. J Bone Joint Surg 47A:313, 1965.
5. Millender, LH, and Nalebuff, EA: Reconstructive surgery in the rheumatoid hand. Orthop Clin North Am 6:712, 1975.
6. Sherrington, CS: The Integrative Action of the Nervous System. Yale University Press, New Haven, CT, 1906.
7. American Academy of Orthopedic Surgeons: Atlas of Orthotics/Biomechanics: Principles and Application. CV Mosby, St Louis, 1975.
8. Malick, MH: Manual on Dynamic Hand Splinting with Thermoplastic Materials. Harmarville Rehabilitation Center, Pittsburgh, PA, 1974, pp 7, 16, 177–183.
9. Fess, EF, and Phillips, CA: Hand Splinting—Principles and Methods. CV Mosby, St Louis, 1987.
10. Boyes, J: Bunnell's Surgery of the Hand, 5th ed. JB Lippincott, Philadelphia, 1970, pp 10–11, 173–175.
11 Melvin, JL: Rheumatic Disease: Occupational Therapy and Rehabilitation. FA Davis, Philadelphia, 1977.
12. Convery, FR, Conaty, JP, and Nickel, VL: Dynamic splinting of the rheumatoid hand. Orthop Prosth, March, 1968, p 41.
13. Nolinske, T: Principles of upper limb orthotics. Physical Disabilities Special Interest Section Newsletter, AOTA, Rockville, MD, 9(2):1.
14. Malick, MH: Manual on Static Hand Splinting. Harmarville Rehabilitation Center, Pittsburgh, PA, 1973.
15. Kiel, JH: Basic Hand Splinting—A Pattern Design Approach. Little, Brown & Co, Boston, 1983.
16. Flatt, AE: Care of the Rheumatoid Hand, ed 3, CV Mosby, St Louis, 1974, p 250.
17. Quest, D, and Cordery, J: A functional ulnar deviation cuff for the rheumatoid deformity. Am J Occup Ther 25:32, 1971.
18. Smith, EM et al: Flexor forces and rheumatoid metacarpophalangeal deformity. JAMA 198:130, 1966.
19. Swanson, AB: Flexible Implant Resection Arthroplasty in the Hand and Extremities. CV Mosby, St Louis, 1973, pp 171–183.
20. Colditz, JC: Low profile dynamic splinting of the

injured hand. Am J Occup Ther 37(3):182–188, 1983.

21. Swanson, AB, Swanson, GG, and Leonard, J: Postoperative rehabilitation program for inflexible implant arthroplasty of the digits. In Hunter, JM, Schneider, LH, Mackin, EJ, and Bell, JA: Rehabilitation of the Hand. CV Mosby, St Louis, 1978.

22. Madden, JW, DeVore, G, and Arem, AJ: A rational postoperative management program for metacarpophalangeal joint implant arthroplasty. J Hand Surg 2:358, 1977.

23. Melvin, J, and Carlson Rioux, J: Compliance and effectiveness of a thumb-CMC-MCP orthosis for OA of the CMC joint (in press).

24. Nalebuff, EA, and Millender, LH: Surgical treatment of the swan neck deformity in rheumatoid arthritis. Orthop Clin North Am 6:733, 1975.

25. Bennett, RL: Wrists and hand slip-on splints. In Licht, E (ed): Arthritis and Physical Medicine. Elizabeth Licht Publishers, New Haven, CT, 1969, pp 484–485.

ADDITIONAL SOURCES

Barr, RN: The Hand: Principles and Techniques of Simple Splint Making and Rehabilitation. Butterworth & Co, Boston, 1975. (Excellent resource. Describes method for making wire outriggers and polyethylene thumb splint.)

Bennett, RL: Orthotic devices to prevent deformities of the hand in rheumatoid arthritis. Arthritis Rheum 8:1006, 1965.

Bergfeld, AJ, Weiker, CG, Andrish, JT, Hall, R: Soft playing splint for protection of significant hand and wrist injuries in sports. Am J Sports Med 10(5):293–296, 1982.

Besser, MI: The conservative treatment of the swan neck deformity in the rheumatoid hand. Hand 10(1):91, 1978.

Biddulph, SL: The effect of the Futuro wrist brace in pain conditions of the wrist. S Afr Med J 60(10):839–891, September 1981.

Biewlawski, T, and Bear-Lehman, J: A gauntlet work splint. Am J Occup Ther 40(3):199, 1986.

Brand, PW: The forces of dynamic splinting: Ten questions before applying a dynamic splint to the hand. In Hunter, JM, Schneider, LH, Mackin, EJ, and Bell, JA (eds): Rehabilitation of the Hand. CV Mosby, St Louis, 1978.

Callahan, AD, and McEntee, P: Splinting proximal interphalangeal joint flexion contractures: A new design. Am J Occup Ther 40(6):408, 1986.

Carlson, JD, and Trombly, CA: The effect of wrist immobilization on performance of the Jebsen Hand Function Test. Am J Occup Ther 37(3):167–175, 1983.

Carr, K: Hand splints for rheumatoid arthritis. Can J Occup Ther 35:17, 1978.

Colditz, JC: Low profile dynamic splinting of the injured hand. Am J Occup Ther 37(3):182–188, 1983.

Convery, RF, and Minteer, MA: The use of orthoses in the management of rheumatoid arthritis. Clin Orthop 102:118, 1974.

Day, L: Splinting the Rheumatoid Hand. LDS Enterprises, Dallas, 1983.

Elliott, RA Jr: Splints for mallet and boutonniere deformities. Plast Reconstr Surg 52:282, 1973.

English, CB, Rehn, RA, and Petzoldt, RL: Blocking splints to assist finger exercise. Am J Occup Ther 36(4):259–362, 1982.

Enos, L, Lane, R, and MacDougal, BA: The use of self-adherent wrap in hand rehabilitation. Am J Occup Ther 38(4):265, 1984.

Falkenburg, SA: Choosing hand splints to aid carpal tunnel syndrome recovery. Occup Health Saf 56(5):60, 63–64, 1987.

Feinberg, J, and Brandt, KD: Use of resting splints by patients with rheumatoid arthritis. Am J Occup Ther 35(3):173–178, 1981.

Fess, EE: Principles and methods of splinting for mobilization of joints. In Hunter et al (eds): Rehabilitation of the Hand, 2nd ed. CV Mosby, St Louis, 1984.

Gumpel, JM, and Cannon, S: A cross-over comparison of ready-made fabric wrist-splints in rheumatoid arthritis. Rheum Rehab 20(2):113–115, 1981.

Hooper, RM, and North, ER: Dynamic interphalangeal extension splint design. Am J Occup Ther 36:257, 1982.

Johnson, BM, Flynn, MJ, and Beckenbaugh, RD: A dynamic splint for use after total wrist arthroplasty. Am J Occup Ther 35(3):179–184, 1981.

Mikic, Z, and Helal, B: The treatment of the mallet finger by the Oakley splint. Hand 6:76, 1974.

Mildenberger, LA, Amadio, PC, and An, KN: Dynamic splinting: A systematic approach to the selection of elastic traction. Arch Phys Med Rehabil 67(4):241–244, 1986.

Moberg, E: Splinting in Hand Therapy. Thieme Stratton, New York, 1984.

Moon, M: Compliancy in splint wearing behavior of patients with rheumatoid arthritis. NZ Med J 83(564):360, 1976.

Nicholas, JJ, Gruen, H, Weiner, G, Crawshaw, C, and Taylor, F: Splinting in rheumatoid arthritis: I. Factors affecting patient compliance. Arch Phys Med Rehabil 63(2):92–94, 1982.

Nicolle, FV, and Pressweell, D: A valuable splint for the rheumatoid hand. Hand 7:67, 1975.

Rayan, GM, and O'Donoghue, DH: Ulnar digital compression neuropathy of the thumb caused by splinting. Clin Orthop May(175):170–172, 1983.

Redford, JB (ed): Orthotics etcetera, 2nd ed. Williams & Wilkins, Baltimore, 1980.

Seeger, MS: Splints, braces, and casts. In Riggs, MA, and Gall, EP (eds): Rheumatic Diseases—Rehabilitation and Management. Butterworths, Boston, 1984.

Souter, WA: Splintage in the rheumatoid hand. Hand 3:144, 1971.

Van Straten, O, and Mahler, D: Four new hand splints. Br J Plast Surg 34(3):345–348, 1981.

Williams, JG: Splints for the rheumatoid hand. Br Med J 1:106, 1970.

Chapter 24

Joint-Protection and Energy-Conservation Instruction

Driving
Standing and Walking
Lifting and Transporting Objects
Counterwork
House and Yard Work
Mopping, Vacuuming, Sweeping, and Raking
Washing of Car, Wall, or Windows
Tub Cleaning
Clothes Washing
Bedmaking
Infant-Child Care
Dressing and Hygiene Activities
Bedrest
Sexual Positioning

Joint protection is a *process* in which the therapist evaluates the patient's total living pattern, his or her psychological response to the arthritis, family or personal support systems, and the patient's willingness to influence his or her arthritis by modifying behavior or adapting his or her environment.

The goal or purpose of joint protection is to *reduce stress and pain* in the involved joints and consequently *to reduce inflammation* and *preserve the integrity of the joint structures.* The incorporation of energy-conservation training helps the patient conserve physical resources and improve functional endurance.

When joint protection was first introduced, it was hoped that diligent application of these principles could prevent deformity.[1] But widespread clinical application demonstrated the difficulty of effecting steadfast patient compliance over long periods of time. This difficulty in achieving long-term compliance has limited our ability to demonstrate the preventive potential of joint-protection methods.

The primary value of joint protection lies in its effectiveness for reducing pain, stress to the joint, and inflammation. Although efficacy studies on joint protection have not been published, the effectiveness of joint-protection techniques can be easily demonstrated in the clinic. If certain techniques are recommended to reduce pain and joint stress, the effectiveness of the technique is generally immediate. This can be demonstrated by having the patient perform a task, such as picking up a saucepan, in a routine fashion and then having the patient repeat the task using joint-protection techniques. When the techniques are used correctly, performing the task *is* less painful. The reduction of inflammation is more variable and may take one to three days to be noticeable to the patient, depending upon the activities eliminated and the amount of stress reduced in the joint. When patients are taught how to monitor the signs and symptoms of inflammation, they are able to appreciate the benefits of joint-protection methods. This provides positive reinforcement that is invaluable for encouraging patients to continue to use joint-protection methods.

PATIENT INSTRUCTION

A wide range of methods for teaching joint-protection instruction has been developed; in fact, almost every clinic has developed its own system. Most programs instruct patients in the principles (and specific techniques) of joint protection as defined by Joy Cordery, OTR, in her original article on the topic and often include a list of dos and don'ts based on these principles for the patient to memorize.[1] While the Cordery principles form the conceptual framework for the joint-protection process, the methods used for incorporating these principles in daily activities are different for each patient.[1] The instructions given need to be specific to each patient's pattern of arthritis.[1] A standard list of dos and don'ts given to all patients negates the importance of individualizing the process for each patient; and if each recommendation requires a behavior change, the list may pose an overwhelming responsibility for the patient, a factor that contributes to noncompliance.

Janet Sliwa, OTR, developed guidelines for instructing patients with systemic polyarthritis in joint-protection methods.[2] These guidelines capitalize on the value of individualized instruction and on teaching concepts rather than rules. Both factors encourage patient participation and problem solving in the joint-protection process. A modified version of these guidelines is included here to demonstrate how these teaching principles can be incorporated into a joint-protection program and to encourage therapists to critically analyze their own teaching methods in relation to these concepts. Sliwa's guidelines for instruction include the following:[2]

1. Explain the rationale and value of joint protection, based on the inflammatory process.

2. Teach the patient how to recognize and monitor the signs and symptoms of inflammation (i.e., pain, warmth, and swelling).

3. Encourage the patient to evaluate disease activity level through recognition of inflammatory signs.

4. Stimulate awareness for the need to modify activities based on disease activity level.

5. Identify activity pacing as the process of balancing activities with rest periods.

6. Explain to the patient that pursuing activities despite pain may cause joint damage and that ignoring the symptoms of fatigue may precipitate an exacerbation of disease.

7. Have the patient describe alternative methods for pacing activities.

8. Identify the consequences of static positioning at rest and dynamic forces during activity.

9. Explain and demonstrate proper and improper joint alignment and the consequences of prolonged malalignment.

10. Have the patient practice correct alignment and methods for reducing stress and pain in activities selected by the patient.

11. During the instruction have the patient identify appropriate principles and their application.

12. Throughout the instruction provide verbal, written, or demonstrative reinforcement when the patient expresses or demonstrates joint-protection concepts correctly.

13. All written handouts or home programs should be designed for the patient's level of understanding.

14. Have the patient describe the relevance and importance of the instruction to his or her overall medical and rehabilitative program.

Additional information on developing patient education programs can be found in Chapter 2.

PRINCIPLES OF JOINT PROTECTION: RATIONALE AND TREATMENT IMPLICATIONS

Respect for Pain

Fear of joint pain can lead to unnecessary inactivity whereas total disregard for joint pain can lead to unnecessary joint damage and increased pain. Patients need to respect pain, that is, to understand the source of joint pain and how to monitor activity appropriately. Decisions about activity should be based on knowledge and understanding, not on fear.

Clients should carry out activities and exercise only up to the point of fatigue or discomfort, before pain occurs. Time or effort spent on an activity should be reduced if pain does occur and lasts *more than 1 hour* after the client discontinues the activity. It is important that the client distinguish between usual arthritic discomfort and pain resulting from excessive stress to a joint. His or her understanding of the two can be facilitated through discussion. Occasionally a patient (not on corticosteroid medication) will have a high pain tolerance or may not perceive the pain because of psychological denial. These processes should be considered when a patient with active synovitis reports doing strenuous activity without a proportional amount of pain. For these patients monitoring swelling and warmth is a more effective guideline than pain is for participating in activity; these patients should not do stressful activity using swollen joints.

For the client who is experiencing pain with activities, it is essential to review activities that are commonly overdone and discuss how to lessen them. For example, if a client does a moderate amount of housework in a two-bedroom home and his or her knees hurt for the following two days, instruction in work simplification to minimize ambulation and knee stress is indicated.

Rest and Work Balance

The efficient and appropriate use of rest during the day's activities is probably the most effective weapon a person with arthritis can use against the demands of the disease. It is also the most difficult to incorporate into the patient's daily life.

Rest is prescribed for three reasons:

1. To help restorative processes in the body combat systemic disease
2. To improve a person's overall endurance for activity
3. To enhance muscle function (See Chapter 5 on fibromyalgia.)

Chronic pain and systemic diseases such as rheumatoid arthritis and systemic lupus erythematosus put a tremendous drain on a patient's physical and psychological resources, resulting in excessive fatigue. Clients with systemic diseases need greater amounts of rest and sleep. *How much?* The consensus of rheumatologists is *10 to 12 hours* per 24-hour period, including a *1- to 2-hour nap* in the afternoon. It is crucial that each client understand the physiologic basis for resting and that suggestions regarding rest are specific to him or her as an individual.

The most effective method to increase functional endurance is *rest before becoming exhausted.* Taking a short 5- to 10-minute rest during activities is difficult but can significantly increase overall functional endurance. The concept of *resting for 10 minutes in the middle of vacuuming* is totally foreign for the majority of housewives. This practice implies lengthening the total time spent doing housework, and the desire to get housework over with is usually a strong one. Resting is also effective during activities such as shopping; sitting for only a few minutes *before* one becomes tired will greatly expand the total endurance for the activity. However, rest breaks during work not only increase endurance but also allow the client more energy later on for the activities he or she enjoys.

The practice of resting before one becomes tired or exhausted is so effective that it should be the number one priority in energy-conservation instruction. Once a person employs this practice the benefits are usually self-evident. With encouragement and some self-discipline the patient (or therapist) can use this process to advantage.

Maintenance of Muscle Strength and Joint Range of Motion

See Chapter 26, Functional Activities, and ROM and muscle strength sections of Chapter 27, Exercise Treatment.

Reduction of Effort

Reducing the effort required in activities is recommended for people with arthritis because reduced effort produces less stress and therefore less pain to involved joints. In addition, it improves total endurance and allows people more energy for activities they enjoy.

An indepth assessment of the work environment for determining appropriate joint-protection and energy-conservation measures is included in Chapter 22.

Principles of energy conservation include (1) avoiding rushing, (2) preplanning and organizing activities, (3) setting priorities, (4) eliminating unnecessary tasks, (5) using good posture and body mechanics, (6) avoiding unnecessary motion or energy expenditures, (7) using assistive devices or appliances to reduce work, (8) incorporating frequent planned rest breaks, and (9) having an appropriate working environment in terms of work area heights, lighting, ventilation, and noise level.[3-6]

The following list of questions (compiled by Ceis Wilden, OTR) has been valuable for training patients to analyze their own activities. The list is not comprehensive, but its simplicity and directness facilitate patient use. It teaches patients an *approach* for questioning and analyzing their daily activities. After using it once patients often identify additional factors not included on the list and this patient participation reinforces the learning process.

Work Simplification: Task Analysis

Questions

1. How many trips were made between any two points?
2. Could the number of trips be reduced?
3. Could the order of performing different parts of the job be reduced?
4. Are materials and needed equipment within easy reach?
5. Do storage areas contain only the needed materials or are they cluttered with seldom used things?
6. Can any part of this be omitted or changed and still produce the desired results?
7. Are good body mechanics used in posture, sitting, standing, lifting? How can they be improved?
8. Are two hands used to the best advantage?
9. Would the use of wheels be helpful?
10. Are sitting facilities comfortable and of the proper height?
11. Are the materials prepositioned and ready for use?
12. Is the rate of work too fast?
13. Should someone else do part of the task?

Avoidance of Positions of Deformity

The patient should avoid external pressure and internal joint stresses that facilitate common deformities.[1] The exact pressures and stresses to avoid depend on the joints involved and the disease entity being treated. This is especially important in cases of (1) metacarpophalangeal (MCP) joint synovitis, where strong grasp can play a significant role in deformity;[1,7] (2) hip and knee involvement, when sleeping with the joints flexed can lead to contracture; and (3) neck involvement, when characteristic deformities of neck flexion and hip flexion can be prevented.

Posture during work, leisure (particularly watching TV and reading), and bedrest are important considerations. (See Chapter 28 on positioning.)

Use of Stronger/Larger Joints

Any given amount of stress is better tolerated by the larger joints.[1] Use of stronger and larger joints includes use of feet to close low drawers and hips to push open doors; lifting packages with forearm and trunk; and use of palms rather than fingers to lift or push.

Proper body mechanics in lifting and daily activities should be observed (described in this chapter under back protection). However, back-protection methods may require modification for patients with hip or knee pain.

Use of Each Joint in Its Most Stable Anatomical and Functional Plane

The patient should learn to use each joint in its most stable anatomical and functional plane.[1] This is especially important in protecting knees, wrists, MCP joints, and back. Using this procedure minimizes excessive stretch on joint ligaments and allows muscle power to be used to the greatest advantage. For example, when rising from a sitting position the client should avoid leaning to either side, since rotational forces may stress knee ligaments, thereby increasing instability.

Avoidance of Staying in One Position

Muscles become fatigued in a static position, and thereby transmit positional stress to the underlying ligaments and related structures. Additionally, prolonged positioning promotes stiffness. Sustained joint compression can cause pressure on damaged articular surfaces. Therefore the patient should avoid staying in one position for a prolonged period of time.[1]

A patient should move frequently enough to avoid stiffness and the pain associated with prolonged static positioning. *It is recommended that patients change position* or stretch about every 20 minutes. This amount varies for each patient. Some can tolerate 30 minutes without stiffness, while others can tolerate only 10 minutes without getting stiff.

Avoidance of Activities that Cannot Be Stopped

Activities must be stopped immediately if they become too stressful.[1] Continuing a task in the presence of sudden or severe pain is likely to cause joint damage. Therefore, the client should be taught to avoid activities that cannot be stopped immediately upon stress (e.g., standing while showering, walking down a long hallway, or carrying a package a long distance). These tasks should be attempted only if there is a way to take a rest break as needed.

Use of Assistive Equipment and Orthoses

This includes functional orthoses and assistive devices or adaptive equipment, ranging from electric can openers to furniture adaptations. Many medical articles recommend that assistive devices should be issued only as a last resort, when the patient cannot perform the activity in any manner. This is valid in some instances; for example, if stretching to reach the toes is good for a person, then a long shoe horn or sock donner may in fact be detrimental. But, for people with arthritis it is also important to consider the use of equipment to protect joints prior to the presence of deformity and not only as a compensation for loss of function. (For further discussion of the use of orthoses and equipment to protect joints, see Chapter 23, Orthotic Treatment for Arthritis of the Hand; Chapter 25, Assistive Devices; and Chapter 22, Evaluation of Activities of Daily Living at Home, Work, and Leisure.)

APPLICATION OF JOINT-PROTECTION PRINCIPLES TO SPECIFIC JOINT INVOLVEMENT

All of the above general principles of joint protection apply to each joint. The following specific principles are suggested as additional measures.

Fingers with Inflammatory Joint Disease

As mentioned earlier, the patient must avoid activities or positions that enhance deformities particular to his or her disease. (See Chapter 19, Hand Pathodynamics and Assessment, for the dynamics of deformities and Part II, Major Rheumatic Diseases, for deformities unique to each disease.) All of the following information pertinent to the hand is applicable to adults with rheumatoid arthritis, psoriatic arthritis, and systemic lupus erythematosus, and to children with late-onset polyarticular JRA who have the potential for developing hand deformities similar to adults. Young children with polyarthritis develop a pattern of deformity that is different from adults. Typically they develop flexion contractures of the MCP, PIP, and DIP joints.[8] Consequently ulnar drift of the MCP joints is uncommon; in fact, radial drift is seen more frequently.[8] Joint-protection instruction needs to be individually designed to meet the needs of each child. See the section on hand and wrist therapy in Chapter 14 for joint-protection instruction for these children.

MCP Involvement

MCP Volar Subluxation and Ulnar Drift. These deformities develop during the active phases of synovitis, when the joint capsule and ligaments not only are weakened by the inflammatory process but also are on stretch as a result of *intra-articular swelling.*[7] The work of Smith and associates demonstrated that almost all normal functional hand patterns, such as power grasp, hook grasp, palmar pinch, and strong lateral pinch, produce stress on the MCP joints that encourage subluxation and drift.[7] (See Fig. 19–22 in Chapter 19.) Consequently, avoidance of hand usage that fosters drift and subluxation is most important during periods of active synovitis. This is difficult because most hand activities facilitate deformity. The most practical way of protecting the joint structures during active synovitis is by orthotic immobilization to minimize the influence of the long finger flexors during functional activities[7] and to teach clients to substitute bilateral prehension and to use their palms instead of fingers during activities. Orthoses for this purpose are described in Chapter 23, Orthotic Treatment for Arthritis of the Hand. When considering orthoses for this purpose it is important to keep in mind that immobilization or restriction of the MCP joints *may* cause additional stress to the PIP joints. See Chapter 19, Hand Pathodynamics and Assessment, for a detailed discussion of the role of flexor tendons in MCP joint deformity.

During periods of remission the value of joint-protection techniques to *prevent* or forestall MCP subluxation and drift is highly questionable. However, joint-protection techniques for the hands during remission can be of value in reducing stress to the joints and thus reducing pain (from biomechanical stress) and improving functional hand strength. (Strength is enhanced by minimizing the pain inhibition factor.)

Methods suggested during periods of synovitis to reduce pain and improve functional strength include the following (Figs. 24–1 to 24–3):

1. Use of the palm, heel of the hand, and lateral edge of the palm whenever possible. These are the strongest, most stable parts of the hand and the least vulnerable to stress. This method applies to lifting, pushing, opening jars, transferring, and manipulating switches and equipment. In addition, this practice serves to strengthen the finger extensors, since the fingers must actively extend to allow palmar contact.

2. Use of two hands instead of one when lifting (bilateral prehension).[1]

3. Use of the forearm for lifting and pulling, whenever possible. For car door and home appliance handles that are difficult to open, stress can be minimized by attaching a strap loop through the handle so the patient can open the door (or drawer) with the forearm (or palm of the hand) by slipping it through the loop.

Swan-Neck Deformities. When swan-neck deformities are due in part to in-

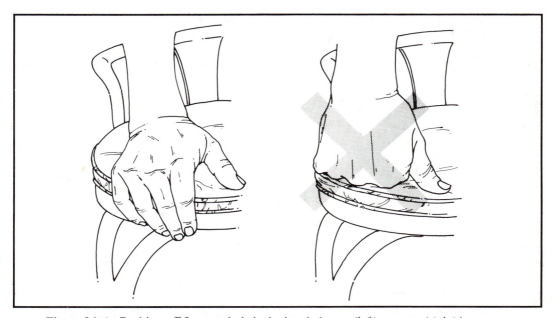

Figure 24–1. Pushing off from a chair is depicted above: *(left)* correct, *(right)* incorrect.

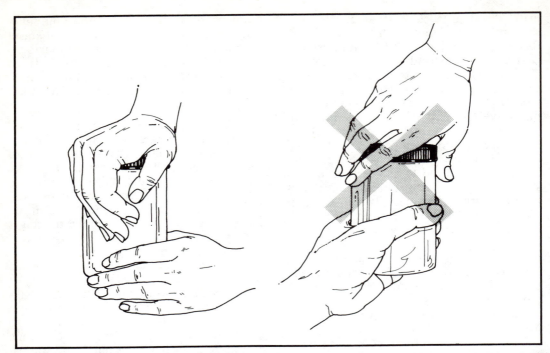

Figure 24–2. Opening a jar is depicted above: *(left)* correct, using heel of hand and avoiding MCP pressure; *(right)* incorrect.

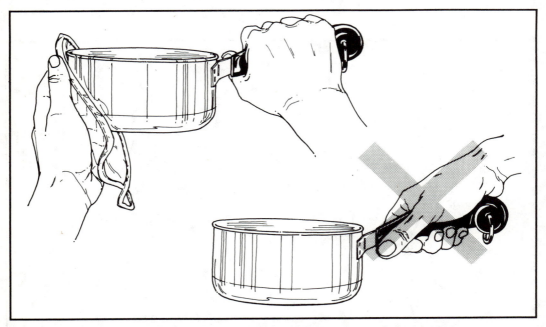

Figure 24–3. Lifting a pan is illustrated: *(above)* correct, *(below)* incorrect.

trinsic muscle tightness, the following is advisable:

1. Avoidance of prolonged intrinsic plus positions (see Fig. 19–34, Chapter 19) such as holding a book while reading, resting the chin on the dorsum of fingers, resting or watching television with the MCP joints flexed and PIP joints extended, and activities such as crocheting, knitting, and hand sewing. (See section on crocheting and knitting in Chapter 26, Functional Activities, for adaptive methods for performing these crafts.)

2. Hand activities or exercises that encourage full PIP flexion while the MCP joints are in extension (intrinsic muscle stretching exercises).

3. Dorsal MCP orthoses to keep the MCP joints in full extension and encourage PIP flexion. Orthoses may be used for positioning during stretching exercises, during functional activities, or all night. (See Chapter 23, Orthotic Treatment for Arthritis of the Hand.)

PIP Involvement

Boutonnière or Flexion Deformities. The three principles of treatment for these deformities are (1) avoidance of keeping fingers in a flexed position at rest; (2) daily ROM exercises; and (3) anti-deformity exercises (i.e., active DIP flexion with the PIP joint stabilized in full extension). It is desirable to maintain joint mobility with these deformities in order to facilitate personal hygiene and the application of gloves.

There have been reports that the use of orthotic immobilization in extension for 6 weeks can reverse mild (less than 20 degrees) boutonnière deformities. However, it is difficult to find patients with early deformity who can tolerate this type of orthotic program. See the section on boutonnière deformity in Chapter 19, Hand Pathodynamics and Assessment, for referenced discussion.

Wrists

Methods suggested for pain reduction and improvement of functional strength in MCP joint involvement of the hands also minimize stress to the wrist. *Activities or positions that enhance volar subluxation and radial deviation of the wrist should be avoided.* (See Chapter 19, Hand Pathodynamics and Assessment, for discussion of pathodynamics.) The following should be avoided:

1. Activities that involve wrist flexion and rotation, such as stirring with the utensil diagonal to the palm (Fig. 24–4).

2. Heavy lifting and traction, such as carrying suitcases and purses with hands forming a hook grasp (Fig. 25–5).

3. Activities that encourage radical deviation of the wrist.

4. Positioning in ulnar deviation at rest.

Reduction of stress is accomplished by using the wrist in straight alignment as much as possible and by using the forearm and trunk to lift items whenever possible. Wrist stabilization orthoses should be used during periods of active synovitis or when pain interferes with hand function. (See Chapter 23, Orthotic Treatment for Arthritis of the Hand.) One of the most effective methods for reducing stress to the wrist is the use of commercial elastic-vinyl gauntlet orthoses, with a removable volar reinforcement bar (e.g., the Freedom splint). These orthoses allow approximately 50 degrees of flexion and extension, but they prevent circumduction, thus reducing considerably rotational stress to the wrist. These orthoses require the patient to use his or her wrists in a neutral, stable alignment during functional activities. The volar reinforcement bar provides greater support for inflamed wrists, but for some patients it is too restrictive for daily use. The orthosis can be effective for joint protection even with the metal support removed.

Shoulders and Elbows

People primarily reduce stress to the shoulder by reducing their range of active motion. When there is acute pain or inflammation, joint protection would involve doing activities with as little pain as possible and having someone perform gentle passive ROM to the shoulder following conscious relaxation. People in this situation can often benefit from a simple review of how to avoid stressful motions such as donning jackets with the painful side first

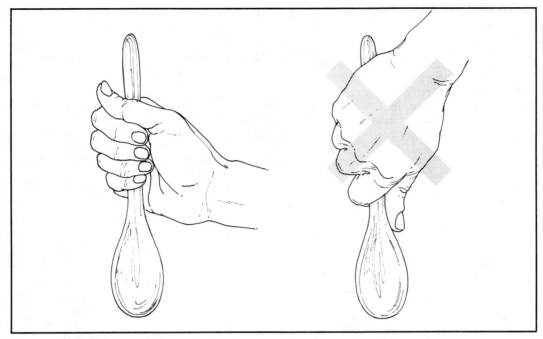

Figure 24–4. Shown here, holding a spoon for stirring: *(left)* correct with wrist in straight alignment; if the person also has MCP synovitis the handle should be built up; *(right)* incorrect.

and doffing with the normal or least painful side first. When limited shoulder motion is the primary problem, joint protection is not an issue; use of assistive devices to improve functional ability is the primary treatment.

For the elbow, treatment is similar, avoiding painful motions during the acute stage and using assistive devices to extend reach or facilitate approximation to the body if limited ROM is a primary problem. Severely limited ROM or instability may make a patient a candidate for surgery. For patients who are not surgical candidates, an elastic elbow sleeve (approximately 10 inches long) can help provide some stability and comfort. A dynamic elbow orthosis is a potential treatment but these orthoses are often not well tolerated by people with severe debilitating RA. Otherwise, treatment focuses more on assistive devices and adaptive methods.

Knees and Hips

Stress to knees may be lessened by using seats of an appropriate height with arm rests. Trauma to osteoporotic hips and ver-tebrae can be reduced if the patient does not plop down when sitting into low seats. Rising from a seat is also less painful and easier if the person moves to the edge of the seat prior to rising. Facilitation of quadriceps strength may be achieved prior to standing by having the patient (1) do a quad set, (2) straighten the knee completely once or twice, (3) flex and extend the knee two to three times in midrange. The choice of facilitation method depends upon which causes the least amount of discomfort since pain inhibits muscle strength.

For patients who are overweight, weight reduction is the most valuable method of joint protection. All overweight patients should receive dietary counseling and encouragement to participate in a weight-reduction program. For patients with OA of the knees, weight reduction alone can often eliminate symptoms.[9]

Other suggestions for reducing knee stress include (1) avoiding walking on rough, uneven ground; (2) going up steps with the good leg first, descending with the most painful knee first; (3) strengthening the knee extensor muscles; (4) using knee supports to help keep the knee warm and to serve as a postural reminder to use the knee

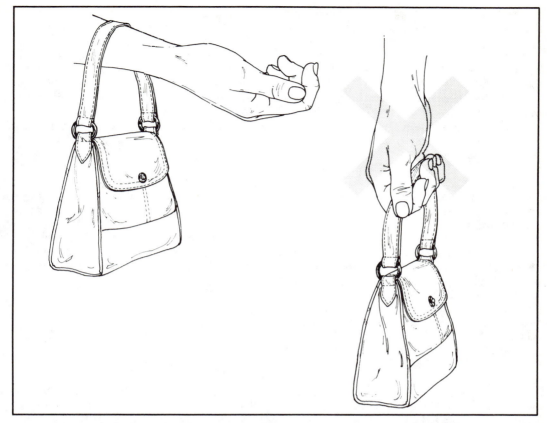

Figure 24–5. This figure depicts the correct and incorrect ways to carry a purse: *(left)* correct, avoiding MCP stress; *(right)* incorrect.

in stable, straight alignment rather than with the body rotated; and (5) wearing good walking or athletic shoes with a strong heel counter or internal custom orthoses to reduce foot pain (this can significantly reduce stress to the knee).

Feet

Patients with early foot involvement should be instructed in foot and toe ROM exercises to prevent insidious contractures secondary to digital muscle spasm.

Appropriate shoes are extremely important. They should be firm and lightweight with a resilient sole, provide good support for the longitudinal arch, have a soft upper with adequate width to accommodate splayfoot and hallux valgus deformity, give adequate depth (patient should be able to curl toes inside the shoe), and have a firm heel counter.[10,11]

The patient who reports that he or she can wear only soft shoes such as slippers should have a medical foot examination to determine if he or she would benefit from shoe adaptations or orthoses.

The following adaptations and orthoses have proven valuable for arthritic foot problems.

1. *Plastazote (¼-inch thick) shoe liners.* Easily cut from sheet Plastazote, these liners help to distribute pressure evenly over the foot and reduce pressure over the metatarsophalangeal (MTP) heads. These are most effective in the course of the disease before subluxation takes place. These are often fitted in occupational therapy (OT).

2. *Plastazote foot orthoses.* These are custom-made and designed to support the longitudinal arch and provide an MTP bar to reduce stress to the MTP joints by shifting the pressure of weight bearing proximal

to the painful metatarsal heads. These orthoses can also be designed to provide accommodation of abnormal valgus. These orthoses are worn inside regular shoes. They are more effective than MTP bars fixed to the sole of the shoe.[10]

3. *Polyprophylene or rigid plastic orthoses (similar to runner's orthoses) with an MTP bar.* These can be made with a heel cup, to reduce inversion and eversion and thereby reduce stress to the subtalar joint, and with a post to stabilize or reduce ankle valgus.[10]

4. *Commercial extra-depth shoes.* These are most effective when the liner is removed and replaced with a Plastazote liner or orthosis.

5. *Custom-made soft leather sandals and shoes.* These are most frequently made to reduce pain that prevents ambulation in patients with severe deformity. The inside conforms to the deformity, distributing pressure over the entire sole of the foot and has a built-in MTP pad. These shoes can also be made with a heel cup to stabilize or reduce hindfoot subluxation.[10]

NECK-PROTECTION INSTRUCTION

The one objective of all neck-protection methods is *to keep the neck in neutral alignment during activities.* Another way to conceptualize this principle is *to keep the back and neck in as straight a line as possible.*[12,13]

Motions or positions that should be avoided include neck extension (hyperextension), *prolonged* forward and lateral flexion or rotation, and repetitious motion in any direction.[12]

The therapist should use a mirror to instruct the patient in proper neck alignment during activities. This is particularly effective because there are no visual body cues regarding neck position when the head is in straight posture alignment.

A soft neck collar can be an excellent training aid for instructing patients in neck-protection techniques. A soft neck collar maintains the neck in neutral alignment. If a patient practices the daily activities below while wearing a soft collar, he or she learns how to position work, reading, and so forth, to accommodate the restriction of

the collar. This is the positioning and alignment the patient should use without the collar. After learning proper body mechanics the patient can discontinue using the collar or save it for specific activities during which it may be too difficult to maintain alignment without an aid. Generally a soft collar needs to be ordered by a physician. Using a collar only as a teaching aid versus having the patient wear one all the time needs to be cleared with the referring physician.

For patients with severe cervical subluxation, a soft or semirigid (Plastazote) collar should be used when indicated, especially during activities with a high risk of neck injury, such as driving. (For patients with limited hand or shoulder involvement it is helpful if the collar can be adapted with a side opening.)

Specific Suggestions for Incorporating the Basic Principles

Sitting and Desk Work

1. Chair type and desk height should facilitate proper posture. When sitting erect in a chair, the desk should be at a height that supports the elbows, with the elbows touching the body or 2 inches away. If the desk is too short, it becomes necessary to slouch to support the elbows. Also the lower the table is the more neck flexion is required to perform desk work.

2. Prolonged writing should be done on an angle, for example, at a drafting table, with a tilted desk top, or through the use of a clip board propped up on an angle. This reduces the neck flexion necessary for horizontal work.[12,13]

Reading

1. Prolonged reading should be done with the book at eye level on an angle with the desk or table. This can be accomplished through the use of an inexpensive book rack propped up on a stack of books or on a file tray.

2. Reading in bed or slumped in a chair is contraindicated since this can require prolonged forward flexion of the neck.

3. Bifocals that require neck hyperextension in order to use the reading portion are

not recommended. Reading glasses or bi-focals with a large lower portion are preferred.[12]

Secretarial Work

1. Typing: Ideally, the copy draft should be placed at eye level directly above the typewriter.* This eliminates the need for repetitive neck rotation and flexion that is necessary when the draft lies flat and to the side of the typewriter.

2. Telephone use: Frequent or prolonged use of a telephone can put a severe stress on the neck muscles. The most efficient method for eliminating this stress is to use a device* (designed like a drafting light) that maintains the receiver at an ear level position, without the use of hands or neck muscles to position it. Another alternative is to use a lightweight headphone.

Driving

1. Place the seat as close to the wheel as possible to facilitate proper spine alignment.

2. Add or adjust mirrors to minimize neck motion. A side mirror on the right side of the car and a bubble mirror attached to the side mirrors can be helpful in reducing the need for turning to see blind spots (a task not possible if the neck muscles are in spasm).

3. Headrests positioned so they do not necessitate neck hyperextension are recommended. Permanent headrests that are set too far back should be built up with foam padding or exchanged for a different type of pad.

Lifting and Transporting Objects

Lifting methods described in the back-protection section also apply to neck protection, because bending the back to pick up something instead of squatting necessitates neck hyperextension. Likewise, reaching for objects overhead instead of using a stepstool requires neck hyperextension.

---

*A draft holder and telephone holder designed for these purposes are produced by Luxo Lamp Corporation, Monument Park, Pt. Chester, NY 10573. Available through most distributors.

Bedrest

1. Sleeping in a side-lying or supine position is recommended; sleeping in a prone position is contraindicated because it maintains the neck in a prolonged rotated position.

2. A firm mattress with a top layer of foam and springs should be used with a bed board as indicated.

3. A round, tubular pillow designed for cervical pain syndromes (Cervipillo) is an important adjunct to neck protection because it maintains optimal neck alignment in both the supine and side-lying positions.[12] These pillows are available at major rehabilitation equipment distributors and have high patient acceptance. Thick multiple pillows are contraindicated since they cause excessive neck flexion. Patients with respiratory difficulty who need head elevation should raise the head of the bed 4 to 8 inches on blocks.

Self-Care Activities

In general, commonly used items should be placed within easy reach.

Dressing. Avoid pullover garments that require neck extension.

Hair Care. Shampoo hair in the shower since this is the only means of maintaining proper neck alignment during hair care.

Facial Hygiene. Use a washcloth while maintaining the neck in good alignment. Rinsing the face without a cloth or brushing the teeth over the sink can put the neck into severe extension. If bending over the sink is necessary it should be done with the chin tucked in. For men, an electric shaver requires less hyperextension than a safety razor.

Drinking. Drinking from bottles, small glasses, or cans should be avoided. Wide-mouth glasses and cups or straws are recommended.

BACK-PROTECTION INSTRUCTION

Prior to about 1983 the literature for patient education on management of back pain was very simplistic and advocated two basic principles, namely reducing the lordotic curve and keeping the spine straight.

Reducing the lordotic curve with a pelvic tilt can be an effective and appropriate technique for certain back conditions, especially specific common forms of ruptured disc. However, the mechanics of the back, posture, and alignment are too complex for a single technique to be appropriate for all patients. For some patients reducing the lordotic curve increases pain and therefore is not appropriate.[14] The rule of "keeping the spine straight," as it refers to alignment, is still appropriate for most patients because when a person tries to sit "straight" he or she tends to move into a more normal posture, which encourages the natural curves of the spine.

Back- or neck-protection programs with simplistic "rules for all" are not very effective. The most effective programs are based on the findings of a comprehensive musculoskeletal assessment, conducted by a physical therapist, of the patient's posture, tone, strength, pain, spasm, alignment, ROM, and movement. The physical therapist should determine the postural guidelines the patient should incorporate and instruct the patient in basic body mechanics. For many patients, learning how to incorporate these measures into daily activities takes actual practice and experience with the activity. This is often most easily done in OT where there are activities of daily living (ADL) or work capacity stations. In these situations the occupational therapist needs to work very closely with the physical therapist.

Posture and alignment, although important, are only two factors that influence back pain. Muscular tension and tightness are also critical factors that strongly influence pain during functional tasks. For example, a person can drive with good alignment with the shoulders and back tight *or* relaxed; or a person can walk with the pelvis rigid and tight or, conversely, relaxed. Helping patients learn to sit, walk, and work with the back relaxed is a major challenge in back (or neck) treatment.

An effective way to teach patients the desired body mechanics is to instruct them in the principles, present them with the activity, and have them problem solve how to accomplish the task incorporating the principles. There are many ways (too numerous to list here) to accomplish each task. Solutions generated by the patient do not have to be taught, only reinforced. This process simplifies the therapist's job and empowers the patient—a win-win situation.

The use of back-protection methods for low back pain syndromes is most effective when done in conjunction with relaxation training and an exercise program in physical therapy to (1) strengthen the abdominal and back musculature and (2) strengthen the quadriceps and arm musculature (to accomplish lifting tasks). Therapists who instruct patients in back-protection techniques should be knowledgeable about the patient's specific pain syndrome and the total conservative management of low back pain. Information on low back pain is available in numerous resources,[14-19] see the references and additional sources listed at the end of this chapter.

The following suggestions reflect the more common techniques employed for reducing strain on the back, especially the low back. They are presented here only as a stimulus for generating ideas on how tasks can be done, not as hard and fast absolute rules.

Principles of Back Protection

1. To practice sitting, standing, sleeping, working postures that minimize stress to the back. For some people this means reducing the lordotic lumbar curve using the pelvic tilt maneuver. For others it means maintaining or encouraging lumbar lordosis.

2. To keep the spine as straight as possible during sitting and lifting activities. Slouching, forward bending, or rotation of the lumbar spine increases pressure on the intervertebral discs.

Specific Suggestions for Incorporating the Basic Principles

Sitting

1. Use straight back chairs with arms rather than overstuffed chairs. Rocking chairs that support the lower back are helpful since they allow motion to ease back tension. Use a pillow to support the lumbar curve, if indicated. (Principle 1)

2. Sit with buttocks as far back into the seat as possible.

3. Keep back as straight as possible when sitting or rising. When rising, pivot to the edge of the chair, lean forward at the hips, and use leg strength to rise. (Principle 2)

4. When sitting, to reduce lumbar curve, keep the knees bent and higher than the hips by using a foot prop or crossing one leg over the other. (Principle 1)

5. Avoid sitting for prolonged periods or take frequent stretch breaks.

Desk or Table Work

1. All the general rules for sitting apply during desk work; a foot prop under the desk or table helps to keep one or both knees above the hips to reduce lumbar curve.

2. The type of desk and seating, working, and lighting arrangements should foster proper posture. If they do not, adaptations are necessary. A pillow may be needed to support the low back.

3. Always directly face the task; for example, if sitting and facing the desk, do not reach to the side to pick up the phone directory. Turn your whole body toward the directory and pick it up using the arm muscles, not the back muscles. A stable swivel chair facilitates repetitive turning. (*Note:* People typically lift moderately heavy desk items with their back muscles and need to be taught how to lift using only the arm muscles.)

Driving

1. Get into the car by sitting on the side of the seat and pivoting into the car, keeping the knees together. (Principle 2)

2. Keep the seat as close to the pedals as possible to increase hip and knee flexion. (Principle 1)

3. Use a seat-back support. There are two kinds, one that provides a rigid or firm surface and one that provides contoured support for the back.

4. For severe back problems, a lumbar corset support may be indicated during distance driving.

5. Use seat belts and shoulder harnesses to minimize danger in the event of sudden stops.

6. Keep shoulders and upper back relaxed while driving.

Standing and Walking

1. Women and men should wear sturdy low-heeled shoes.

2. During prolonged standing, shift weight from one foot to the other. Flatten the lower back by tightening the abdominal muscles and by tucking the buttocks under. Also keep knees slightly flexed. Avoid locking the knees in extension.

3. Avoid prolonged standing when possible.

4. Open doors wide enough to walk through comfortably. People in the acute or postacute phase may want to avoid crowded conditions, sports events, and theaters, which often necessitate turning sideways while walking through areas, or at least be conscious about back alignment in such situations. The safest solution is to wear a lumbar corset in these situations.

Lifting and Transporting Objects

1. When lifting items below waist height (e.g., on a low shelf or on the floor), face the object with feet about 12 inches apart and one foot forward and squat down, keeping the back straight (as if doing a deep knee bend). Place hands underneath the object if possible. Then, keeping the back straight, tighten the stomach and back muscles. Raise your body and the object using only the leg (quadriceps) muscles. This is the only recommended method of lifting. Lifting with the back by keeping the legs straight and bending at the waist is contraindicated because the mechanical stress to the third to fifth lumbar vertebrae is excessive and approximately 150 percent greater than with the leg-lift method. (*Note:* the recommended method of lifting with the legs is included in all body mechanics literature; however, a person needs strong quadriceps muscles and good knee joints to carry out this advice. Professional furniture movers and truck drivers with low back problems probably would have no trouble, but the average housewife or sedentary worker will probably need quadriceps strengthening to benefit from this method. Patients often need quite a bit of practice to incorporate this method spontaneously.)

2. Assistance should be sought to lift any items that cannot be lifted in the recommended manner.

3. Heavy items *should not* be lifted overhead. When removing lightweight items from a high shelf (1) use a stepstool whenever possible, (2) place one foot on a sturdy step to ease low back muscle tension, or (3) place one foot forward and reach for the object with body weight on the forward foot and transfer weight to the back foot as you bring the object down, keeping the back as straight as possible. Reverse the process for placing an object on the shelf. (Do not keep feet even or parallel when reaching high.)

4. Carry objects as close to the body as possible because stress to the spine increases proportionately to the distance of the carrying lever arm.

5. Avoid carrying heavy objects that necessitate leaning backwards for balance, since back hyperextension increases spinal pressure considerably. (Principle 1)

6. Slide objects instead of lifting whenever possible, keeping the back straight. (Principle 2)

7. Avoid carrying unbalanced loads (e.g., one heavy suitcase with one arm and nothing with the other). Consider substituting a nylon carrying bag with shoulder strap in lieu of a heavy briefcase or purse. (Principle 2)

8. When pushing an object keep one foot forward with knees bent, tighten the back muscles to keep the spine straight, and then use the leg (quadriceps) muscles to move the object.

Counterwork

1. Keep frequently used items within easy reach or at counter level. (Principle 2)

2. Use a high stool with back support and footrest or footbar to keep one or both knees flexed if it is desired to reduce the lordotic curve. (Principle 1)

3. When standing for a prolonged period, keep one foot on a stepstool or an opened lower drawer to ease back muscle tension. (Principle 1)

House and Yard Care

1. Alternate tasks and incorporate short rest periods to avoid fatigue.

2. Use adaptive equipment to avoid bending (e.g., extended handles, dusters, bathbrushes, toilet brushes, and dustpans).

3. Eliminate unnecessary motions and tasks.

4. Kneel or light fireplace from a low stool, using long fireplace matches.

Mopping, Vacuuming, Sweeping, and Raking

1. Use equipment with handles long enough to avoid stooping. (You may adapt handles with extensions.)

2. Face the material or area being cleaned. Do the work in front, not to the side, to minimize twisting. Keeping the knees slightly bent while working also helps reduce the tendency to twist.

Washing of Car, Wall, or Windows

1. For portions above head level, keep one foot on a stepstool or use a stepladder, keeping feet at different levels. Reach with one arm at a time. (Principle 1)

2. For lower portion, kneel (as described for lifting), keeping the back straight.

3. Keep water bucket or cleansing materials on a chair or stool to avoid bending.

Tub Cleaning

1. Kneel and use an extended handle toilet brush for cleaning.

2. After bathing, put a strong washing detergent in the water to reduce or prevent tub ring, thereby reducing the necessity for scrubbing.

Clothes Washing

1. A front-loading washer is preferred over a top-loading one because it allows loading from a kneeling or squatting position or from a low stool. The top loader necessitates bending. (Principle 2)

2. Wash laundry frequently rather than once a week or every two weeks.

3. Transfer multiple small loads rather than single large ones.

4. Lower clothesline to shoulder height. Elevate wash basket on a chair. (Principle 2)

Bedmaking

1. Raise the bed 3 to 4 inches on blocks to miminize back stress. If this is not sufficient or possible, an alternate method is making the bed while on one's knees. (Principle 2)

2. Straightening the covers while in bed before arising will minimize this daily chore.

3. Have bed away from wall or on coasters for easy moving.

Infant-Child Care

1. Always use arm or leg muscles rather than back muscles when lifting an infant.

2. Have the child stand on a chair or stepstool while you are dressing or performing facial hygiene for small children. (Principle 2)

3. Kneel while washing a child in the tub. (Principle 2)

4. Wash, change, and dress the infant at counter height. (Principle 2)

Dressing and Hygiene Activities

1. Lower extremity dressing (including shoes) should be done from a sitting position, bending the knees (one at a time) instead of the back. If dressing in this manner is not possible, devices such as long-handled shoe horns, dressing sticks, and stocking aids are helpful. (Principle 2)

2. Comfortable garments with front openings should be used to minimize the need for twisting during upper extremity dressing. (Principle 2)

3. During bathing or showering a cloth back scrubber (one pulled from side to side) is preferable over a long-handled brush for back washing. The long-handled back-brush, however, is helpful for lower extremity washing.

4. Hair washing is best done in the shower.

5. Bending over the sink for washing the face, brushing the teeth, and shaving can be accomplished by bending the knees and hips and keeping the back straight (instead of bending at the back).

6. An electric shaver is preferable over a safety razor for men since it does not require bending to use the sink. (Principle 2)

Bedrest

1. Recommended sleeping positions* for reducing the lordotic curve are:
   a. Side lying with knees and hips flexed (fetal position)
   b. Supine with pillow under knees

2. If the goal is to maintain or increase the lumbar curve, a lumbar roll may be helpful.

3. Lying prone is not recommended. If, for some reason, it is essential, a small pillow should be placed under the pelvis to reduce the lordotic curve.

4. When lying in bed, do not reach overhead or rest both arms behind your head since this increases the lordotic curve and spinal pressure.

5. When rising from a lying position, roll to the side and move to the edge of the bed, keeping the back straight and the hips and knees bent. Use the arms to push up to a sitting position while lowering the feet to the floor.

6. A firm mattress with a top layer of foam and firm box springs should be used. A bed board (¾-inch plywood) should be used only as a last resort when it is not possible to purchase a firm bed.

7. The value of a water bed for back pain is uncertain and appears to depend on the individual. The supportive effect depends a great deal on how much it is filled. An air-filled or padded bumper facilitates transfer in and out of bed. Water beds have been reported to enhance the maintenance of a stationary position, thereby reducing the need to change positions.

8. Electric blankets are often helpful since they provide consistent warmth and are lightweight and easy to manage.

Sexual Positioning

The recommended positions are those that allow hip and knee flexion (e.g., the lower position in the traditional missionary position or various side lying positions). Many, if not most, patients are able to alter

---

*These positions are contraindicated for people with arthritis of the hips or knees.

their positioning to accommodate back pain without any advice. However, there are many patients who use only the traditional position and may need to hear advice from an authoritative medical person to consider alternative methods.

REFERENCES

1. Cordery, JC: Joint protection: A responsibility of the occupational therapist. Am J Occup Ther 19:285, 1965.
2. Silwa, J: Performance objectives for joint protection instruction. AHP Newsletter, Arthritis Foundation, 12(4), Winter, 1978–1979.
3. Gilbert, D: Energy expenditures for the disabled homemaker: Review of studies. Am J Occup Ther 19:321, 1965.
4. Fish, HU: Take It Easy, Nos. 1, 2, and 3. American Heart Association, New York. (Pamphlets on work-simplification methods for the homemaker. Also in the *Heart in the Home* booklet.)
5. Rusk, HA et al: A Manual for Training the Disabled Homemaker. Rehabilitation Monograph VIII, 2nd ed. Institute of Rehabilitation Medicine, New York University Medical Center, New York, 1961. (Excellent section on work simplification.)
6. Zee, E, Feit, L, Jallo, L, Stewart, J, Warner, K, and Wood, B: Manual on Motion Economy. Occupation Therapy Department, City of Hope Medical Center, 1500 East Duarte Road, Duarte, CA 91010. (In English or Spanish)
7. Smith, EM, Juvinall, R, Bender, L, and Pearson, J: Role of the finger flexors in rheumatoid deformities of the metacarpophalangeal joints. Arthritis Rheum 7:467, 1964.
8. Chaplin, D, Pulkki, T, Saarimaa, A, and Vainio, K: Wrist and finger deformities in juvenile rheumatoid arthritis. Acta Rheum Scand 15:206, 1969.
9. Templeton, CL et al: Weight control group approach for arthritis clients. J Nutrition Educ Vol. 10, January–March 1978.
10. Wood, B: The painful foot. In Kelley, WM et al (eds): Textbook of Rheumatology. WB Saunders, Philadelphia, 1981.
11. Ishmael, WK, and Shrobe, HB: Care of Your Feet. JB Lippincott, Philadelphia, 1967.
12. Jackson, R: The Cervical Syndrome, 4th ed. Charles C Thomas, Springfield, IL, 1977.
13. Ishmael, WK, and Shrobe, HB: Care of Your Neck. JB Lippincott, Philadelphia, 1966.
14. McKenzie, RA: The Lumbar Spine: Mechanical Diagnosis and Therapy. Spinnal Publications, Waikanae, New Zealand, 1981.
15. Berland, T, and Addison, RG: Living with Your Bad Back. Bantam Books, New York, 1972.
16. Ishmael, WK, and Shrobe, HB: Care of Your Back. JB Lippincott, Philadelphia.
17. Macnab, I: Backache. Baltimore, Williams & Wilkins, 1977.
18. Finneson, BE: Low Back Pain. JB Lippincott, Philadelphia, 1973.
19. Preston, GM: Advice on housework for patients with low back pain. Occup Ther (Br) p 24, March 1976.

ADDITIONAL SOURCES

Adler-Korbel, M: A Joint Effort. The Western Washington Chapter, Arthritis Foundation, Dextor Horton Building, Seattle, WA 98104.

Blakeney, AB: Occupational therapy intervention in chronic pain. OT Health Care 1(3), 1984.

Bluestone, R: The patient who hurts all over: Practical approach to diagnosis and management. Postgrad Med 72(6):71–79, 1982.

Caruso, LA, and Chan, DE: Evaluation and management of the patient with acute back pain. Am J Occup Ther 40(5):347–351, 1986.

Day, NR: Back to Backs: A Guide to Preventing Back Injury. PAS, Daly City, CA, 1983.

Deyo, RA: Conservative therapy for low back pain. JAMA 250(8):1057–1062, 1983.

Flor, H, and Turk, DC: Etiological theories and treatments for chronic back pain. I. Somatic models and interventions. Pain 19(2):105–121, 1984.

Flower, A, Naxon, E, Jones, R, and Mooney, V: An occupational therapy program for chronic back pain. Am J Occup Ther 35(4):243–248, 1981.

Furst, GP, Gerber, LH, Smith, CC, Fisher, S, and Shulman, B: A program for improving energy conservation behaviors in adults with rheumatoid arthritis. Am J Occup Ther 41(2):102–111, 1987.

Gottlieb, HJ: Low back pain comprehensive rehab program—Follow up study. Arch Phys Med Rehabil 63:458–461, 1982.

Grahame, R (ed): Low back pain. Clin Rheum Dis 6(1), 1980.

Haviland, N, Kamil-Miller, L, and Sliwa, J: A Workbook for Consumers with Rheumatoid Arthritis. American Occupation Therapy Association, Distribution Center, 1383 Piccard Drive, Rockville, MD 20850.

Holmes, D: The role of the occupational therapist-work evaluator. Am J Occup Ther 39(5):308–313, 1985.

Johnson, EW, and Wolfe, CV: Bifocal spectacles in the etiology of cervical radiculopathy. Arch Phys Med Rehabil 53:201, 1972.

Joint Protection and Energy Conservation for the Early Rheumatoid Arthritis Patient. A slide-tape presentation with a patient teaching booklet. Graphic Plus Associates, 214 Boulevard of the Allies, Pittsburgh, PA 15222.

Lytel, RB, Botterbusch, KF: Physical demands job analysis: A new approach. University of Wisconsin, Stout Vocational Rehabilitation Institute, Menomie, WI, 1981.

Matheson, L, Ogden, LD, Violette, K, and Schultz, K: Work hardening: Occupational therapy in industrial rehabilitation. Am J Occup Ther 39(5):314–321, 1985.

Mayer, TG: Rehabilitation of the patient with spinal

pain. Orthop Clin North Am 14(3):623–637, 1983.

McCloy, L: The biomechanical basis for joint protection in osteoarthritis. CJOT 49:85, 1982.

Parent, LH: Energy: The illusive factor in daily activity. OT Health Care 3(1), 1986.

Rosenbusch, DF: Psychic energy—The activator of the low energy patient. OT Health Care 3(1), 1986.

Saunders, HD: Evaluation, Treatment and Prevention of Musculoskeletal Disorders. Viking, Minneapolis, 1985.

Stephenson, V: Occupational therapy and the nurse. Nursing (Oxford) 2(31):912–913, 1984.

White, AA, and Gordon, SL: Synopsis: Workshop on ideopathic low back pain. Spine 7(2):141–149, 1980.

Work Practices Guide for Manual Lifting. US Department of Commerce, National Technical Information Service, Springfield, VA, 1981.

Work Simplification. (A patient instruction booklet.) Bellin Memorial Hospital, 744 South Webster Avenue, PO Box 1700, Green Bay, WI 54305.

Chapter 25

Assistive Devices

This chapter discusses the specific considerations needed in assistive equipment for people who have arthritis. Within this context equipment or adaptive methods are used as a treatment modality to achieve the following goals:[1]

1. Reduce pain and preserve joint integrity by minimizing extraneous stress
2. Increase the patient's independence in a task that otherwise could not be performed because of a physical limitation

FACTORS TO CONSIDER WHEN EVALUATING AND ORDERING EQUIPMENT

The evaluation of the patient's equipment needs is part of the activities of daily living (ADL) assessment. For employed people the ADL assessment and equipment

recommendations should extend to the workplace. (See Chapter 22.) When selecting or designing equipment for patients with arthritis, it is important to keep the following considerations in mind:[1]

1. The patient's equipment needs in the morning may differ from those in the afternoon; they may also differ during periods of exacerbation and remission.

Example: Many patients are dependent during the first 2 to 4 hours in the morning but become independent in the afternoon as their morning stiffness wears off. A portable raised toilet seat would allow easy removal by the patient when it is not needed in contrast to a permanent seat that cannot be removed easily.

2. The equipment may affect other joints of the body.

Example 1: One of the most common situations is the issuance of a cane, crutch, walker-aid, or wheelchair to protect the lower extremities without consideration of the deforming stresses that the ambulation aid can cause to the wrist, hand, or shoulder.

Example 2: Assistive devices ordered for shoulder or elbow range limitations frequently have long lever arms and can cause severe stress to the hands (e.g., extended-handle brushes or reachers).

3. Activities and equipment involving strong grasp are contraindicated for patients with active MCP involvement.

Solution: For patients with active MCP synovitis, MCP subluxation, or tight intrinsic muscles, options include doing the task bimanually using the palms; using an orthosis to maintain MCP extension during the activity; adapting handles to keep the MCP joints in extension. This should also include adaptation of cane, crutch, and walker-aid handles. Adapted handles to keep the MCP in extension can be of three shapes: rectangular, cone, and elliptical cone. (*Note:* Patients with protective ulnar drift splints frequently need handles built up to facilitate grip.)

4. Some patients with wrist or hand involvement are unable to grip standard transfer assist equipment.

Solution: Order grab bars or transfer bars that attach to the edge of the tub or floor-to-ceiling poles so the patient can hook his or her forearm around the bar for leverage. Bars may need to be padded. Also, patients with thumb carpometacarpal (CMC) adduction contractures may not have sufficient motion to grasp transfer bars or ambulation aids adequately. For these patients a narrow or thinner bar may be needed to allow functional grasp.

5. Convenience appliances are not always convenient for patients with arthritis.

Example: Many electrical appliances such as electric can openers, knives, and toothbrushes operate with buttons that are too difficult for patients with hand involvement to use or they can be too heavy for a patient to hold long enough to complete the task required. Therefore, it is imperative that the therapist be familiar with the strength and dexterity required to operate an appliance before ordering it for a patient.

6. A change in ambulation aids requires instruction in ADL.

Example: If there is a decrease in ambulation status and the patient needs to use a crutch, walker, or wheelchair, it is important that he or she receive retraining as to how to do work with the required aids.

7. Patient equipment needs may be temporary or long term.

Example: A patient with rapid progressive joint destruction may be unable to schedule surgery for 3 months, and the equipment needed prior to surgery may be unnecessary afterwards. For short-term equipment needs, consider purchasing equipment that is less elaborate or less expensive than the top-of-the-line models. But if the equipment is needed for a long period of time, more expensive or sturdier equipment may last longer and be more cost-effective over time.

8. Lower extremity dressing aids sometimes do more harm than good.

Example: If a patient with ankylosing spondylitis (AS) or osteoarthritis can just barely don his or her socks independently and without pain, it is preferable to have him or her continue doing the task without an aid. The movements involved in putting on one's socks help maintain hip and spinal flexion. Even though using an aid makes the job easier, it may contribute to further disability. Conversely, a patient with acute AS and spinal muscle spasms should use an aid to reduce the stress on the acute spinal muscles. Use gentle methods, such as pool therapy, to maintain flexibility.

COMMON FUNCTIONAL LIMITATIONS AND POSSIBLE SOLUTIONS

In an outpatient setting it is common to treat people early in the course of their illness; for example, patients who have only hand or knee involvement. In these cases the problem solving for adaptive solutions is initiated by the site of the arthritis. For this reason adaptive devices and methods are organized by level of involvement.

In an inpatient or long-term care setting it is common to treat people with severe arthritis in multiple or all joints. The goal in these cases is often to improve functional ability in self-care of a specific area of ADL. For this reason I have included the work of Helen Schweidler, OTR, which organizes adaptive aids for arthritis by functional activity.[2]

The following material will familiarize therapists with some of the equipment or methods used for certain physical limitations and functional activities. Not all problems are included nor is the solution list exhaustive. It is designed to stimulate thinking and to acquaint therapists new to arthritis patient care with some of the equipment and adaptive solutions commonly used.

Therapists working in this area of practice should also be familiar with the following three excellent resources.

1. *The Self-Help Manual,* produced by the Arthritis Health Professions Section of the Arthritis Foundation.[3] It includes a comprehensive review with photos of assistive equipment for people with arthritis.

2. Beverly Bingham, OTR, a master chef who also happens to have arthritis. Her text, *Cooking with Fragile Hands,*[4] is an excellent resource on kitchen equipment and planning and organizing cooking. She also publishes a newsletter called *ADL Update.*

3. The *ABLEDATA System,*[5] a program of the National Institute of Disability and Rehabilitation Research, can provide computerized listings of commercially available aids and equipment for disabled people. Manufacturers for all of the equipment listed in this chapter can be located through this system.

4. Sefra Pitzele, a writer, poet, and woman with systemic lupus erythematosus (SLE) who has written an outstanding book, *We Are Not Alone: Learning to Live With Chronic Illness.*[6] It includes a section on adaptive living strategies. (See References at the end of this chapter for ordering information.)

Hand Involvement

Active inflammation, swelling, and pain can limit one's ability to apply strength. Wrist tenosynovitis may impair flexor tendon gliding and reduce applied power of the profundus and sublimis flexor muscles. Flexor muscle weakness not due to pain can diminish ability for grasp and object manipulation. Loss of finger flexion due to contractures makes it difficult to apply power when grasping thin or narrow handles. Consequently if the person loses extension in the MCP or thumb CMC joints he or she will have difficulty grasping large objects. If a person has a severe CMC adduction contracture, handles on ambulation aids and other devices often have to be reduced or narrowed. Loss of lateral pinch can severely limit hand skills. Severe wrist flexion or ulnar deviation contractures can create compensatory stress to the elbow, shoulder, and spine. Because systemic sclerosis can result in such severe loss of hand function, adaptation for this condition is reviewed separately in Part II.

See Table 25–1 for aids for hand involvement.

Elbow Involvement

Loss of elbow flexion can severely interfere with ability to feed or wash or touch one's face. Loss of extension can interfere with ability to touch feet and perform lower extremity dressing, as well as to push off from chairs. Rheumatoid nodules may be aggravated by pressure or repetitive trauma. Severe bilateral limitations are extremely disabling and an indication for surgery.

See Table 25–2 for elbow involvement aids.

Shoulder Involvement

A considerable amount of shoulder range of motion (ROM) (approximately 50 percent) can be lost before causing significant restriction to functional activities. People with 90 degrees of shoulder flexion or less generally need some aids to assist with reach or dressing. Painful shoulders can reduce the ability of the upper extremity in all strength tasks such as lifting, carrying, and pushing.

See Table 25–3 for shoulder limitation aids.

Neck Involvement

In the early stages, inflammation of the facet joints can be aggravated by repetitive motion or posture in extremes of range

Table 25–1 Hand Involvement Aids

Devices	Comments
Joint protection for hands	See Chapter 24.
Adapted, built-up, or narrowed handles	Adhesive foam, foam tubing, or custom handles made out of orthotic material are the most common methods. On forearm crutches the plastic handle can be removed and the narrow stem lightly padded.
Nonslip pads or plastic sheets (e.g., Dycem mats)	To reduce force required to stabilize items (e.g., when used under a dinner plate), a person only has to cut food, not cut and press down to stabilize.
Faucet turners	When possible it is worth investing in lever fixtures for taps or faucets.
House or car key adaptations	Commercial key holders that increase leverage are available. If only 1 or 2 keys are a problem, this can be adapted by sealing the end between 2 pieces of orthotic material. *Caution:* Custom adaptions may not fit recessed area for ignition keys.
Lamp switch extenders and switches in extension cords	
Soaped runners on kitchen drawers for easier sliding	Silicon Spray (e.g., WD40) can ease operation of sliding doors, locks, and hinges.
Lightweight kitchen utensils	
Electric can opener	Therapists should be familiar with the amount of strength required to operate openers before ordering.
Jar opener	Wall-hung or under-counter openers that allow bilateral palmar holding of the jar are the best for people with active hand inflammation.
Bowl holders	There are now round bowls with a rubber stabilizing ring that allows the bowl to be positioned at any angle.
Saucepan stabilizers	If a full tea kettle is kept on the stove the saucepan can be stabilized against it while stirring.
Spring-loaded clipping scissors	
Suction bottle/glass brushes	These fit into the bottom of the sink and are very helpful if there is no dishwasher.
Electric scissors	These take practice to learn to use easily.
Cutting boards with stainless steel nails to stabilize vegetables for cutting	
Strap loops for forearm for oven doors, drawers, sliding door	Allows one to slip forearm through loop to open door. In the kitchen they can be made out of attractive sturdy ribbon or colored webbing.
Shoulder strap for handbags, suitcases, shopping bags	Commercial shoulder pads for straps are available at luggage stores.
Blanket cradles or ribbon handles sewn on blankets	To make blanket manipulation easier.
Electric blankets	To minimize bulk as well as an aid for reducing morning stiffness.
Sheet tucker (small wooden paddle)	
Universal cuff to hold brushes, silverware, pencils	
Book racks	To hold books upright at an angle without manually holding them. Plastic ones are available for cookbooks.

Table 25–1 Hand Involvement Aids *Continued*

Devices	Comments
Newspaper holders	
Pen or pencil holding devices	There are many styles. My favorite for reducing hand strain is sticking the pen or pencil through the center of a small (2-inch diameter) firm (not hard) foam ball.
Electric shaver holders	
Cup holders, lightweight mugs, mugs with open handles	Open handle can accommodate deformity.
Button hooks	Again, depending on the hand problem, these may need to be built up or narrowed, padded, or firm.
Soap on a rope (for shower or tub)	Prevents soap from falling.
Car door openers	Styles available to open all doors.
Aerosol can holders	These allow grip pressure to press spray knob.
Plastic open handles for milk cartons and large soda bottles	
Pop-top and screw-cap openers	
Plastic bag and box top openers	
Luggage carrier	Can also be used around the house.

Table 25–2 Elbow Involvement Aids

Devices	Comments
Elbow sleeve pads	These can be worn to bed to reduce pressure on nodules or sensitive skin when people use elbows for stability during movement or transfers. They can also be used during the day as a treatment to reduce nodules aggravated by or resultant from pressure. They are made with a loose net sleeve (Diamond) that is easy to don with weak hands or a tighter cotton knit (Heelbo).
Extended-handle tableware for feeding	
Extended straws	
Lower extremity dressing aids	
Adapted chairs, easy to stand up from	

such as forward flexion while reading. In cases of severe involvement (e.g., juvenile rheumatoid arthritis [JRA] or AS), neck immobility restricts visual range. This is particularly critical where safety is a concern, such as during driving or child care. An immobile neck also makes it difficult to participate in conversation in a group setting, where conversation may originate from different directions, because the person has to turn the entire body to view someone. If ankylosis is inevitable, aids should be considered to help maintain optimal alignment.

See Table 25–4 for neck involvement aids.

Knee Involvement

Knee pain inhibits muscle strength of the knee extensors, reducing ability for rising from a sitting position, standing, and ambulation. Greater than a 30-degree loss of extension can severely limit ambulation. A minimum of 100 degrees of knee flexion is needed to sit in a chair or climb steps comfortably.

See Table 25–5 for knee involvement aids.

Table 25–3 Shoulder Involvement Aids

Devices	Comments	Devices	Comments
Extended handles with enlarged grip on hairbrushes, combs, toothbrushes, tableware, backbrushes	*Caution:* Extended handles increase the forces on the hand and wrist. Use lightweight devices.	Reachers	*Caution:* These increase forces on the hand and wrist. Use lightweight devices. Also helpful for reaching, pulling, or pushing items other than clothing.
Long cloth back scrubbers	Preferred over backbrushes. Often available at notions counters.	Dressing sticks (cup hook on one end, adapted coat hook on other end)	
Extended drinking straws		Front-opening clothes	
Coat holders	Available from European companies. Bracket with clips holds coat while donning, foot pedal release.	Sponges and dustpans with extended handles for floor care	
		One-handed hair rollers (Velcro-like covering holds hair in place without clips)	
Lightweight down winter coats			

Hip Involvement

A minimal hip flexion can create physical problems such as encouraging knee flexion contractures or compensatory spinal changes such as lordosis. These in turn reduce efficiency in gait and movement. It may impede participation in sports but not prevent functional activities. A moderate contracture increases the above problems and would make it difficult for the person to lie supine.

Loss of hip flexion (an extension contracture) creates more functional limitations.

Table 25–4 Neck Involvement Aids

Devices	Comments
Chairs that swivel	Neck stiffness or immobility requires turning the entire body to see to the sides. Swivel chairs allow the patient visual range without getting up. Executive office chairs can have wheels removed and be used in the living room.
Wide-angled, rearview mirror	Available at most auto-part stores.
Expandable/mounted mirrors	Allow adjustment to create correct angle for viewing.
Typing draft holder	Holds typing directly above typewriter; eliminates need for repetitive turning to side.
Adjustable book holders	For students, I recommend using a single wire holder on top of a stack of books to bring the book to eye level. (Works well in the library.)
Cervical contour pillows (available from medical distributors)	The Jackson Cervipillo is a good one to start with. It also works well in the car against the neck rest.
Telephone receiver holders	For people who work on the telephone, a lightweight headset receiver is a worthwhile investment. Contact your local telephone company for resources.
Stepstool and reachers for upper cabinets	Stepstool reduces need to hyperextend neck.

Table 25–5 Knee Involvement Aids

Devices	Comments
Elevated chairs in the living room, kitchen, at work (and in the clinic)	Sofas and office waiting room chairs can be adapted by setting them on top of a 3-inch carpeted platform.
High kitchen stool	It is important that these are lightweight as well as sturdy so they can be moved easily.
Raised toilet seat	If possible it is worth having an elevated toilet installed. If an attachment has to be removed frequently, its weight and ease of attachment should be considered.
Arm bars for toilet	
Shower bench	Benches that block shower curtain closure allow water to get on the floor. The ability of the patient to clean up the water must also be a consideration. A hand-held shower head may be helpful.
Tub grab bars	
Walking aids	Canes should have wide rubber tips that are replaced when worn. There are several adaptations for using a cane on icy streets.
"Half step" or short steps	Steps can be adapted so they are half the height of regular steps.
Tea cart for transporting dishes and other such utensils	If this will be used a lot, a sturdy cart is recommended.
Shopping carts	

Ninety degrees of hip flexion is necessary to sit in a regular chair comfortably. If a person has less, the back will press into the chair. (This can become a source of back pain.) Severe loss of flexion (e.g., 45 degrees) makes it impossible to sit normally in a chair. Shallow seats or sitting on the edge of a seat may provide a solution in some situations. For any person with this type of problem, who is not a candidate for surgery, obtaining comfortable seating is a critical part of therapy. If proper seating would make a difference on the person's employment or attendance in school, the state department of rehabilitation may be able to assist in funding for equipment.

Equipment for this problem includes specially adapted chairs and toilet seats that allow the patient to sit upright with the hips in less than 90 degrees of flexion.

Hip, Back, or Elbow Involvement

See Table 25–6 for adaptive devices for use in hip, back, or elbow involvement that limits hand to foot or floor range.

Dressing Limitations

Limited range in proximal upper and lower extremity joints may make it difficult to get clothing over the feet or over the head. Poor grasp strength and loss of fine

Table 25-6 Hip, Back, or Elbow Involvement Aids*

Devices	Comments
Reachers	
Sock donners	Also available for pantyhose.
Elastic shoe strings	
Boot jack	To catch heel of boot, to help pull it off.
Dressing sticks	
Pants dressing poles	
Extended shoe horns	
Double-faced carpet tape on the end of a stick	To pick up small items like pills or broken glass.

*If involvement limits hand to foot or floor range.

prehension skills create problems in manipulating fasteners. Upper extremity weakness interferes with putting on coats or jackets.

See Table 25–7 for dressing aids.

Grooming Limitations

Decreased proximal upper extremity range impedes hair care, applying makeup, shaving, and dental hygiene. Loss of hand dexterity also interferes with these tasks as well as with nail grooming. Temporomandibular joint disease may complicate dental care.

See Table 25–8 for grooming aids.

Table 25–7 Dressing Aids

Devices	Comments
Dressing stick	
Reaching devices	Reachers are appropriate for individuals who have no arthritic hand and wrist involvement. The lightweight passive reacher may solve upper extremity problems.
Shoe/sock aids	
Stocking donner	
Long-handled shoe horn	
Boot jack	
Adaptive closures	A wide variety of commercial and home-made styles. Shoes can be adapted with Velcro, zippers, and clip-style closures.
Elastic shoelaces	
Button hook	
Zipper pull	
Zipper loop or ring	
Zipper tab	
Adapted clothing	Patterns or specially made garments may be purchased. Difficult closures may also be replaced with simpler fasteners or Velcro strips. Clothing may be selected with elasticized waists, front closures, and for wraparound style.

Table 25–8 Grooming Aids

Devices	Comments
Enlarged or extended handles on toothbrush, comb, razor	Lightweight materials to build up handles include cylindrical foam, adhesive foam, small wooden doweling, and aluminum tubing. Plastic coating or applications of low-temperature plastic splinting materials foster better grip.

Dental hygiene aids
  Electric toothbrushes
  Water jet appliances
  Floss and toothpick holders
  Toothpaste tube key
	Careful selection of these devices is advised as some are heavy, have clumsy grip, or require too much pinch.

Nail care devices: electric nail files, buffers	Compensate for weakness and loss of fine pinch. Clippers may be mounted on a wooden block or extensions may be placed on the handles.
Adaptations for cosmetic containers	Attachment for aerosol spray can provides lever to press spray button. Cosmetics may be selected for accessible containers (push-up lipsticks, deodorants with larger tops).

Bathing Limitations

Limitations in ambulation and transfer skills may make getting in and out of the tub or shower fatiguing, unsafe, or impossible. Loss of upper extremity strength and range interferes in managing faucets, washcloths, soap, shampoo, and so on. Limited range in proximal upper and lower extremity joints creates problems in reaching body parts, and fatigue could prevent the person from completing a bath independently.

See Table 25–9 for bathing aids.

Table 25–9 Bathing Aids

Devices	Comments
Safety aids	
Safety mats	Aid transfer. Increase safety.
Grab bars	Vertical pole or bars that attach to tub assist weak grasp since forearm may be substituted.
Tub/shower seats	Aid transfer. Increase safety. Wide variety of styles and heights available.
Lever faucet handles	Aid limited upper extremity strength and range.
Tap-turning devices	Reduce joint stress.
Hand-held shower heads	Aid limited range. Save energy. May be mounted at side of tub for easier access.
Bathing supplies	
Shower caddies	Aid limited strength and range. Wide variety available.
Tub trays	
Soap dispensers	
Washing and drying	Aid limited range in proximal joints. Long-handled sponges impractical if wrists/hands involved. Mitts aid limited grasp. Terry cloth robe saves energy required for drying after bath.
Long-handled sponge	
Wash mitts	
Adapted washcloths	
Terry cloth robes	

Table 25–10 Toileting Aids

Devices	Comments
Elevated toilet seats	Wide variety of temporary and permanent adaptations possible.
Commodes	Aid transfer and increase safety.
Grab bars	
Dressing	See dressing section.
Adapted clothing	
Dressing aids	
Toilet paper holder	Device holds paper and extends reach for cleaning after elimination.

range in proximal upper and lower extremity joints or loss of hand skills may interfere with managing toilet paper as well as cause problems in dressing and undressing for toileting.

See Table 25–10 for toileting aids.

Toileting Limitations

Limitations in knee and hip flexion and extension and in transfer skills create difficulty getting on and off a toilet. Decreased

Housekeeping Limitations

Aids and adaptations may be necessary due to problems in mobility, proximal upper and lower extremity ROM and strength, or hand problems. As noted in meal preparation, it is important to consider aids that will promote early joint protection and energy conservation.

See Table 25–11 for housekeeping aids.

Table 25–11 Housekeeping Aids

Devices	Comments
Kitchen or utility carts	Conserve energy, reduce joint stress, compensate for limited strength. Wheeled carts eliminate lifting and carrying with many items carried in one trip.
Lightweight sweepers	Conserve energy. Reduce joint stress. Lightweight sweepers may be used to reduce frequency of heavier vacuuming.
Self-propelled vacuums	
Shortened handles on broom and dustpan for wheelchair use	
Laundry aids	Compensate for strength and range limitations. Automatic washers and dryers should be selected for accessibility and easy-to-operate controls; clothes for easy care, little ironing.
Platforms to raise washer/dryer height	
Lowered clothes racks and lines	
Adjustable-height ironing board	
Lightweight "travel" iron or plastic regular iron	

Table 25–12 Meal Preparation Aids

Devices	Comments
Lightweight utensils, cookware, and dishes	Less strength and energy are required; reduce joint stress. Ceramic plates may range in weight from 24 oz to 11 oz each.
Devices to open containers: jar openers, can openers	Compensate for weak grasp and/or loss of fine prehension. Electric appliances must be selected so that controls are easy to operate.
Aids for cutting and chopping	These compensate for weak grasp and loss of fine hand skills as well as reduce joint stress. Knives and scissors should be maintained with sharp cutting edges to reduce the force required in cutting. Spring-style scissors are less stressful to joints. Cutting board may be adapted with rustproof nails to hold food.
Labor-saving appliances	Generally lessen joint stress, because less strength and energy are required. Examples include microwave ovens, electric skillets, blenders, and food processors. Appliances should be selected so that controls are easy to operate and parts that must be lifted are lightweight.
Adaptations for storage: pegboard, vertical storage, pull-out shelves	Conserve energy. May compensate for loss of range and strength. Work areas should be arranged so that tools and equipment are stored at the place where they are first used. Adaptations may be permanent and built-in, or temporary commercially available items.

Meal Preparation Limitations

The person with arthritis may need special aids to compensate for impaired mobility, limited range in reaching and bending, or lack of strength and endurance. Because many kitchen tasks are resistive or repetitive, it is especially important to consider joint protection and energy conservation.

See Table 25–12 for meal preparation aids.

Eating Limitations

Limited proximal upper extremity range may impair the person's ability to get food to the mouth and lack of supination or fine prehension, the ability to manipulate utensils. Weakness may make it difficult to cut food or lift a glass or cup.

See Table 25–13 for eating aids.

Transportation and Shopping Limitations

The ability to drive and ride in a car and to manage social and recreational outings and shopping may be limited by problems in mobility and transfer, upper extremity strength and range, and endurance.

See Table 25–14 for transportation and shopping aids.

Table 25–13 Eating Aids

Devices	Comments

Adapted utensils
  Enlarged or extended handles
  Utensil cuffs
  Swivel forks and spoons
	Attractive utensils are commercially available with enlarged handles. Handles or cuffs of standard utensils may be enlarged with foam or plastic to eliminate tight grasp of utensil. Swivel handles compensate for loss of supination.

Aids for drinking
  Long straws
  Lightweight and spillproof cups
  Thermal mugs
  Trays
  Table height adjustments
	Thermal mugs with wide handles allow both hands to be used with MCP joints in less stressful position. Severely disabled or hospitalized patients may need meals served at more accessible table height.

Table 25–14 Transportation and Shopping Aids

Devices	Comments
Car door openers	Reduce stress on thumb. Devices are commercially available or may be simply constructed.
Key holders	Compensate for weak lateral pinch by providing leverage.
Seat cushions	Aid transfer. Covered in slick materials, these facilitate sliding and pivoting. Catapult cushions may be placed sideways on car seat to aid standing.
Wide-angle rearview mirrors	Compensate for limited neck range.
Devices for loading and unloading wheelchair	Wide variety available. May be needed by individual or the person who assists him.
Seat canes	Conserve energy and provide means to rest periodically during long walk or long period of standing.
Wheeled shopping carts	Conserve energy and compensate for loss of strength. Attention should be given to height of the handle to allow erect posture.
Shoulder bags	Reduce joint stress of prolonged grasp by allowing larger joints to carry items; also free hands for ambulation aids.
Back packs	
Ambulation aids	Canes, crutches, walkers, and wheelchairs need to fit the individual and instruction in their proper use must be given. It may be appropriate to use a wheelchair for safety or energy conservation during outings even though the individual can ambulate. Powered chairs such as the "Amigo" are useful for long distances and uneven terrain. (They can be rented when traveling.)

REFERENCES

1. Melvin, JL: Rheumatic Disease—Occupational Therapy and Rehabilitation. FA Davis, Philadelphia, 1977.
2. Schweidler, H: Assistive devices, aids to daily living. In Riggs, G, and Gall, EP (eds): Rheumatic Diseases and Management. Butterworth, Boston, 1984.
3. Self Help Manual. Arthritis Foundation
4. Bingham, B: Cooking with Fragile Hands. Creative Cuisine, Inc, Box 518, Naples, FL 33939, 1985. (Also, *ADL Update,* a quarterly newsletter.)
5. ABLEDATA System, National Institute of Disability and Rehabilitation Research (NIDRR). (Computerized database on products and manufacturers [not distributors]. It is accessible through any institution that subscribes to Bibliographic Retrieval Service [BRS]—medical libraries, hospitals, some public libraries. If you need assistance in organizing your search, call NIDRR for advice (call 1-800-555-1212 for current number). If you know how to search ABLEDATA, call 1-800-555-1212 for local BRS.)
6. Pitzele, S: We Are Not Alone: Learning to Live with Chronic Illness. Thompson & Co, Minneapolis, 1985.

ADDITIONAL RESOURCES

Services

Access Travel: A Guide to Accessibility of Airport Terminals. US General Services Administration, Washington, DC, 20405.

Air Travel for the Handicapped. TWA, 605 Third Ave, New York, NY 10016.

Air Travelers Fly Rights. Office of Consumer Affairs, Civil Aeronautics Board, Washington, DC 20428.

American Automobile Association, 1712 G Street, NW, Washington, DC 20015. (Free list of automobile hand-control manufacturers.)

American Foundation for the Blind, 15 W 16th Street, New York, NY 10011. (Provides talking book services.)

American Heart Association, 7320 Greenville Ave, Dallas, TX 75321.

American Home Economics Association, 2010 Massachusetts Ave, NW, Washington, DC 20036.

Appliance Information Service (AIS), Whirlpool Corporation, Administration Center, Benton Harbor, ME 49022. (Ask for *Designs for Independent Living* and other booklets.)

Consumer Product Information Service, Public Documents Distribution Center, Pueblo, CO 81009.

Medic Alert Foundation International, PO Box 1009, Turlock, CA 95380, 209-634-4917 (call collect). (A confidential 24-hour medical information service providing emergency information related to members' medical conditions; free medical information bracelet or necklace provided with membership fee.)

National Arthritis and Musculoskeletal and Skin Diseases Information Clearinghouse (formerly the Arthritis Information Clearinghouse), PO Box 9782, Arlington, VA 22209, 703-558-8250. (Provides current bibliographies on assistive devices at no charge.)

National Center for a Barrier Free Environment, 1140 Connecticut Ave, NW, Suite 1006, Washington, DC 20036.

National Library, Services for Blind and Physically Handicapped, Library of Congress, 1291 Taylor, NW, Washington, DC 20542.

National Odd Shoe Exchange, Rural Route 4, Indianoala, IA 50125.

Randall, M: Locating rehabilitation product information through ABLE DATA. Occup Ther Health Care 1(4), Winter 1984. (Rehabilitation International, USA, Box PR, 1123 Broadway, New York, NY 10010. Write for *International Directory of Access Guide* for disabled travelers; send stamped, self-addressed, business envelope.)

US Government Printing Office, Washington, DC 20402. (Ask for list of topics related to an illness, including *Clothing Tips for the Woman with Arthritis.*)

Distributors and Manufacturers

AARP Home Care Special-log, Retired Persons Services, Inc, One Prince Street, Alexandria, VA 22314.

Abbey Rents and Sells, 933 East Sandhill, Carson, CA 90746, 800/262-1327 (toll-free number in California), 800/421-5126 (toll-free number in other states).

Alda Industries, Inc, 214 Harvard Ave, Boston, MA 02134. (E-Z up chair to help people who have difficulty with sitting and getting out of a chair.)

Alimed, Inc, 297 High Street, Dedham, MA 02026.

Amigo Sales, Inc, 6693 Dixie Highway, Bridgeport, MI 48603.

Bird and Cronin, Inc, Home Health Care Centers, 508 Jackson Street, St Paul, MN 55101. (Write for "Home Health Care" catalog.)

Birkenstock Shoes, 46 Galli Drive, Vorato, CA 94947. (Write for current shoe catalog.)

Bolz, AR, 3939 Cloverhill Road, Baltimore, MD 21218. (Sleeves to filter ultraviolet light from fluorescent lights.)

Brookstone Company, 127 Vose Farm Road, Peterborough, NH 03458. (Write for catalog on hard-to-find tools and other fine things.)

Cleo Living Aids, 3957 Mayfield Road, Cleveland, OH 44121. (Write for catalog on daily living aids, including bath and shower devices.)

Comfortably Yours, 52 West Hunter Ave, Maywood, NJ 07607. (Write for catalog on aids for easier living.)

Cosco Home Products, 2525 State Street, Columbus, IN 47201.

Dixson, Inc, PO Box 1449, Grand Junction, CO 81502. (Designer, manufacturer, and marketer of a full line of aids for daily living.)

Earl's Stairway Lift Corporation, 2513 Center Street, Highway 218 North, Cedar Falls, IA 50613.

Elder Ensembles, 7400 Metro Boulevard, Suite 410, Edina, MN 55435.

Enrichments, Inc (Division of Fred Sammons, Inc), 145 Tower Drive, Burr Ridge, IL 60521. (Full-color catalog contains a complete selection of independent living aids.)

Everest and Jennings, 3233 E Mission Oaks Boulevard, Camarillo, CA 93010. (Wheelchairs, home, and hospital medical supplies.)

Fashion-Able, Inc, Box S, Rock Hill, NJ 08553. (Write for adaptive clothing catalog, mail order clothes for women.)

Fred Sammons Inc, Box 32, Brookfield, IL 60513. (Catalogs on daily living aids for professions; Enrichments catalog, above, for patients.)

Grass Roots Promotions, Department W, 322 West Roosevelt Street, Freeport, IL 61032. ("Rest-stop" seat to put on walker.)

Guardian Products, PO Box C-4522, Arleta, CA 91331.

Hammacher Schlemmer, 145 East 57th Street, New York, NY 10022. (Catalog of gadgets and aids for living.)

Handi-Ramp, Inc, 1414 Armour Boulevard, Mundelein, IL 60060.

Help-Yourself Aids, Mail Order Catalog 103, PO Box 289, Elmhurst, IL 60126. (Wide variety of aids to help independence.)

Helping Hand Service for the Handicapped, Greyhound Lines, Greyhound Towers, Phoenix, AZ 85077.

Independence Factory, PO Box 597, Middletown, OH 45042.

Independent Living Aids, Inc, 11 Commercial Court, Plainview, NY 11803.

Joan Cook, 3200 SE 14th Ave, Ft Lauderdale, FL 33316. (Gadgets and aids.)

Lumex, Inc, 100 Spence Street, Bayshore, NY 11706.

Madack, Inc, Pequannock, NJ 07440. (Write for catalog of home health-care equipment, *Special Products for People with Special Needs.*)

McKay's Arthritis Specialties, 1421 Hamilton, Janesville, WI 53545.

Miles Kimball, Kimball Building, 41 West 8th Ave, Oshkosh, WI 54901. (Catalog of gadgets and practical devices.)

Montgomery Ward, Albany, NY 12201. (Write for home health-care catalog or call local store.)

North Coast Medical, 450 Salmar Ave, Campbell, CA 95008. Excellent catalog.

Para Medical (Distributors), 2020 Grand Ave, PO Box 19777, Kansas, MO 64141.

Prentke Romich Co, 1022 Heyl Road, Wooster, OH 44691. (Excellent environmental controls.)

Rehabilitation Equipment and Supply, 1823 West Moss Ave, Peoria, IL 61606.

Rubbermaid, Inc, 1147 Akron Road, Wooster, OH 44691. (Kitchen and other household equipment.)

Sears Roebuck and Co, 4640 Roosevelt Boulevard, Philadelphia, PA 19321. (Write to headquarters or call the catalog desk of your local store.)

Spencer Gifts, Atlantic City, NJ 08411. (Gadgets and aids for living.)

Sunset House, 12800 Culver Boulevard, Los Angeles, CA 90066. (A gadget catalog for easier living plus fun items.)

Swedish Rehabilitation Products Corp, 17 Briar Cliffe Drive, Scotch Plains, NJ 07076. (Excellent catalog.)

Velcro Corporation, 681 Fifth Ave, New York, NY 10022. (Write for a catalog on the uses of Velcro.)

Ways and Means Capability Center, 28001 Citrin Drive, Romulus, MI 48174.

Zim Manufacturing Co, 2850 West Fulton Street, Chicago, IL 60612. (Write for a catalog including the Zim jar opener.)

Adaptive Clothing and Dressing Aids

Bare, C, Boetke, E, and Waggoner, N: Self Help Clothing for Handicapped Chidren. National Easter Seal Society for Crippled Childred and Adults, 1962. (Cost: 75 cents.)

Dallas, MJ, and White, LW: Clothing fasteners for women with arthritis. Am J Occup Ther 36(8):515–518, 1982.

Clothing Designs for the Handicapped. Accent Special Publications, Box 700, Bloomington, IL 61701. (Designs for men, women, and children. Section on aids, directions for altering clothing and patterns. Cost: $15.)

Exceptionally Yours, Inc, 22 Prescott Street, Newtonville, MA 02160. (Designs and manufactures selection of adaptive casual wear for children and adults with disabilities and special needs.)

Flexible Fashions: Clothing Tips for Women with Arthritis. US Department of Health, Education, and Welfare, Publ No. 1814, 1982.

Goldworthy, M: Clothes for Disabled People. 1981. Available from David & Charles, Inc, North Pomfret, VT 05053. (Cost: $11.95.)

Kennedy, ES: Dressing with Pride: Clothing Changes for Special Needs. 1981. Available from PRIDE Foundation, Inc, 1159 Poquonnock Road, Groton, CT 06340. (Cost: $9.50.)

Kreisler, N, and Kreisler, J: Catalog of Aids for the Disabled. McGraw-Hill, New York, 1982.

Moratz, VA: Adapting shirts to fit over a halo vest. Am J Occup Ther 33(8):524–525, 1979.

Ober, B: Clothing for the Aging Woman. Available from the Center for Studies in Aging Resources, North Texas State University, PO Box 13438, Denton, TX 76203. (Cost: $2.50.)

On the Rise: Clothing for Special People with Special Needs. 1982. On the Rise, 2282 Four Oaks Grange Road, Eugene, OR 97405.

Adapted Kitchen and Cooking Methods

Bingham, B: Cooking with Fragile Hands. Creative Cuisine, Inc, PO Box 578, Naples, FL 33939.

Kaufman, M: Fare and feeding for patients with arthritis. Am J Occup Ther 19(5):281, 1965.

Klinger, JL: Mealtime Manual for People with Disabilities and the Aging. Available by writing to Mealtime Manual, Box 38, Ronks, PA 17572.

McCullough, HE, and Farnham, MB: Kitchens for

Women in Wheelchairs. Illinois University Extension Service, Circular No. 841, 1961.

Moore, JW: Adapted knife for rheumatoid arthritis. Am J Occup Ther 32(2):112–113, 1978.

Adaptive Seating

Bendix, T, and Biering-Sorenson, F: Posture of the trunk when sitting on forward inclining seats. Scand J Rehab Med 15(4):197–203, 1983.

Boothby, B: Seating by design. Physiotherapy 70(2):44–47, 1984.

Chamberlain, MA, and Munton, J: Designing chairs for the disabled arthritic. Br J Rheumatol 23(4):304–308, 1984.

Ellis, MI, Sedom, BZ, Amis, AA, Dowson, D, and Wright, V: Forces in the knee joint while rising from normal and motorized chairs. Eng Med 8:33–40, 1979.

Fink, GL: Adaptive equipment design and fabrication: The 'seven F' guide for occupational therapists. Occup Ther Health Care 1(4), Winter 1984.

Flaherty, PT, and Jurkovich, SJ: Transfer for Patients with Acute and Chronic Conditions. Rehab Publ No. 702. Sister Kenny Institution, Minneapolis, 1970.

Haworth, RJ: Use of aids during the first three months after total hip replacement. Br J Rheumatol 22(1):29–35, 1983.

McPhee, B: Occupational health—Work chairs and seating. Aust J Physiother 28(5):30–33, 1982.

Munton, J: Seating for the arthritic. Rep Rheum Dis 77–78, July 1981.

Munton, JS, Ellis, MI, Chamberlain, MA, and Wright, V: An investigation into the problems of easy chairs used by the arthritic and the elderly. Rheumatol Rehabil 20(3):164–173, 1981.

Ross, T: Are you sitting comfortably? Nurs Times 79(51):8–10, 1983.

Watkin, B: Are you sitting comfortably? Health and Safety at Work 5(10):29–30, 1983.

Assistive Devices and Aids

Aids and Adaptations. Compiled by the Occupational Therapy Department, Canadian Arthritis and Rheumatism Society, British Columbia Division, Vancouver, Canada. Available from The Arthritis Society, 920 Yonge Street, Suite 420, Toronto, Ontario, M4W 3J7 Canada. (Contains designs and instructions for fabrication. Cost: $2.50.)

Breuer, JM: A Handbook of Assistive Devices for the Handicapped Elderly: New Help for Independent Living. Haworth Press, New York, 1982.

Casamassimo, P: Toothbrushing and Flossing: A Manual of Home Dental Care for Persons Who Are Handicapped. (Covers techniques, aids, and adaptations. Cost: $1.50.) Also, Helping Handicapped Persons Clean Their Teeth. (Cost: 15 cents.) National Easter Seal Society for Crippled Children and Adults, 2023 West Ogden Ave, Chicago, IL 60612.

Chamberlain, MA: Aids and equipment for the arthritic. Practitioner 224(1339):65, 1980.

Chamberlain, MA, Thornby, G, and Wright, V: Evaluation of aids and equipment for bath and toilet. Rheum Rehab (Br) 17(3):187, 1978.

Davies, H: Spotlight on children: A disabled mother. Nurs Times 77(25) (P Suppl 2), 1981.

Davis, W: Aids to Make You Able. Available from Beaufort Books, Inc, 9 E 49th Street, New York, 1981.

Ellis, ST: Adapted inhaler designed for hand-impaired people. OT Week February 5, 1987, p 3.

Erving, E (ed): Green Pages Rehab Sourcebook, 4th ed. Sourcebook Publications, Winter Park, FL, 1982.

Lorig, K, and Fries, JF: The Arthritis Helpbook. Addison-Wesley, Reading, MA, 1980.

Maddus, S: Infant handling and childcare techniques for the physically disabled parent. Occup Ther Forum 2(25):18–19, June 18, 1986.

Patricelli, J, and Eckroth, J: Adapted knife for partial hand amputation patients. Am J Occup Ther 36(3):193–194, 1982.

Redmond, L: Reading, Writing and Other Communication Aids for Visually and Physically Handicapped Persons. 1981. Available from Reference Section, National Library Service for the Blind and Physically Handicapped, Library of Congress, Washington, DC 20542.

Rusk, HA, and Lowman, EW: Self-Help Devices. Rehabilitation Monograph XXI. Institute of Rehabilitation Medicine, New York University Medical Center, New York, 1965.

Self Help Device Catalogs, Vols 1, 2, and 3. The Independence Factory, PO Box 597, Middletown, Ohio 45042. (Manufactures and/or provides fabrication plans.)

Self-Help Manual, 2nd ed. Arthritis Health Professions Association, Arthritis Foundation, 3400 Peachtree Road, NE, Atlanta, GA 30326, 1980. (Cost: $4.95. Excellent resource.)

Solomonow, M, and Feder, T: Simple living aids for the arthritic patient. Bull Prosthet Res 10–35:60–63, Spring 1981.

Veterans Administration: Directory of Living Aids for the Disabled Person. 1982. Available from Superintendent of Documents, USGPO, Washington, DC 20402.

General Adaptations for Living and Occupational Therapy References

Cruzic, K: Disabled? Yes. Defeated? No. Resources for the Disabled and their Families, Friends, and Therapists. Prentice-Hall, Englewood Cliffs, NJ, 1982.

Fastow, K: Adapted fitted bed sheets. Am J Occup Ther 31(6):393, 1977.

Hale, G: The Source Book for the Disabled. Grosset & Dunlap, New York, 1979.

Hodgeman, K, and Warpeha, E: Adaptations and Techniques for the Disabled Homemaker. Rehab Publ No 710, 1973. Sister Kenny Institution, 1800 Chicago Ave, Minneapolis, MN 55404. (Cost: $1.75.)

Institute for Information Studies: Rehabilitation Engineering Sourcebook. 1979. Available from National Technical Information Service, 5285 Port Royal Road, Springfield, VA 22161.

Institute for Information Studies: Rehabilitation Engineering Sourcebook, Supplement I. 1980. Available from National Technical Information Service, 5285 Port Royal Road, Springfield, VA 22161.

Institute for Information Studies: Rehabilitation Engineering Sourcebook, Supplement II. 1982. Available from Institute for Information Studies, 400 N Washington Street, Suite 202, Falls Church, VA 22046.

Lunt, S: A Handbook for the Disabled: Ideas and Inventions for Easier Living. Scribner's Sons, New York, 1982.

May, EE, Wagonner, NR, and Hotte, EB: Independent Living for the Handicapped and Elderly. Houghton-Mifflin, Boston, 1974.

Montgomery, MA: Resources of adaptation for daily living: A classification with therapeutic implications for occupational therapy. Occup Ther Health Care 1(4), Winter 1984.

Pitzele, SK: We Are Not Alone—Learning to Live with Chronic Illness. Thompson & Co, Inc, Minneapolis, 1985. (This excellent book has a chapter on adaptive living strategies.)

Rehabilitation Engineering and Product Information Resource Guide. Department of Education #E8022015, Room 3106 Switzer Building, 330 C Street SW, Washington, DC 20202.

Sargent, JV: An Easier Way: Handbook for the Elderly and Handicapped. Iowa State University Press, Ames, 1984.

Schweidler, H: Assistive Devices, Aides to Daily Living. In Riggs, GK, and Gall, EP: Rheumatic Diseases: Rehabilitation and Management. Butterworth, Boston, 1984.

Taira, ED: An occupational therapist's perspective on environmental adaptations for the disabled elderly. Occup Ther Health Care 1(4), Winter 1984.

Wade, CS, and Kramer, RM: The relationship between arthritic adults and furniture usage: A study. Rehabil Lit 45(3–4):80–84, 1984.

Washburn, MG: Designing environments for the elderly. Occup Ther Health Care 3(1), Spring 1986.

Wright, V, and Moll, JMH: Seronegative Polyarthritis. Elsevier, North-Holland Press, Amsterdam, 1976, pp 411–415. (Includes a section on aids for patients with fused necks. Describes a unique right angle mirror for driving that allows patients to see traffic approaching from the side.)

Chapter 26

Functional Activities

THERAPEUTIC CRAFTS AND GAMES
    Crocheting and Knitting
LEISURE ACTIVITIES
ACTIVITIES OF DAILY LIVING

Functional activities refer to crafts, games, and activities of daily living so structured as to achieve a specific therapeutic goal, such as increasing range of motion (ROM), strength, or dexterity. When these activities are performed with rheumatic disease patients, the following points are important to keep in mind.

1. *When the activity is designed for treatment of a specific area, it is important to be aware of the effect of the activity on other body parts.* The severity of synovitis can vary from joint to joint. An activity effective for strengthening the elbow may aggravate the shoulder or wrist.

2. *Home carry-over is a crucial factor in the treatment of chronic conditions.* Selection of activities should be relevant to the follow-up home program. For example, floor loom weaving may be effective for maintaining a patient's upper extremity strength during hospitalization, but it is not as effective for ensuring home follow-through as, perhaps, frame weaving or caring for house plants.

3. *Joint-protection principles should be applied to activities.* For example, a patient with metacarpophalangeal synovitis should not perform activities involving strong grip or pinch (handles should be built up or splints worn as indicated), and the patient prone to joint stiffness should stand up or stretch during prolonged sitting activities. (For additional joint-protection methods, see Chapter 24, Joint-Protection and Energy-Conservation Instruction.)

4. *The basic treatment principles in using functional activities for restoration of ROM or strength are the same as those used for exercise* (see Chapter 27). The functional activity program needs to be coordinated with the physical therapy program to avoid overexertion of specific muscle groups.

THERAPEUTIC CRAFTS AND GAMES

Crafts and games can be used specifically for physical restoration, but in general they play a minor role in rheumatic disease rehabilitation. Even though they can be an effective method for strengthening, increasing ROM, and improving endurance, they frequently are not as efficient as an exercise, and rising medical costs mandate efficient treatment. However, in certain instances, they can be both an effective and efficient modality.

Example 1: For an inpatient on a progressive shoulder-strengthening program, additional strengthening can be achieved in the evening or on the weekend with the use of elevated crafts and weighted arm cuffs. (Weights are not indicated for grade 2 (poor) muscles as gravity offers sufficient resistance.) For example, frame weaving and macrame used in this manner can play a significant role in physical restoration.

Example 2: For strengthening finger extensors, frame weaving in which the patient packs the weft with the dorsum of the fin-

452

gers is an effective treatment method. The project should have a loose weave; the amount of resistance is graded by the thickness of the weft.

Example 3: Peg games can be used to encourage motion of the metacarpophalangeal (MCP) joint when the proximal interphalangeal (PIP) joint is immobilized with a temporary splint. This can be a particularly helpful activity following MCP implant arthroplasty.

The efficiency of crafts in rheumatological rehabilitation is a highly individualized matter. Therapeutic crafts and games effective for one patient may not be helpful for another. The use of crafts for general mental diversion has definite value but is *not* within the realm of current occupational therapy practice in rheumatology except when psychological responses, such as depression, are thwarting the medical regimen. Therapists should keep an open mind toward the use of crafts and games because additional exploration and experimentation are needed in this area.

Crocheting and Knitting

Crocheting and knitting are considered separately from other crafts because of the special role they play as avocations for many women confined by disease to a sedentary life. Both crocheting and knitting are unique in that they are traditional crafts which are easily learned, require minimal and available equipment, and are productive; that is, they produce a usable, functional product. In addition they are crafts that can be performed by patients with severe hand limitations. Many therapists advise patients against performing these activities because of the effects that prolonged static positioning in an intrinsic plus position may have on the joints. However, the psychological benefit of being productive and making something that is useful, stylish, and valued by others is of great importance for rheumatic patients. Careful consideration must be made in advising patients with regard to these activities.

In general the only hand conditions in which knitting and crocheting may cause harm are (1) active MCP synovitis, (2) beginning swan-neck deformities caused in part by intrinsic tightness, and (3) OA of the carpometacarpal (CMC) joint of the thumb.

Crocheting and knitting can have an adverse effect for a patient with active MCP synovitis by facilitating ulnar drift and MCP volar subluxation. Crocheting and knitting involve power pinch in a prolonged static intrinsic plus position and place ulnar deviating pressure on the MCP joints. (See Chapter 24, Joint-Protection and Energy-Conservation Instruction, for detailed discussion.) A patient, however, can perform crocheting and knitting without an adverse effect by wearing a hand orthosis that prevents the ulnar deviating pressures such as the orthosis shown in Figure 23–10 in Chapter 23, Orthotic Treatment for Arthritis of the Hand.

For the patient with beginning or mild swan-neck deformities caused in part by intrinsic muscle tightness, crocheting and knitting may increase the degree of intrinsic tightness by maintaining the fingers in a static intrinsic plus position. Any adverse effects resulting from participation in these crafts can be prevented by (1) wearing a hand orthosis that keeps the MCP joints in extension (as described above) or (2) performing intrinsic stretching exercises in addition to the crocheting and knitting.

The patient with OA of the thumb will probably find crocheting and knitting painful. However he or she can perform these activities without any adverse effect by using a thumb CMC stabilization orthosis (described in Chapter 23, Orthotic Treatment for Arthritis of the Hand).

Generally, a patient with typical OA (in the fingers), progressive systemic sclerosis, or severe chronic inactive rheumatoid arthritis hand deformities would *not* be adversely affected by crocheting and knitting with the exception that prolonged positioning may cause increased joint stiffness when the activity is stopped. This patient usually is aware of this kind of problem and avoids increased stiffness by taking frequent rest breaks or doing the activity for short periods only.

An additional point to consider when advising patients about crocheting and knitting is that the psychological benefit of being productive and making something that is useful, stylish, and valued by others may be of greater importance to the patient than whatever amount of hand function *might* be retained by not doing the craft (or doing the craft without adequate protection).

LEISURE ACTIVITIES

Counseling on leisure activities to help patients develop avocational interests that are within their capabilities can play a valuable role in helping patients cope with disability and the restrictions it places on their life-style. This kind of counseling, like other interventions, is not needed by all patients. However, many patients, discouraged by their inability to participate in favorite hobbies or activities, need encouragement and a realistic plan for participating in alternative activities.

Occupational therapists by virtue of their training are in a unique position to provide this service to patients, for they are the only members of the health care team knowledgeable in the three areas of rheumatology, kinesiology, and activity analysis. When patients have severe disabilities, expertise in all of these areas is needed to develop a viable, successful, avocational program that the patient will enjoy and continue over a period of time.

Resources on leisure activities suitable for patients with arthritis involvement are listed at the end of this chapter. An increasing number of resources are available on gardening, since this is a popular activity for adults and children alike.

ACTIVITIES OF DAILY LIVING

Because the rheumatic diseases are chronic, it is especially important to minimize debilitation that occurs secondary to disuse and bedrest. One method for counteracting this problem is to have the patient perform activities of daily living to tolerance during hospitalization. For a patient with an acute condition, this may mean only feeding and facial hygiene, but for a patient on a rehabilitation service, activities could include making his or her bed, dressing and bathing daily, and attending a dining room for meals.

The use of activities of daily living as a therapeutic medium for patients with rheu-

matic disease is the same as for patients with other physical disabilities. The main role of these activities in physical restoration is in maintaining muscular tone and improving endurance.

To improve endurance, it is necessary to graduate the length of time the patient is able to participate in selected activities, for example, cooking or personal hygiene (hair brushing, shaving). The activity selected should incorporate joint-protection principles and should allow the patient to stop readily as pain and tolerance dictate.

ADDITIONAL SOURCES

Occupational Therapy and Activities

Barish, H: Introduction to Acrylic Painting—An Approach to Encourage Creative Expression in Older Adults. Potentials Development Inc, 775 Main Street, Buffalo, NY 14203.

Bissell, JC, and Mailloux, Z: The use of crafts in occupational therapy for the physically disabled. Am J Occup Ther 35(6):3669–3674, 1981.

Cohen, J: Occupational therapy following hand tendon surgery. In Symposium on Tendon Surgery in the Hand. American Academy of Orthopaedic Surgeons. CV Mosby, St Louis, 1975, p 292.

Collins, E: Occupational therapy with rheumatoid arthritis. Am J Occup Ther 11:266–270, 1948.

Cynkin, S: Occupational Therapy: Toward Health Through Activities. Little, Brown & Co, Boston, 1979, 157 pp.

DiJoseph, LM: Independence through activity: Mind-body and environment interaction in therapy. Am J Occup Ther 36(11):740–744, 1982.

Edwards, B: Drawing on the Right Side of the Brain. (A course in enhancing creativity and artistic confidence.) JP Tarcher Inc, Los Angeles, 1979, 204 pp.

English, C, and Nalebuff, EA: Understanding the arthritic hand. Am J Occup Ther 25:352, 1971.

Eyler, R: Treatment of flexion contractures. Am J Occup Ther 19:86, 1965.

Hale, G (ed): The Source Book for the Disabled. Paddington Press, New York, 1979, 288 pp. (Includes a chapter on a wide range of leisure and recreational activities and an excellent section on gardening.)

Matsutsuyu, JS: The interest check list. Am J Occup Ther 23:323, 1969.

Nystrom, EP: Activity patterns and leisure concepts among the elderly. Am J Occup Ther 28:337, 1974.

Phillips, EL and Wiener, DN: Writing therapy: A new approach to treatment and training. In Short-Term Psychotherapy and Structured Behavior Change. McGraw-Hill, New York, 1966.

Richards, M: Centering in Pottery, Poetry, and the Person. Wesleyan University Press, Middletown, CT, 1964.

Rosenthal, I: The Not-So-Nimble Needlework Book.

Grosset & Dunlap, New York, 1977. (Includes projects and self-help aids and techniques.)

Spelbring, LM, Kirchman, MM, and Muller, RB: The use of activities in rheumatic disease. Am J Occup Ther 19(5):259–262, 1965.

Walker, A: A treatment program for rheumatoid arthritis. Am J Occup Ther 14:207, 1960.

White, RW: The urge towards competence. Am J Occup Ther 25:271, 1971.

Yerxa, E: Authentic occupational therapy. Am J Occup Ther 21:1, 1967.

Gardening

Chaplin, M: Gardening for the Physically Handicapped and Elderly. Royal Horticultural Society, London, 1978, 144 pp.

Gardening in Containers. A Sunset Book. Lane Publishing, Menlo Park, CA, 1977.

The Easy Path to Gardening. Available from the Disabled Living Foundation, 346 Kensington High Street, London, W14 8NS.

Chapter 27

Exercise Treatment

The occupational therapist applies the principles of exercise through functional activities for physical restoration. However, direct therapeutic exercise is also an essential part of effective occupational therapy for many specific clinical situations.

EXERCISE FOR RANGE OF MOTION

Range-of-motion (ROM) exercises are those in which the patient or the therapist moves the patient's body part through complete available range of motion. These exercises are utilized to *maintain* joint mobility and prevent limitations. When active or passive stretch is incorporated at the end of range, these exercises can be used to *increase* joint mobility.

The occupational therapist is most likely to be responsible for ROM exercises for the hand and upper extremity and occasionally for the foot. Generally, physical therapy is responsible for ROM of the other joints.

The hand poses the most challenge for determining the source of limitations because of its functional complexity and the effect that extrinsic tendon involvement at one level can have at other levels on joints controlled by the tendon.

When prescribing ROM exercises, five issues need consideration: (1) how joint disease affects ROM, (2) the type of exercise to use, (3) the minimal number of repetitions necessary to maintain or increase mobility, (4) the time of day the exercises should be done, and (5) follow-through (achieving patient cooperation).

How Joint Disease Affects Joint Mobility

Before recommending an exercise program it is critical to evaluate the musculoskeletal involvement and accurately determine the source of joint limitations. ROM can be limited by any of the following:

Joint synovitis/effusion
Tenosynovitis
Decreased tendon excursion
Muscle spasm
Muscle weakness (nerve entrapment)
Tendon attenuation/rupture
Edema
Soft tissue contractures (fibrosis)
Bone erosions
Bony ankylosis

Chapter 19, on hand assessment, describes how to determine if the conditions listed above are the source of joint limitation.

When inflammation is present, anti-inflammatory measures must be taken in addition to ROM exercise.

When deciding on a program for a particular patient, several factors need to be considered:

1. Synovitis not only weakens the joint capsule and supportive ligaments but also creates intra-articular swelling, placing these structures on stretch.[1] When a joint is swollen, exercise needs to be gentle, as passive pressure would further stretch and traumatize the joints.
2. Periarticular or extra-articular swelling causes joint compression and this by itself tends to cause range limitations; hence there is a need to reduce edema.
3. Pain induces spasms in the flexor-adductor muscles surrounding the joint (protective muscular splinting), limiting joint extension.[2]
4. Bedrest or inactivity secondary to pain increases the risk for adhesions, musculotendon shortening, and muscle weakness.

The interrelationship of these factors varies depending on the phase of arthritis present. In the acute and subacute phases, there is a greater risk of losing ROM because of periarticular edema, disuse, and muscular spasm. In the chronic-active phase dynamic forces acting upon weakened and overstretched supporting structures are the major threat to joint integrity. In noninflammatory joint disease ROM is often limited by bony growth (osteophytes).[3]

Types of Exercise: Force or No Force

The philosophy regarding active versus passive exercise for patients with arthritis is one of the most misunderstood concepts in rheumatological rehabilitation. Physicians, fearful that therapists will apply strenuous exercise, often request active-assistive exercise, believing it is less strenuous than passive exercise. This may not always be the case. A patient can exert more stress on a joint by attempting active motion than he or she would exert during gentle passive motion. When a person has acute synovitis with associated pain and muscle spasm, active exercise increases the tension in the muscle and increases joint compression forces. Often in the presence of active synovitis, greater and less painful mobility can be achieved with gentle passive exercise. In certain joints such as the wrists, elbows, and ankles, active exercises may be the most effective and the easiest to carry out. For the larger joints, such as the shoulders, knees, and hips, passive exercise that incorporates muscle relaxation is often preferable for maintaining mobility during acute or active synovitis. In instances in which there is a lag in motion, for example, due to tenosynovitis or weakness, passive ROM exercises are the only type recommended.

There are three forms of ROM exercises:

1. **Active ROM:** Patient moves body part through full joint range without assistance, using the muscles related to the joint.
2. **Active-assistive ROM:** Active motion through partial range with assistance from an external force to complete range. External forces include:
   a. Gravity-assist through positioning
   b. Equipment such as deltoid aid and pulleys
   c. Functional exercises such as finger ladder climbing, cone stacking, and wand exercises
   d. Water (for ROM in hydrotherapy or in the tub)
   e. Verbal cues (encouragement) or visual feedback during exercises
   f. Another person (manual assistance)
   g. Use of muscles other than those involved in the motion of this act (self ROM)

3. **Passive ROM:** The body part is moved through complete ROM solely by an external force.[4]

The terms used to prescribe ROM exercises, that is, *active* or *passive,* describe how the motion should be done but state nothing about the amount of force that should be used. If you want a patient to perform only active exercise without stretch, the procedure needs to be carefully demonstrated. Many patients become overzealous and think that if a little is good more is better, thus causing joint damage with inappropriate stretching.

The duration of pain is a guide for prescribing exercise. *Pain or discomfort resulting from the exercise should not last for more than one hour following the exercises.* If joint pain lasts for several hours or the patient feels excessive joint discomfort the following day, the exercises were too stressful and should be reduced.[5]

Stretch at the end of ROM is recommended to increase ROM in the chronic-active or chronic-inactive phases. Gentle pressure at the end of ROM may be indicated for the subacute phase to ensure that *complete* ROM is being achieved. However, *stretch is not recommended in the acute phase.* This is primarily because it induces pain facilitating protective muscle spasm and puts additional stress on structures already on maximal stretch due to intra-articular swelling. Trauma at this point can cause additional scarring.[6]

How Much? How Often?

There is no hard and fast rule regarding the number of repetitions necessary to maintain or increase mobility. Some patients (e.g., those with stable, chronic conditions) may need to perform *only one complete ROM daily* for maintenance, while patients in an acute or subacute phase (when there is more periarticular swelling and less physical activity) *may need to perform two complete ROMs per day.*[7] Although this sounds simple, keep in mind that it may take two to five warm-up reaches for a person to achieve a complete ROM.[8]

To increase joint mobility, positioning of the joint to allow gentle-sustained passive stretch is the most effective method. This procedure takes advantage of muscle relaxation and lengthening of both the agonists and antagonist muscles.[9] For fixed contractures sustained stretch requires the use of progressive or serial splinting or casting.

When Exercises Should Be Done

Exercises should be done at the best time of the day for a patient, when he or she feels the most limber and following adequate analgesic medication. For some patients doing the exercises in or following a warm shower or bath is the ideal time. For other patients specific application of heat or cold prior to exercising may be indicated.[8]

Follow-Through

The self-ranging maintenance program of the patient is a major treatment concern because most forms of arthritis are chronic. I believe it is essential that all home programs be written out for the patient. If there is questionable comprehension or if there are follow-through problems, the exercise emphasis should be placed on the one or two joints most crucial to functional independence.

I have found it effective to start instruction of the home ROM program on the first day of treatment for inpatients, usually completing instruction by the third session. Subsequent ROM treatment during hospitalization consists of having the patient perform his or her ROM program under observation (patient is allowed to refer to the written program). This method does not guarantee follow-through, but it at least guarantees that the patient *can* perform his or her program independently at the time of discharge. It also allows time to modify the program.

The other instructional method I have found particularly effective is to use exercises that provide visual feedback of progression or regression for the patient. Treatment is directed toward having the patient monitor and alter his or her treatment as indicated between follow-up appointments.

1. *Shoulder and elbow ROM:* Instead of having the patient reach as high as possible,

have him or her face a wall, stand as close as possible, then reach as high as comfortably possible with each arm, and mark the wall at that point. A maintenance ROM exercise for shoulder flexion and elbow extension would be to touch each mark once a day with each hand.

2. *Finger hyperextension range:* Have the patient place palms together, keep metacarpophalangeal joints touching, and hyperextend the fingers. While fingers are separated, patient can hold them to a ruler and measure opening span to monitor progression. (Maintenance of hyperextension ROM is not critical to function; however, it is the first motion lost in the presence of metacarpophalangeal joint involvement. This exercise helps maintain the extensibility of the volar structures.)

3. *Thumb web space:* With hand flat on a paper and thumb extended, have patient trace web space. Subsequent tracings can be done in a different color to mark improvement or maintenance.

4. *Finger abduction:* This can also be monitored with tracings of the hand while the hand is palm down on paper.

5. *Temporomandibular excursion:* Have patient measure aperture between upper and lower teeth (with a ruler or marked index card in front of a mirror). This is especially important for progressive systemic sclerosis patients. It allows them to monitor jaw range and increase their exercises as needed.

EXERCISE FOR MUSCLE STRENGTH AND ENDURANCE

Basic Principles

When strengthening exercises are being employed for rheumatic disease clients, the following factors need consideration:

1. **Does the client have a systemic disease?** If so, the client's total daily activity regimen must be considered to avoid overexertion.

2. **What is the extent of joint involvement in individual joints:** acute, subacute, chronic active, or chronic inactive? The degree of inflammatory involvement can change from day to day. It is important to be aware of the effect a specific exercise may have on adjacent joints or body parts; for example, exercise to strengthen the external rotators of the shoulder may aggravate elbow involvement.

3. **Is the joint painful?** When pain is a factor, all exercises should be done with the joint or body part positioned in the least painful position. All efforts should be made to minimize discomfort during treatment.

4. **What is the goal of strengthening:** grade 5, grade 4, or grade 3 strength; grade 5 or grade 4 strength may be impossible for muscles associated with a damaged or inflamed joint. (See grading system defined in Chapter 21.)

5. **How will the goal be determined?** By muscle test, a plateau of strength gains, functional ability? Having a definite program that gives the client visible feedback of progress can be a significant motivation factor.

6. **How will strength be maintained once the goal is obtained?** A definite program for maintaining achieved strength is essential.

7. The muscle groups treated should demonstrate some fatigue at the end of treatment, but not overfatigue. *If pain brought on by exercise persists for over an hour after the activity is stopped or limits function, the amount of exercise should be decreased the following day.*

Type of Exercise

Exercise for strengthening muscles takes two forms: **isometric** and **isotonic.** The method of choice for clients with joint disease is the method that induces the least amount of pain since pain inhibits strength.[10] Isometric exercises are usually the least painful for clients with joint disease since they eliminate motion, which is frequently a direct source of pain in damaged joints.

Isometric exercise can be as effective or more effective than isotonic resistive exercise for both maintaining and improving muscle strength and endurance in clients with rheumatoid arthritis.[11,12] Resistive isotonic exercise had been hailed as the superior strengthening method in the past, because it is the most efficient technique for increasing muscle bulk.[11] However, there is *no direct positive correlation* between muscle bulk and muscle strength.[10] A muscle can have severe atrophy and the patient can still demonstrate grade 4 or 5 strength. This is a common phenomenon in rheumatoid arthritis, particularly in the intrinsic musculature of the hand. (Disuse weakness is not the same as disuse atrophy.) Specifically, because of this phenomenon, strengthening exercises should be directed toward the recovery of function rather than normal muscle structure or form.

Although isometric exercise is preferred when pain is a factor, isotonic exercise has a definite place in rheumatological rehabilitation and is of particular value when motor function is being relearned (e.g., in tendon transplants and other postoperative treatment).

Amount of Exercise

The amount of exercise needed depends upon the specific treatment goal.

To Counteract Disuse Weakness

The amount of exercise for this goal is based on studies that demonstrate that (1) the strength of a normal muscle decreases at a rate of 3 to 5 percent per day during inactivity, and (2) a single daily contraction at 50 percent maximal strength is sufficient to maintain normal muscle strength.[13] A reasonable exercise protocol to maintain strength or counteract disuse weakness for clients with physical dysfunction and normal muscle innervation would be a single maximal strength contraction per day for each muscle group.

In addition to exercise, an important adjunct to combating disuse weakness and maintaining general conditioning is to have the client perform activities of daily living to tolerance.

To Improve Muscle Strength and Endurance

One exercise program is needed to improve both strength and endurance. Clinically it has been shown that clients on exercise programs to improve endurance (i.e., low resistance-high repetition) demonstrate gains in strength, and clients on programs to increase strength (i.e., high resistance-low repetition) demonstrate gains in endurance.[11,14,15]

Several studies that evaluate strengthening techniques have been conducted for both normal subjects and people with rheumatoid arthritis.[11,12,13,16] In these studies, it has been demonstrated clinically that as little as six isometric contractions per day can significantly increase muscle strength. Two to four isometric exercises per day could constitute a strengthening program for the severely weak patient, while the client with grade 4 or 5 strength may need more repetitions to improve strength and endurance. Again, there is no hard and fast rule regarding the number needed. Probably the best guide is the number of repetitions necessary to bring on just fatigue (not pain).

To Maintain Strength Gained in Treatment

The optimal maintenance program is highly dependent upon the client's total daily regimen once maximal or the desired amount of strength is achieved. Sedentary patients may need to do a daily isometric exercise program, while more active clients may only need to do specific strengthening exercises once a week for maintenance. It has been demonstrated in normal subjects that maximal strength can be maintained with exercise as seldom as once every two weeks.[13]

Methods of Strengthening

Isometric Exercise

Definition. Maximal muscle contraction without joint motion. Often called **muscle setting.**

Positioning. The muscle or muscles being strengthened should be positioned slightly shorter than their resting length[17] (the point of maximal muscle tension during contraction). When it is not possible to stabilize the joint in this position, position the muscle at its shortest length. If this position causes pain, the joint should be positioned in a manner that produces the least amount of discomfort.[10]

Procedure. Have the client contract the

muscle as tightly as possible without moving the joint and hold for 6 seconds (count of eight), or the desired amount of time, and then relax for 6 seconds. Repeat procedure for the prescribed number of repetitions. Studies in Poland have demonstrated that exercises done with a consistent rhythm are more effective than those done in a haphazard manner.[14]

Progressive Resistive Exercises (PRE)

Definition. A strengthening technique using isotonic exercise and definite grading of resistance. The type of resistance can vary from very gentle manual pressure to the application of heavy weights.

Indications. Indications for PRE are

1. Postsurgical treatment when retraining of the motor unit and strengthening of the maximal number of muscle fibers is desired (e.g., tendon transfers)
2. To specifically increase muscle bulk
3. In general, when joint pain is not a factor

Precautions. Muscles need to be able to hold against slight resistance or more (grade 3.5 strength) to use this method.

Procedure. The following procedures are suggested:

1. Assess the client's maximal resistance level. This is determined by trial and error. It is the maximal amount of resistance the client can move steadily and smoothly through active ROM and return to resting. If the client trembles, starts fast, uses momentum, or releases fast, it is too much weight.
2. Begin the strengthening program with less than the maximal resistance tolerated. The right amount is that which causes slight muscle fatigue but does not overfatigue the muscle or cause pain that lasts for longer than one hour after the end of exercise.
3. The starting position is with the muscle lengthened. Have the client move the resistance smoothly and steadily through available ROM.
4. The number of repetitions depends upon the treatment goal. Two to six repetitions per muscle group a day are sufficient to increase strength.

Active-Assistive Exercise Using a Deltoid Aid

Definition. Treatment involving isotonic exercise through active ROM with assistance from a counterbalance weight mechanism to complete range of motion.

Indications. To strengthen shoulder flexors and abductors with grade 2 strength. (*Note:* Equipment also provides resistive exercise to shoulder extensors and adductors.) This method can be incorporated during self-care activities, such as feeding, or with therapeutic crafts.

Procedure. Establish the minimum assistive weight, that is, the minimum amount of weight necessary to assist the arm through the desired amount of abduction or flexion. Begin the program with *more than* the minimum amount of weight necessary, reducing the assistance as strength improves.

Muscle Re-education

Definition. Therapeutic exercise during the period of initial return of voluntary motor control.

Indications. Primarily for postoperative cases (e.g., tendon transplants, arthroplasties), neuropathies, and peripheral nerve injuries.

Procedure. *Positioning* is the same as for individual muscle testing. Directions for this are given in *Muscle Testing: Techniques of Manual Examination* by Daniels and Worthingham.[18]

Restoring mental awareness of motor function is accomplished by demonstrating passive motion (visual), giving verbal description of motion and action (auditory), and stroking point of insertion of prime muscles (tactile). Robert Bennett gives an in-depth discussion of muscle re-education in Chapter 10 in Licht's book, *Principles of Therapeutic Exercise.*[19]

Developing muscle function:

1. The therapist manually assists the part through full available range while requesting maximum active contraction from the client. Palpate and decrease assistance as patient gains control of motion.
2. The patient should not use substitute muscles. If this occurs (especially if the patient is trying too hard), eliminate those

muscles by increasing the amount of assistance.

3. It is important to establish good patterns of motion (control) before decreasing assistance.

4. Cutaneous stimulation techniques such as tapping, vibration, and brushing can be utilized to facilitate motor response.

REFERENCES

1. Understanding Inflammation—A Giant Step. A reprint from the 1969 Arthritis Foundation Annual Report. Available from the Arthritis Foundation, 475 Riverside Drive, New York, NY 10027.
2. Swezey, RL, and Fiegenberg, DS: Inappropriate intrinsic muscle action in the rheumatoid hand. Ann Rheum Dis 30:619, 1971.
3. Arthritis Manual for Allied Health Professionals. Arthritis Foundation, New York, 1973, Chap 2. (Available, no charge.)
4. Toohey, P, and Larson, CW: Range of Motion Exercise: Key to Joint Mobility. Rehab Publ 703. Sister Kenney Institute, Minneapolis, MN, 1968. (Resource for how to do passive ROM.)
5. Kendall, PH: Exercise for arthritis. In Licht, S (ed): Therapeutic Exercise, 2nd ed. Elizabeth Licht Publications, New Haven, CT, 1965, pp 702–720.
6. Flatt, A: Care of the Rheumatoid Hand. CV Mosby, St Louis, 1974, p 37.
7. Mead, S, and Knott, M: Ice therapy in joint restriction, spasticity and certain types of pain. Gen Prac 1961, p 16.
8. Swezey, RL: Essentials of physical medicine and rehabilitation in arthritis. Semin Arthritis Rheum 3:352, 1974.
9. Flatt: Care of the Rheumatoid Hand, p 44.
10. Kendall: Exercise for arthritis, pp 715–718.
11. Liberson, WB, and Asa, MM: Further studies of brief isometric exercises. Arch Phys Med Rehabil 40:330, 1959.
12. Machover, S, and Sapecky, AJ: Effects of isometric exercise on the quadriceps muscle in patients with rheumatoid arthritis. Arch Phys Med Rehabil 47:737, 1966.
13. Muller, EA: Influence of training and inactivity on muscle strength. Arch Phys Med Rehabil 51:449, 1970.
14. Personal communication from M Musar, PhD, RPT, Department of Rehabilitation, Rheumatological Institute, Warsaw, Poland.
15. DeLateur, BJ, Lehmann, JF, and Fordyce, WE: A test of the DeLorme axion. Arch Phys Med Rehabil 49:245, 1968.
16. Rose, DL, Radzyminski, SF, and Beatty, RR: Effect of brief maximal exercise on the strength of the quadriceps femoris. Arch Phys Med Rehabil 38:157, 1957.
17. Darling, RC: Physiology of exercise and fatigue. In Licht, S (ed): Therapeutic Exercise, 2nd ed. Elizabeth Licht Publications, New Haven, CT, 1965, p 33.
18. Daniels, L, and Worthingham, C: Muscle Testing: Techniques of Manual Examination. WB Saunders, Philadelphia, 1972.
19. Bennett, R: Principles of therapeutic exercise. In Licht, S (ed): Therapeutic Exercise, 2nd ed. Elizabeth Licht Publications, New Haven, CT, 1965, pp 472–485.

ADDITIONAL SOURCES

Banwell, BF: Exercise and mobility in arthritis. Nurs Clin North Am 19(4):605–616, 1984.

Collins, E: Occupational therapy with rheumatoid arthritis. Am J Occup Ther 11:266–270, 1948.

Danneskiold-Samse, B, Lyngberg, K, Risum, T, and Telling, M: The effect of water exercise therapy given to patients with rheumatoid arthritis. Scand J Rehab Med 19(1):31–35, 1987.

Flor, H, Haag, G, and Turk, DC: Long-term efficacy of EMG biofeedback for chronic rheumatic back pain. Pain 27(2):195–202, 1986.

Olivo, JL: Developing an exercise program for the elderly with osteoarthritis. Ortho Nurs 6(3):23–26, 1987.

Panush, RS, and Brown, DG: Exercise and arthritis. Sports Med 4(1):54–64, 1987.

Van Deusen, J, and Harlowe, D: The efficacy of the ROM Dance Program for adults with rheumatoid arthritis. Am J Occup Ther 41(2):90–95, 1987.

Vasudevan, S, and Melvin, J: U.E. edema control: rationale of the techniques. Am J Occup Ther 33(8):520, 1979.

Books for Patients

Adams, RC: Games, Sports, and Exercises for the Physically Handicapped, 3rd ed. Lea & Febiger, Philadelphia, 1982.

Carr, R: Arthritis: Relief Beyond Drugs. Harper & Row, New York, 1981.

Dial, S, and Sexton, A: A New Twist to Living: Wise Exercise for People with Arthritis. University of Alabama, Birmingham, 1978.

Garnet, ED: Movement is life: A holistic approach to exercise for older adults. Princeton Book Co, Princeton, NJ, 1982.

Hart, FD: Overcoming Arthritis: A Guide to Coping with Stiff or Aching Joints. Arco Publishing Co, New York, 1981.

Jamieson, RH: Exercises for the Elderly. Emerson Books, New York, 1982.

Lorig, K, and Fries, JF: The Arthritis Helpbook: What You Can Do for Your Arthritis. Addison-Wesley, Reading, MA, 1980.

Lupus Foundation of America: Hands, Feet, and Elbow Exercises; Hip and Knee Exercises. Tampa Area Chapter, 305 S Hyde Park Ave, Tampa, FL, 1982.

Rosenberg, AL: Living With Your Arthritis: A Home Program for Arthritis Management. Arco Publishing Co, New York, 1979.

Wiggins, P, Freeman, L, and Collier, M: Arthritis: Fighting the Wear and Tear—A Patient Guide to Self-Management. Available from Medical University of South Carolina, Department of Medicine, 171 Ashley Ave, Charleston, SC, 1980.

Water Exercises

Arthritis Foundation: Water Exercise for Persons With Arthritis. Metropolitan Washington Chapter, 1901 Ft Myer Drive, Suite 507, Arlington, VA, 1984.

Arthritis Foundation: Pool exercise educational program for persons with rheumatoid arthritis. Nebraska Chapter, 120 N 69th, Omaha, NE, 1980.

Jetter, J, and Kadlec, N: The Arthritis Book of Water Exercise. Holt, Rinehart & Winston, New York, 1985.

McDuffie, FC, and Boutaguh, M: Pool exercise programs for people with arthritis. Clin Rheum Prac 3(4):168–169, 1985.

Wilson, K: Twinges in the Hinges. Available from YMCA of Greater Whittier, 12817 E Hadley Street, Whittier, CA, 1980.

Chapter 28

Positioning and Lying Prone

In a rehabilitation hospital with a rheumatic disease unit, bed positioning and prone positioning will probably be carried out by nursing personnel. However, in hospitals without a specific arthritis rehabilitation section, it is often up to therapists to instruct the patient, family, and staff nurses in the proper positioning procedure for specific rheumatic diseases.

POSITIONING

Positioning for joint disease involves standard positioning procedures to achieve natural anatomical alignment and the addition of some specific orthoses. With joint disease, however, positioning is a primary treatment. The speed with which contractures can develop and the severity of the contractures necessitate efficient preventive care.

The Bed

At Night

The bed should be flat. Patients who have difficulty with reflux esophagitis or hiatus hernia should have the entire head of the bed, not just the mattress, raised 8 inches on blocks to aid esophageal motility and peristalsis, without encouraging hip flexion contractures.

The mattress should provide good, even support, with no sagging, and have a layer of foam on top to reduce pressure on bony prominences. The foam can be built into the mattress or added under the sheet. At home, eggcrate pads or 1½ inches of high-quality foam sheeting can be used. (Fire safety must be taken into consideration when purchasing these items.) Hospitals have very specific regulations about the types of pads that can be used. If the mattress sags, a bed board (¾-inch plywood) may improve support.

During the Day

For adjustable or hospital beds, if the patient has active knee or hip arthritis, the knee gatch should not be raised because this contributes to knee and hip flexion contractures. Patients with hip involvement who are in a sitting position for prolonged periods should have prone lying as a part of their daily program.

For patients with active arthritis, knee flexion in bed is permissible as long as it is alternated with periods of knee extension and range of motion (ROM) is maintained.

It is common practice in hospitals to raise the knee portion of the bed slightly (technically called the **semi-Fowler position**) when the patient is sitting up, so the patient will not slide in bed. Ideally a footboard should be used that can be moved toward the center of the bed, so the patient can sit up in bed with knees straight and feet against the board.

Head and Neck

The first objective of cervical positioning is to support the cervical muscles, thereby allowing complete relaxation, and consequently reducing muscle spasm, pain, and stiffness; the second objective is to maintain the normal lordotic curve of the cervical spine. The method selected should be comfortable, and the occipital bone, or back of the head, should be touching or close to the mattress. Sleeping with a regular pillow or without a pillow causes flexion of the spine and flattening of the lordotic curve and tension on the cervical ligaments and joints.[1]

To determine the depth of the lordotic curve of the neck, have the patient stand with his or her back against a wall, head level, and occipital bone touching the wall. The distance between the back of the neck and the wall indicates the depth of the curve (providing the patient does not have marked thoracic kyphosis). A proper cervical support will fill this space and maintain this alignment.

The objectives of cervical support can be achieved by several methods: a cervical pillow; a soft, thin down pillow that can be shaped around the neck; or a soft towel or foam roll. The method does not matter as long as the objectives are achieved.

For people with ankylosing spondylitis proper neck positioning is critical and can prevent deformity. They should use a soft neck roll or adapted cervical pillow that supports and maintains the normal lordotic curve of the neck but that allows the occipital skull to touch the mattress. (See Chapter 8, Ankylosing Spondylitis.)

Spine

Ideally proper positioning should support and preserve the anatomical lordotic curve of the lumbar spine. A small flat pillow or foam roll may be used under the low back. For people with early ankylosing spondylitis (AS), proper cervical and lumbar positioning must be considered together. Patients must be responsible enough to ensure proper positioning. If the patient with AS is unreliable, it may be better to simplify the rules and recommend sleeping without any pillows. For patients with AS, the home mattress (with foam pad) should have the amount of support that encourages straight alignment of the spine while sleeping in the side-lying position.

Elbows

Patients with elbow nodules, sensitive skin, or ulnar nerve sensitivity often find hospital sheets or synthetic sheets irritating to the dorsum of the elbow. Slip-on elbow protectors, the type with a foam pad inside a knit sleeve, can greatly improve comfort during bedrest. These are particularly helpful to patients who rely on their elbows for mobility in bed. Currently there are two different brands of elbow protectors on the market. Both are excellent but have different qualities. The Heelbo has a stronger, more durable knit sleeve. It works well for children and patients with thin arms, because it fits more snugly and is less bulky. However, the snug fit makes it difficult for patients with painful hand involvement to pull on. Heelbo works well for people who need protection during the day, while they are working, since it is less bulky, fits under clothing, and has a less obtrusive appearance. Another brand, Diamond, is less expensive and has more padding and greater bulk; however, its loose knit sleeve allows independent donning by most people with arthritis. It is helpful to have both brands available to meet the needs of all patients.

There are also fiber-fill sleeves now on the market. These may work for people *not* at risk for losing elbow extension. But these sleeves or any (such as lamb's wool elbow protectors) that have a contour design that encourages flexion or are made of material that restricts extension are not recommended because they can produce elbow flexion contractures. The inexpensive thin foam protectors, available in bulk, are simply ineffective.

A volar positioning orthosis or bivalved cast may be the only solution for progressing elbow contractures or isolated elbow involvement. Care must be taken to maintain both flexion and extension ROM. Orthotic straps over the olecranon should be padded with fleece to avoid pressure over the ulnar nerve, which is more vulnerable when the elbow is flexed. The fleece padding also helps to keep the strap in place.

Hands and Wrists

In the hand, the only adequate means of positioning joints with acute synovitis is with a hand orthosis. The orthotic design may support the entire hand and forearm (wrist–hand orthosis), only the wrist, or only the MCP joints.

Positioning the Wrist

All wrists should be positioned in 10 degrees of ulnar deviation if possible, because this is the center of functional deviation. Positioning for extension depends on the nature of involvement.

1. *Active wrist synovitis or tenosynovitis.* Splint in 10 degrees of extension to maximize the carpal tunnel and reduce the risk of carpal tunnel syndrome.
2. *Muscle weakness, not joint involvement, limits extension.* Splint in 30 degrees of extension, the standard functional position.
3. *Severe involvement with high risk of* *ankylosis* (there has been rapid loss of ROM):
    a. *Unilateral.* I splint in 10 degrees of extension because after discontinuing the orthosis, flexor forces tend to pull the wrist down to neutral (now considered the best position for function).[2]
    b. *Bilateral.* Many surgeons advocate the ideal positions for bilateral ankylosis to be dominant or preferred hand in neutral to 10 degrees of extension and the nondominant hand in 10 degrees of flexion. Some advocate bilateral neutral position. Slight flexion in the nondominant hand facilitates self-care, toileting, touching the body, and activities such as buttoning. Slight extension of the dominant hand can facilitate writing or desk activities. One study found neutral to be the single most functional position in normal hands.[2] Hand deformities must be taken into account when deciding the ideal position for ankylosis for a patient. Swan-neck deformities and an intrinsic plus posture may require 10 to 20 degrees of wrist extension for optimal function. Mutilans deformity may require more flexion. A patient at risk for bilateral ankylosis needs careful assessment, custom orthoses, and frequent monitoring to ensure optimal functional outcome. (See instructions for use of specific hand splints in Chapter 23, Orthotic Treatment for Arthritis of the Hand.)

Hips

The ideal position for prolonged positioning is in neutral, full extension, zero rotation. Hip rotation can be controlled either by towel or blanket rolls placed on the lateral side of the hip, knees, and ankles, or by an orthosis with a **rotation stop bar** attached to the heel. People with active hip arthritis or tight hip flexors from prolonged sitting should have prone lying as a part of their daily program. (See section on prone positioning later in this chapter.)

Knees

The ideal position for prolonged positioning is full extension, because even minor knee flexion contractures of 10 to 30 degrees are an impediment to ambulation. In addition, they can encourage hip flexion and ankle plantar flexion deformity. Thermoplastic, plaster, or aluminum full-length leg-resting orthoses should be considered for beginning or progressing contractures.

It is highly recommended that children with chronic knee inflammation wear thermoplastic full leg–foot orthoses at night. Incorporating the foot in the splint usually increases wearing comfort and avoids pressure areas around the ankle. If the patient complains of pressure from the top (proximal) edge of the orthosis, it usually means the orthosis is too short and needs a longer thigh length.

Ankles

The ankles should be kept in 90 degrees of dorsiflexion. There are several methods for maintaining this position. The most effective is a posterior, ankle–foot orthosis or bivalved cast (with or without a rotation stop bar). These orthoses allow the patient the most freedom to move in bed.

A footboard is essential for holding up the bedcovers so they do not rest on the feet, thus pulling them down into plantar flexion. The footboard is also helpful in teaching the patient daily ankle ROM, because the patient can press against the board until both the heel and ball of the foot touch the board. However, a footboard is not recommended as the only means of preventing footdrop because a footboard becomes ineffective if the patient moves at all.

Whenever an occupational therapist fits a patient with an ankle orthosis, it is recommended that skin status and ankle ROM be carefully documented in the medical chart at the time of application. Frequently, patients develop pressure sores or flexion contractures that have gone unnoticed or undocumented prior to the application of the orthosis. These conditions may later be unjustly blamed on the orthosis and the occupational therapist who applied it.

Lamb's wool or knit sleeve protector pads (described earlier for the elbows) can help reduce the risk of pressure sores on the base of the heel. In this instance the contour of the lamb's wool pad is not a limitation since ankle dorsiflexion is encouraged.

Another method of positioning that can be used with patients who do not have active ankle synovitis is to position a pillow under the entire lower leg (but not under the knee or heel). This method, commonly used following knee surgery, allows gravity to assist knee extension, and it elevates the foot to reduce edema and eliminates pressure on the heel. Care must be taken that this position does not encourage a plantar flexion contracture when an orthosis is not being used.

PRONE POSITIONING

Prone positioning is a specific therapeutic procedure for stretching the hip into full extension. The hip is a large joint with a strong capsular structure. Hip flexion contractures are the most common sequela to arthritis of the hip. Several factors contribute to hip flexion contractures. Hip flexion and external rotation is the position that relaxes the joint and reduces intra-articular pressure, so it is the position the patient assumes when there is hip pain. Most patients with hip pain sit as much as possible. All sitting and most sleeping postures maintain the hip in flexion. For many patients their hips are maintained in a flexed position 24 hours a day. For some patients hip pain causes spasm of the associated hip flexors and adductors, further reducing active motion. There is a strong Y-shaped ligament along the anterior capsule that can become contracted in the presence of chronic flexion positioning.

Patients with hip involvement should be encouraged to develop a routine for lying prone every day. There is no hard and fast rule to the length of time spent lying prone. Some major rehabilitation centers advocate a goal of 90 minutes per day. Some patients can start right off with 3 sessions of half an hour each, while others can start with only 10 minutes per day and then build up tolerance. Prone lying is a critical treatment for children with hip arthritis (see Chapter 14).

Procedures

Have the patient lie prone on a firm bed *with feet hanging over the edge* (to prevent pressure into plantar flexion and to encourage knee extension). Small children can be strapped to a padded rectangular coffee-table in a manner that allows them to play games or watch television. Small pillows should be used under the shoulders to increase comfort, straighten shoulders, and make breathing easier. Any amount of pillows can be used to improve comfort as long as they do not interfere with hip extension.

Caution: Regarding Patients with Low Back Pain

Lying prone and lying supine with knees straight frequently aggravates low back pain by increasing the lordotic spinal curve. These positions are usually contraindicated or impossible for the patient with low back pain.

In fact, a patient with low back pain is advised to sleep with pillows under his or her knees or to sleep side-lying with knees bent. Obviously, this is a problem for the patient with concomitant knee or hip arthritis. This particular patient needs to be diligent in ROM exercise programs to prevent hip and knee contractures. The preferred hip ROM method for these patients is by stretching one hip at a time with the ipsilateral knee bent and the contralateral hip slightly flexed. ROM and positioning programs need to be individually tailored for these patients.

REFERENCES

1. Jackson, R: The Cervical Syndrome, 4th ed. Charles C Thomas, Springfield, IL, 1978.
2. Speltz, S, Schutt, A, and Beckenbaugh, RD: Functional wrist position for wrist arthrodesis. J Hand Surg 8:627, 1983 (abstr).

ADDITIONAL SOURCES

Bergstrom, D, and Coles, CH: Basic Positioning Procedures. Rehab Publ No. 701. Sister Kenny Institute, 1800 Chicago Ave, Minneapolis, MN 55404, 1971.
Nursing Care of the Skin, revised ed. Rehab Publ No. 711. Sister Kenny Institute, 1800 Chicago Ave, Minneapolis, MN 55404, 1975.
Welles, C: Body mechanics of the bed patient as related to occupational therapy. Am J Occup Ther 1952. (Excellent resource.)

PART VI

SURGICAL REHABILITATION

The late 1960s ushered in the era of total joint replacements, and successful versions of all the joint replacement prostheses were introduced between 1965 and 1978. The 1970s were the decade of prosthetic design development. The 1980s are providing the first opportunity to assess short-term and moderate-term results of these surgeries on a large scale. The longest follow-up period is 20 years—total hip replacement was introduced in England in 1965 and in the United States in 1968. Otherwise, only short-term and moderate-term follow-up results exist.

Overall, the reports that have come in, mostly during the past 5 years, have shown excellent short-term results and good moderate-term results in terms of pain relief and improved function. Loosening of the cement–bone interface remains the main complication of cement-fixated lower extremity prostheses. These findings have spurred the development of cementless and press-fit prostheses, which encourage biological fixation through a porous-coated surface. So far, this type of prosthesis has been created for the hip, knee, and wrist.

For the wrist and metacarpophalangeal silastic arthroplasty, the development of metal intermedullary canal grommets (sleeves) is a major advance. The grommets protect the stems from rough bone ends, which often fracture and cause these implants to fail.

Historically, orthopedic surgery has been considered a last resort, to be tried after all else has failed, or reserved for joints that are nonfunctional. This is no longer true. Reconstructive surgery is now considered a part of total care for the person with chronic destructive joint disease. Consultation with an orthopedic surgeon early, before severe joint destruction occurs, allows the patient more surgical options and optimal timing of both preventive and corrective surgery.

The decision to perform surgery for arthritis must take into account a series of factors. The criteria common to all major surgery must be considered, including the patient's age, the diagnosis, secondary diagnoses, pain tolerance, postoperative complications, medications, family support, life-style, and psychological response to surgery. Ideally, all of these conditions should be favorable to the surgery being considered. In addition to these factors the decision to operate is based on several factors specific to the nature of chronic rheumatic disease.

The number of joints involved, the severity of the joint disease, and how the surgery will affect adjacent or contralateral joints all have critical implications for the decision regarding surgery for arthritis. For patients with polyarticular joint involvement, staging of multiple surgeries is a critical consideration for successful results. For example, the ability to ambulate and perform knee-strengthening exercises is critical to the success of total knee replacement surgery. If the patient also has painful hip disease that prevents ambulation or participation in therapy, he or she may not achieve satisfactory results from the knee surgery, resulting in extensor lag, instability, or a flexion contracture. To encourage optimal rehabilitation it would be preferable to operate on the hip first and the knee second. This can be done during either one or two hospitalizations.

The extent of associated systemic involvement (particularly cardiac, pulmonary, and peripheral vascular systems) may preclude major surgery or the use of general anesthesia. In many facilities upper extremity surgery is performed under a regional block, and lower extremity surgery, including total hip and knee replacement surgery, can be carried out under a spinal anesthesia, without the risks of a general anesthesia. Anesthesia provided in this manner makes surgery possible for adults and children who have severe cervical spine or TMS disease and cannot be safely intubated for general anesthesia. It reduces the surgical risk for patients having multiple surgeries; it eliminates the unpleasantness of recovering from general anesthesia; and it is attractive to many patients who are fearful of being made unconscious.

Most surgeries require the active participation of the patient in postoperative therapy to achieve the desired results. There has been little research evaluating psychological factors in relation to the outcome of orthopedic surgery. Several years ago, a study of patients receiving total knee surgery at Rancho Los Amigos Hospital demonstrated that patients with significant depression attained poorer results than patients without depression.

To encourage or ensure appropriate patient motivation for surgery, orthopedic surgeons generally do not try to convince patients to have surgery. They explain the options—risks and gains—*and require the patient to make the decision.* If a patient waits until the joint is so painful that he or she "can no longer stand it," surgery is often viewed as a positive experience; the patients looks forward to life without debilitating pain. A patient *talked* into surgery when he or she has only moderate pain may view the pain and stress of surgery with less enthusiasm. Sometimes this process encourages patients to wait too long for surgery and the destruction from the disease becomes so severe it makes rehabilitation more difficult.

A question that often arises is "How early should surgery be performed?" Although the specific timing is different for each surgery, most surgeons are in agreement that surgery should be performed only after all conservative measures have been given a fair trial and the patient is stabilized on a medication regimen. In a traditional sense, appropriate conservative treatment for rheumatoid arthritis would include adequate trials of both nonsteroidal anti-inflammatory drugs and disease-modifying drugs, intra-articular corticosteroid injections, orthoses, thermal modalities, exercise, and joint-protection training. From a holistic perspective, conservative management would include developing a positive psychological/emotional approach for working with the illness, nutrition for optimal health, physical fitness training, and a relaxation or stress management process for improving the immune system and overall health. Patients who have persistent synovitis and pain for 3 to 6 months, despite conservative measures, are considered possible candidates for joint surgery.

The role of the therapist in surgical treatment varies widely among medical facilities. Occupational therapists play a primary role in (1) *functional evaluation,* before and after surgery; (2) *rehabilitation,* before and after surgical procedures for the upper and lower extremities, through orthotic treatment, exercise, and selected functional activities; (3) *patient education,* regarding joint protection, the use of splints, edema reduction, safety measures, and assistive equipment; (4) *activities of daily living (ADL) training,* instruction and practice in methods for incorporating postoperative precautions, and restrictions in ADL.

The protocols for occupational therapy (OT) and physical therapy (PT) surgical assessment vary across the country. In some facilities, the referral to therapy occurs on the day intervention is required; in other facilities, the surgical protocol includes a preoperative OT and PT assessment with intervention scheduled as indicated. Having a routine preoperative assessment enables the therapist to evaluate the patient's preoperative functional ability and to appreciate the severity of the joint involvement and the impact that the surgery will have on the patient's functional ability. The preoperative assessment of range of motion (ROM) of the nonoperative joints provides a rational goal for postoperative ROM and edema reduction. More importantly, the preoperative assessment enables the therapist to develop a rapport with the patient and to orient the patient to postoperative exercises and protocols when the patient is not experiencing surgical pain. This greatly enhances the patient's ability to learn exercises following surgery.

The chapters in Part VI outline the timing for postoperative management. *These programs are designed to provide general guidelines and not to provide a ready-made treatment protocol. Each treatment program should be modified to answer the patient's individual needs or to suit the personal philosophy of the surgeon.* It is essential that the surgeon and therapist have direct communication and that together they establish the procedures, precautions, and specific timing for preoperative and postoperative therapy.

A treatment protocol written by both therapist and surgeon is one of the most effective tools for establishing communication and clarity regarding postoperative management. If your facility does not have written protocols, I encourage you to use the ones in this section as a starting point; feel free to photocopy them. The surgeon may modify these protocols according to his or her philosophy and techniques. Add your input and a final consensus approval, and you will have protocols tailored to your specific approach, philosophy, and patient population.

RECOMMENDED RESOURCES ON REHABILITATION MANAGEMENT OF THE SURGICAL PATIENT

Avioli, LV (ed): The Osteoporotic Syndrome: Detection, Prevention, and Treatment. Grune & Stratton, New York, 1985.

Boswick, JA (ed): Advances in Upper Extremity Surgery and Rehabilitation. Aspen, Rockville, MD, 1986.

Clum, GA, Scott, L, and Burnside, J: Information and locus of control as factors in the outcome of surgery. Psych Rep 45:867–873, 1979.

Farrell, J: Illustrated Guide to Orthopedic Nursing, 2nd ed. JB Lippincott, Philadelphia, 1982.

Garner, RW, Mowat, AG, and Hazleman, BL: Wound healing after operations on patients with rheumatoid arthritis. J Bone Joint Surg 55B:134–144, 1973.

Inglis, AE (ed): Symposium on Total Joint Replacement of the Upper Extremity. CV Mosby, St Louis, 1982.

Jackson, O (ed): Physical Therapy of the Geriatric Patient. Churchill-Livingston, New York, 1983.

Kay, NRM, and Noble, J: Complications of Total Joint Replacement. WB Saunders, Philadelphia, 1986.

Kelley, WM, Harris, E, Ruddy, S, and Sledge, CB (eds): Textbook of Rheumatology. WB Saunders, Philadelphia, 1985.

Moskowitz, RW, Howell, D Goldberg, VM, and Mankin, AJ: Osteoarthritis: Diagnosis and Management. WB Saunders, Philadelphia, 1984.

Nickel, VL (ed): Orthopedic Rehabilitation. Churchill-Livingston, New York, 1982.

Chapter 29

Hand, Wrist, and Forearm Surgery

Since most of the muscles in the upper extremity cross more than one joint, there is considerable synchronization of function throughout the upper extremity. Arthritis in a single joint affects all other joints to a greater or lesser degree. For example, decreased mobility in wrist flexion/extension or forearm supination/pronation alters the biomechanics imposed on the elbow and shoulder during functional activities. Thus, if a patient cannot supinate his or her wrist, he or she can only position the palm by abducting and externally rotating the shoulder. All surgical and orthotic procedures must take into account the effect the process will have on adjacent joints. The wrist is often the most frequent site of involvement in rheumatoid arthritis (RA) and juvenile rheumatoid arthritis (JRA) and a common site in psoriatic arthritis (PA), systemic lupus erythematosus (SLE), and systemic sclerosis (SS). The wrist provides the foundation for hand function. Pain solely in the wrist can severely limit grip, pinch, dexterity, and functional use of the fingers. Often one of the goals of wrist surgery is to improve function of the fingers.

Hand and wrist surgery for RA can be divided into five groups: (1) synovectomy, (2) tenosynovectomy, (3) tendon surgery, (4) arthroplasty, and (5) arthrodesis.[1] Forearm surgery is limited to resection and replacement of the distal end of the ulna and the proximal end of the radius. Resection of the distal ulna is usually done in conjunction with wrist surgery and is discussed in this section, whereas radial head resection is frequently combined with elbow synovectomy and is reviewed in Chapter 30, Elbow Surgery.

The most extensive surgery is often performed on patients with RA; therefore, RA is used as a prototype for discussing hand surgery in this chapter. Patients with other diagnoses may require only one or a few of the surgeries used for RA. The surgeries in this chapter are listed according to the type of procedure and the level of the lesion, distal to proximal (i.e., hand, wrist, forearm). This is done only to impart some sense of order and not to imply that surgery is necessarily performed in this sequence.

PSYCHOLOGICAL CONSIDERATIONS

All patients facing surgery have apprehension and fear about the procedure, anesthesia, the risks, and achieving desired results. The fear of surgery is mediated considerably if the procedure has predictable results and is clearly going to improve function (e.g., repair a ruptured tendon, realign a dislocated wrist). In these cases the patient often looks foreward to the surgery as a positive solution. When the surgical outcome is not so predictable (e.g., metacarpophalangeal [MCP] or proximal interphalangeal [PIP] arthroplasty, flexor tenosynovectomy), the patient is less optimistic and the risks are often in clearer focus than the gains. For women, who comprise the majority of arthritis hand surgery patients, a special concern is the aesthetic appearance of the hand, as well as function. The more disabled a person is the more function takes precedence over cosmesis. But one cannot overlook the impact the appearance of the hand has on a person's self-esteem. The hospital experience, the immediate recovery period, and the rehabilitation/immobilization period all elicit unresolved issues around being dependent and crippled. For people with polyarthritis, postoperative immobilization brings to reality the fear of being more disabled, having to depend on others, and often not being able to carry their share of work fully—not being a contributing, productive person. Yes, it may only be for 6 weeks, and intellectually patients understand it is temporary, but the fear and anxiety around dependency and disability run deep and their presence postoperatively can influence the patient's systemic health as well as the patient's participation and follow-through with therapy. The various emotional contingencies around surgery especially in the immediate postoperative days can cause patients to misinterpret instructions, especially those involving exercise or procedures that may cause pain. Anxiety can often amplify the perceived postoperative disability.

The most effective way a therapist can help reduce the emotional stress of surgery and prevent problems resulting from misinterpreted instructions is to see the patient preoperatively as an outpatient for a hand assessment and postoperative planning. For many hand surgeries, knowing the preoperative range of motion (ROM), strength, sensation, and function is invaluable for determining postoperative treatment goals.

The **preoperative assessment** allows the therapist an opportunity to

1. Review the goals of surgery with an emphasis on how it will improve function.
2. Review the postoperative rehabilitation program and scheduling of therapy.
3. Help the patient plan realistically for assistance with transportation, housework, and adaptive methods for accomplishing activities of daily living (ADL) during immobilization.
4. Instruct the patient in joint-protection methods for arthritis of the nonsurgical hand. (Increased use of this hand during the postoperative period frequently exacerbates inflammation in the hand.)
5. Give the patient a chance to talk about his or her fears and concerns related to surgery. I often ask my patients "What is your greatest fear about the surgery?" This gives me an opportunity to provide reassurance, make recommendations, or direct the patient to appropriate sources that address the major concern(s).

A clear understanding of the upcoming procedures and realistic planning help make the patient a part of the team. It gives the patient a greater sense of control, reduces anxiety and stress, and makes the entire postoperative phase calmer and more organized.

Patients have so much on their minds when preparing for surgery, and there is so much planning and reorganizing that needs to be done that it is very difficult for them (or anyone) to keep all the instructions straight, *so provide as many instructions, schedules, and educational material in writing as possible.*

SYNOVECTOMY

Pannus or hypertrophic synovial tissue has both a mechanical and biomechanical impact on the surrounding structures. The tissue mass itself distends the capsule and ligaments mechanically, contributing to their elongation. In addition, it may become trapped between the bones, blocking motion; or in the case of the flexor sheaths, it may restrict tendon gliding or adhere the sublimis to the profundus, preventing independent gliding of these tendons. Each synovial cell contributes to the inflammatory process and enzymatic destruction of the cartilage and capsule. So the more tissue present, the more biochemical damage possible. Removal of the synovium eliminates (at least temporarily) the inflammation, reduces intra-articular pressure, and eliminates tension placed on surrounding structures.[2]

Clearly, the most rampant inflammation is associated with synovitis. But it is important to keep in mind that RA and all chronic, inflammatory arthritides are systemic diseases, and, therefore, that every cell in the body is affected to some degree. In the hand, all of the structures outside of the joint or tendon sheath (e.g., tendons, muscles, and skin) reflect degenerative changes. These changes are visible when one observes tissue directly in surgery.

Synovectomy cannot prevent progression of disease, but it can play an important role in relieving symptoms and forestalling joint destruction in selected patients. This operation appears to be the most valuable to patients with low-grade, uncontrolled inflammation and minimal or no destruction of cartilage and bone.[2]

Indications
1. Pain and decreased function secondary to persistent, uncontrolled boggy synovitis of at least 3 months' duration that is nonresponsive to corticosteroid injection and shows *no* evidence of cartilage destruction.
2. To protect joint structures.

Occurrence
All inflammatory arthritides.

Surgical and Functional Goals
Postsurgical expectations are relief of pain, decreased inflammation and swelling, return of ROM loss due to the swelling, and improved function due to the elimination of pain.

Surgical Prerequisites
1. Smooth joint motion, absence of crepitus, or x-ray changes of cartilage destruction.
2. Absence of infection.

Wrist Synovectomy

Surgical Procedure
1. Approach: Dorsal, slightly curved, or longitudinal incision.
2. Dorsal retinaculum is reflected.
3. Dorsal tenosynovectomy is performed as necessary.
4. Transverse capsular incision is made.
5. Synovium is removed from the radiocarpal and involved intercarpal joints. (Total or complete synovectomy is not possible due to anatomical restraints.)
6. A portion of the retinaculum is relocated deep to the extensor tendons.
7. A drain is used for 24 hours to prevent hematoma.

Postoperative Management
Average hospitalization: 2 to 3 days.

1. Initially, the hand is in a voluminous compression bandage and elevated to reduce edema. A plaster splint is used to immobilize the wrist in neutral to allow capsular healing; it should not interfere with MCP joint or thumb motion.
2. Second or third day: Bandage is reduced. Active and passive finger ROM is started. Patient may have difficulty with active finger extension due to swelling around the tendons.
3. After discharge: Patients with bilateral arthritis will need instruction in joint-protection techniques and assistive devices for the nonsurgical hand. Patients may be afraid to move the fingers and need encouragement to do active ROM to avoid stiffness and tendon adherence.
4. Approximately seventh to tenth day: Dressing and sutures are removed. Gentle active and passive wrist ROM is started. (ROM is done to tolerance; it is not as critical to push for full ROM in the wrist as it is in the digits.) Warm water soaks facilitate motion. Lotion massage reduces swelling and induration, improves skin tone, and helps decrease skin sensitivity. Patient may use a thermoplastic or commercial wrist orthosis as needed for comfort.

Metacarpophalangeal Joint Synovectomy

Surgical Procedure
1. Approach: Transverse incision is used for multiple joints and a longitudinal incision is used for single joint.
2. Extensor mechanisms are incised along the ulnar border.
3. The ulnar intrinsic muscles are released if they are tight.
4. Extensor tendons are retracted radialward.
5. Joint capsules are incised longitudinally.
6. Synovium is removed; attention is given to the areas deep to the collateral ligaments.
7. Capsules are closed. This may be combined with a radial collateral ligament repair or shortening.
8. Extensor tendons may be centralized if necessary.
9. A drain is used for 24 hours to prevent a hematoma.

Postoperative Management
Average hospitalization: 2 to 3 days (depends on number of joints operated on).

1. Initially, the hand is in a voluminous compression dressing with a volar plaster orthosis. The orthosis should maintain the wrist in approximately 20 to 30 degrees of

extension and the MCP joints in approximately 30 degrees of flexion; it should not block PIP joint or thumb motion.

2. Second day:

(a) Gentle active and passive ROM is started for the MCP, PIP, and distal interphalangeal (DIP) joints. During hospitalization, the patient should have exercises supervised by a therapist 2 or 3 times a day. The orthosis can be removed during the exercises. When the orthosis is on, the patient is encouraged to actively move the PIP joints as much as possible to help reduce edema.

(b) A dynamic MCP extension orthosis may be used to support the digits in extension and radial deviation if necessary. Care should be taken not to position the fourth and fifth MCP joints in full extension, since maintaining full flexion is critical in these joints for tight grasp. The dynamic orthosis is used during the day, and the plaster splint is used at night. A dynamic orthosis is the most effective way to maintain alignment and encourage motion. (See Chapter 25 for information on postsurgical orthotic treatment.)

4. After dischage: Patients with bilateral arthritis will need instruction in joint-protection techniques and assistive devices for the nonsurgical hand.

5. Seventh to tenth days: Dressing and sutures are removed. Warm water soaks and massage can be added to the program to increase mobility. ROM and strengthening exercises should progress as tolerated. The goal of therapy is full active and passive ROM.

Proximal Interphalangeal Joint Synovectomy

Surgical Procedure

1. Approach: Exposure of the PIP joint is more difficult than exposure of the MCP joint due to the extensor mechanism and snug collateral ligaments. The extensor mechanism can be divided longitudinally or reflected along one margin. Some surgeons routinely divide a collateral ligament and spread the joint laterally to facilitate exposure.[3] (This method would necessitate a delay in beginning active postoperative motion.)

2. Synovectomy is performed.

3. Divided and incised structures are repaired, and the wound is closed.

Postoperative Management

Average hospitalization: outpatient surgery (single digit) or 2 to 3 days (multiple digits).

1. Initially, the hand is in a voluminous compression dressing with the joint held in slight flexion (approximately 10 to 15 degrees).

2. Second day: Dressing is reduced.

a. Active motion is encouraged but is usually limited by pain and swelling. Active and passive exercises are delayed until pain and swelling decrease and the exercises can be tolerated.

b. The main risks of this surgery are stiffness (i.e., loss of active motion because of immobilization and swelling) and lack of full extension because of damage to or stretching of the extensor mechanism. Flexion is usually regained more easily than extension, so the goal of early therapy is to regain extension and then focus on gaining flexion.

c. For patients with an extensor lag, a dynamic PIP joint extension orthosis (such as an LMB Spring Extension Splint[4]) is used during the day, and an aluminum and foam static splint or custom thermoplastic extension orthosis is used at night.

d. Gentle ROM and strengthening exercises are progressed to tolerance. Strengthening of both the extensor communis muscle and the interosseous muscles should be done.

3. After discharge: Patients with bilateral arthritis will need instruction in joint-protection techniques and assistive devices for the nonsurgical hand. Twelfth to fourteenth day: Stitches are removed. Finger orthoses are used until extensor lag is resolved.

References (Synovectomy)

1. Nalebuff, EA: Present status of rheumatoid hand surgery. Am J Surg 122:304, 1971.
2. Geschwend, N: Synovectomy. In Kelley, WM et al (eds): Textbook of Rheumatology, 2nd ed. WB Saunders, Philadelphia, 1985.
3. Lipscomb, PR: Synovectomy of the distal two joints of the thumb and fingers in rheumatoid arthritis. J Bone Joint Surg 49A:1135, 1967.
4. LMB Hand Rehab Products, Inc., PO Box 1181, San Luis Obispo, CA 93406.

TENOSYNOVECTOMY

Tenosynovectomy is considered preventive as well as corrective surgery. Several large series have supported the use of tenosynovectomies to prevent tendon rupture and other complications of chronic tenosynovitis.

There are four locations in the hand where the tendons pass through synovial-lined sheaths. The purpose of the sheath is to facilitate gliding, particularly where the tendon must slide over several joints. The four locations are the dorsum of the wrist, the volar aspect of the wrist, flexor surface of the fingers, and the volar aspect of the thumb, which contains the sheath for the flexor pollicis longus. The clinical symptoms vary at each site due to the anatomical differences at each level.[5]

The synovium lining the tendon sheaths is similar to the synovium in the joints and subject to the same changes. When synovitis occurs, excess fluid builds up in the sheath. The sheath has a closed double wall construction, and the fluid becomes trapped between the inner and outer walls. If the synovitis becomes chronic, the synovium will become thickened and hypertrophied. The inflammatory process through an enzymatic process weakens the integrity of the tendons, making them more susceptible to rupture. In confined areas, the excess tissue may cause sufficient pressure to compromise the vascular supply to the tendon, resulting in ischemic areas. Additionally, chronic synovitis can result in granulomatous plaques (tendon nodules) forming on the surface of the tendons. These plaques can invade the inner substance of the tendons, causing tendon disruption and increasing the risk of rupture.[5-7]

Dorsal Wrist Tenosynovectomy

At the dorsum of the wrist, the finger and wrist extensor tendons pass through six separate compartments. The tendons in each compartment are surrounded by a synovial sheath, which extends approximately one-half inch proximal and distal to the retinaculum. The dorsal retinaculum ligament forms the dorsal surface of the tendon compartments. Vertical septa extend from the retinaculum to the radius and ulna, forming the walls of the tendon compartments.[6] Tenosynovitis can occur in a single compartment or in all six. In the early stages, the swelling usually conforms to the boundaries of each sheath. Tenosynovitis of compartments two through five is generally *not painful.*[7] (If a person has wrist pain, it is usually due to concomitant radiocarpal or radioulnar joint pain.) However, tenosynovitis of the first compartment (de Quervain's syndrome) or the sixth compartment *can* be very painful. It is believed that these two compartments are painful because they are adjacent to the dorsal branches of the radial and ulnar nerves. Dorsal tenosynovitis is readily apparent because the skin is looser directly over the tendon sheaths so it conforms to the swelling. (See Fig. 19–41.)

The main consequence of chronic dorsal tenosynovitis is rupture of the finger and thumb extensors. The tendons most frequently ruptured are the extensor digiti quinti, extensor communis (four and five), and extensor pollicis longus. Rupture results from infiltration of the disease into the tendons and attrition or wearing away of the tendon over bony spurs or rough edges of subluxed joints. Most extensor tendon ruptures occur at the wrist level.[8]

Chronic tenosynovitis of the compartment threatens the integrity of the extensor carpi ulnaris tendon, considered a key tendon for maintaining the stability of the wrist.[9] If the ligaments that maintain the alignment of the tendon become stretched, the tendon can migrate volar to become a strong flexor force contributing to volar subluxation of the carpus.[9]

Dorsal tenosynovectomy with retinacular relocation is considered the treatment of choice for persistent dorsal tenosynovitis. Ideally, it should be performed before tendon rupture occurs.[7]

A recent study of 38 wrist surgeries combining dorsal tenosynovectomy with dorsal wrist synovectomy validated the effectiveness of this surgery for people with RA. The results showed 95 percent had pain relief with no recurrence of synovitis and minimal subsequent tendon rupture. On the negative side there was a significant loss of wrist ROM although range was in a functional arc. Carpal translocation occurred in 44 percent of the patients. Only 5 wrists required on arthroplasty and 3 wrists an arthrodesis. Overall these are considered excellent results.[10]

Indications

1. Persistent dorsal tenosynovitis despite 3 to 6 months of adequate medical management.

2. Extensor tendon rupture.

3. Rapid proliferation of the tenosynovitis.

Occurrence

RA and JRA.

Surgical and Functional Goals

Prevention of further destruction by removing the inflamed tenosynovium and protection of the tendons by relocating the synovial-lined retinacular ligament beneath the tendons.[8]

Postsurgical expectations are: decrease in swelling, improved comfort (particularly if combined with a wrist synovectomy), improved appearance, and possibly an increase in wrist ROM.

Surgical Prerequisites

No specific prerequisites.

Surgical Procedure

This procedure may be combined with a wrist synovectomy, wrist fusion, extensor tendon repair, or excision of the distal ulna.

1. Approach: Slightly curved longitudinal incision over the dorsum of the wrist.

2. Dorsal retinacular ligament is reflected.

3. Diseased tenosynovium is removed from around the extensor tendons and from beneath the retinacular ligament.

4. Synovium is removed from the wrist joint.

5. Dorsal retinacular ligament is placed beneath the extensor tendons to protect them from further damage.

6. Distal ulna may be resected at the same time (Darrach procedure). Silastic ulnar head prosthesis may or may not be implanted.

Postoperative Management

Average hospitalization: 3 to 5 days.

1. Initially, the hand is immobilized in a compression dressing with a volar plaster orthosis to hold the wrist in extension and the MCP joints in 40 degrees of flexion.

2. Second day: Dressing is reduced. Active and passive MCP extension, PIP, DIP, and thumb ROM is started.

3. After discharge: Patients with bilateral arthritis will need instruction in joint-protection techniques and assistive devices for the nonsurgical hand. Tenth to fourteenth day: Sutures and dressing are removed. Active wrist flexion, extension, pronation, and supination exercises are started. Exercise is modified if additional surgical procedures are carried out simultaneously. If a patient has an MCP extension lag, consider using a dynamic MCP extension orthosis. (See Chapter 23.) Care should be taken not to position the ring and little fingers in full extension.

4. Third to fourth week: If a wrist synovectomy was also done, a volar wrist orthosis should be used between exercise periods.

Wrist Volar Tenosynovectomy

At the wrist level, the nine long flexor tendons of the fingers and thumb are enclosed in tendon sheaths as they pass through the narrow carpal tunnel. The tunnel is formed by a concave formation of the carpal bones on three sides and the transverse carpal ligament on the fourth or volar surface.[7] The tunnel is very narrow and affords a passageway for the four flexor digitorum profundus tendons and four tendons of the flexor digitorum superficialis enclosed in one sheath as well as the flexor pollicis longus and the median nerve. The position of the median nerve between the flexor tendons and the unyielding volar carpal ligament makes it very susceptible to compression or entrapment (carpal tunnel syndrome), if there is any swelling in the carpal tunnel.[11] Hypertrophy of the tenosynovium can cause sufficient pressure to compromise the blood supply to the nerve, resulting in ischemia and loss of nerve function.[11] Distal to the transverse carpal ligament, the recurrent motor branch on the median nerve supplies the abductor pollicis brevis and the opponens pollicis, the flexor pollicis brevis (superficial head). The sensory branch supplies the volar aspect of the thumb, index, and middle fingers and the radial half of the ring finger. Damage to this nerve can severely reduce hand dexterity and function. The ulnar nerve is superficial to the transverse carpal ligament and, therefore, is not vulnerable to compression from flexor tenosynovitis.

The transverse carpal ligament is covered by the volar carpal ligament and thick palmar fascia at the distal edge. Therefore, tenosynovitis in the palmar sheaths or deep in the tunnel can be extensive without the obvious swelling. Tenosynovitis generally occurs without pain. If there is wrist pain, it is usually due to concomitant radiocarpal synovitis or compression of the median nerve.[7] In addition to nerve entrapment, chronic tenosynovitis can invade the tendons and result in tendon rupture. The flexor pollicis longus and profundus tendons are the most likely to rupture. This is often due to attrition from bony spurs that form on the scaphoid.[12] However, rupture of the flexor tendons is less common than rupture of the extensor tendons.[7]

A common and often overlooked complication of flexor tenosynovitis is limited tendon excursion or "bound down" tendons. If this occurs, it can limit *active flexion* or *passive extension.* If excursion in a proximal direction is limited, the person will have incomplete active flexion but greater or possibly full passive flexion. Whenever a person has a ROM lag in all four digits, binding of the finger flexors at the wrist level should be evaluated. If excursion of the tendons is limited in a distal direction, the patient will not be able to achieve full active or passive extension of all digit and wrist joints. The patient will have a tenodesis action in the hand (e.g., the digits will be able to extend fully only when the wrist is flexed). If this problem is not treated promptly, first by conservative measures (i.e., steroid injection and ice compresses) or by surgery, the muscle can become fibrosed in a shortened position and the digits can develop fixed contractures due to the lack of active motion.

Flexor tendon excursion can become limited at the wrist level or at the digit level. When all four digits are limited, the problem can usually be traced to the wrist. If only one or two fingers are limited, the problem is most likely in the digital sheath.

The most frequent problem that necessitates flexor tenosynovectomy is median nerve entrapment (carpal tunnel syndrome).[13] Initially, patients complain of tingling and numbness at night. They should be treated by conservative measures in the early phase[11] (i.e., orthoses with or without corticosteroid injections). A patient is a candidate for surgery if a 3-month trial of conservative measures has not alleviated the symptoms of tenosynovitis; if the symptoms are constant day and night; if there is diminished 2-point discrimination; and if there is weakness of the abductor pollicis brevis muscle (this muscle will show motor impairment first) or a tendon rupture occurs. Once the impingement is severe enough to cause motor or significant sensory loss, conservative measures will not help. Prompt surgery improves the possibility of full return of nerve function.

Indications
1. Carpal tunnel syndrome, secondary to flexor tenosynovitis, that is nonresponsive to conservative treatment or presents with thenar atrophy.
2. Rupture of a long flexor tendon at the wrist level.
3. Decreased excursion of the flexor tendons.
4. Decreased excursion of the flexor pollicis longus tendon secondary to wrist flexor tenosynovitis.

Occurrence
RA and JRA.

Surgical and Functional Goals
To relieve pressure on the median nerve. When nerve impairment has not been of long duration, full sensory and motor recovery is expected. The surgery can prevent further destruction or rupture of the tendons by removing the diseased synovium.[7]

Surgical Prerequisites
Carpal tunnel syndrome needs to be clearly established. Nerve impingement at the cervical spine level needs to be ruled out as a possible cause of sensory and motor loss in the hand.

Surgical Procedure (for Rheumatoid Arthritis)
1. Approach: Curved incision along the thenar crease with a zigzag incision proximal to the wrist (to minimize scarring across transverse wrist crease).
2. Palmar fascia divided longitudinally. (Terminal branches of the palmar cutaneous nerve should not be cut; damage may result in persistent local tenderness.)[14]

3. Median nerve identified proximal to wrist.

4. Transverse carpal ligament divided along the ulnar border, exposing contents of carpal canal.

5. Diseased synovium removed from the superficialis tendons. They are cleaned sufficiently to allow independent action. Adhesions between the profundus tendons may not be extensively removed, since independent action is less important in these tendons.

6. Internal neurolysis of the median nerve may be carried out for severe cases of compression.

7. Any bony spicules are removed from the floor of the canal.

8. Traction is applied to individual tendons to evaluate digital tendon motion. If the tendons are not pulling through, a digital flexor tenosynovectomy may be done.

9. The transverse carpal ligament is *not* repaired, so pressure cannot recur in the canal.

10. The wound is closed and a drain is used for 24 hours to prevent a hematoma.

Postoperative Management

Average hospitalization: 1 to 3 days. (Patients are usually kept in the hospital until swelling has decreased and the tendons are moving smoothly.)

1. Initially, the hand is in a voluminous compression bandage with a plaster orthosis. The orthosis should maintain the wrist in approximately 25 degrees of extension to keep the flexor tendons in the carpal tunnel and thus prevent bowstringing during the healing process.

2. Second postoperative day until discharge: Dressing is reduced. Active and passive finger motion is started three times a day to tolerance. Excessive bleeding occasionally occurs and can delay exercises, although some gentle motion should be done each day. The profundus and superficialis tendons for each finger should be exercised individually. (This is done by using the same positioning procedures as for individual muscle testing.)

3. After discharge: Patients with bilateral arthritis will need instruction in joint-protection techniques and assistive devices for the nonsurgical hand. Tenth to twelfth day: Dressing and sutures are removed. Warm water soaks and massage to increase mobility can be started. Light strengthening exercises can be started, using a soft sponge ball or soft Thermaplast. A Freedom Splint (prefabricated elastic gauntlet type) or thermoplastic wrist orthosis is recommended for a few weeks for support and comfort.

Digital Flexor Tenosynovectomy

The tendon sheaths for the long finger flexors start at the volar aspect of the MCP joints and extend the length of the finger. The sheath for the flexor pollicis longus extends the entire length of the tendon from the interphalangeal (IP) joint of the thumb to 1 inch proximal to the volar carpal ligament.[15]

The sheath and tendons are held in place by fibrous bands. At the point where the tendons cross the digit joints, the bands become thick and are referred to as **annular ligaments** or pulleys. Their primary function is to prevent bowstringing of the tendons during pinch and grip activities.[15,16]

Granulomatous masses (nodules) may form on the surface of the tendons with or without tenosynovitis. These nodules can be particularly troublesome, since they can catch on annular ligaments during tendon motion and prevent tendon excursion, a condition commonly referred to as **trigger finger.** Tendon nodules or excessive tenosynovium can get caught in the annular ligaments and cause the digit to painfully lock in flexion or extension. This occurs most frequently at the level of the MCP joint, but it can occur at the PIP level in the fingers and the IP level in the thumb.[16,17]

In the early stages of tenosynovitis, just the sheath effusion alone can limit full excursion of the profundus tendon. Patients may have swollen fingers, *without* pain or warmth, and may not be able to actively flex their DIP joints fully. If the condition becomes chronic, the tenosynovium hypertrophies and crepitus with motion is common. The excess diseased tissue may prevent the tendon from gliding or it can infiltrate the tendon and result in a rupture.[7]

It is not uncommon for people with normal PIP joints to develop PIP joint contractures secondary to the flexor tenosynovitis. These contractures remain after the tenosynovitis resolves.[18]

Conservative management should be tried before a tenosynovectomy is considered. The most common approach is simply a steroid injection. If swelling is present, ice compresses or contrast baths should be added (heat is contraindicated because it increases swelling).

The combination of injection and orthotic immobilization has shown about the same success rate (70 percent) as steroid injection alone (67 percent).[19,20] Patients with single-digit involvement and less than 4 months' duration have the highest response rate to conservative management (98 percent) compared to those with multiple digits or long duration (41 percent).[19]

Indications

1. Persistent, painful, or dysfunctional trigger finger that does not respond to conservative treatment.

2. Marked tenosynovial hypertrophy, resulting in limited tendon excursion. (This is demonstrated by a discrepancy in active and passive ROM.)

Occurrence

RA and JRA.

Surgical and Functional Goals

For trigger finger, the goal is to relieve pain and restore function. For chronic tenosynovitis, the goal is to improve ROM and function and to protect the tendons from further damage and prevent tendon rupture.[7]

Surgical Prerequisites

Intact tendons.

Surgical Procedure

1. Approach: For multiple digits, an incision is made along the distal palmar crease (see Fig. 23–1) to expose the tendons. It may be possible to remove sufficient synovium from this incision; if not, a zigzag incision is made along the volar aspect of the digit to expose the tendon distally.

2. The tendon sheath is opened, and diseased tenosynovium and adhesions between the tendons are removed. Any nodules (localized granulomas) are also removed.

3. If both flexor tendons are severely involved, it may be necessary to sacrifice (cut) one slip of the sublimis tendon to ensure smooth gliding of the profundus.[16]

Postoperative Management

Average hospitalization: 2 to 3 days.

1. Initially, the hand is in a voluminous compression dressing with a volar plaster orthosis. The orthosis should maintain the wrist in approximately 20 degrees of extension and the MCP joints in about 30 degrees of flexion. The MCP joints should be blocked to encourage tendon function at the PIP joints. If this is not done, patients tend to flex their MCP joints using their intrinsic muscles and then have difficulty using their long flexors in this position.

2. Second day to discharge: Dressing is reduced. Active and passive ROM exercises are started for the PIP and DIP joints. Slight resistance to flexion, applied at the finger pad, provides additional proprioceptive feedback and encourages active motion. The profundus and superficialis tendons should have active ROM exercise separately for each. This is performed in the same manner as individual muscle testing.

3. The orthosis should be removed at least three times a day for ROM of the wrist and MCP joints. Tendon ROM exercises are progressed to tolerance.

4. After discharge: Patients with bilateral arthritis will need instruction in joint-protection techniques and assistive devices for the nonsurgical hand. Tenth to twelfth day: Dressing and sutures are removed. Warm water soaks and massage are added to the program to encourage motion. The orthosis is discontinued. An MCP block may be used during the exercise sessions. Strengthening exercises are progressed to tolerance. Exercises are continued until there is no lag in digit motion and grip strength is at an appropriate level for the patient.

References (Tenosynovectomy)

5. Nalebuff, EA: Present status of rheumatoid hand surgery. Am J Surg 122:304, 1971.
6. Linscheid, RL, and Dobyns, JH: Rheumatoid arthritis of the wrist. Orthop Clin North Am 2:3, 1971.
7. Millender, LH, and Nalebuff, EA: Preventive surgery: Tenosynovectomy and synovectomy. Orthop Clin North Am 6(3):76, 1975.
8. Kessler, L, and Vainio, K: Posterior (dorsal) synovectomy for rheumatoid involvement of the hand and wrist. A follow-up study of six procedures. J Bone Joint Surg 48:1048, 1966.

9. Flatt, A: The Care of the Rheumatoid Hand, 3rd ed. CV Mosby, St Louis, 1974, pp 102–103.
10. Thirupathi, RG, Ferlic, DC, and Clayton, ML: Dorsal wrist synovectomy in rheumatoid arthritis—A long term study. J Hand Surg (Am) 8(6):848–856, 1983.
11. Phalen, GS: Reflection on 21 years of experience with carpal-tunnel syndrome. JAMA 212:1365, 1970.
12. Mannerfelt, L, and Norman O: Attrition ruptures of flexor tendons in rheumatoid arthritis caused by bony spurs in the carpal tunnel. J Bone Joint Surg 51B, 1969.
13. Clawson, DK, and Convery, FR: Surgery of rheumatoid arthritis of the wrist. In Cruess, R, and Mitchell, N (eds): Surgery of Rheumatoid Arthritis. JB Lippincott, Philadelphia, 1971.
14. Nalebuff, EA, and Smith, J: Preservation of terminal branches of the median palmar cutaneous nerve in carpal tunnel surgery. Orthopedics 2(4):370, 1979.
15. Dyle, JR: Anatomy of the flexor tendon sheath and pulleys of the thumb. J Hand Surg 2(2):149, 1977.
16. Ferlic, DC, and Clayton, ML: Flexor tenosynovectomy in the rheumatoid finger. J Hand Surg 3(4):364, 1978.
17. Seradge, H, and Kleinert, HE: Reduction flexor tenoplasty. Treatment of stenosing flexor tenosynovitis distal to the first pulley. J Hand Surg (Am) 6(6):543–544, 1981.
18. Millis, MB, Millender, LH, and Nalebuff, EA: Stiffness of the PIP joints in rheumatoid arthritis. J Bone Surg 58A(6):801, 1976.
19. Rhoades, CE, Gelberman, RH, and Manjarris, JF: Stenosing tenosynovitis of fingers and thumbs. Results of a prospective trial of steroid injection and splinting. Clin Orthop 190:236–238, November 1984.
20. Kolind-Sorenson, V: Treatment of trigger fingers. Acta Orthop Scand 41:428, 1970.

Additional Sources (Tenosynovectomy)

Denman, EE: The anatomy of the incision for carpal tunnel decompression. Hand 13(1):17–28, 1981.
Kessler, FB: Complications of the management of carpal tunnel syndrome. Hand Clin 2(2):401–406, May 1986.

TENDON SURGERY

Surgical procedures performed on or with tendons are considered restorative or corrective procedures, since they are performed *after* a specific deformity occurs. **Synovectomy** and **tenosynovectomy** are considered prophylactic surgical procedures when they are done to prevent certain consequences of chronic synovitis.[21]

Restorative tendon surgery for arthritis includes tendon relocation, tendon repair and adjacent suture, tendon transfer, tenotomy, and tendon release.[21]

Extensor Tendon Relocation

Migration or dislocation of the long finger extensor tendons into the ulnar valleys between the MCP heads is a common sequela of chronic synovitis of the MCP joints. When this occurs, the extensor tendons become ulnar deviators of the MCP joint and lose their mechanical leverage for extending the joint.[22] Once the tendons have slipped volar to the axis of the MCP joint, the patient is unable to actively extend the fingers at this level. However, the patient *is* able to maintain the joints in active extension, if the joints are passively aligned. Having the patient maintain passive extension then becomes a specific maneuver or test for ruling out the possibility of ruptured extensor tendons, the primary differential diagnosis.

If this migration process occurs in a patient with moderate MCP ulnar drift, the ulnar placement of the tendons can become a major dynamic force contributing to severe ulnar drift. In most cases the tendon slippage occurs after severe ulnar drift is in existence. In these cases, it is considered a consequence of MCP ulnar drift, not a causal factor.[23] (Prior to 1960 and E. M. Smith's work[23] on the role of the flexor tendons in ulnar drift, ulnar dislocation of the extensor tendons was erroneously thought to be a prime *causal* factor of MCP ulnar drift.)

Indications
Tendon relocation as a sole surgical procedure is done in a selected group of patients who have well-preserved joint cartilage and in whom the condition can easily be passively corrected.[1]

Occurrence
RA, SLE.

Surgical Prerequisites
Intact tendons and well-preserved joint surfaces and easy passive correctability.

Surgical Procedure[21,22,24]
This surgery is often combined with MCP synovectomy.

1. Dorsal transverse or longitudinal incision.

2. Shortened transverse fibers on the ulnar side of the extensor mechanism are divided.

3. The ulnar intrinsic insertion is released.

4. Extensor tendons are relocated and held in position by reefing stitches in the elongated radial transverse fibers.

5. In severe cases of MCP ulnar drift, the radial collateral ligaments are shortened.

6. In certain cases, extensor tendons may be sutured to the base of the proximal phalanx.

7. A drain is used only if the surgery is done in conjunction with a synovectomy.

Postoperative Management
Average hospitalization: 2 to 3 days.

1. First day to discharge: Immobilization in a compression dressing with a volar plaster orthosis to support the MCP joints in maximal or neutral extension and the PIP joints in moderate flexion.

2. Gentle active assistive ROM to all hand and wrist joints.

3. After discharge: Patients with bilateral arthritis will need instruction in joint-protection techniques and assistive devices for the nonsurgical hand. Dynamic MCP extension assist orthosis is applied to maintain the MCP joint in extension during the day. This orthosis is recommended for at least 6 weeks. A thermoplastic wrist MCP stabilization orthosis should be used for 6 to 8 weeks at night to support the MCP joints in a functional position and prevent prolonged full flexion.

Tendon Repair and Transfer

The most frequent causes of tendon rupture are tenosynovitis compromising the integrity of the tendons (attenuation or compression) or attrition over rough edges of carpal bones (Fig. 29–1).[24]

Rupture of the finger extensors usually occurs at the distal end of the ulna. The extensor pollicis longus tendon commonly ruptures at Lister's tubercle, where the tendon turns toward the thumb. Flexor tendons most frequently rupture over the scaphoid bone. However, they can rupture at the digit or palm level.[24,25] (See Fig. 29–1.)

The following tendons have the highest

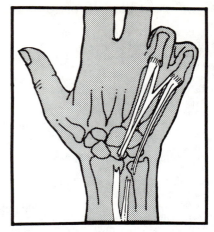

Figure 29–1. The digit extensor tendons typically rupture at the wrist level because of attrition. The extensor digiti quinti and the extensor communis tendons to the little and ring fingers are often the first to rupture.

incidence of rupture (listed in order of most frequent occurrence): extensor digitorum quinti (EDQ), extensor communis (EC) (fifth and fourth are the most frequent), extensor pollicis longus (EPL), flexor pollicis longus (FPL), flexor digitorum profundus (FDP) to the index finger. Rupture of the extensor indicis proprius (EIP) is rare.[25]

In some cases, it is possible to complete an end-to-end repair of the ruptured tendon. But in most cases, the rupture is too long-standing, the gap between the ends cannot be reduced, or the proximal motors adhere or retract with loss of their normal excursion. For these reasons, in RA, tendon function is restored by attaching the distal stump to a healthy adjacent tendon or by transferring another musculotendon unit to the distal stump. With either procedure, a tenosynovectomy is also performed to protect the repaired tendon and adjacent tendons from further damage.[25]

Adjacent suture is the method of choice for single extensor tendon ruptures. Tendon transfers provide a better solution when multiple tendons are ruptured.[25]

One of the most commonly used tendon transfers is the use of the EIP. The EIP is ideal since it is expendable, has independent action, and can reach any digit including the thumb. It also can be used for extensor tendon ruptures of the fourth and fifth digits. The EIP tendon is transferred to the distal stump of the EDQ tendon and the

EC tendon of the ring finger is sutured to the adjacent intact extensor of the middle finger.[25] It is not uncommon to find patients who have ruptured the EDQ and the third and fourth EC tendons. In these cases, one of three transfers might be considered: an FDS tendon can be used; if the patient has limited wrist motion or is to have a wrist fusion, the extensor carpi radialis longus tendon is a possibility; or if the thumb MCP joint requires fusion, the EPL can be spared.

Ruptures of the flexor tendons pose special problems because of the tendency for tendon adhesions to form within the tendon sheath. If one of the profundus tendons ruptures and the proximal end retracts, it may not be possible to perform an end-to-end repair. In these cases, the treatment of choice may be to excise the FDP tendon and fuse the DIP joint. For a rupture of the sublimis tendon in the digit sheath, the treatment of choice is to excise the remaining FDS tendon and perform a synovectomy of the tendon sheath to protect and ensure smooth gliding of the healthy profundus tendon. (In these cases, repair of the FDS may only increase the risk of adhesions, while not improving function.)[25]

Rupture of both the FDP and FDS tendons can occur, usually in the index finger, and results in loss of control of the index PIP and DIP joints. Patients with this problem tend to have severe hand involvement. The most reasonable approach may be to fuse the PIP and DIP joints in a functional position and strengthen the intrinsic muscles for MCP flexion. This provides the patient with a stable post for writing, pinch prehension, and so forth. If fusion is not desired, a two-stage tendon graft or tendon transfer can be performed. But these procedures are complex and generally reserved for trauma cases and rarely indicated in RA.[25]

Extensor Tendon Repair and Transfer

Indications
Ruptured or attenuated tendon.

Occurrence
Primarily RA.

Surgical and Functional Goals
The extensor mechanism is restored by reattaching the distal stump to an adjacent intact musculotendon unit or by transferring another musculotendon unit to the distal stump.

Postsurgical expectation is restoration of active joint extension.

Surgical Prerequisites
1. Normal or functional passive extension of the joints distal to the rupture.
2. Intact adjacent musculotendon units or units that can be transferred.
3. Patient motivation to follow through with an exacting, often slowly progressive, rehabilitation course.

Surgical Procedure
There are several surgical options for repair, depending on the status of adjacent tendons or available motor units for transfer. These options include suture to an adjoining tendon, tendon transfer, or tendon graft.[25]

1. For rupture of the extensor communis tendon:
   a. Approach: Dorsal, slightly curved or longitudinal incision.
   b. Dorsal tenosynovectomy (the removal of synovium from around the extensor tendons and relocation of synovial-lined retinacular ligament beneath tendons to avoid recurrence).
   c. Suture of the distal stump of the ruptured tendon to an adjacent musculotendon unit or transfer of another tendon to the ruptured distal stump.
   d. Procedure is frequently combined with complete or partial resection (modified Darrach procedure) of the ulnar head and wrist joint synovectomy when rupture was due in part to attrition by the distal ulna.
2. For rupture of the EPL: The EIP is transferred to the EPL and sutured over the dorsum of the thumb MCP joint.

Postoperative Management
Average hospitalization: 1 to 3 days or outpatient surgery.

1. First 3 to 4 weeks after discharge (protective stage):[26]
   a. For extensor and EDQ repairs, initial immobilization: short arm cast or orthosis with wrist in moderate (approximately 25 degrees) extension and MCP joints in slight flexion.
   b. For extensor pollicis repairs, immobilize wrist in slight ulnar deviation and

extension, and the thumb in midrange between abduction and extension.

c. During this stage, it is important to minimize edema and to provide an ROM program to prevent stiffness in the elbow and shoulder joints. Patients with bilateral arthritis will need instruction in joint-protection techniques and assistive devices for the nonsurgical hand.

2. About fourth week (mobilization stage):

a. Orthosis can be removed intermittently to begin therapy when the tendon junctures are strong enough to withstand muscle contractions.

b. When surgery involves tendon transfer, muscle re-education is started with repetitive active extension (with or without orthosis). The amount of muscle re-education required depends upon the tendon transferred. If the flexor digitorum superficialis is transferred to an extensor, re-education can be extensive. (See section on muscle strengthening in Chapter 27, Exercise Treatment, for specific techniques.) Active or passive flexion is avoided. Electrical stimulation may be helpful if there is excessive scarring. Electromyogram (EMG) biofeedback can facilitate the re-education process but is rarely needed.

3. About fifth week:

a. Muscle re-education is continued.

b. Active motion can be started.

c. Use of the resting orthosis may be continued between exercise sessions and at night.

4. About sixth week:

a. Orthosis is discontinued.

b. Hand can be used in light functional activities.

c. Muscle re-education may or may not still be needed.

d. Functional activities are gradually increased. Strong resisted flexion and extension should be avoided for an additional 2 to 3 weeks. For transfers of the EDC tendons, activities such as transferring with pressure on a dorsum of the hand should always be avoided.

e. Active and light resistive exercises to strengthen the repaired tendons. Depending on the nature of the repair and the surgeon's preference, resistive strengthening exercises may be delayed until the eighth week.[26]

References (Tendon Surgery)

21. Millender, LH, and Nalebuff, EA: Preventive surgery—Tenosynovectomy and synovectomy. Symposium on Rheumatoid Arthritis. Orthop Clin North Am 6(2):765, 1975.
22. Flatt, A: The Care of the Rheumatoid Hand, 3rd ed. CV Mosby, St Louis, 1974, pp 72–74.
23. Smith, EM, Juvinall, R, Bender, L, and Pearson, J: Role of the finger flexors in rheumatoid deformities of the MCP joints. Arthritis Rheum 7:467, 1964.
24. Boyes, JH: Tendons. In Boyes, JH (ed): Bunnell's Surgery of the Hand, 5th ed. JB Lippincott, Philadelphia, 1970, pp 393–436.
25. Nalebuff, EA: The recognition and treatment of tendon ruptures in the rheumatoid hand. American Academy of Orthopedic Surgeons: Symposium on Tendon Surgery in the Hand. CV Mosby, St Louis, 1975, pp 255–269.
26. Toth, SE: Therapist's management of tendon transfers. In Mackin, ED (ed): Hand Clinics. WB Saunders, Philadelphia 1986.

Additional Sources (Tendon Surgery)

Baxter, PL, and Carter-Wilson, M: Management of tendon transfers. In Hunter, JM, Schneider, LH, Mackin, EJ, and Callahan, AD (eds): The Hand: Another Decade of Tendon Surgery. CV Mosby, St Louis, 1985.
Beasley, RW: Principles of tendon transfer. Orthop Clin North Am 1(2), 1970.
Brand, PW: Mechanics of tendon transfers. In Hunter, JM, Schneider, LH, Mackin, EJ, and Callahan, AD (eds): Rehabilitation of the Hand, 2nd ed. CV Mosby, St Louis, 1984.
Cohen, J: Occupational therapy following hand tendon surgery. In American Academy of Surgeons: Symposium on Tendon Surgery in the Hand. CV Mosby, St Louis, 1975, p. 292.
Green, DL: Operative Hand Surgery, Vol 2. Churchill-Livingston, New York, 1982.
Koumban, SL: Pre-operative and post-operative management of tendon transfers. In Hunter, JM, Schneider, LH, Mackin, EJ, and Callahan, AD (eds): Rehabilitation of the Hand, 2nd ed. CV Mosby, St Louis, 1984.

SURGERY FOR BOUTONNIÈRE DEFORMITY

When it is associated with arthritis, the boutonnière deformity results from synovitis in the PIP joint altering the tendon balance in the finger. The complete deformity has three components: (1) PIP joint flexion, (2) DIP hyperextension, and (3) MCP joint hyperextension.[27]

Synovial hypertrophy stretches the extensor mechanism. The central slip becomes unable to support the PIP joint in full extension. The lateral bands become displaced volarly and result in shortening of the transverse retinacular ligaments. This secondary shortening leads to distal joint hyperextension and limited flexion. When the PIP flexion deformity becomes marked, the patient compensates by hyperextending the MCP joint.[27]

In the early stages, functional loss is related as much to the lack of full DIP joint flexion as to the lack of PIP joint extension. Severe deformity resulting in the inability to extend the PIP joint to grasp objects becomes the major hindrance. The recommended surgical procedures vary, depending on the severity of the deformity.

Early Boutonnière

An **extensor tenotomy** (tendon division) is a simple procedure that can correct the DIP joint hyperextension component of the deformity and aids extension of the PIP joint by altering the balance of forces.[28] The procedure is done under local anesthesia and involves a longitudinal incision over the middle phalanx. The extensor mechanism is divided obliquely or transversely. Postoperative management includes active antideformity exercises (i.e., DIP joint flexion with the PIP joint supported in extension); daytime dynamic splinting of the PIP joint with a reverse knuckle bender type of splint for 4 to 6 weeks; and night splinting of the PIP joint in extension with an aluminum finger splint. If there is a lag in DIP joint extension immediately postoperatively, it can usually be corrected with splinting in extension.

Moderate Boutonnière

Once the patient loses 40 to 50 degrees of extension of the PIP joint, functional loss becomes more significant. The deformity may be reducible or fixed in this stage. The objective of surgery is to restore PIP joint extension by tightening the central slip and relocating the lateral bands. This extensor reconstruction is combined with an extensor tenotomy to correct DIP joint limitations.[27]

If there is PIP joint synovitis, a preoperative trial of corticosteroid injection and gentle dynamic orthotic treatment is done to shrink the capsular structures and to stretch out soft tissues that restrict extension.[27]

The surgery involves a dorsal longitudinal curved incision over the PIP joint. The central slip is divided distally and separated from the lateral bands proximally. Approximately one quarter of an inch of the central slip is excised and the remaining portion is reattached to the base of the middle phalanx.[27] Two releasing incisions are made just volar to the lateral bands. These divide the transverse retinacular ligaments and make it possible to bring the lateral bands dorsally so they can be sutured to the central slip or to each other.[27] A tenotomy is done, which essentially places all of the extensor forces at the PIP joint level.[28] The action of the oblique retinacular ligament is considered responsible for preventing a mallet finger from occurring.[29] Following the reconstruction, it should be possible to passively flex the PIP joints 70 or 80 degrees; the remainder is gained in postoperative therapy.[29] A Kirschner wire is placed across the PIP joint to maintain full extension during the early postoperative phase, which lasts 3 to 4 weeks.

Postoperative management includes active DIP joint motion; daytime PIP orthosis with dynamic extension assist for 3 to 6 weeks following removal of the wire; night positioning with a padded aluminum splint; and after the fourth week, heat and gentle sustained passive flexion are started.

Severe Boutonnière

This stage includes deformities with greater than a 60-degree loss of PIP joint extension; these deformities are not passively correctable.[27] Surgery to restore the extensor mechanism cannot be done unless the joint can be passively extended without tension. Surgical options for these patients include serial casting of the digit to regain extension followed by extensor mechanism reconstruction and tenotomy, PIP joint arthroplasty with Silastic implant,[30] and PIP joint fusion in a functional position.

The methods for serial finger casting

were developed by Judy Bell, OTR, and can be found in two publications.[31]

PIP joint arthroplasty is particularly appropriate for deformities of the ring and little fingers in which PIP joint flexion is critical for functional activities.[30] Arthroplasty may not be feasible in patients with small or osteoporotic phalanges. When the procedure is done for a boutonnière deformity, it is combined with reconstruction of the extensor mechanism as described above.[30]

The position of fusion varies according to the digit involved. Nalebuff and Millender use approximately 25 degrees of flexion for the index finger and gradually increase the flexion to about 40 degrees for the small finger.[27]

The surgical procedures and postoperative management for arthroplasty and fusion are described in separate sections later in this chapter.

References (Boutonnière Surgery)

27. Nalebuff, EA, and Millender, LH: Surgical treatment of the boutonniere deformity in rheumatoid arthritis. Orthop Clin North Am 6:733, 1975.
28. Dolphin, JA: Extensor tenotomy for chronic boutonniere deformity of the finger: Report of two cases. J Bone Joint Surg 47A:161, 1965.
29. Littler, JW, and Eaton RG: Redistribution of forces in the correction of the boutonniere deformity. J Bone Joint Surg 49A:1267, 1969.
30. Swanson, AB: Flexible implant arthroplasty for arthritic finger joints. J Bone Joint Surg 54A:435, 1972.
31. Bell, J: Plaster cylinder casting for contractures of the interphalangeal joints. In Hunter, JM, Schneider LH, Mackin, EJ, and Bell, JA (eds): Rehabilitation of the Hand, 2nd ed. CV Mosby, St Louis, 1984. (This information is also available in a booklet from the Hand Rehabilitation Center, Philadelphia, PA.)

SURGERY FOR SWAN-NECK DEFORMITY

Until 1982 it was postulated that the swan-neck deformity was the end result of muscular imbalance caused by synovitis in the MCP, PIP, or DIP joint. It now appears that wrist synovitis and carpal collapse may also contribute to this deformity. The complete deformity consists of three components: (1) PIP joint hyperextension, (2) DIP joint flexion, and (3) MCP joint flexion.[32,33]

The extent of functional loss due to a swan-neck deformity correlates with the loss of *PIP joint flexion,* not the degree of PIP hyperextension present.[32] Patients with severe (40 degrees or more) PIP joint hyperextension but full flexion will have no functional limitations due to the swan-neck deformity. Conversely, a patient with 10 degrees of hyperextension but only 50 degrees of flexion could be limited in functional activities.

Nalebuff has devised a classification system for swan-neck deformities based on the degree of PIP joint flexion and PIP joint integrity present.[32] This classification provides an organized approach for delineating the myriad of surgical options available for correcting these deformities. Swan-neck deformities are complex because they can appear similar in appearance but can have very different causal factors and functional consequences.

Type I: Swan-Neck with Full PIP Joint Flexion[32]

Deformities included in this group generally originate at either the DIP joint or the PIP joint. DIP joint involvement produces a partial or complete rupture of the distal attachment of the EDC tendon, resulting in a flexion deformity of the DIP joint secondary to hyperextension imbalance at the PIP joint. If the deformity originates at the PIP joint, it is usually due to synovitis stretching the volar capsule or attenuation of the FDS tendon. These patients usually do not have severe MCP joint disease.[32]

The objective of surgery for these patients is to prevent or correct PIP joint hyperextension or restore DIP joint extension or both. Surgical options include

1. DIP joint fusion in a functional position, approximately 5 to 10 degrees of flexion.
2. **Dermadesis.** Removal of a wedge of skin over the volar aspect of the PIP joint to use skin tightness as a means of restricting hyperextension.[32] (This method can be used only in very mild cases.)
3. **Flexor tenodesis.**[34] A slip of the sublimis tendon is cut proximally and attached to the proximal phalanx with the PIP joint in 20 degrees of flexion. The slip then acts

as a checkrein to prevent full extension. The objective is to create a slight flexion contracture. Postoperatively, the patient is positioned with an orthosis in a manner that allows full flexion but limits extension to −20 degrees.

4. Retinacular ligament reconstruction.[35] In this procedure, the ulnar lateral band is cut proximally and left attached distally. The band is then brought volar to Cleland's fibers and to the axis of PIP joint motion and sutured to the fibrous sheath under approximate tension to restore DIP extension and prevent PIP hyperextension. It is effective for increasing DIP joint extension when the primary problem is in the PIP joint and not the DIP joint.

Type II: Swan-Neck with PIP Flexion Limited by Intrinsic Tightness[32]

It is theorized that pain and swelling in the MCP joints elicit a reflex spasm of the associated interosseous muscles. In addition, carpal collapse can further diminish extrinsic power, encouraging an intrinsic imbalance.[33] Chronic spasm or imbalance can result in fibrosis of the muscle in a shortened position. Decreased excursion of the intrinsic muscles impedes PIP flexion when the MCP joints are in extension. Full PIP flexion becomes possible only when the MCP joints are flexed. The insertion of the interosseous muscles exerts force directly on the lateral bands to extend the PIP joints. If there is damage to the PIP joint or natural laxity of the volar plate, intrinsic spasm can become a major dynamic force contributing to PIP hyperextension or swan-neck deformity.

In these patients, it is not sufficient to restrict PIP joint hyperextension. It is necessary to correct the intrinsic tightness and the MCP joint disorder that initiates and prolongs the muscular imbalance in the finger. This is accomplished by intrinsic release (digital) in patients without active MCP synovitis and with well-preserved MCP joints, and by MCP joint arthroplasty and intrinsic release in others.

Digital intrinsic release (Littler procedure)[36] is carried out through a dorsal ulnar longitudinal incision over the proximal phalanx. The oblique fibers of the intrinsics are resected from the extensor mechanism. A triangle wedge is removed from the dorsal mechanism to lessen the chances of recurrence. This procedure results in improved PIP flexion with the MCP joint extended or radially deviated. This procedure may be combined with a DIP fusion, dermadesis, or flexor tenodesis to further restore balance to the PIP and DIP joints.

An MCP joint arthroplasty (Swanson) with resection of the metacarpal heads lengthens the intrinsic muscles. However, some surgeons, in addition, resect the ulnar intrinsic muscles to reduce the risk of recurrent intrinsic tightness and ulnar drift of the fingers.

Type III: Swan-Neck with PIP Joint Contracture and Intact Cartilage[32]

Initially, it was thought that PIP joint stiffness was due to severe PIP joint disease and the only recourse for correction was arthroplasty or fusion.[37] It is now apparent that many patients are limited by secondary soft tissue changes and the options for treatment of these contractures have expanded. Swan-neck deformity with limited flexion but well-preserved joint surfaces is delineated as type III. Those with severe PIP joint damage are classified as type IV.[32]

The first objective of surgery is to restore *passive motion* by using one of several release procedures. If the flexor tendons are intact and moving freely, postoperative strengthening exercises will be sufficient for restoring full active motion. However, if the flexor tendons are adherent, it is necessary to perform a second procedure such as a tenosynovectomy or tenolysis before full functional ROM can be achieved.

If the contracture is long standing, there is usually fibrosis in all of the surrounding joint structures.[32] The extensor mechanism collateral ligaments and the skin are key structures that restrict passive flexion and are amenable to surgery.[32] If there are additional deformities at the MCP or DIP joints contributing to the swan-neck process, these will have to be corrected with additional surgeries such as arthroplasty, intrinsic release, or fusion. Otherwise, the PIP joint limitation is likely to recur.[32]

PIP Joint Manipulation and Skin Release[32]

The patient's PIP joint is *gently* manipulated under anesthesia. In many cases, it is possible to achieve 80 or 90 degrees of flexion. The joint is then fixed with a Kirschner wire for 2 weeks. This is followed by heat and active and passive exercises to increase both flexion and extension and to improve the strength and excursion of the long flexor tendons. Orthotic positioning that maintains the PIP joint in flexion should be continued until the patient can maintain flexion without them, as determined by 1-, 2-, or 3-day trials without the orthoses. The orthoses may be needed for as long as 8 to 12 weeks. Taping the finger to padded aluminum splints or using LMB wire-foam Flexion Springs[4] is generally well tolerated by patients. This procedure is often combined with MCP arthroplasty. The temporary fixation of the PIP joint encourages flexion of the MCP joints during the postoperative exercise program.[32]

Excessive tension on the skin over the PIP joint can cause ischemia and secondary necrosis. A skin release is done just distal to the PIP joint to reduce tension on the skin during temporary fixation in flexion of a previously stiff joint.[32] The incision is left open and it gradually closes over a 2- to 3-week period.

Not all patients are candidates for joint manipulation. Patients with severe osteoporosis are prone to fractures. If patients cannot be *gently* manipulated into flexion, they are considered for a soft tissue release.[32]

Lateral Band Mobilization

In a swan-neck deformity the lateral bands migrate dorsal and become contracted, losing their ability to shift lateral and volar with flexion. These contracted bands can prevent passive flexion during manipulation. Freeing the lateral bands from the central slip can often make manipulation possible without releasing the collateral ligaments or lengthening the central slip.[38–40]

If the surgery is done under local anesthesia the success of the release can be determined during surgery. The lateral bands should shift during active flexion and extension. If the release of the bands is not sufficient to allow desired flexion, it may be necessary to release the collateral ligaments and central slip as well.

Following the surgery, the patients are splinted or fixed with a Kirschner wire for two weeks. Then active and passive exercises are started to restore ROM, strength, and dexterity. Night taping the PIP joint in flexion should be continued until patients can maintain flexion without the tape. This may take as long as 2 to 3 months.

Type IV: Swan-Neck with PIP Joint Contracture and Damaged Cartilage

The surgeries described for swan-neck deformities Types I to III require an intact PIP joint to be successful. If there is evidence of cartilage destruction, these procedures will not work and a salvage procedure such as arthroplasty or fusion needs to be considered. The criteria and procedures for these surgeries are discussed in separate sections of this chapter.

References (Swan-Neck Surgery)

32. Nalebuff, EA, and Millender, LH: Surgical treatment of the swan-neck deformity in rheumatoid arthritis. Orthop Clin North Am 6:733, 1975.
33. Shapiro, JS: Wrist involvement in rheumatoid swan-neck deformity. J Hand Surg 7(5):484–491, 1982.
34. Swanson, AB: Surgery of the hand in cerebral palsy and the swan-neck deformity. J Bone Joint Surg 42A:951, 1960.
35. Littler, JW: Restoration of the oblique retinacular ligament for correction of hand contractures. G.E.M. Nol, Paris, L'Epansion, 1966.
36. Littler, JW: Quoted by Harris, C Jr, and Riordan, D: Intrinsic contracture in the hand and its surgical treatment. J Bone Joint Surg 36A:10, 1954.
37. Flatt, AE: The Care of the Rheumatoid Hand. CV Mosby, St Louis, 1968.
38. Nalebuff, EA: Surgical treatment of finger deformities in the rheumatoid hand. Surg Clin North Am 49:833, 1969.
39. Leach, RE, and Baumgard, SH: Correction of swan-neck deformity in rheumatoid arthritis. Surg Clin North Am 48:661, 1968.
40. Gainor, BJ, and Hummel, GL: Correction of rheumatoid swan-neck deformity by lateral bank mobilization. J Hand Surg (Am) 10(3):370–376, May 1985.

ARTHROPLASTY

Once there is cartilage loss, instability, and deformity, joint restoration is no longer possible. It then becomes necessary to choose between two salvage procedures—**arthroplasty** (joint reconstruction) and **arthrodesis** (joint fusion). Both surgeries relieve pain, provide stability, correct or reduce deformity, and improve function. The arthroplasty provides the additional benefit of motion. The surgery of choice depends on the joint level, integrity of the bone, and the function of the digits.[41]

The first metal hinge finger prostheses were developed in the late 1950s. They were metal hinges, originally created to provide a solution for swan-neck deformities of the PIP joint and later adapted for the MCP joint. The metal prostheses for the MCP joints eventually proved unsatisfactory.[42]

The advent of synthetic materials that could be used in the body opened up the field of implant development and revolutionized joint surgery. Alfred Swanson developed the first flexible Silastic digit implants in 1962.[43] They became available to surgeons in major medical centers around 1969. There are other digit implants available, but the Swanson implants are the most widely used and have the most extensive follow-up. The fact that they have been used in over a quarter of a million patients attests to the worldwide acceptance of this procedure.[43] Since the success of the digit implants, a number of flexible Silastic implants have been developed. Implants for the wrist, thumb, carpal bones, and radioulnar joints have gained the widest acceptance.[43] In 1968, Niebauer created a digit prosthesis similar in design to the Swanson implant but added a Dacron mesh to the stems to encourage scarring or fixation of the stems for greater stability.[44] This is in contrast to the Swanson design, in which the stems are loose in the canal and glide slightly during flexion and extension, allowing the hinge to reposition relevant to the axis of rotation, creating a more ideal distribution of forces over a broader section.[43] The Niebauer prostheses are also effective and widely used.[44]

The term **implant** is used to describe these devices because they are spacers rather than artificial joints. They function as a hinge and do not perform all of the intricate gliding and rotational motions of a normal joint.[45]

Prior to 1970, the only surgery available to correct severe pain or deformity of the MCP joints was a resection arthroplasty, in which the heads of the metacarpals were removed. A short period of fixation followed surgery to encourage tightening of the soft tissues. For many patients, this was an excellent surgery that resulted in pain-free mobile joints.[46] However, results were often unpredictable and ulnar drift frequently recurred.[46] Swanson developed his implant as a "dynamic spacer" that acts as an interpositional material for resection arthroplasty to make results more predictable, reproducible, and durable.[43]

In addition to providing a spacer for the resected bone, the flexible implant provides support for the capsuloligamentous system that develops around it. The collagen, scar-like tissue that forms around the joint following surgery (encapsulation process) can be shaped or trained during the formation process to enhance motion or stability in certain planes as desired. Shaping the capsule is a key aspect of splinting, particularly in the MCP joints.[43,47-49]

This encapsulation process is a major component of the flexible implant arthroplasty and critical to postoperative management.[49] Prostheses that use cement fixation do not rely on the capsule or ligamentous structures for stability. Therefore, the surgical and postoperative protocols for flexible implants are different from those for cemented implants.

Since flexible implants are widely used and require the most postoperative therapy, they will be reviewed in this section.

Wrist Implant Arthroplasty

Over the past 16 years, many different prostheses have become available for replacement of the radiocarpal joint. Currently there are four different design modes being used:[50] (1) the Swanson-designed Silastic flexible hinged spacer,[51] (2) the Volz-designed cement fixated semiconstrained prosthesis with a single distal prong,[52] (3) the Meuli-designed cement fixated ball joint prosthesis (no longer recommended due to high reoperation rate within 5 years),[50,53] and (4) the spherical triaxial constrained ball-and-socket design with cement fixation from the Hospital for Special Surgery.[54] Each prosthesis has advantages and disadvantages, which is evident in the continued search to find the ultimate prosthesis, one that provides long-term pain-free stability and mobility.

The Swanson-designed flexible implant spacer introduced in 1970 has been the most popular because until recently it was the only one that did not use cement for fixation and could be easily removed if an infection occurred or replacement was needed. The major complication has been fracture of the implant secondary to tears from sharp bone ends. Also, since it rides loosely in the bones and is not fixated, it is highly dependent on soft tissue encapsulation for stability.[43] To reduce the risk of fracture, wrists are immobilized for 6 weeks postoperatively to encourage capsular/soft tissue stability, and postoperative ROM is limited to 30 degrees of flexion and 30 degrees of extension. Swanson has recently attempted to resolve the problem of fractures by using metal (titanium) grommets (bone liners) to protect the implant from the bone ends.

The Volz prosthesis, introduced in 1974, is the most popular of the cement fixated prostheses. There has been good short-term and moderate-term follow-up results. A problem with ulnar deformity was resolved with a design change in 1977.[50,52] Recently the prosthesis has been modified to allow press-fit (cementless) fixation with good short-term results on a limited number of patients.[55] If this is successful it will allow the surgeon another cementless option, one with greater stability and ROM and less dependence on soft tissue encapsulation as compared to the flexible Silastic implant.

In addition to the radiocarpal joint, there are Silastic replacement implants for the scaphoid and lunate bones. These are used primarily to relieve pain secondary to trauma or aseptic necrosis (Kienböck's disease) of these carpal bones and nonunion of the scaphoid.[43]

Radiocarpal Joint (Swanson Flexible Hinged Implant)

The radiocarpal flexible hinged implant is a one piece intramedullary stemmed hinge fabricated from high-performance Silastic material. The proximal stem of the implant fits the intramedullary canal of the radius and the distal stem passes through the capitate and fits the intramedullary canal of the third metacarpal.[47,51,56] The implant is available in 5 anatomical sizes.

Indications[41,51]
1. Chronic wrist synovitis with subluxation or dislocation unresponsive to conservative treatment.
2. Stiffness or fusion in a nonfunctional position.
3. Stiffness in which movement is required for function.

Occurrence
RA, JRA, PA, and traumatic arthritis.

Surgical and Functional Goals
The ideal outcome is a pain-free, stable joint with approximately 30 degrees of flexion and 30 degrees of extension and slight radial and ulnar deviation.[41,43]

Surgical Prerequisites
1. Adequate quality bone stock to hold the implant. (Patients with mutilans of the carpal bones are not good candidates.)
2. Intact wrist extensor tendons.
3. Adequate capsular and soft tissue to secure the prosthesis.

Surgical Procedure[51,56]
1. Dorsal curved longitudinal incision.
2. Capsule and ligaments are preserved.
3. Contractures are released.
4. Distal end of the radius is resected and the scaphoid, lunate, part of the triquetrum, and base of the capitate are removed. (The end of the ulna may also be removed if forearm rotation is limited; Fig. 29–2.)
5. A trial implant is fitted to determine correct size. The distal stem is trimmed so it does not extend beyond the base of the third metacarpal.
6. Proximal and distal grommets are inserted; implant is fitted.
7. The capsuloligamentous repair is firmed to allow 30 degrees of passive flexion and 10 degrees of ulnar and radial deviation.
8. The wrist extensors and retinacular construction are balanced. A strip of retinaculum is placed over extensor tendons to prevent bowstringing.
9. Ruptured digital extensor tendons are repaired if present.

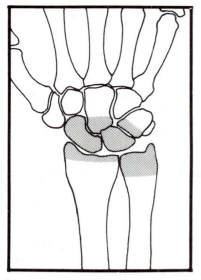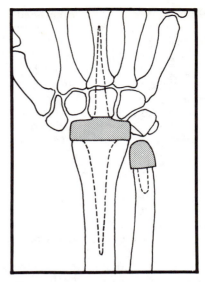

Figure 29–2. Bone resection is required for placement of the Swanson wrist implant and radial head replacement. The dotted line indicates the stem on the implant inside the bones.

Postoperative Management

Average hospitalization: 3 to 5 days.

1. Initially, the hand is in a voluminous dressing with palmar or palmar and dorsal plaster orthosis and elevated. Dynamic MCP extension assists are used if the extensor tendons are repaired.

2. Second day:

    a. Compression dressing is reduced. Some surgeons use a short-arm cast.

    b. It is necessary to immobilize the wrist for 4 to 6 weeks to allow capsular healing.

    c. The goal of surgery and therapy is a pain-free stable joint with approximately 30 degrees of flexion and 30 degrees of extension.

    d. Begin daily ROM to digital and proximal joints.

3. After discharge: The cast is removed (approximately 4 to 6 weeks): Gentle wrist ROM exercises are started. A thermoplastic orthosis or commercial elastic canvas wrist gauntlet is worn as needed to protect the wrist during functional activities and to relieve discomfort. It should be gradually discontinued over a period of 8 to 10 weeks. Some surgeons believe a wrist orthosis should be used indefinitely during heavy tasks. If the patient has excessive lateral motion when the cast is removed, he or she should be fitted with a wrist-hinge orthosis that would allow flexion and extension for use during the daytime for an additional 2 to 4 weeks.[57]

4. If the patient has less than 30 degrees of flexion or extension, then gentle passive exercises can be added. *Caution:* During postoperative therapy, ROM should be restricted to 30 degrees of flexion and 30 degrees of extension. Patients who gain greater motion have a higher risk of implant fracture.

5. Patients with bilateral arthritis will need instruction in joint-protection techniques and assistive devices for the nonsurgical hand.

Radioulnar Joint—Distal Ulnar Resection and Replacement (Darrach Procedure)

Chronic synovitis of the radioulnar joint weakens the supporting ligaments and can result in a subluxation between the ulna and radius. (This is incorrectly referred to as *dorsal subluxation of the ulna.* The ulna is the more stable bone. It is more likely that the hand is pulling the radius into volar subluxation on the ulna.) If the subluxation is severe, it can limit supination and pronation. In addition, synovial hypertrophy can limit forearm rotation.

Resection of the ulna eliminates the distal radioulnar joint, thereby eliminating distal radioulnar joint pain and any block to forearm motion. The ulnar head implant is made of Silastic material and is of one-piece construction with an intramedullary stem. (See Fig. 29–2.) The replacement is designed to preserve the anatomical relationship and the physiology of the distal radioulnar joint. Swanson reports that, with the use of the replacement, less bone needs to be removed and the physiologic length of the ulna is maintained to help prevent ulnar carpal shift and provide greater wrist stability.[43,47] The cap can help achieve these goals for some patients but it is not a guarantee. In a 4-year follow-up of 33 Darrach procedures, Gainor and Schaberg found that both patients with and without caps manifested considerable carpal collapse, carpal translocation, rotational change of the wrist, and radial shift of the wrist. Four wrists had dislocated ulnarly. They report that some patients developed an osseous carpal stabilizer and that this was a good prediction of stability. Patient selection based on the surgical prerequisites below is critical to reducing the above complications.[48]

An ulnar head replacement implant made of Silastic material designed to preserve the anatomical relationship and physiology of the distal radioulnar joint is available. However, recent reports of bone resorption and implant subluxation have made this a less popular procedure.

Indications
1. Pain secondary to destructive arthritis of the distal radioulnar joint.
2. Dorsal subluxation of the ulnar head, threatening the overlying extensor tendons.
3. Limitation of forearm rotation secondary to distal radioulnar joint disease or dorsal subluxation of the ulna.

Occurrence
RA, traumatic arthritis, JRA, and PA.

Surgical and Functional Goals
Postsurgical expectations are decreased wrist pain and improved forearm rotation.

Surgical Prerequisites
Stable radiocarpal joint (radioscaphoid-lunate joint), preferably without joint disease, with absence of ulnar displacement of the carpus on the radius.[56]

Surgical Procedure
This procedure may be combined with a dorsal clearance, extensor tendon repair, or a wrist fusion.

1. Approach: Slightly curved incision over the dorsum of the wrist or an ulnar midlateral incision.
2. Last ½ to ¾ inch of distal ulna is excised. Bone end and canal are prepared.
3. Radioulnar joint synovectomy.
4. Silastic ulnar head prosthesis may be implanted and end sutured in place (only in selected cases).
5. Periosteum around the last inch of the ulna is closed (not necessary if an implant is used).
6. Soft tissue closure to prevent volar migration of the radius. If the extensor carpi ulnaris tendon has displaced volarly, it may be relocated dorsally and held in place with a checkrein ligament fabricated from the retinaculum.[51]

Postoperative Management
Average hospitalization: 2 to 3 days.

1. Immobilization in a compression dressing with a short arm plaster orthosis or cast that extends to the proximal palmar crease and allows full flexion of the MCP joints and thumb. (If an ulnar prosthesis is implanted, a dorsovolar cast that encloses the elbow [a sugar-tong cast] to prevent wrist rotation may be used.) During hospitalization the arm is elevated and digit ROM exercises are started. The patient is instructed in a home program for edema control and digit ROM. (Patients with bilateral arthritis will need instruction in joint-protection techniques and assistive devices for the nonsurgical hand.)
2. After removal of cast (3 to 6 weeks):
   a. Active ROM exercises of the wrist are started with emphasis on supination and pronation.
   b. Gradually functional use is increased.
   c. Use of a static orthosis that holds the wrist in slight ulnar deviation (10 degrees) to prevent increasing ulnar displacement of the carpus on the radius, which results in radial deviation and wrist deformity. (See Chapter 19, Hand Pathodynamics and Assessment, for detailed discussion of the dynamics of wrist subluxation and dislocation.)

Metacarpophalangeal Joint Implant Arthroplasty (Swanson Silastic Implants)

Prior to the advent of the flexible implant, the most frequent procedure carried out for MCP joint pain and deformity was a resection arthroplasty. This procedure involved resection of the metacarpal head, soft tissue reconstruction, and temporary internal fixation. Resection arthroplasty was often successful but the results were at best unpredictable and inconsistent. The flexible implant resolved these shortcomings by providing an internal splint to control the encapsulation process (Fig. 29–3). The MCP implant arthroplasty is a reliable procedure for relieving pain, correcting deformity, and preserving motion (Fig. 29–4).

The goal of this surgery is to have a pain-free functional arc of motion; 70 degrees of flexion is considered desirable for the fourth and fifth fingers, but 60 to 65 degrees is considered good for the index and middle fingers. Too much motion leads to instability and possible recurrence of deformity, especially in the index finger, which is especially vulnerable to ulnar pressure. There is always a risk of less than ideal outcome (e.g., an extension lag and less than 70 degrees of flexion). There is also the risk of implant fracture (failure) and infection. Also people with chronic rheumatic diseases often face the trauma of multiple surgeries during the course of their illness. So no surgery should be done unless it is essential.

In light of these considerations the current practice is to recommend this surgery only if the ideal or even less than ideal results will improve function. In other words, it is not done just for appearance (cosmesis) or solely for ulnar drift if the hand is otherwise strong and functional.

If a person had severe MCP ulnar drift and volar subluxation, but no pain and near normal flexion and extension, he or she would probably have good functional ability (barring any PIP problems). This surgery would put such a person at risk of losing ROM and function.

Similar to the wrist implant the main complication of this surgery is fracture of the implant midsection due to propagation of tears initiated by sharp bony edges or subluxing bone ends.[56] To prevent this problem press-fit titanium grommets (bone liners) have been used since 1982 with good follow-up results so far.[56]

Indications
1. Pain secondary to destructive arthritis of the MCP joints.
2. Ulnar drift not amenable to soft tissue repair alone.
3. Subluxation or dislocation of MCP joints that severely limits function.
4. Stiffness or ankylosis and functional loss of MCP joints.

Occurrence
Primarily in RA; occasionally in traumatic arthritis.

Surgical and Functional Goals
Postsurgical expectations are relief of pain, increased joint stability, increased

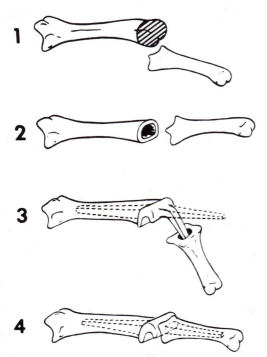

Figure 29–3. Resection of the metacarpal head and insertion of a Silastic Swanson design implant are shown here. The stems of the implant are inserted into the intramedullary canals. (Cement is not required.) A comprehensive soft tissue release procedure is necessary to obtain adequate space for the prosthesis. (From Swanson, AB: Silastic finger joint prosthesis. Dow Corning Bulletin, 1972, with permission.)

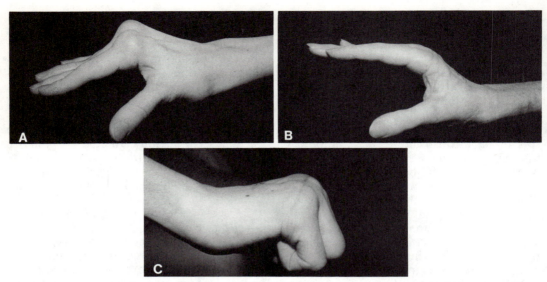

Figure 29–4. MCP arthroplasty and thumb CMC arthroplasty with thumb arthrodesis are shown here. (*A*) Preoperative status: Patient with RA has limited MCP extension (−70 degrees) resulting from marked MCP subluxation. Her ability for grasp is reduced because of a type IV thumb deformity with CMC joint adduction contracture and lateral instability of the thumb MCP joint. (*B*) Postoperative extension: Her ability for grasp and prehension is significantly improved. MCP extension has gained 40 degrees (now −30 degrees). (*C*) Postoperative flexion: Patient has functional, nearly full flexion, although she has lost some flexion compared with her preoperative ROM. This is consistent with the goal of the MCP implant arthroplasty to provide a more functional arc of motion rather than simply to increase excursion or achieve normal ROM. The patient's grasp strength and dexterity skills also improved. Thumb prehension skills are enhanced by the stability provided by the MCP arthrodesis.

mobility (ideally a 60- to 70-degree arc of motion), improved hand function, and improved cosmetic appearance. Many patients find they are not able to do more or different hand tasks postoperatively, but are able to do the same tasks, especially tasks requiring improved dexterity, with greater ease and without pain.

Surgical Prerequisites[43]

1. Intact neurovascular supply.
2. Intact flexor and extensor tendons.
3. Patient capable and motivated to follow precise postoperative splinting and exercise routine.
4. Absence of infection.
5. Adequate bone density to accept implant.

Surgical Procedure[43]

1. Approach: Transverse incision over the dorsum of the MCP joints or dorsal longitudinal incisions between the metacarpal heads.

2. Extensor hood and the joint capsule are incised.
3. Metacarpal heads are excised, and all cartilage is removed.
4. Synovectomy of the MCP joints is performed.
5. Contracted soft tissues are released (collateral ligaments, volar capsule [volar plate if necessary], ulnar intrinsic muscles with possible transfer to radial intrinsic muscle). The ulnar intrinsic to the index finger is preserved if possible to prevent pronation tendency. The abductor digiti minimi is sectioned.
6. Intramedullary canals of the proximal phalanx and metacarpal bones are broached.
7. Appropriate prosthesis size is selected; proximal and distal grommets and implant are placed.
8. Capsular closure is performed.
9. Reefing (pleating) of the radial fibers of the extensor hood is done to maintain alignment of the extensor tendon.

Postoperative Management[43,49,58]

> "The positioning and control of movement through dynamic orthotics and therapy during the first 6–8 weeks after reconstruction are as important as surgery."
>
> Alfred Swanson[56]

General Considerations

1. Before working with patients having this surgery, therapists should be familiar with encapsulation theory and process. (See above, introduction to arthroplasty surgery.)

2. Patients with bilateral arthritis will need instruction in joint-protection techniques and assistive devices for the nonsurgical hand.

3. Therapists should have a copy of the booklet *Postoperative Care for Patients with Silastic Finger Joint Implants* by Dr. Alfred Swanson. It is available through his office.[56]

4. Some patients will gain ROM with this surgery whereas others will have the same ROM, but the arc of motion will be in a more functional range. For example, preoperatively the patient may have a 45-degree arc between 45 to 90 degrees of flexion; postoperatively he or she may continue to have a 45-degree arc but between 10 to 60 degrees of flexion. This change alone often results in a more functional range. It is not clear why this happens in some patients, despite excellent surgery and optimal postoperative care. It seems to occur more frequently in patients with MCP deformities of long duration.

Considering this phenomenon, the following question needs to be answered with regard to each digit. If a person is going to have a limited postoperative arc of motion, what would be the most functional range to have the arc in?

Positioning of the ring and little fingers. Relevant to the above question, it is important to consider that in the normal hand full flexion of the ring and little fingers is more critical for grasp than full flexion of the radial digits; however, extension of the index and middle fingers is more important for opposition to the thumb and nonprehension dexterity. If the ideal postoperative arc of motion is 0 to 70 degrees, then in the little finger it would be more important to have the arc between 10 to 80 degrees. This would also be the best for the ring finger. The goal is not to achieve full motion, because in some cases this can create a greater risk of instability and recurrent deformity. Postoperative extension is determined by the tension and placement of the extension assists.

5. Another factor that influences the positioning of the extensor assists is the presence of extensor tendon lag. Prolonged fixed flexion deformity can result in lengthening of the extensor tendons. In the initial postoperative days one might adjust all extensor assists for neutral alignment if there is significant extensor lag, then reduce the tension on the ring and little fingers as the lag is diminished.

6. The fact that the flexors to the little finger are weaker than those to the other digits also influences the decision to use less tension on the fifth digit assists compared to the other digits.

7. It is important that patients do not apply lateral pinch force to the index finger during the encapsulation process. Swanson applies a thumb outrigger to prevent patients from accidentally using the thumb in this manner.

Protocol

Average hospitalization 3 to 5 days.

1. First to third day: The hand is in a voluminous compression bandage, elevated to reduce edema, with MCP joints extended and IP joints slightly flexed. Shoulder and elbow should receive daily ROM.

2. Second to third day: The compression bandage is replaced with a smaller dressing.

3. Third to seventh (op) day:

   a. Postoperative orthosis is fitted over a lightly padded dressing. (See Chapter 23, Orthotic Treatment for Arthritis of the Hand, for different types of postoperative orthoses and specific fitting instructions.) The orthosis should be worn all the time except for ROM of the wrist and hand hygiene.

   b. Extensor outriggers should keep the index, middle, and ring (if desired) fingers in zero extension and slight radial deviation. For the index finger this means about 10 degrees ulnar deviation, because the normal alignment of the index finger is 20 degrees ulnar deviation. The little finger should be maintained in 15 degrees of flexion and slight radial deviation. Tension assists should be tight enough to maintain desired extension but allow full *active* flexion.

 c. To increase MCP joint motion, active sustained flexion and extension exercises of the MCP joints should be performed 4 to 6 times each day for 15 to 20 minutes. These exercises need to be carefully defined and monitored in order that PIP flexion is not substituted for MCP flexion. Digital cylinder orthoses can be used to maintain PIP extension during exercises (see Chapter 23).

 d. To avoid recurrent intrinsic contracture, active PIP joint exercises with the MCP joints maintained in full extension should be performed 4 to 6 times each day.

4. Between the tenth and fourteenth day, and then the sixth to eighth week postoperative

 a. Use of flexion assists may be started if necessary with about one-half hour flexion alternated with an hour and a half extension and gradually increasing flexion to 1 hour.

 b. The optimal ratio of flexion positioning versus dynamic extension positioning depends upon the range of active motion. Ratio is increased in favor of the range with the greatest deficit.

 c. Splinting procedure is continued about 6 to 8 weeks with a full hand orthosis used at night; the amount of time spent in the orthosis during the day is gradually reduced, depending on the degree of active motion of the MCP joints, with the dynamic orthosis discontinued at about the tenth week. (Additional resources: Detailed guides by Dr. Swanson on postoperative treatment are available.[49,56] Madden, DeVore, and Arem have published an excellent article describing a comprehensive postoperative rehabilitation program.[59])

Proximal Interphalangeal Joint Implant Arthroplasty

For stiff swan-neck deformities with cartilage damage, the choice of surgery is between arthroplasty or a fusion. When possible the mobility provided by an arthroplasty is preferred for the ring and little fingers, where flexion is needed for strong grip. In the index and middle fingers, lateral stability is needed for strong pinch. If the surrounding joint structures are strong enough to ensure lateral stability, an arthroplasty is recommended. If the structures are weak or the bones are small, a fusion is often done in the index and middle fingers.[41,60,61]

Indications[60,61]
1. Pain secondary to destructive arthritis of the PIP joints.
2. Instability associated with destructive arthritis of the PIP joints.
3. Stiffness and functional loss of the PIP joints.
4. Stiff swan-neck deformity, when adjacent joints and tendons are intact.
5. Boutonnière and lateral deviation deformities.

Occurrence
RA, OA, traumatic arthritis, and PA.

Surgical and Functional Goals
Pain is diminished by the complete removal of the articular surfaces and diseased synovium. Function is improved by realignment of the joints, increased motion and stability, and decreased pain.[41]

Postsurgical expectations are relief of pain, increased stability or increased mobility (depending upon initial status), improved functional use, and improved cosmetic appearance.[61]

Surgical Prerequisites[61]
1. Intact neurovascular supply.
2. Intact extensor and flexor tendons.
3. Absence of recent infection (6 months minimum).
4. Absence of significant MCP joint flexion deformity. (MCP flexion deformity should be corrected prior to PIP surgery.)

Surgical Procedure
1. Approach: Dorsal, volar, or midlateral incision.
2. Extensor tendon mobilized; capsule incised.
3. Excision of the head of the proximal phalanx (synovectomy if indicated).
4. Intramedullary canals reamed and shaped to receive the prosthesis.
5. Selection of appropriate prosthesis and installation.
6. Capsular closure and extensor tendon reconstruction as indicated.

Postoperative Management[43,49,58]
Average hospitalization: 3 to 5 days

1. First to fifth day: The hand is in a voluminous compression bandage and ele-

vated to reduce edema. ROM of the upper extremity should be done daily.

2. Second to fifth day:

a. Compression bandage is removed.

b. Active ROM is started several times per day.

c. *The exercise program needs to be modified depending on whether or not extensor tendon reconstruction was also performed.* Early motion is contraindicated when tendon surgery is done.

d. Joint is positioned in extension with a small dorsal aluminum splint, except during exercise periods. If there has been prior swan-neck deformity or stiffness, the joint might be positioned into slight flexion. In severe swan-neck deformities, the joint can also be taped into flexion at night.

e. Flexion can be encouraged by stabilizing the MCP joint in extension during active finger flexion, using either an orthosis or a device like a Bunnell block.

3. After discharge: Patients with bilateral arthritis will need instruction in joint-protection techniques and assistive devices for the nonsurgical hand. Third to fourth week: Orthosis can be discontinued during the day if the joint is stable; it is usually retained for protective night positioning.

4. About sixth to eighth week: Orthosis can be discontinued.

Thumb Carpometacarpal Joint Arthroplasty

The trapeziometacarpal joint is a common site of primary OA. Cartilage thinning and osteophyte formation can block motion and result in subluxation or dislocation of the CMC joint.[62]

Pain in this joint can be severely debilitating, since 45 percent of hand function is attributed to the thumb.[43]

Patients with episodic pain often are satisfied with using a CMC-MP stabilization (short opponens) orthosis during painful periods. Once the pain becomes unrelenting or is not relieved by corticosteroid injection or orthosis, surgery is indicated.

There are several surgeries available for this problem (e.g., resection arthroplasty[57] and hemiarthroplasty). The trapezium implant is one of the most widely used. The trapezium implant is similar to other spacers in that it is designed to preserve the anatomical relationships of the basal joints of the thumb after resection arthroplasty. The stem of the implant fits into the intramedullary canal of the first metacarpal. The trapeziometacarpal joint is eliminated and motion then occurs between the implant and the trapezoid and scaphoid bones.[47,62-66]

Indications[62]

1. Persistent pain of the CMC joint that is nonresponsive to conservative management. (X-ray changes alone without symptoms are not sufficient indication for surgery.)

2. Decreased motion that reduces prehension.

Occurrence

OA, RA, and traumatic arthritis.

Surgical Prerequisites

Intact carpal bones (scaphoid).

Surgical and Functional Goals

Ideally, pain and crepitus are relieved by elimination of the damaged joint. ROM and strength are improved but the final outcome depends on the extent of the preoperative deformity, atrophy, and limitation. (See Chapter 20, Evaluation of Range of Motion, for special techniques for measuring CMC joint motion.)

Postoperative Management

Average hospitalization: 2 to 3 days.

1. Immobilization in a thumb spica short arm cast for 6 weeks. The cast should not block digit MCP flexion.

2. After discharge: Patients with bilateral arthritis will need instruction in joint-protection techniques and assistive devices for the nonsurgical hand. About the sixth week: Begin program of warm water soaks, active and passive ROM exercises to increase ROM in all planes. Wrapping the thumb into flexion with Coban tape can provide an effective gentle stretch for increasing flexion. Therapy could be continued until there is a plateau in progress. The length of therapy depends on how much stiffness develops during the 6 weeks of immobilization.

References (Arthroplasty)

41. Nalebuff, EA, and Millender, LH: Reconstructive surgery and rehabilitation of the hand. In Kelley,

WM, et al (eds): Textbook of Rheumatology, Vol II. WB Saunders, Philadelphia, 1981.

42. Flatt, A: The Care of the Rheumatoid Hand, 3rd ed. CV Mosby, St Louis, 1974, pp 195–221.

43. Swanson, AB: Flexible Implant Resection Arthroplasty in the Hand and Extremities. CV Mosby, St Louis, 1973.

44. Neibauer, JJ: Dacron-silicone prosthesis for the metacarpophalangeal and interphalangeal joints. In Cramer, LH, and Chase, RA (eds): Symposium on the Hand, Vol 3. CV Mosby, St Louis, 1971, pp 96–105.

45. Swanson, AB, deGroot Swanson, G: Flexible implant resection arthroplasty for the rheumatoid hand. Ann Chirurg Gynaic 74 (Suppl): 198:54–69, 1985.

46. Robinson, HS, Kokan, PB, and Patterson, FP: Functional results of excisional arthroplasty for the rheumatoid hand. Can Med Assoc J 108:1495, 1973.

47. Swanson, AB: Reconstructive Surgery in the Arthritic Hand and Foot. Clinical Symposia, Vol 31, No. 6, 1979. Medical Education Division CIBA Pharmaceutical Co, Summit, NJ.

48. Gainor, BJ and Schaberg, J: The rheumatoid wrist after resection of the distal ulna. J Hand Surg 10(6 Pt 1):837–844, 1985.

49. Postoperative Care for Patients with Silastic Finger Joint Implants (Swanson Design): MCP and IP Joints. Compiled by J Leonard, OTR, A Swanson, MD, and G dG Swanson, MD, 1985. Dow Corning Wright, 5677 Airline Road, Arlington, TN 38002. (This is a detailed postoperative guide.)

50. Levy, RN, Volz, RG, Kaufer, H et al: Progress in arthritis surgery. Clin Ortho Rel Res 200:299–321, 1985.

51. Swanson, AB, Swanson, G, and Maupin, BK: Flexible implant arthroplasty of the radiocarpal joint: Surgical technique and long-term study. Clin Orthop 187:94, 1984.

52. Volz, RG: Total wrist arthroplasty: A clinical review. Clin Orthop 187:112, 1984.

53. Meuli, HC: Meuli total wrist arthroplasty. Clin Orthop 187:107, 1984.

54. Ranawat, CS, Green, NA, Inglis, AE, and Straub, LR: Spherical-triaxial total wrist replacement. In Inglis, AE (ed): Symposium on Total Joint Replacement of the Upper Extremity. CV Mosby, St Louis, 1983, pp 265–272.

55. Coony, WP, Beckenbaugh, RD, and Linscheid, RL: Total wrist arthroplasty. Clin Orthop 187:121, 1984.

56. Swanson, AB: Treatment Considerations and Resource Materials for Flexible (Silicone) Implant Arthroplasty, 1985. Booklet available from Orthopedic Research Department, Blodgett Memorial Medical Center, 1900 Wealthy, SE, Suite 290, Grand Rapids, MI 49506.

57. Johnson, BM, Flynn, MJG, and Beckenbaugh, RD: A dynamic splint for use after total wrist arthroplasty. Am J Occup Ther 35:79–84, 1981.

58. Swanson, AB, Swanson, G dG, and Leonard, J: Postoperative rehabilitation program in flexible implant arthroplasty of the digits. In Hunter, JM, Schneider, LH, Mackin, EJ, and Bell, JA (eds): Rehabilitation of the Hand, 2nd ed. CV Mosby, St Louis, 1984.

59. Madden, JW, DeVore, G, and Arem, AJ: A rational postoperative management program for meta-carpophalangeal joint implant arthroplasty. J Hand Surg 2:358, 1977.

60. Nalebuff, EA, and Millender, LH: Surgical treatment of the swan-neck deformity in rheumatoid arthritis. Surgical treatment of the boutonniere deformity in rheumatoid arthritis. Orthop Clin North Am 6:733, 1975.

61. Swanson, AB, Maupin, BK, Gajjar, NV, and Swanson, GD: Flexible implant arthroplasty in the proximal interphalangeal joint of the hand. J Hand Surg 10(6 Pt 1):796–805, 1985.

62. Swanson, AB, and Swanson, G dG: Disabling osteoarthritis in the hand and its treatment. In Symposium on Osteoarthritis. CB Mosby, St Louis, 1976.

63. Beckenbaugh, RD, Dobyns, JH, Linscheid, RL, and Bryan, RS: Review and analysis of silicone-rubber MCP implants. J Bone Joint Surg 58A:483, 1976.

64. Dell, PC, Brushart, MD, and Smith, RL: Treatment of trapeziometacarpal arthritis: Results of resection arthroplasty. J Hand Surg 3(3):243, 1978. (Also includes a discussion on conservative management.)

65. Millender, LH, Nalebuff, EA, Amadio, P, and Phillips, CA: Interpositional arthroplasty for rheumatoid carpometacarpal joint disease. J Hand Surg 3(6):533, 1978.

66. Swanson, AB, and de Groot Swanson, G: Arthroplasty of the thumb basal joints. Clin Orthop 195:151–160, 1985.

Additional Sources (Arthroplasty)

Blair, WR, Shurr, DG, and Buckwalter, JA: Metacarpophalangeal joint implant arthroplasty with a Silastic spacer. J Bone Joint Surg (Am) 66(3):365–370, 1984.

Bowers, WH: Distal radioulnar joint arthroplasty: The hemiresection interposition technique. J Hand Surg (Am) 10(2):169–178, 1985.

Brase, DW, and Millender, LH: Failure of silicone rubber wrist arthroplasty in rheumatoid arthritis. J Hand Surg 11(2):175–183, 1986.

Burton, RI: Complications following surgery on the basal joint of the thumb. Hand Clin 2(2):265–269, 1986 (review).

Davis, RF, Weiland, AJ, and Dowling, SV: Swanson implant arthroplasty of the wrist in rheumatoid patients. Clin Orthop 166:132, 1982.

DeVore, GL: Preoperative assessment and postoperative therapy and splinting in rheumatoid arthritis. In Hunter et al (eds): Rehabilitation of the Hand, 2nd ed. CV Mosby, St Louis, 1984.

Dryer, RF, Blair, WF, Shurr, DG, and Buckwalter, JA: Proximal interphalangeal joint arthroplasty. Clin Orthop 185:187–194, 1984.

Ferlic, DC, Turner, BD, and Clayton, ML: Compression arthrodesis of the thumb. J Hand Surg 8:207–210, 1983.

Flatt, A: Care of the Rheumatoid Hand, 4th ed. CV Mosby, St Louis, 1983.

Greetchko, J, Richard, MA, and Blatt, G: Postoperative management of the caropmetacarpal arthroplasty of the thumb. J Hand Surg 7:308, 1982.

Hagert, CG, Branemark, PI, Albrektsson, T, Strid, KG, and Irstram, L: Metacarpophalangeal joint replacement with osseointegrated endoprostheses. Scand J Plast Reconstr Surg 20(2):207–218, 1986.

Ho, PK, Jocobs, JL, and Plark, GL: Trapezium implant arthroplasty: Evaluation of a semiconstrained implant. J Hand Surg (Am) 10(5):654–660, 1985.

Hook, WE, and Stanley, JK: The early experience of silastic trapezium implants. J Hand Surg (Br) 1(1):93–97, 1986.

Inglis, AE, Hamlin, C, Sengelmann, RP, and Straub, LR: Reconstruction of the metacarpophalangeal joint of the thumb in rheumatoid arthritis. J Bone Joint Surg (Am) 54(4):704–712, 1972.

Iyer, KM: The results of excision of the trapezium. Hand 13(3):246–250, 1981.

Iyer, KM, and Whitehouse, GH: Arthrography of the metacarpo-scaphoid joint following excision of the trapezium. Hand 13(3):251–256, 1981.

Kleinert, JM, and Lister, GD: Silicone implants. Hand Clin 2(2):271–290, 1986 (review).

Kuarnes, LN, and Reikeras, O: Osteoarthritis of the CME joint of the thumb: An analysis of operative procedures. J Hand Surg (Br) 10(1):117–120, 1985.

Nalebuff, EA: The rheumatoid thumb. Clin Rheum Dis 10(3):589–607, 1984.

Nalebuff, EA, and Garrod, KJ: Present approach to the severely involved rheumatoid wrist. Orthop Clin North Am 15(2):369–380, 1984.

Pellegrini, VD Jr, and Burton, RI: Surgical management of basal joint arthritis of the thumb. Part I. Long-term results of silicone implant arthroplasty. J Hand Surg 11(3):309–324, 1986.

Swanson, AB, and deGroot-Swanson, G: Arthroplasty of the thumb basal joints. Clin Ortho 195:151–160, 1985.

Swanson, AB, and deGroot-Swanson, G: Flexible implant arthroplasty in the rheumatoid metacarpophalangeal joint. Clin Rheum Dis 10(3):609–629, 1984.

Swanson, AB, and deGroot-Swanson, G: Osteoarthritis in the hand. Clin Rheum Dis 11(2):393–420, 1985 (review).

Taleisnik, J: The Wrist. Churchill-Livingston, New York, 1985.

Wilson, RL: Rheumatoid arthritis of the hand. Orthop Clin North Am 17(2):313–343, 1986.

ARTHRODESIS AND PARTIAL FUSIONS

Arthrodesis, or surgical fusion of a joint, is one of the oldest operations for arthritis and, prior to flexible implants, was often the only alternative for severely damaged joints.

So much time and energy are spent trying to maintain mobility in the hand that the idea of an operation that prevents motion permanently often elicits a negative reaction from patients and health professionals alike. But following arthrodesis patients are generally pleased and find that they can do more with a pain-free stable joint than they could with a painful or unstable joint.

Arthrodesis is the treatment of choice in several circumstances and can improve function in severely disabled hands. In cases of mutilans deformity, arthrodesis can prevent the resorption process and maintain the integrity of the bone stock.[67]

In current practice, arthrodesis may be the appropriate procedure to relieve pain, provide stability, and correct nonfunctional deformity in the wrist, PIP, DIP, and thumb joints. In the MCP joints arthrodesis is not recommended because of the need for mobility in these joints and the success of arthroplasty at this level.[68]

Wrist

Arthrodesis of the wrist eliminates flexion and extension but does not affect forearm rotation.[69] The relief of pain and stability of the wrist often result in improved hand function and grip strength. There are basically two clear-cut indications in which arthrodesis is preferred over an arthroplasty: when damage to the carpal bones is so extensive that they cannot accept a prosthesis and when there is loss or rupture of the wrist extensor tendons.[69]

In JRA, arthrodesis is the most common wrist procedure because the intermedullary canals are often not developed and therefore do not have the capacity to accept the prosthesis. Additionally, these patients often develop intercarpal ankylosis, which makes arthrodesis a logical procedure for a severely damaged radiocarpal joint.[70]

If the patient has sufficient bone stock to receive a prosthesis and adequate motor control, the indications for an arthrodesis versus an arthroplasty are factors external to the joint and based on the surgeon's personal preference. Both advantages and disadvantages of the stability provided by an arthrodesis and the mobility afforded by an arthroplasty need to be carefully considered and evaluated in light of the patient's physical status and functional needs.[68,69] For example:

1. If the wrist is painful and has lost considerable mobility an arthrodesis may be considered over an arthroplasty.

2. When both wrists are involved it may be advisable to do an arthrodesis in one wrist for stability and an arthroplasty in the other for motion—although for some pa-

tients it may be preferable to have either procedure bilaterally.

3. For patients who work in vocations with manual labor the stability of a fusion may be desired.

4. If the digital joints are stiff or the proximal upper extremity joints are limited, the motion provided by an arthroplasty may enhance function more than an arthrodesis.

5. For patients who are limited to ambulation with crutches, the stability provided by an arthrodesis is often preferred.

Indications (Definite)

1. Debilitating wrist pain with severe joint destruction.
2. Loss of the wrist extensor muscles.

Occurrence

RA, traumatic arthritis, JRA, and PA.

Surgical Prerequisites

No specific prerequisites.

Surgical Procedure

1. Approach: dorsal longitudinal incision.
2. Synovectomy of the extensor tendons.
3. Excision of cartilage from the distal radius and between the carpal bones.
4. If the procedure is unilateral the wrist is usually fused in neutral. When the procedure is bilateral, one wrist is generally fused in neutral and the other is fused in slight flexion to facilitate self-care.
5. A Steinmann pin or Ross rod is inserted between the second and third metacarpals (or within the third metacarpal), across the carpals, and into the intramedullary canal of the radius. Supplementary fixation (staple) and bone graft may be added.
6. The procedure may be combined with an ulnar head resection (with or without an ulnar head prosthesis) to improve forearm rotation.

Postoperative Management

Average hospitalization: 3 to 5 days.

1. First to third day: Initial immobilization compression bandage with a volar short arm plaster splint. If a drain is used it is removed on the first day.
2. Third day:
   a. Compression bandage exchanged for a forearm cast that allows full flexion of the MCP joints, fingers, and thumb.
   b. Active finger motion is encour-

aged. Techniques for reducing digital edema are applied if needed.
   c. Instruction in ROM exercises for shoulder and elbow.
   d. Patients with bilateral arthritis will need instruction in joint-protection techniques and assistive devices for the nonsurgical hand.
3. Third week:
   a. Short arm cast is converted to a volar plaster or thermoplastic orthosis.
   b. Active finger motion is continued.
   c. Orthosis is worn until roentgenography shows evidence of bony consolidation.

Proximal Interphalangeal Joints

Mobility of the PIP joints is important for dexterity and every effort is made to maintain it. The decision to fuse the PIP joint is based on the type and severity of deformity, the digit involved, the condition of the adjacent joints, and the status of the extensor and flexor tendons and structures.[68]

In the boutonnière and swan-neck deformities the extent of soft tissue contractures is often the determining factor for an arthrodesis. In the early stages, boutonnière deformities may be reducible and correctable with an arthroplasty. However, if the deformity progresses and becomes fixed in flexion greater than 70 to 80 degrees, shortening of the volar structures may prevent joint restoration, and arthrodesis in a functional position may be the only alternative. Similarly, in swan-neck deformity, fibrosis of the surrounding soft tissue may be so severe that restoration of balanced motion may not be possible and surgical fusion in a functional position is the most practical solution.[68]

The digit affected can also influence the surgical decision. Flexion of the PIP joint becomes increasingly important in the digits in a radial to ulnar direction. A primary function of the index finger is pinch prehension against the thumb; it also provides a stable post for thumb opposition in lateral pinch. Both of these functions require only slight to moderate flexion in addition to stability. For each of the consecutive fingers slightly increasing flexion is utilized to maximize functional grasp. Flexion of the ulnar fingers plays a more critical role in tight grasp. For these reasons fusion of the index finger may be less of a handicap than fusion of the little finger.

Another factor that can influence the surgical choice is the degree of mobility present in the MCP joints and secondarily in the DIP joints. The less mobility present in these joints the greater the need for mobility in the PIP joints. The prospect of MCP joint arthroplasty must also be taken into account. When a patient has severe involvement of both the MCP and PIP joints and an MCP implant arthroplasty is indicated (or potential), the length and capacity of the medullary canal is a critical factor and may not be of sufficient length to accommodate prostheses at both levels, necessitating fusion of the PIP joints. Even when it is possible to insert a prosthesis at both levels, most surgeons choose to fuse the destroyed PIP joint when the MCP joint is in need of a replacement.[68]

Indications (Definite)
1. Severe fixed boutonnière or swan-neck deformities.
2. Ruptured flexor tendons.
3. Severe joint or ligamentous destruction.
4. Beginning mutilans deformity.

Occurrence
RA, JRA, traumatic arthritis, PA, and occasionally gout.

Surgical and Functional Goals
Stable motion and relief of pain.

Surgical Prerequisites
No specific prerequisites.

Surgical Procedure
1. Approach: Dorsal curved incision; care is taken to preserve the delicate veins over the PIP joint.
2. The extensor mechanism is split and the collateral ligaments are detached.
3. The bone ends are prepared to achieve contact in the desired position.
4. The bones are fixed with K wires, usually two crossed pins.

Postoperative Management
Average hospitalization: 2 to 5 days (depending on the number of digits involved and the associated procedures).

1. First to third day: Initial immobilization in a volar plaster splint. If multiple digits are operated on, a full hand resting orthosis may be used. Dressing is changed.
2. Protective aluminum splints are worn for 4 to 6 weeks. Volar splints provide the greatest protection but limit function, whereas dorsal splints provide sufficient protection and allow the patient to grasp objects.
3. Activity is limited until there is x-ray evidence of bony consolidation, approximately 8 to 10 weeks.
4. The K wires may be left in the bones indefinitely if they do not cause local tenderness.

Distal Interphalangeal Joints

Arthrodesis is the most frequent surgical procedure performed on the DIP joints. It is used to correct deformity, relieve pain, and provide stability for pinch prehension. It is the procedure of choice in the following conditions.[68]

1. Synovitis can cause bone erosion and laxity of the collateral ligaments resulting in lateral deviation deformity. It can also cause attenuation of the distal attachment of the extensor tendon creating a mallet deformity and possibly a secondary swan-neck deformity.
2. A severe boutonnière deformity can result in a hyperextension deformity of this joint.
3. Rupture of the flexor pollicis longus may render the distal phalanx of the thumb useless for prehension if the joint is hypermobile.
4. Osteophyte formation in osteoarthritis is generally painless, but occasionally it can present with inflammation, severe pain, and limited motion.
5. In osteoarthritis, destruction of the cartilage and formation and collapse of mucoidal cysts may occur on one side of the joint and result in unsightly lateral deviation deformities.

Arthrodesis of the DIP joint is carried out through a dorsal incision and primarily includes removal of articular cartilage from the bone ends and removal of osteophytes in a manner that allows the bones to be approximated at the desired angle (neutral or in 5 to 10 degrees of flexion). The position is maintained with wire fixation until the bone ends fuse together. Distal joint fusions are often performed under digital block anesthesia on an outpatient basis.

Arthrodesis has been the only procedure discussed for the DIP joint because it is the most common. It is possible to perform an arthroplasty on this joint and a condylar prosthesis has been developed; however, its use to date has been limited.

Thumb

When thumb deformities progress to a point at which there is marked instability, relentless pain that limits prehension, or MCP/CMC contractures that limit grasp, an arthrodesis is an effective surgical option.

For the IP joint with severe instability or angulation deformity, arthrodesis in a straight or slightly flexed position is the procedure of choice.[68] An IP joint fusion prevents tip to tip pinch, but the gain in stability usually increases the patient's overall functional ability.

For the MCP joint, it is possible to do an arthroplasty. The decision between this procedure and a fusion depends on the status of the adjacent joints. When there is isolated MCP involvement, a fusion in approximately 15 degrees of flexion provides excellent, pain-free stability for function. However, if there is associated IP joint involvement, then an arthroplasty may be preferred to avoid having a fusion in two adjacent joints.[68]

For the CMC joint, there are several successful arthroplasties available that make fusion of the CMC joint a fairly uncommon procedure. A fusion may be considered for this joint in patients with isolated CMC damage as in cases of traumatic arthritis or severe OA, particularly if the bones are not adequate for an arthroplasty. A fusion may also be considered for patients who have a strenuous vocation in which thumb stability is a key consideration.

In RA, isolated CMC joint involvement is rare. An arthroplasty is generally performed to preserve mobility, in the event the patient may need subsequent fusions of the distal joints. The trapezium implant that works well for OA tends to cause subluxation in patients with RA because of the loss of bone stock in the carpus. For this reason, an alternative type of arthroplasty is performed on the patient with RA. This can be a hemiarthroplasty in which either the base of the metacarpal or part of the trapezium is removed and a Silastic spacer is inserted; or a simple resection of the trapezium is performed to improve the alignment of the metacarpal. Any patient limited by thumb instability or deformity should consider surgical options. The functional outcome is usually excellent.

The postoperative management for arthrodesis of the thumb joints is the same as for fusion of the DIP and PIP joints of the fingers described earlier in this section.

References (Arthrodesis)

67. Nalebuff, EA, and Garrett, J: Opera-glass hand in rheumatoid arthritis. J Hand Surg 1(3):210, 1976.
68. Nalebuff, EA, and Millender, LH: Reconstructive surgery and rehabilitation of the hand. In Kelley, WM et al (eds): Textbook of Rheumatology. WB Saunders, Philadelphia, 1981.
69. Millender, LH, and Nalebuff, EA: Arthrodesis of the rheumatoid wrist. An evaluation of sixty patients and a description of a different surgical technique. J Bone Joint Surg 55A:1026, 1973.
70. Nalebuff, EA, Millender, LH, and Yerid, G: The incidence and severity of wrist involvement in juvenile arthritis. J Bone Joint Surg 54A(4):905, 1972.

Additional Sources (Arthrodesis)

Clayton, ML, and Ferlic, DC: Arthrodesis of the arthritic hand. Clin Orthop 187:89–93, 1984.
Mannerrfelt, L: Surgical treatment of the rheumatoid wrist and aspects of the natural course when untreated. Clin Rheum Dis 10(3):549–570, 1984.
Rayan, GM: Wrist arthrodesis. J Hand Surg 11(3):356–364, 1986.
Speltz, S, Schutt, A, and Beckenbauch, RD: Functional wrist position for wrist arthrodesis. J Hand Surg 8:627, 1983.
Taleisnik, J: Combined radiocarpal arthrodesis and medicarpal (lunocapital) arthroplasty for treatment of RA of the wrist. J Hand Surg 12A:1–8, 1987.
Vahvanen, V, and Tallroth, K: Arthrodesis of the wrist by internal fixation in rheumatoid arthritis: A follow-up of forty-five consecutive cases. J Hand Surg (Am) 9(4):531–536, July 1984.
van Gemert, JG: Arthrodesis of the wrist. A clinical, radiographic, and ergonomic study of 66 cases. Acta Orthop Scand (Suppl) 210:1–146, 1984.

Chapter 30

Elbow Surgery

ULNAR NERVE COMPRESSION
ELBOW SYNOVECTOMY AND RADIAL HEAD RESECTION
  AND REPLACEMENT
TOTAL ELBOW REPLACEMENT SURGERY
CAPITELLO-CONDYLAR ELBOW ARTHROPLASTY
EXCISION OR FASCIAL ARTHROPLASTY

The synovial lining in the elbow is common to both the elbow (humeroradioulnar) joint and the proximal radioulnar joint. Pain and swelling prompt the patient to keep the arm in a comfortable position of flexion and pronation. The typical consequences are contractures of both joints that limit extension and supination. With severe pain and swelling, motion becomes restricted in all planes. (See Chapter 6, Rheumatoid Arthritis, for a discussion on the relationship of elbow contractures to functional ability.)

In the early phases, elbow synovitis is treated conservatively with systemic medications and local steroid injection.[1] For acute flares, ice compresses and orthotic immobilization can be effective for reducing inflammation. When chronic painful synovitis limits function, a person is a candidate for a synovectomy.[1] It can be performed alone but is commonly carried out in conjunction with a radial head resection.[2] Recent studies have shown that in approximately 70 percent of cases, elbow synovectomy is successful in relieving pain and improving function for one to three years. Then, radiographic evidence of joint destruction frequently begins to appear. A synovectomy can buy time, but it is not considered a long-term solution.[2-4]

The total elbow replacement is no longer experimental and has been very successful, especially when performed by surgeons experienced in this area of surgery. However, this procedure has a high rate of complications compared to other joint replacement surgeries and further improvements are needed to make this a more widely predictable and accepted procedure.

Excision arthroplasty, once a common surgery for arthritis, is being done only rarely today and is being supplanted by total joint replacement. It is considered a salvage procedure that relieves pain and allows function (mobility) but reduces stability.[5]

ULNAR NERVE COMPRESSION

One of the consequences of chronic elbow synovitis and a complication of elbow surgery is entrapment of the ulnar nerve.[5-7] Evaluation of ulnar nerve status is important both before and after surgery. Generally, but not always, one of the first indications of nerve compression is the patient's report of paresthesias along the ulnar nerve distribution, palmar and dorsal surfaces of the little finger, the medial half of the ring finger, and ulnar side of the hand.[8] Sensation to the dorsum of the little finger is the key area to test to distinguish between elbow and wrist compression of the ulnar nerve, because the dorsal cutaneous branch is proximal to the wrist. Thus, if the dorsal sensation is diminished, the lesion is at the elbow. If only volar sensation is altered, the compression is at Guyon's canal or more distal. Static and moving 2-point discrimination on the ulnar innervated fingers should be equal to the median innervated digits (providing the patient does not have carpal tunnel syndrome). Postoperative swelling may decrease 2-point sensitivity, but it should affect all digits equally.[9] (On the finger pads, each person has his or her own norm; generally, it is 3 mm, 4 mm, or 5 mm.) In some patients the ulnar fingers have greater sensitivity than the index and thumb digits, which may have thickened skin from pinch prehension. Compression of the ulnar nerve at the elbow can result in weakness of the following muscles: adductor pollicis, flexor pollicis brevis (deep head), all interossei, third and fourth lumbricals, flexor digiti quinti, opponens digiti quinti, abductor digiti quinti, palmaris brevis, flexor digitorum profundus (ring and little finger), and the flexor carpi ulnaris.[6] If there is weakness, one of the first noticeable signs is weakness in pinch and the inability to *adduct* the little and ring fingers and/or slight clawing of these digits. The easiest function to monitor is thumb and index pinch and adduction of the little finger. (See section on ulnar nerve entrapment in Chapter 19, Hand Pathodynamics and Assessment.)

ELBOW SYNOVECTOMY AND RADIAL HEAD RESECTION AND REPLACEMENT

This procedure relieves pain and enhances joint motion by diminishing the humeroradial joint and by removing the diseased synovium from the humeroulnar and proximal radioulnar joints.

Supination and pronation can be limited by either the proximal or distal radioulnar joint. Resection of the radial head improves forearm rotation by eliminating restrictions and incongruities between the radial head and its articulation, the ulna.[2] Swanson has developed a Silastic radial head replacement that reduces the amount of instability that often occurs with this surgery; however, the replacement is not universally used.[9]

Indications

1. Persistent painful synovitis of the elbow joint.

2. Marked limitations of supination and pronation secondary to proximal radioulnar joint disease.

3. Painful subluxation of the head of the radius.

Occurrence

Rheumatoid arthritis, juvenile rheumatoid arthritis, rheumatoid variants, and traumatic arthritis.

Surgical Prerequisites

1. Absence of severe destructive changes in the humeroulnar joint.

2. Collateral ligament stability.

3. The ability and motivation to follow through with postoperative rehabilitation.

Postoperative Management

Average hospitalization: 3 to 6 days.

1. First postoperative day: Initial immobilization with compression bandage and posterior plaster splint or elbow immobilizer positioning the forearm to neutral rotation and the elbow in 90 degrees of flexion.

2. Second day:

a. Active assisted ROM exercises can be started in flexion-extension or pronation-supination.

b. Posterior plaster splint or elbow immobilizer may be used for positioning at night and between exercise periods. A sling may be used during the day for comfort.

c. Active use of the arm is encouraged.

d. Active sustained ROM exercises can be continued in all planes of motion.

e. Active assisted shoulder and hand exercises are started.

TOTAL ELBOW REPLACEMENT SURGERY

Since the 1920s, there have been numerous attempts to relieve pain and increase mobility and function by replacing either the end of the humerus (hemiarthroplasty) or both the end of the humerus and ulna with metal or synthetic material (total elbow replacement [TER]).[2] The hemiarthroplasties have proven more successful with traumatic elbow problems than with chronic arthritis that affects all joint surfaces, and are currently not being used with patients with rheumatoid arthritis.[2] The advent of methylmethacrylate fixation cement in the 1960s expanded the options for securing the prostheses, and now the development of TERs dominates the field.

There are a wide variety of prosthesis designs currently being developed and evaluated in medical centers around the world. Design categories include (1) fully constrained metal hinge replacement; (2) fully constrained metal-to-plastic hinge replacements; (3) flexible elbow replacement; (4) semiconstrained metal to plastic; (5) nonconstrained metal to plastic (with and without intramedullary stems). These are the most common TERs and include the capitello-condylar TER.[2] All of these have proven effective in *some* patients and all have a higher than desirable rate of complications.[10] The main complications continue to be deep wound infections, dislocations, ulnar nerve palsies, and loose prostheses. It is not clear why the elbow is prone to infection, but such factors as corticosteroid therapy, previous surgeries, injections, and the subcutaneous location of the elbow joint all contribute to the risk for infection.[10,11]

Thus, at this time the TER is a viable alternative in the hands of experienced surgeons, but the complication rate needs to be reduced before TER can be widely utilized. Some designs are so new that sufficient long-term follow-up has not been possible, and most are still undergoing design revisions.[2] Therapists interested in a detailed discussion of the above replacements are referred to recent reviews by Morrey[12] and Ewald.[2]

Indications

1. Intractable pain.
2. Destroyed joint.
3. Limitations of elbow motion that prevent self-care.

Occurrence

Rheumatoid arthritis, juvenile rheumatoid arthritis, rheumatoid variants, traumatic arthritis.

CAPITELLO-CONDYLAR ELBOW ARTHROPLASTY

The capitello-condylar TER was developed at the Robert B. Brigham Hospital in 1974. The rehabilitative protocol developed for this surgery has been used for over 8 years and is appropriate for all types of non-hinge TER replacement surgeries (Fig. 30–1).[2] The capitello-condylar TER is a nonconstrained design and requires an intact, soft tissue capsule for stability. A constrained or hinge prosthesis would not have this requirement.

Surgical Prerequisites[2]

1. Sufficient capsular and ligamentous support to maintain alignment. (Patients with a prior excisional or fascial arthroplasty are not candidates for a nonconstrained TER.)
2. Sufficient muscular strength to control the joint.
3. Absence of infection for one year.
4. Adequate bone stock. (Patients with severe osteoporosis or resorption are not candidates.)

Surgical and Functional Goals

The main objective is to have a stable, pain-free elbow with functional ROM. To

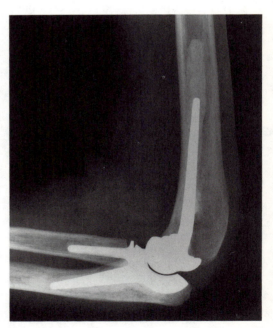

Figure 30–1. Postoperative x-ray film shows placement of a capitello-condylar elbow prosthesis with a radial head replacement. The three intramedullary stems are fixed with acrylic cement. The ulnar component is metal with a polyethylene surface opposing the metal humeral head. On x-ray film the polyethylene appears as a gap between the components. The radial head replacement is not used in all total elbow arthroplasties. (Photo courtesy of Dr. Robert Poss and the Journal of Bone and Joint Surgery.)

date, the average postoperative ROM has been 116 degrees arc. A limitation in extension of 20 to 30 degrees is expected. The ROM should be in the most functional arc.[2] Often the greatest postoperative gains are seen in flexion and pronation rather than extension and supination.[2]

Surgical Procedure[2]

1. Lateral approach between the anconeus and extensor mass.
2. Triceps is partially detached from its ulnar insertion.
3. The extensor mass is elevated from the lateral epicondyle along with the ulnar collateral ligament.
4. The radial head is excised, and synovectomy is performed.
5. The humerus is reamed to accept the fixation stem of the metal component.
6. The ulnar medullary canal is entered and reamed to accept the fixation runners of the polyethylene ulnar replacement.
7. Both components have three major fixation points. These are cemented in place with regard for proper rotation.
8. The soft tissues are reflected back over both epicondylar prominences. The capsule is repaired and the elbow should be able to be flexed to 120 degrees without rupture of the capsule repair.
9. The wound is closed in layers. The triceps is reattached. Both superficial and deep drains are used for 24 hours.

Postoperative Management

Average hospitalization: 5 to 8 days

1. Initially, the elbow is in a compression dressing and positioned with a prefabricated orthosis in comfortable flexion (30 to 40 degrees) and a sling to hold the arm in adduction. The elbow is elevated on pillows to decrease edema.
2. Second or third postoperative day:
   a. Dressing is changed and reduced.
   b. Hand and wrist ROM is started (no forearm rotation). The ulnar nerve is at high risk for being traumatized during surgery or compressed due to swelling or positioning after surgery. Ulnar nerve status should be monitored throughout the postoperative period. (See section on ulnar nerve assessment earlier in this chapter.)
   c. If wound is healing well and drainage has stopped, active assisted elbow ROM exercises (flexion, extension, forearm rotation) are started. During the exercises,

the arm is kept between neutral and internal rotation with the elbow at the side of the body (adduction). The exercises are done out of the sling and orthosis twice a day. Guidelines for supination and pronation vary depending on the surgery. Instruction in relaxation techniques can be helpful in reducing trunk and upper extremity guarding of the surgical extremity. The ultimate ideal goal of therapy is full flexion with no more than a 30-degree flexion contracture. However, this may not be possible if there was a severe preoperative flexion contracture.
   d. Monitor skin integrity daily.
   e. Supine shoulder exercises are started.
3. At the surgeon's discretion the orthosis is used only at night. The sling is continued during the day for comfort only. The arm is allowed out to swing naturally. The most stressful force that can be applied to the prosthesis is lateral torque. This occurs when one reaches out (in abduction), lifts an item, and transports it toward the body with internal rotation of the arm; or when one pushes something away from the body with the hand or forearm using external rotation of the arm. It is lateral torque that is believed to be one of the main causes for loosening of the prosthesis. To reduce stress to the prosthesis and to allow capsular repair during the vulnerable healing period, patients are instructed not to do any activities that can produce lateral torque for 6 weeks. That is, they are instructed to face objects to be lifted and not reach to the side. Specifically, they are instructed to use the surgical extremity with the upper arm in an adducted position; thus, they cannot reach out to the side to pick up something. Methods for dressing, feeding, bathing, and doing housework that incorporate this precaution are reviewed. Depending on the patient, it may take one to four sessions before the patient can demonstrate observance of appropriate precautions without verbal cues from the therapist. It is important that nurses and therapists reinforce precautions with the patient and family.
4. The patient is instructed how to monitor ulnar nerve function and is discharged with a written home program.
5. Sutures are removed. This may be done on an outpatient basis.
6. Some patients prefer to use the sling

during the daytime as a reminder not to reach out. Following a TER, the patient is restricted from returning to racket sports, golf, baseball, and other competitive sports or heavy labor.

7. Most motion is gained through functional use. Home occupational/physical therapy is seldom necessary. Home therapists should be given specific instruction (e.g., no resistance should be applied to the elbow).

EXCISION OR FASCIAL ARTHROPLASTY

This surgery involves excision of the ends of the humerus and the ulna. The raw bone ends are either left exposed or covered with fascia lata from the thigh, skin, or synthetic interpositional material.[5] There is also a Silastic implant (Swanson) that is used as a spacer in conjunction with this surgery.[13] The joint is immobilized for a couple of months postoperatively to encourage tightening of the soft tissues.[13]

It is a radical surgery and in the past was done primarily to restore motion and function to ankylosed joints or to relieve intractable pain. The surgery has worked well for many patients, particularly post-traumatic ankylosis.[14] The main problems with the surgery are that it is difficult to predict the outcome and the joint lacks stability sufficient for crutch or cane ambulation or for strenuous work. Thus, it is not an ideal surgery for patients with lower extremity involvement who may need ambulation aids.[5]

Currently, the treatment of choice for an ankylosed joint is a TER.[2] The excision arthroplasty has current significance in that this procedure is the alternative the patient is left with if a TER fails, for example, due to sepsis, and the prosthesis has to be removed. However, for a patient to have results at least as good as an excision arthroplasty, following failure of a TER, there has to be sufficient length in the bone ends, capsule, and ligaments present.[2] If too many structures have been removed to accommodate the design of the prosthesis, the patient will be left with a completely unstable elbow, which is very difficult to brace.

REFERENCES

1. Geschwend, N: Synovectomy. In Kelley, WM et al (eds): Textbook of Rheumatology, 2nd ed. WB Saunders, Philadelphia, 1985. (Excellent review.)
2. Ewald, FC: Reconstructive surgery and rehabilitation of the elbow. In Kelley, WM et al (eds): Textbook of Rheumatology, 2nd ed. WB Saunders, Philadelphia, 1985.
3. Arthritis Foundation Committee on Evaluation of Synovectomy: Multicenter evaluation of synovectomy on the treatment of rheumatoid arthritis. Arthritis Rheum 20:765, 1977.
4. Brumfield, RH Jr, and Resnick, CT: Synovectomy of the elbow in rheumatoid arthritis. J Bone Joint Surg (Am) 67(1):16–20, January 1985.
5. Dickson, RA, Stein, H, and Bentley, G: Excision arthroplasty of the elbow in rheumatoid disease. J Bone Joint Surg 56B:227, 1987.
6. Nakano, KK: Entrapment neuropathies. In Kelley, WM, et al (eds): Textbook of Rheumatology, 2nd ed. WB Saunders, Philadelphia, 1985.
7. Broudy, AS, Leffert, RD, and Smith, R: Technical problems with ulnar nerve transposition at the elbow: Findings and results of reoperation. J Hand Surg 3(1):85, 1978.
8. Dellon AL: The moving two-point discrimination test: Clinical evaluation of the quickly adapting fiber-receptor system. J Hand Surg 3(5):474, 1978.
9. Bell, JA: Sensibility evaluation. In Hunter, JM, Schneider, LH, Mackin, EJ, and Bell, HA: Rehabilitation of the Hand. CV Mosby, St Louis, 1978, pp 280–283, 289.
10. Levy, RN, Voltz, RG, Kaufer, H et al: Progress in arthritis surgery. Clin Ortho Rel Res 200:299–321, 1985. (Review up to 1985.)
11. Morrey, BF, and Bryan, RS: Infection after total elbow arthroplasty. J Bone Joint Surg 65A:330, 1983.
12. Morrey, BF: The Elbow and Its Disorders. WB Saunders, Philadelphia.
13. Swanson, AB: Flexible Implant Resection Arthroplasty in the Hand and Extremities. CV Mosby, St Louis, 1973.
14. Dee, R: Total replacement arthroplasty of the elbow for rheumatoid arthritis. J Bone Joint Surg 54B:88, 1972.

ADDITIONAL SOURCES

Brumfield, RH, and Volz, RG: Total elbow arthroplasty: A clinical review of 30 cases. Employing the Mayo and HHSC prosthesis. J Clin Orthop 158:137–141, 1981.
Clayton, MK, and Ferlic, DC: Surgery in RA: The elbow. In Boswick, JA Jr (ed): Upper Extremity Surgery and Rehabilitation. Aspen, Rockville, MD, 1986.

Chapter 31

Shoulder Surgery

SHOULDER SYNOVECTOMY, BURSECTOMY, AND
  ACROMIOPLASTY
TOTAL SHOULDER REPLACEMENT

The shoulder is comprised of four joints: **glenohumeral, sternoclavicular, acromioclavicular,** and **scapulothoracic.** Motion is the result of fourteen muscles acting upon the humerus, scapula, and clavicle.[1,2] Mechanically, the shoulder is extremely complex. None of the joints moves independently. They all move together in a synchronous, rhythmic pattern.[2,3] Because of this complexity and the interdependence of the musculoskeletal structures, the postoperative rehabilitation program is critical to the success of the operative procedure. The role of surgery is also influenced by the range of the shoulder motion used in functional activities, the problems inherent in multiple joint involvement and preoperative range of motion (ROM).[4] Approximately 90 degrees of shoulder flexion and abduction and sufficient internal rotation to reach the midline of the body and the opposite axilla are necessary for most functional activities; thus, a person can lose up to 50 percent of shoulder mobility before he or she becomes limited in most activities of daily living. Another factor is that in rheumatoid arthritis, synovitis of the shoulder often comes later in the disease after there is involvement of the hands, feet, and knees.[4] The greatest gains in improving the patient's functional ability often come from surgery of hands and weight-bearing joints. By the time the patient is most concerned about the shoulder, there is severe loss and damage not only to the joint but also to the surrounding musculotendinous support structures.[4]

For patients with rheumatoid arthritis, the functional limitations imposed by a painful and disabled shoulder are dependent upon the involvement of the neck, elbow, and wrist. If these joints have good mobility, the patient will probably be able to do all self-care and daily activities in which reach and lifting can be done unilaterally (e.g., driving). Most patients with shoulder limitations are able to feed themselves, wash their face, shave, and do hair care as long as they have good neck and elbow mobility. If there is severe bilateral shoulder involvement and cervical spine limitations the patient will probably have difficulty in some self-care activities. For patients with multiple joint involvement there is no way of predicting the functional limitations imposed by a painful shoulder without evaluating their actual performance.

Currently, the most common surgeries being performed for problems of the shoulder related to arthritis include synovectomy, bursectomy (with or without an acromioplasty), and total joint arthroplasty.[2,4]

Most cases of bursitis and tendinitis respond to conservative management consisting of anti-inflammatory medication, ice/heat therapy, phonophoresis, and steroid injections.[3] Occasionally, some patients develop a severe proliferative synovitis in their subacromial bursa. If the glenohumeral joint is spared, patients can receive excellent results from a bursectomy.[4] In some patients, rheumatoid disease weakens the rotator cuff so that the humeral head continually rides up and impinges upon the acromion, causing pain and further wear on the rotator cuff. Partial removal and shaping of the acromion (acromioplasty) can eliminate this impingement process. In rheumatoid arthritis an acromioplasty is usually done in conjunction with a bursectomy, synovectomy, or total joint replacement.[2,4]

Total shoulder replacement (TSR) surgery is recommended for patients with severe damage to both surfaces of their glenohumeral joints, the most common sequela in adult or juvenile rheumatoid arthritis.[4] A humeral head replacement is available for patients who have damage to the humeral surface only, for example, secondary to trauma or osteonecrosis (aseptic necrosis).[4]

SHOULDER SYNOVECTOMY, BURSECTOMY, AND ACROMIOPLASTY

This procedure is limited to the patient with severe, predominantly bursal shoulder involvement without damage to the surfaces of the glenohumeral joint. The subacromial bursa normally provides a cushion between the head of the humerus and the acromion process. Chronic bursitis may result in swelling and thickening and the production of fibrin bodies within the sac separating the humerus from the acromion, thus preventing elevation of the humerus. The surgery eliminates pain from this source and improves motion and function.[4] Neer recommends a 6-month postoperative exercise program to obtain optimal results.[4]

If there is also weakness of the rotator cuff, an acromioplasty is also done.

Indications
1. Thickened subacromion bursa that is nonresponsive to conservative management.

Occurrence
Rheumatoid arthritis, juvenile rheumatoid arthritis, osteoarthritis, and rheumatoid variants.

Surgical Prerequisites
1. Preserved glenohumeral joint cartilage.

Surgical Procedure (Neer Method)[4]
1. Approach: Across the shoulder from the acromion to the coracoid.
2. The deep fascia is incised and the anterior deltoid is split longitudinally. Part of the deltoid is detached from the acromion.
3. If there is involvement of the acromioclavicular joint, 2 cm of the clavicle may be removed.
4. The clavipectoral fascia is divided.
5. Traction is placed on the arm so the rotator cuff can be inspected and any sharp edges or spurs on the acromion can be detected.
6. If the rotator cuff appears damaged from impingement against the acromion, an anterior acromioplasty is performed (removal of the anterior edge with beveling of the undersurface).
7. The bursa is excised. (The axillary nerve is at the greatest risk in this surgery.)
8. The subscapularis is detached. The inferior capsule is released and synovectomy of the glenohumeral joint and the sheath of the long head of the biceps is performed.
9. The subscapularis is reattached but may be lengthened by a Z-plasty if it is contracted.
10. The capsule is left open and the deltoid is repaired. The wound is closed and a drain is used for 24 hours.

Postoperative Management[2,4]
Average hospitalization: 5 to 7 days.

1. Initially, the patient is in a voluminous dressing. Patients with preoperative shoulder stiffness are placed in an abduction orthosis.
2. Second day: Dressing is changed and reduced. ROM exercises to the hand and elbow are started.
3. First week (approximately): When wound healing permits, passive ROM to maintain shoulder rotation and elevation are started two to three times a day. Pendulum exercises with the orthosis on are begun when tolerated.
4. Second week: Gentle isometric exercises are started. Active and resistive exercises are delayed until the reattached muscles have fully healed, approximately three weeks.
5. Third week: The orthosis can be discontinued if ROM can be maintained.

TOTAL SHOULDER REPLACEMENT

Total joint replacement surgery is indicated when chronic pain and immobility secondary to glenohumeral joint destruction limit functional ability.[5]

The joint prosthesis most frequently used in this country is the Neer prosthesis (nonconstrained), originally developed in 1973. The Neer prosthesis consists of a metal humeral head with intramedullary fixation stem. The glenoid component is made of polyethylene and fixed with acrylic cement. New metal-backed glenoid components with polyethylene liners have recently been developed to provide greater humeral contact for severely damaged joints. They function for the humeral head in an acetabulum-like manner (Fig. 31–1).[4]

In the shoulder, neither shape of articulation (bone) nor ligaments provide stability. The function of the shoulder after the prosthesis is implanted depends upon the muscles.[4] The glenoid and humeral components are not connected. Therefore, the stability and function of the shoulder following arthroplasty are dependent upon soft tissue reconstruction and rehabilitation to achieve results.[6]

In patients with mild to moderate rheumatoid arthritis in the shoulder and with good rotator cuff as well as surrounding muscles, the hoped-for results are pain-free stable motion, near-full functional use, ROM (flexion and abduction) of about 150 degrees, and nearly full rotation. For patients with severely damaged shoulders, pain relief and functional ROM are hoped-for results.[4] However, for some of these patients, only pain is relieved and active motion may remain severely limited.

Neer reports that only 4 of 194 patients with TSRs felt they had not benefitted from

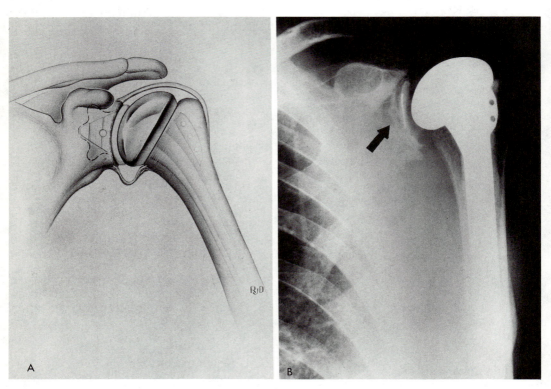

Figure 31–1. The illustration (*A*) and the x-ray film (*B*) show the standard long head total shoulder resurfacing unit. The polyethylene glenoid component is anchored with acrylic cement (*arrow*). The metal humeral head has an intramedullary fixation stem, which does not require cement. The humeral stem is available in three diameters and lengths. (From Neer, CS II,[4] with permission.)

the surgery. The main complications were postoperative dislocation in 4 patients and rotator cuff tears in 5 patients.[7] Cofield, on the other hand, did not have any dislocations in his follow-up of 73 patients receiving the Neer prosthesis. However, loosening of the glenoid component was a problem in 8 patients and 80 percent of all patients had radiographic evidence of lucent lines around the glenoid component, suggesting fixation problem.[8]

Indications

Debilitating pain and damage to both the humeral head and glenoid articular surfaces.

Occurrence

Rheumatoid arthritis, juvenile rheumatoid arthritis, osteoarthritis, traumatic arthritis, avascular necrosis, radiation necrosis, and rotator cuff arthropathy.[7,9]

Surgical Prerequisites[4]

1. Absence of infection.
2. Adequate bone stock to hold the prosthesis.
3. Absence of neurological impairment to the shoulder muscles. (If there is neurological impairment, the goals of surgery are reduced to simply pain relief.)

Surgical Procedure

1. Approach: The incision is over the deltopectoral groove, from the clavicle to near the deltoid insertion.
2. The deltoid is retracted, clavipectoral fascia is divided, and the subscapularis tendon is divided.
3. The capsule is released anteriorly and inferiorly. (The biceps is left intact.)
4. The humeral head is rotated into the wound. Diseased synovium is removed from the capsule and bursa. The humeral head is excised at the margin of the articular surface. (On rough edges, osteophytes or granulation tissue is removed from the bicipital groove at this time.)
5. The medullary canal of the humerus is reamed to receive the fixation stem. A trial prosthesis is used to determine proper

fit, length, and angle of retroversion (40 degrees).
6. Acromioplasty and acromioclavicular arthroplasty are carried out if needed.
7. The rotator cuff tendons are released from adhesions.
8. The humeral head is inserted; ideally, it fits snugly and cement is not required. In patients with severe rheumatoid arthritis, the medullary canals are often too soft to hold the stem firmly.
9. The soft tissue repair around the implant is considered of equal importance to the orientation and seating of the prosthesis. The rotator cuff and subscapularis tendons are reattached. (If the subscapularis is tight, it may be lengthened with a Z-plasty.) The wound is closed and two drains are used for 24 hours to prevent hematoma.

Postoperative Management[4,10−12]

Average hospitalization: 5 to 10 days.
1. Initially the shoulder is in a voluminous compression bandage. An abduction orthosis may be used if the rotator cuff is repaired. If the splint is of thermoplastic material, it is usually made preoperatively so that it can be fitted by the surgeon in the operating room.
2. The postoperative rehabilitation program is the same as that described for synovectomy and acromioplasty except for the following:
    a. If the deltoid is *not* detached from the clavicle, active shoulder exercises can be started during hospitalization.
    b. If one of the larger glenoid components is used, the abduction orthosis is not indicated.
3. a. By discharge day, patients are performing a daily exercise program, including supine exercises, isometric exercises, self-assisted pulleys, and pendulum exercises.
    b. A sling may be used for comfort.
    c. There may be some restrictions to external rotation due to subscapularis repair.
    d. Patients often make gains up to 1 year postoperatively. The slow rate of progress can be frustrating for them.

REFERENCES

1. Bateman, JE: The Shoulder and Neck. WB Saunders, Philadelphia, 1972.
2. DePalma, AF: Surgery of the Shoulder, 2nd ed. JB Lippincott, Philadelphia, 1973.
3. Bland, JH, Merrit, JA, and Boushey, DR: The painful shoulder. Semin Arthritis Rheum 7(1), 1977.
4. Neer, CS II: Reconstructive surgery and rehabilitation of the shoulder. In Kelley, WM et al (eds): Textbook of Rheumatology, 2nd ed. WB Saunders, Philadelphia, 1985.
5. Herdon, JH, and Hubbard, LF: Total joint replacement in the upper extremity. Surg Clin North Am 63:715, 1983.
6. Levy, RN, Voly, RG, and Jaufer, H: Progress in arthritis surgery. Clin Ortho Rel Res 200:299–321, 1985.
7. Neer, CS, Watson, KC, and Stanton, FJ: Recent experience in total shoulder replacement. J Bone Joint Surg 64A(3):319–337, 1982.
8. Cofield, RH: Total shoulder arthroplasty with Neer prosthesis. J Bone Joint Surg 66A:899, 1984.
9. Neer, CS, Craig, EV, and Fukuda, H: Cuff tear arthroplasty. J Bone Joint Surg 65A:1232, 1983.
10. Neer, CS II: Arthroplasty of the Shoulder: Neer Technique. (Illustrated guide for surgical and postoperative therapy.) Available from 3M Corporation, Orthopedic Products—Surgical Products Division, 3M Center, St Paul, MN 55101.
11. Hughes, MA, and Neer, CS II: Glenohumeral joint replacement and postoperative rehabilitation. Phys Ther 55:850, 1975.
12. Paradis, DK, and Ferlic, DC: Shoulder arthroplasty in RA. Phys Ther 55:157, 1975.

ADDITIONAL SOURCES

Amstutz, HC, Sew Hoy, AL, and Clarket, IC: UCLA anatomical total shoulder arthroplasty. Clin Orthop 155:7–20, 1981.

Clayton, ML, Ferlic, DC, and Jeffers, PD: Prosthetic arthroplasties of the shoulder. Clin Orthop April(164):184–191, 1982.

DeJean, J, Berg, PJ, and Gottlieb, R: Total shoulder replacement: Therapeutic considerations. OT Forum 2(10):19–22, March 5, 1986.

Ferlic, DC, and Clayton, ML: Rheumatoid disease of the shoulder. In Boswick, JA Jr (ed): Upper Extremity Surgery and Rehabilitation. Aspen, Rockville, MD, 1986.

Neer, CS: Unconstrained shoulder arthroplasty. Instructional Course Lecture 34:278–286, 1985.

Nitz, AJ: Physical therapy management of the shoulder. Phys Ther 66(12):1912–1919, 1986.

Resnick, D: Shoulder pain. Orthop Clin North Am 1:81–97, January 1983 (review).

Souter, WA: The surgical treatment of the rheumatoid shoulder. Ann Acad Med Singapore 12(2):243–255, April 1983.

Swanson, AB, deGroot-Swanson, G, Leonard, J et al: Upper limb joint replacement. In Nickel, V (ed): Orthopaedic Rehabilitation. Churchill-Livingston, New York, 1982, pp 525–547.

Swanson, AB, deGroot-Swanson, G, Maupin, BK, Wei, JN, and Khalil, MA: Bipolar implant shoulder arthroplasty. Orthopedics 9(3):343–351, March 1986.

Chapter 32

Spinal Surgery

CERVICAL SPINE
ATLANTOAXIAL SUBLUXATION
THORACIC AND LUMBAR SPINE

CERVICAL SPINE

Subluxation of the cervical spine is common in rheumatoid arthritis and juvenile rheumatoid arthritis.[1] This is in contrast to degenerative joint disease in which the most frequent condition seen is osteophytic formation impinging on the neural structures or limiting apophyseal motion.

Fortunately, in the inflammatory arthritides, the majority of problems related to subluxation can be managed with conservative measures such as medications, pillows, joint protection, exercise, relaxation techniques, collars, and traction.[2] Surgical fusion is indicated when **myelopathy** (spinal cord disorder) is present and not responsive to conservative measures or if there is persistent debilitating pain.[1,2] When osteophytes create neurological impairment, surgical removal of the osteophytes or spinal fusion is indicated. Patients with ankylosing spondylitis occasionally develop cervical ankylosis in a nonfunctional position, necessitating a cervical osteotomy to correct or reduce the deformity.[1]

ATLANTOAXIAL SUBLUXATION

The unique anatomy of the **atlantoaxial joint** makes it particularly vulnerable to damage and subluxation in the presence of inflammatory joint disease.[1]

There are two **synovial joints** between the occipital bone and the atlas (C-1). These joints primarily permit nodding of the head. Rotation of the head and atlas takes place upon the **axis** (C-2) by means of four articulating surfaces—two large joints on each lateral mass and two small joints on the anterior and posterior sides of the odontoid process (dens) between the atlas and the transverse ligament that maintains the alignment of the **odontoid process** within the atlas. These two small **atlanto-odontoid joints** are critical because their location allows synovitis directly to erode and weaken the odontoid process and the adjacent transverse ligament that secures the position of the odontoid process.[3] If this ligament becomes stretched or attenuated (ruptured), subluxation of the atlas on the axis occurs. The **atlas** differs from other vertebrae, in that it is simply a ring of bone. Within that ring, the spinal cord occupies one-third of the space, the odontoid and transverse ligament occupy one-third of the space, and the remaining one-third of the space is unoccupied. This extra amount of space allows a considerable amount of subluxation to take place before the odontoid actually impinges on the spinal cord (Fig. 32–1).[3]

Patients with atlantoaxial subluxation present with pain and tenderness in the upper cervical spine and radiation of pain to the suboccipital area, aggravated by full neck flexion or extension. They may have paresthesias or Lhermitte's sign (electricity-like pain radiating into the extremities with neck flexion).[1,2] They may also have a feeling of weakness and instability.[2] Occasion-

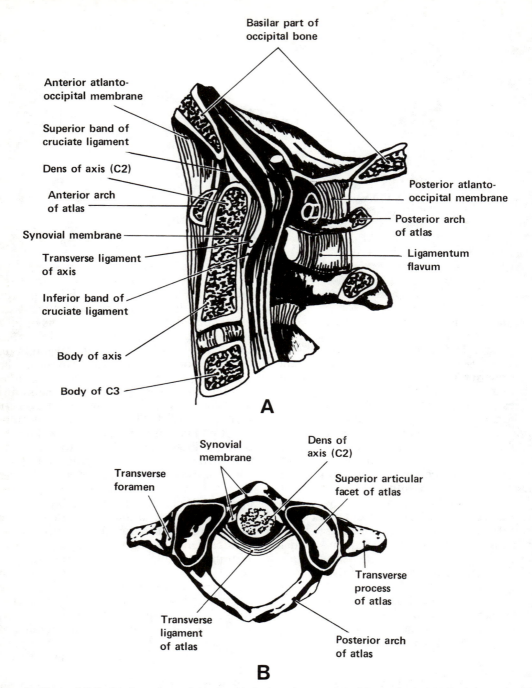

Basilar part of
occipital bone

Anterior atlanto-
occipital membrane

Superior band of
cruciate ligament

Dens of axis (C2)

Anterior arch
of atlas

Synovial membrane

Transverse ligament
of axis

Inferior band of
cruciate ligament

Body of axis

Body of C3

Posterior atlanto-
occipital membrane

Posterior arch
of atlas

Ligamentum
flavum

A

Synovial
membrane

Dens of
axis (C2)

Transverse
foramen

Superior articular
facet of atlas

Transverse
process
of atlas

Transverse
ligament
of atlas

Posterior arch
of atlas

B

Figure 32–1. *(A)* Sagittal section of the first (atlas) and second (axis) cervical vertebrae is depicted here. Note how the dens of the axis fits into the atlas. *(B)* Superior view of the articulation of the atlas and the dens of the axis is illustrated. The transverse ligament of the atlas maintains the alignment of the dens. Inflammatory infiltration of this ligament and subsequent weakening can result in C1-2 subluxation and impingement of the dens on the spinal cord. (From Polly, H, and Hunder, G: Physicial Examination of the Joints, 2nd ed. WB Saunders, Philadelphia, 1978, with permission.)

ally, the patients are able to feel the bones sublux, stating it feels like their head will "slip off."[2] Compression of either of the vertebral arteries may cause visual disturbance (diplopia, blurring), loss of equilibrium, tinnitus, dizziness, or lightheadedness.[4,5] Neurological symptoms do not have to be present.[6] If they are present, they can be multiple and varied, and may include any of the following: occipital neuralgia, upper motor neuron symptoms, altered reflexes, or quadriparesis.[4-8] Subjective sensation may be altered, producing feelings of paresthesia, numbness, heat, and cold. (These symptoms need to be distinguished from fibromyalgia, anxiety, and carpal tunnel syndrome.) Bulbar disturbance can be sudden and fatal or it may present with abnormal swallowing or phonation.[4]

Once frank symptoms of cord compression are evident, the only measures that will help are skeletal halo traction and cervical fusion.[4,6,7] Cervical collars and intermittent halter traction are usually not sufficient to reduce subluxation. Halo traction is used preoperatively on a frame bed or in a halo wheelchair to reduce subluxations and myelopathic changes.[4,7]

If the subluxation can be reduced, the patient may need a cervical collar for 3 to 4 months following surgery. However, if the bones cannot be realigned through grafting, wiring, or cementing, it may be necessary for the patient to wear a halo vest apparatus to provide adequate immobilizaion of the fusion.[2,4,7] Occupational therapy assessment of function while the patient is in halo traction is often critical for determining the position of fusion in severely disabled patients. Postoperative therapy includes gentle active range-of-motion (ROM) muscle strengthening, ambulation training, and possibly dexterity and sensory re-education. Patients in collars may need assistive activities of daily living (ADL) equipment for self-care to allow accommodation of the neck restriction. For example, a patient with severe shoulder limitations may not be able to comb his or her hair with the neck erect. Because patients with rheumatoid arthritis are often severely involved throughout at the time of cervical fusion, the ability to reach the hand to the mouth can be affected when straightening the neck in halo body jacket apparatus. These patients may require mobile arm supports to regain this function during the postoperative period.

Fortunately, the halo and vest traction devices are seldom needed, for they can be very restrictive, especially to someone disabled in other areas. Patients with these devices often need advice, equipment, and counseling in all areas of ADL. Acquiring a comfortable sleeping position is often a major challenge. Some patients have found it helpful to place a Trueze Cervipillo between their neck and the posterior two bars for support.

Devices such as reading racks can make reading a feasible and comfortable leisure activity. It is important to keep in mind that patients with fused necks have a restricted peripheral view, so they must turn their entire body to see to the side. This is not only inefficient energy-wise, but also painful for those with stiff joints or limited ROM. One of the most valuable home aids for these patients is a comfortable, safe chair with a swivel base. This provides an effortless rotational ability to participate in conversations and to view activities around the house. In other words, a swivel chair in the living room would allow these patients to turn and see what was happening in the kitchen without having to get up. This is particularly helpful for patients with small children or grandchildren in their care. (Executive office chairs with the casters removed work well for this purpose and often can be purchased at reasonable cost at used office furniture stores.) If the patient returns to driving, a wide extension for the rear-view mirror and side mirrors need to be used to ensure adequate peripheral vision. (These can be purchased at auto part and supply stores.)

THORACIC AND LUMBAR SPINE

In patients with spondyloarthropathies, severe dysfunctional spinal deformity can often be corrected with **spinal osteotomy.** Other than this procedure, surgery for the lower spine is the same as for nonrheumatic conditions such as degenerative or herniated disc.

REFERENCES

1. Simmons, EH: Surgery of the spine in rheumatoid arthritis and ankylosing spondylitis. In Cruss, RL, and Mitchell, NS (eds): Surgery of Rheumatoid Arthritis. JB Lippincott, Philadelphia, 1971.
2. Thomas, WH: Surgical management of the rheumatoid cervical spine. Orthop Clin North Am 6(3):793, 1975.
3. Jackson, R: The Cervical Syndrome, 4th ed. Charles C Thomas, Springfield, IL, 1977.
4. Lipson, SJ: Rheumatoid arthritis of the cervical spine. Clin Ortho Rel Res (182):143–149, 1984.
5. Fielding, JW, and Bjorkengren, AG: Surgery for arthritis of the cervical spine, Chapter 121. In Kelley, WM et al: Textbook of Rheumatology, 2nd ed. WB Saunders, Philadelphia, 1985.
6. Pellicci, PM, Ranawat, CS, Tsairis, P, and Bryan, WS: A prospective study of the progression of rheumatoid arthritis of the cervical spine. J Bone Joint Surg 63A:342, 1981.
7. Conaty, JP, and Mongan, ES: Cervical fusion in rheumatoid arthritis. J Bone Joint Surg 63A:1218, 1981.
8. Weiner, S, Bassett, L, and Spiegel, T: Superior, posterior and lateral displacement of C1 in rheumatoid arthritis. Arthritis Rheum 25:1378, 1982.

Ferguson, RJ, and Caplan, LR: Cervical spondylitic myelopathy. Neurol Clin 3(2):373–382, 1985 (review).
Fisher, SV et al: Cervical orthoses effect on cervical spine motion: Roentgenographic and goniometric method of study. Arch Phys Med Rehabil 58:109, 1977.
Hart, DL, Johnson, RM, Simmons, EF, and Owen, J: Review of cervical orthoses. Phys Ther 58(7):857, 1978.
Johnson, RM et al: Cervical orthoses: A study comparing their effectiveness in restricting cervical motion in normal subjects. J Bone Joint Surg 59A(3), April 1977.
Komusi, T, Munro, T, and Harth, M: Radiologic review: The rheumatoid cervical spine. Semin Arthritis Rheum 14(3):187–195, 1985 (review).
Liddel, DB: Anterior cervical discectomy—A basis for planning nursing care. J Neurosci Nurs 18(1):29–35, 1986.
Ranawat, CS et al: Cervical spine fusion in rheumatoid arthritis. J Bone Joint Surg (Am) 61(77):1003, 1979.

ADDITIONAL SOURCES

Althoff, B, and Goldie, IF: Cervical collars in rheumatoid atlanto-axial subluxation: A radiographic comparison. Ann Rheum Dis 39:485, 1980.

Chapter 33

Hip Surgery

TOTAL HIP ARTHROPLASTY

The **hip joint** is a large joint highly dependent upon the shape of the articulation for stability, rather than ligamentous support like the knee or muscular support like the shoulder.[1]

Chronic synovitis of the hip results in increased intra-articular pressure pain and diminished cartilage. Hypertrophic synovium (pannus) gets trapped between the joint surfaces, increasing cartilage wear and limiting motion. Secondary muscle spasm and fibrosis of the capsule limit motion even further.[2] Subchondral cysts may appear and then collapse, leaving irregularities in the femoral head. In severe rheumatoid arthritis (RA), the head of the femur may push the softened acetabulum into the pelvic cavity, a condition referred to as **protrusio acetabulae.**[2] In both osteoarthritis (OA) and RA, osteophyte formation occurs and can restrict motion.[2]

Flexion, adduction, and external rotation contractures are the most common deformities seen in the hip, and they can result from four factors: flexion, adduction, and external rotation of the hip is the position that reduces intra-articular pressure and provides the greatest comfort, and therefore it is the position assumed at rest;[2] hip pain can produce spasm of the associated flexor and adductor muscles; patients with hip pain avoid walking or standing and all sitting activities encourage a flexion deformity; constant flexion positioning allows the strong anterior iliofemoral ligament (referred to as the "Y" ligament) to become contracted in a shortened position. Full hip extension may occur only when the patient does specific stretching exercises. Lying prone daily (see Chapter 28) is a valuable conservative as well as postoperative measure for maintaining or improving hip extension.[3]

In the hip, the weight-bearing forces are the primary stress factors that aggravate the synovitis in RA and wear out the cartilage in OA.[1] It is estimated that a force equal to four times body weight is exerted at the hip joint when a person is weight bearing on one extremity, for example, during ambulation and climbing stairs. Therefore, a critical aspect of conservative management is body weight reduction and the use of ambulation aids to relieve stress across the joint.[1,2]

All health professionals (and patients) should be aware that the cane or crutch should be used in the hand *opposite* the painful hip (or knee). Thus, when a person leans to use the cane, the center of gravity is shifted over the good hip, reducing the weight borne by the affected hip. If the cane is used on the painful side, body weight is shifted over the painful joint during ambulation, increasing pain and producing a more abnormal gait.[1,2]

Patients with progressive hip pain that interferes with daily activities despite proper medication and physical therapy are considered candidates for hip surgery.

TOTAL HIP REPLACEMENT ARTHROPLASTY

The total hip replacement arthroplasty (THR) is by far the most common hip surgery for arthritis. There are now three types of fixation available for the femoral component of the total hip prosthesis: (1) cemented, (2) porous-coated prosthesis (referred to as the cementless THR), and (3) press-fit fixation (also without cement). The acetabular component may be cemented or press fit in place. The only other common surgery for arthritis of the hip is an osteotomy done for selected patients with OA. Synovectomies are rarely done because of the high risk of osteonecrosis of the femoral head[3] and the fact that they need to be done early to be effective. Most patients with severe hip pain show radiographic cartilage changes.

The **total hip replacement (THR)** with cemented metal femoral stem and plastic acetabular component (Fig. 33–1) was developed in England by Sir John Charnley in 1961. It was first performed in the United States in 1968.[3] It was estimated that during 1985 between 300,000 and 400,000 THRs were performed worldwide, with approximately 100,000 of these occurring in the United States.[4] THR competes with coronary bypass surgery as the most successful surgical procedure for relieving pain and disability on a major scale.[4] It is considered to have an overall success rate of greater than 90 percent. In one British review of 1,000 patients, 97 percent reported that they were highly satisfied.[5] In another study comparing work disability before and after THR, it was found that 54 percent of the patients who were totally disabled before the surgery were fit to return to work after the surgery.[6]

The main complications of the THR are loosening of the components, particularly loosening years after the surgery, and infection.[7] When loosening occurs, an attempt is made to revise the surgery. This is successful approximately 70 to 80 percent of the time.[7] Since micromotion of an implant within its skeletal bed can give rise to pain with usage, pain is the first clinical sign of the component loosening.[4] A radiolucent line around the component is often the first harbinger of the loosening process. If a person continues to have pain and loosening after multiple revisions with loss of bone stock, there may be no further options and the patient is left with a painful hip. If deep sepsis occurs, the component usually has to be removed. In the past, this precluded revision and the patient was left with a totally unstable hip, referred to as **Girdlestone procedure.** Ambulation was ungainly and possible only with a crutch or cane.[7] In most cases it is now possible to reimplant a prosthesis successfully after the infection is gone. For some people with OA postoperative heterotropic bone formation around the component has created restrictions. The use of radiation treatment postoperatively has proven successful in preventing formation of heterotropic bone.[8,9]

The success of the THR is greatly influenced by patient selection. Clearly, elderly patients who are less active due to another disability of age put less strain on the components and have the best results.[10] Men under the age of 60 with monoarticular hip OA have a high rate of failure because once the problem joint is fixed many become unrestricted in their activities and resume an active life-style.[11,12] Obesity also creates a risk for loosening of components.[4]

If the femoral stem becomes loose, removal of the prosthesis and the cement is a difficult procedure and, as mentioned, does

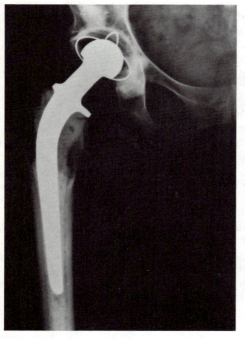

Figure 33–1. Postoperative x-ray film shows placement of total hip prosthesis. The metal femoral head articulates with a polyethylene acetabular component. Both the femoral stem and acetabular cup are cemented in place. (Courtesy of Dr. Robert Poss and the Journal of Bone and Joint Surgery.)

not have as high a success rate as the primary surgery. In the younger patient, under 60 years of age, the odds are that the cemented THR will not last a lifetime and will require a difficult revision in 10 to 20 years.

The use of the porous-coated femoral stem is the latest attempt to develop a prosthesis that will biologically fixate in the bone without the use of cement. The porous covering allows tissue ingrowth, creating the fixation. This surgery is considered experimental and is controlled by the Federal Drug Administration at this time because it is new (the first ones were used in the late 1970s), and there is limited information on long-term results. However, it is considered the surgery of choice for younger patients since failure leaves the option of using a cemented stem.[13–16] The main complications of the surgery are incomplete or insufficient fixation and infection. As this prosthesis is used on younger people, questions arise about the effect of natural changes in the medullary canals caused by aging and the long-term impact of the metallic ions from the coating being released into adjacent tissue.[4] Postoperative rehabilitation takes longer than for the cemented prosthesis, requiring 12 weeks of partial weight bearing. This means that it also takes longer for total relief of pain.

Total hip surface replacement was an alternative to THR that received attention a few years ago.[17] This procedure involves capping the femoral head with a metal surface and enlarging and resurfacing the acetabulum with plastic. However, it is no longer being performed by most orthopedists in the United States because of poor results. The major risks are osteonecrosis of the femoral head under the metal cap and loosening of the acetabular component.

Functional and Surgical Goals[3,18]

Postsurgical expectations include relief of hip pain, joint stability, and increased range of motion (ROM; ideally zero degrees extension and 100 degrees flexion). Restoration of hip motion improves gait and alleviates stress from the back and knees.

Surgical Prerequisites

1. Adequate bone stock for seating of the prosthesis. (If inadequate it can be autografted or allografted.)

2. No current sepsis anywhere else in the body.

3. Competent abductor mechanism.

4. Intact joint sensation.

Surgical Procedure

1. Approach: lateral, posterior, or a combination incision. (Rarely is an anterior approach used; the anterior approach requires different postoperative precautions.)

2. Capsulectomy or capsulotomy.

3. Greater trochanter may or may not be removed. (It is typically not removed in primary surgeries and is removed in revisions.)

4. Acetabulum remodeled: polyethylene prosthetic cup may be cemented or press fit in place.

5. Femoral head is excised, the shaft is broached, and the metal prosthesis is cemented in place with methylmethacrylate (acrylic cement) or press fit in place.

6. If greater trochanter is osteotomized, it is reattached with wire sutures or bands.

7. When bilateral THR is indicated, a 1- to 2-week interval between surgeries is recommended.[2,18] This period is longer for cementless THRs.

Postoperative Physical Therapy [3, 19–23]

For adult THR with posterolateral approach, average hospitalization: 5 to 7 days.

1. First postoperative day:

   a. Initiation of isometric strengthening exercises for knee and hip extensors (taught in the preoperative strengthening program).

   b. Instruction in proper postoperative positioning. Bed positioning varies; some facilities use a balanced suspension or pillow suspension for 24 hours. Other facilities use an abduction pillow.

   c. Instruction in calf-pumping exercises to prevent venous stasis.

2. Second day to discharge:

   a. Instruction in postoperative precautions:

   (1) No side-lying on nonoperated side without pillow between legs to prevent adduction.

   (2) No hip adduction past neutral.

   (3) No hip flexion past 90 degrees. (Some facilities advocate 60 degrees as the limit to provide some interpretive leeway with the expectation that the patient will not exceed 90 degrees during functional ac-

tivities. Others recommend the "knee should never be higher than the hip.")

    b. Hip ROM exercises are started.

    c. The patient begins sitting at the side of the bed, feet dangling.

    d. Instruction in transfer training. Sitting to tolerance in a chair at least 24 inches high. (This is for an average-height person; it is too high for a short person.)

    e. Independent partial weight bearing (≤ 50 percent). Ambulation with assistive equipment on level ground and on stairs. If the trochanter is removed or a cementless prosthesis is used, weight-bearing on the operated side is limited. Patients are instructed to use ambulation aids to ensure partial weight bearing on the surgical hip for 2 to 3 months.

    f. Exercises to increase ROM and strengthen the hip and knee muscles are started. Patients are instructed in prone lying and home programs.

    g. Stationary bicycles may be used to increase ROM and strength. (Items d and e may be done on an outpatient or home therapy basis.)

    h. Patients are discharged partial weight bearing. Patients with cemented THRs may be progressed to a cane at 6 weeks. Patients with cementless THRs remain partial weight bearing for 12 weeks.

    i. Ideally, the patient is independent in performing ROM and strengthening exercises, prone lying, partial weight bearing ambulation, and self-care. When this is not possible, a family member may be instructed how to assist the patient, or home or outpatient therapy may be indicated.

After Discharge

Home program for graded strengthening of hip flexors, extensors, and abductors and to maintain ROM. Use of a stationary bicycle is encouraged.

For THR (Cement Fixation) for Children with Juvenile Rheumatoid Arthritis

THR for children is not a common procedure. Children's Hospital in Los Angeles has the largest series of children with this procedure. The postoperative protocol, developed by the physical therapy department and Dr. Joseph Isaacson, differs from the one described above in the following: (1) flexion is restricted to 45 degrees initially and to 60 degrees at the end of the first week. (2) At approximately 5 to 7 days, children with severe involvement are transferred to the rehabilitation service for an additional 6 to 8 weeks of therapy, where pool therapy is an important part of their treatment. (3) All instruction and therapy activities are age related.

Postoperative Occupational Therapy[24-26]

    1. Preoperative: Evaluation, instruction in postoperative precautions, and issuance of assistive equipment.

    2. Second or third day to discharge:

    a. Instruction in functional activities is initiated. The type of training needed depends upon the precautions for each patient, which are determined by the surgical approach, type of prosthesis and fixation, muscle tone, degree of postoperative ROM, the patient's daily activities, and the nature of the surgical procedure, that is, whether or not the trochanter was removed. Instruction involves training in adaptive methods or use of assistive equipment to avoid (1) excessive hip flexion, adduction, and internal rotation in combination (this is the most common cause of dislocation), and (2) hip flexion beyond 90 degrees (to protect the posterior incision and repair). Training should include methods for toilet, chair, tub, bed, and car transfers; stair climbing (taught in physical therapy, reinforced in occupational therapy); shoe and sock dressing on the surgical extremity; adaptive methods of washing and drying the foot as well as nail care on the surgical side; and sexual positioning.

    b. An important aspect of postoperative ADL training is counseling the patient and spouse or the person or persons living with the patient about postoperative precautions and how this will affect the patient's ability to participate in household responsibilities.

    For the severely limited patient, responsibilities may not be very different. For a young patient with OA who is used to doing a lot around the home, use of ambulation aids and partial weight bearing for 3 months can markedly shift the household work to the spouse or other household members. Realistic discussions about daily work—caring for pets, taking out trash, shopping, yard care, cooking, and so forth—and how this will affect the spouse or family member's life can be very helpful in reducing postoperative emotional stress and family discord.

    c. Precautions until first postoperative visit (6 to 8 weeks): Night positioning to prevent hip flexion, adduction, and internal rotation. (Some of these precautions may be needed indefinitely, depending on the patient.)

3. Suggestions for incorporating postoperative precautions in daily activities.

a. *Sitting*:

- The chair should be high enough so the patient can sit and rise with less than 90 degrees of hip flexion. Low chairs, sofas, and toilets may require more than 90 degrees of flexion. If a person has knee involvement or weak hands, a higher seat facilitates transfer.
- The patient should not bend to pick something off the floor while sitting because this tends to flex the hip greater than 90 degrees.
- The patient should not sit in a chair with a footstool under the operative leg because this can increase flexion greater than 90 degrees.
- *As a general rule, the knee should never be higher than the hip when sitting.*
- While sitting, the patient should not cross the operative leg over the nonoperative leg at the knee or ankle.
- When sitting or rising from a chair, bed, or toilet, arm supports should be used to support the body weight.
- The knee on the operated leg should be kept extended to avoid full weight bearing on the hip and prevent excessive flexion of the hip when rising from a seat.

b. *Ambulation with a walker*:

- Patients must be taught how to partial weight bear on the surgical hip. Bilateral ambulation aids are used until the patient has sufficient abductor strength to prevent Trendelenburg gait with a unilateral aid.
- The walker should be used straight ahead of the person—not put to the side before turning—to avoid hip rotation.
- Patients should use the arms on chairs for rising, not the walker, for stable support and more efficient rising.
- The walker should be used in a stable manner with all four feet on the ground, not tilted so that only two of the feet touch the floor.

c. *Bath and shower transfer*:

- To bathe, patients should use a shower seat or chair for safety while partial weight bearing. Transfer should be done as above with the knee of the operated leg extended.
- Bathing is accomplished using a shower hose and extended-handle sponge to avoid excessive flexion of the hip while washing feet.

d. *Bed transfer*:

- If the patient's bed is low, it should be raised on blocks.
- Transfer is facilitated if the bed is firm or a bed board is used under the mattress. A top layer of foam (e.g., an egg crate cushion) may make sleeping more comfortable.
- Platt and co-workers[26] recommend the following procedure: (1) have the patient sit on the bed two-thirds of the way down; (2) enter the bed leading with the operated side; and (3) then have the patient lie flat on his or her back and try to move the body as a whole with the legs apart; (4) to get out of bed reverse this process—start with the unoperated side, and keep the body straight and use the elbows for support.

e. *Bed positioning*:

- The patient should sleep with pillows between the legs to prevent the hip from adducting, rotating inward.
- If the patient sleeps on his or her side, it is best to sleep on the operated side only after sufficient wound healing.

f. *Car transfer*:

- In the early stages, the patient should sit semireclined in the back seat of the car.
- To get into a car, the patient should first back up to the back

door on the side that will allow the operated leg to rest against the car seat, then back onto the seat and slide the buttocks back so that he or she is sitting in a semireclined position.

- Some cars have a reclining front seat that allows proper positioning. Each car is different. Transportation home from the hospital and car transfers need to be reviewed with the patient and family prior to hospitalization and again prior to discharge.

g. *Dressing*:
- Patients should get dressed while in a seated position and frequently will require the assistance of an adaptive dressing device.
- Slacks and underwear can be slipped over the feet and pulled up to the knees with a dressing stick. The patient should then stand with the walker in front and pull the pants all the way up.
- Dress the operated leg first; reverse the procedure while undressing.
- It is recommended that men and women wear knee-high socks or stockings; a stocking aid helps the patient slide the socks on and off.
- Slip-on shoes or elastic shoe

laces that don't require bending down to tie them facilitate dressing independence.
- A dressing stick or a shoe horn with a long handle can be used to help put on and take off the shoes.

h. *Homemaking*:
- Some patients wear an apron with many pockets or attach a bag to the walker to carry around frequently needed items.
- Patients with systemic diseases or poor endurance should incorporate energy-conservation measures such as minimizing physical efforts whenever possible (e.g., sliding objects along a countertop instead of carrying them, and sitting down while working).
- Scatter rugs should be removed from the floor to prevent accidents.
- The patient should never bend down to pick up objects from the floor; use a reacher stick instead or bring the operated leg behind to reach down to the floor, if able. Doubled-faced tape on the end of a stick allows retrieval of smaller delicate objects (e.g., pills, broken glass, and so on).

REFERENCES

1. Singleton, MC, and LeVeau, B: The hip joint: Structure, stability and stress—A review. Phys Ther 55(9):957, 1975.
2. Sledge, CB: Correction of arthritic deformities in the lower extremity and spine. In McCarty, DJ (ed): Arthritis and Allied Conditions. Lea & Febiger, Philadelphia, 1979.
3. Poss, R, and Sledge, CB: Surgery of the hip in rheumatoid arthritis. In Kelley, WM et al (eds): Textbook of Rheumatology. WB Saunders, Philadelphia, 1981.
4. Levy, RN, Volz, RG, and Kaufer, H et al: Progress in arthritis surgery. Clin Ortho Rel Res 200:299–321, 1985.
5. Kay, A, Davidson, B, Bradley, E, and Wagstaff, S: Hip arthroplasty and patient satisfaction. Br J Rheum 22: 243, 1983.
6. Nevitt, MC, Epstein, WC, Masem, M, and Murr, WR: Work disability before and after total hip arthroplasty. Assessment of effectiveness in reducing disability. Arthritis Rheum 27:310, 1984.
7. Turner, RH, and Scheller, AD Jr (eds): Revision Total Hip Arthroplasty. New York, Grune & Stratton, 1982.
8. Conventry, MB, and Scanlon, PW: The use of radiation to discourage ectopic bone. A nine year study in surgery about the hip. J Bone Joint Surg 63A:201–208, 1981.
9. Parkinson, JR, Evarts, CM, and Hubbard, LF: Radiation therapy in the prevention of heterotopic ossification after total hip arthroplasty. Orthop Trans 61:441, 1982.
10. Beckenbaugh, RD, and Ilstrip, DM: Total hip arthroplasty: A review of three hundred and thirty-three cases with long term followup. J Bone Joint Surg 60A:306, 1978.
11. Collis, DK: Cemented total hip replacement in patients who are less than 50 years old. J Bone Joint Surg 65A:353, 1984.
12. Ranawat, CS, Atkinson, RF, Salvati, EA, and Wilson, PD: Conventional total hip arthroplasty for degenerative joint disease in patients between the

ages of 40 and 60 years. J Bone Joint Surg 66A:745, 1984.

13. Morscher, EW: Cementless total hip arthroplasty. Clin Orthop 181:76, 1983.
14. Lord, G, and Bancet, P: The Madriporic cementless total hip arthroplasty: New experiment data and a seven year clinical followup study. Clin Orthop 176:67, 1983.
15. Engh, CA: Hip arthroplasty with a Moore prosthesis with porous coating: A five-year study. Clin Orthop 176:52, 1983.
16. Amstutz, HC, Graff-Radford, A, Gruen, TA, and Clark, IC: Thaires surface replacements: A review of the first 100 cases. Clin Orthop 134:2, 1978.
17. Amstutz, HC, Thomas, BJ, and Jinnah, R: Treatment of primary osteoarthritis of the hip and comparison of total joint and surface replacement arthroplasty. J Bone Joint Surg 66A(2):228–241, 1984.
18. Jergensen, HE, Poss, R, and Sledge, CB: Bilateral total hip and knee replacement in adults with RA: Evaluation of function. Clin Orthop 137:120, November–December 1978.
19. Richardson, RW: Physical therapy management of patients undergoing total hip replacement. Phys Ther 55(9):984, 1975.
20. Wiesman, HJ, Simon, SR, Ewald, F, Thomas, WH, and Sledge, CB: Total hip replacement with or without osteotomy of the greater trochanter: Clinical and biomechanical comparisons in the same patients. J Bone Joint Surg 60A:203, 1978.
21. Physical Therapy Total Hip Protocol. Childrens Hospital of Los Angeles, 4650 Sunset Boulevard, Los Angeles, CA 90027.
22. Thielen, PL, and Mueller, KH: Immediate postoperative management of patients with total hip replacement. Phys Ther 53(9):949, 1973.
23. Myers, MH, McNelly, DB, and Nelson, K: Total hip replacement: A team effort. Am J Nurs 78(9):1485–1488. (Description of the nursing and physical therapy programs at Rancho Los Amigos Hospital.)
24. Seeger, M, and Fisher, L: Adaptive equipment used in rehabilitation of hip arthroplasty patients. Am J Occup Ther 36(8):503–508, 1982. (Detailed description of THR program at UCLA and survey of patient use of assistive equipment.)
25. Todd, RC, Lightowler, CDR, and Harris, J: Low friction arthroplasty of the hip joint and sexual activity. Acta Orthop Scand 44(6):690, 1973.
26. Platt, JV, Hahn, R, Kessler, S, and McCarthy, DQ: Daily activities after your hip surgery. American Occupational Therapy Association, 1383 Piccard Drive, PO Box 1725, Rockville, MD 20850-4376. (Call 1-800-the-AOTA to order.)

ADDITIONAL SOURCES

Adair, F: Nursing care study: Hip replacement. Nurs Mirror 158(5):39–40, 1984.
Baldursson, H: Hip replacement with the McKee-Farrar prosthesis in rheumatoid arthritis. Acta Orthop Scand 51(4):639–648, 1980.
Baldursson, H, and Brattstrom, H: Multiple operations in the rehabilitation of patients with rheumatoid arthritis. Scand J Rehabil Med 12(2):87–90, 1980.

Bombelli, R: Osteoarthritis, 2nd ed. Springer-Verlag, Berlin, 1982.
Burton, KE, Wright, V, and Richards, J: Patient's expectations in relation to outcome of total hip replacement surgery. Am Rheum Dis 38:471, 1979.
Charnley, J: Low Friction Arthroplasty of the Hip: Theory and Practice. Springer-Verlag, Berlin, 1979.
Fischer, P: Girdlestone's operation. Nurs Mirror 157(2) (Suppl iv–vii), 1983.
Harris, WH: Current status of noncemented hip implants. Hip 251–256, 1987.
Haworth, RJ: Use of aids during the first three months after total hip replacement. Br J Rheumatol 22(1):29–35, 1983.
Haworth, RJ, Hopkins, J, Ells, P, Ackroyd, CE, and Mowat, AG: Expectations and outcome of total hip replacement. Rheumatol Rehabil 20(2):65–70, 1981.
Hedley, AK, and Dorr, LD (eds): Cementless total hip revisions. Techniques in Orthopaedics 2(1), April 1987.
Hedley AK, Gruen, TA, Borden LS, Hungerford, DS, Habermann, E, and Kenna, RV: Two-year follow-up of the PCA noncemented total hip replacement. Hip 225–250, 1987.
Inman, VT, Ralston, HJ, and Todd, F: Human Walking. Williams & Wilkins, Baltimore, 1981.
Kim, WC, Grogan, T, Amstutz, HC, and Dorey, F: Survivorship comparison of THARIES and conventional hip arthroplasty in patients younger than 40 years old. Clin Orthop January (214):269–277, 1987.
Liang, MH, Cullen, KE, and Poss, R: Primary total hip or knee replacement: Evaluation of patients. Ann Intern Med 97(5):735–739, 1982.
Pipino, F, Patella, V, Bancale, R, and Moretti, B: The present-day value of simple displacement osteotomy in surgical treatment of osteoarthritis of the hip. Orthopedics 9(10):1369–1378, 1986.
Ranawat, CS (ed): Bone ingrowth hip arthroplasty. Techniques in Orthopaedics 1(3), October 1986.
Reikeras, O: Rehabilitation by total hip replacement in patients with osteoarthritis. Scand J Rehabil Med 14(4):197–198, 1982.
Suman, RK, and Freeman, PA: Bilateral hip and knee replacement in rheumatoid arthritis. J Arthroplasty 1(4):237–240, 1986.
Wilcock, GK: A comparison of total hip replacement in patients aged 69 years or less and 70 years or over. Gerontology 27(1–2):85–88, 1981.
Yoshino, S, Fujimori, J, Morishige, T, and Uchida, S: Bilateral joint replacement of hip and knee joints in patients with rheumatoid arthritis. Arch Orthop Trauma Surg 103(1):1–4, 1984.

Total Hip Replacement for Children and Adolescents

Garcia-Morteo, O, Maldonado-Cocco, JA, and Babini, JC: Ectopic ossification following total hip replacement in juvenile chronic arthritis. J Bone Joint Surg 65A(6):812–814, 1983.
Herring, JA: Destructive arthritis of the hip in juvenile rheumatoid arthritis. J Pediatr Orthop 4(2):259–261, 1984.
Lachiewicz, PF, McCaskill, B, Inglis, A, Ranawat, CS, and Rosenstein, BD: Total hip arthroplasty in ju-

venile rheumatoid arthritis. Two to eleven-year results. J Bone Joint Surg 68A(4):502–508, 1986.

Mogensen, B, Svantesson, H, and Lidgren, L: Surface replacement of the hip in juvenile chronic arthritis. Scand J Rheumatol 10(4):269–272, 1981.

Roach, JW, and Paradies, LH: Total hip arthroplasty performed during adolescence. J Pediatr Orthop 4(4):418–421, 1984.

Ruddlesdin, C, Ansell, BM, Arden, GP, and Swann, M: Total hip replacement in children with juvenile chronic arthritis. J Bone Joint Surg 68B(2):218–222, 1986.

Scott, RD, Sarokhan, AJ, and Dalziel, R: Total hip and total knee arthroplasty in juvenile rheumatoid arthritis. Clin Orthop (182):90–98, January–February 1984.

Chapter 34

Knee Surgery

INFLAMMATORY ARTHRITIS OF THE KNEE
OSTEOARTHRITIS OF THE KNEE
KNEE SYNOVECTOMY
TOTAL KNEE REPLACEMENT ARTHROPLASTY (WITH
  NON-HINGE PROSTHESIS)

INFLAMMATORY ARTHRITIS OF THE KNEE

The knee joint is a frequent site of involvement in all of the rheumatic diseases. In rheumatoid arthritis (RA), the most common consequence of chronic synovitis is knee flexion contractures. Unfortunately, many contractures develop because patients have not received appropriate instruction, orthotic treatment, or physical therapy early enough. When the knee is inflamed, a position of slight flexion provides the greatest comfort. However, patients who sleep with pillows under their knees for comfort frequently then cannot regain extension after the inflammation subsides. It is also theorized that pain and tension of the capsule cause a reflex spasm of the knee flexor muscles and inhibition of the extensors, which encourages a flexed position.[1,2] A flexion contracture greater than 15 degrees impairs functional ability by decreasing quadriceps efficiency and increases the energy cost of ambulation. If possible, knee flexion contractures greater than 30 degrees should be reduced through serial casting, traction, and exercise prior to surgery. If a contracture is nonresponsive to traction, due to shortening of the muscles and posterior capsule, a posterior lateral soft tissue release may be performed although in current practice a release is rarely done because a total knee replacement can help correct this problem.[3,4]

For patients with persistent synovitis and beginning flexion deformity, but with minimal cartilage changes, a synovectomy is a feasible short-term solution for relieving pain and forestalling joint damage. The benefits of synovectomy typically last for 1 to 3 years but can last longer in some patients.[5] The predictably short-term benefits of synovectomies make this an unpopular surgical choice for long-term chronic disease.

In the moderate stages of RA, synovitis erodes all of the articulating surfaces equally, causing a symmetric reduction in the height of the joint. The loss of height creates laxity in the supporting ligaments and knee instability. With progression and severity of the disease, asymmetric erosions and collapse of the cartilage can occur, producing valgus; however, varus rotational deformities and posterior subluxation of the tibia are also seen.[4]

For either moderate or late destruction, the **total knee replacement (TKR)** is considered the treatment of choice. The TKR is designed to replace the joint surfaces and to restore height to the joint so the ligaments can be at appropriate tension to provide stability. If valgus or varus deformity is present, the tibial components can be adjusted to correct angulation. Rotation deformity or posterior subluxation requires additional soft tissue reconstruction.[3,4]

Prior to the advent of modern arthroplasty, **arthrodesis,** or fusion of the knee,

527

was a common solution to severe destruction of the knee. However, the functional limitations of a stiff knee and the abnormal biomechanical forces it places on the body over time make this a procedure to use as a last resort. The one rare exception would be severe destruction of the knee due to chronic infection, where arthrodesis might be used as a primary procedure. In the management of arthritis, arthrodesis is considered a salvage procedure used after the failure of a TKR and usually after multiple revisions.

OSTEOARTHRITIS OF THE KNEE

The problems encountered in osteoarthritis (OA) of the knee are very different from those seen in RA. In OA, the cartilage destruction is often unilateral, involving one compartment of the knee, and typically produces a varus (bow-leg) deformity. These patients often have monoarticular involvement and are more active than patients with RA and, therefore, would place greater demands on the surgical repair.[3]

Surgical options for patients with OA include the following:

1. **Debridement.** This includes removing osteophytes, degenerated menisci, and loose cartilage bodies; shaving degenerated cartilage; and drilling eburnated bone. This procedure can provide satisfactory pain relief, particularly in younger patients. This procedure has become increasingly popular with the advent of surgical arthroscopy.[6]

2. **Osteotomy.** For patients with unicompartmental destruction and varus deformity, a thin wedge of bone is removed from the tibia beneath the unaffected compartment to shift weight-bearing forces to the unaffected lateral side. This prolongs the integrity of the joint by decreasing the weight-bearing pressure on the affected compartment. It is effective for mild (10-degree) varus deformities.[7] For marked valgus deformity, a femoral osteotomy or a unicompartmental arthroplasty is often used.[3] This is the treatment of choice for younger patients with early disabling arthritis whose functional demands would exceed the TKR.

3. **Total knee replacement.** This is indicated with patients with persistent pain and decreased range of motion (ROM) who are not candidates for an osteotomy or debridement procedure.[3]

KNEE SYNOVECTOMY

Indications
Persistent painful synovial mass, intermittent or constant effusion that has not responded to at least 4 to 6 months of adequate medical treatment. It is the primary treatment for pigmented villonodular synovitis.[8] Synovium can be removed by arthroscopic surgery, rendering the surgical synovectomy uncommon in current practice.

Occurrence
Primarily RA, JRA, and rheumatoid variants, and chronic infectious arthritis.

Surgical and Functional Goals
1. Relief of pain.
2. Increase in active ROM of knee from 0 degrees to at least 90 degrees of flexion.
3. Delay in the progression of joint destruction.[4]

Surgical Prerequisites
1. Absence of cartilage destruction on preoperative x-ray studies.
2. Flexion contracture of less than 15 degrees.
3. Ligamentous stability.
4. Competent quadriceps mechanism.
5. Motivation to participate in an extensive postsurgical rehabilitation program. No significant presurgical depression.

Surgical Procedure
1. Approach: Anteromedial.
2. The deep fascia and capsule are incised.
3. As much synovium as possible is excised.

Postoperative Physical Therapy
Average hospitalization: 7 to 10 days.

Isometric quadriceps-strengthening exercises are started preoperatively. Continuous passive motion (CPM) is initiated in the recovery room or when available. Schedule of use depends on activity and progress but it is generally used until the patient achieves 90 degrees of flexion.

1. First postoperative day to discharge: Isometric quadriceps-strengthening exercises are re-established, and assisted

straight leg-raising exercises are initiated. Neuromuscular electrical stimulation may be started and continued until the quadriceps muscle is a 3.5-strength grade.

2. A knee immobilizer is worn when the patient is at rest or off of CPM throughout the postoperative period.

3. Active assisted ROM exercises are started.

4. Isometric quadriceps-strengthening exercises are started when the quadriceps are a grade 3.5 on a 5-point scale (fair +).

5. Ambulation guideline: Beginning about the third postoperative day, partial weight bearing for approximately 6 weeks. The knee orthosis is used until quadriceps control is sufficient to control the knee.

6. Joint manipulation under anesthesia is considered if the expected amount of flexion has not been achieved.[4]

Postoperative Occupational Therapy

When the patient is ready for sitting, instruction in joint-protection techniques and use of assistive equipment can be started if indicated. (See Chapter 24, Joint-Protection and Energy-Conservation Instruction, and Chapter 25, Assistive Devices.)

TOTAL KNEE REPLACEMENT ARTHROPLASTY (WITH NON-HINGE PROSTHESIS)

There have been over 300 different prostheses designed in the past 30 years. Currently, the most successful replacements fall into two categories:[4,9]

1. **Nonconstrained:** The tibia and femoral components resurface the joint and restore height. They have gliding contact and are dependent upon the ligamentous integrity for stability (Fig. 34–1). These components make it possible to replace only the damaged surfaces. The unicondylar, total condylar, and kinematic prostheses are in this category.

2. **Semiconstrained:** These provide greater stability because of their highly congruent surfaces and a tibial peg or protrusion that fits loosely into the femoral component compensating for the damaged cruciate ligaments. The variable axis and Install-Burstein posterior stabilizer prostheses are in this category.

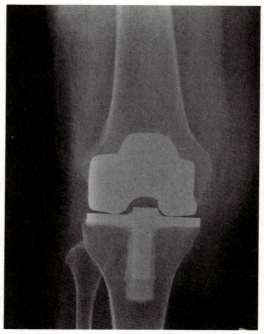

Figure 34–1. Postoperative x-ray film of a non-constrained total knee arthroplasty. The femoral component is all metal and secured with cement. The tibial component is metal with a 6-mm thick polyethylene surface to articulate with the femoral component. The angle of this film does not show the plastic tibial surface clearly and gives the impression that the two metal surfaces are touching. (Courtesy of Dr. Robert Poss and the Journal of Bone and Joint Surgery.)

There have been several attempts to develop a full hinge prosthesis that would provide full stability for the severely destroyed joint. The all metal hinges (Wallidius, Shiers, Guepar) are no longer used because of a high rate of infection and loosening and the possible consequence of an arthrodesed or totally unstable knee in the event of failure.[4,9]

The most recent advance in knee surgery for arthritis has been the advent of a cementless TKR in the early 1980s. So far short-term results of femoral fixation have been very promising; however, ingrowth into the tibial component has been unpredictable. If this technique shows results over the long term it will make the surgery simpler and revision surgery easier.

At this time there is no single prosthesis that can be recommended over all others. The most popular prostheses share the following: one-piece femoral unit; one-piece tibial unit; a provision for total resurfacing of the patellofemoral joint; high-density polyethylene on polished-metal bearing surfaces and provision for controlled triaxial motion. Other variables that influence a surgeon's choice are cement versus cementless fixation; desire to spare or to sacrifice the posterior-cruciate ligament; the degree of constraint; and the effect of metal-reinforced plastic versus all plastic components.[10]

Since good results have been achieved with many different designs it has become clear that patient selection and surgical technique are more important determinants of quality and long-term outcome than are design variables. However, for some patients design may be the critical factor. To address these needs, some hospitals are now creating custom computer-designed prostheses.

Indications
Persistent debilitating pain associated with joint destruction or limited joint motion impairing functional ability.[9]

Occurrence
RA, OA, and other arthropathies due to trauma, gout, or hemophilia.[9]

Surgical and Functional Goals
Ideally, this surgery will result in pain relief, joint stability, and an increase in range of motion from 0 to 90 degrees or more of flexion. It is hoped the patient will have 120 degrees of flexion.

Surgical Prerequisites[9]
1. Intact extensor mechanism.
2. Ligamentous stability. (Completely unstable joints require a hinge prosthesis.)
3. Intact joint sensation (not for neuropathic joints).
4. Flexion contractures should be less than 15 degrees. (Contractures between 15 and 40 degrees should be considered for serial casting prior to surgery.)
5. Adequate bone stock on which to seat the prosthesis or potential for bone grafting.
6. Motivation to participate in an extensive postsurgical rehabilitation program. Absence of severe depression.

Surgical Procedure
1. Approach: Anteromedial incision.

2. Synovectomy, if active synovitis is present.
3. Resection of bone ends and cementing of components in place.
4. Repair of capsule and quadriceps mechanism.

Postoperative Physical Therapy[3,4,9,11]
Possible complications that need to be observed are infections anywhere in the body, peroneal nerve compression, and patella fractures during activities.[4,12,13]

Average hospitalization: 5 to 10 days.

1. First postoperative day:
   a. Initial immobilization—compression dressing, knee immobilizer or cast, or application of a continuous passive motion device in the recovery room.[14,15]
   b. Isometric gluteal and quadriceps exercises and straight leg-raising exercises (taught to the patient in the preoperative strengthening program) are initiated.

2. Second to third day:
   a. Compressive dressing is changed; if a posterior splint or cast is used, this is changed to a knee immobilizer.
   b. Gentle, active, and active assisted flexion and extension ROM exercises are started.
   c. Quadriceps and hamstring exercise programs are started. (Some surgeons do not start strengthening exercises until approximately the third week and are adament against the use of weights for strengthening.[4])
   d. Instruction in transfer methods.
   e. When the knee has approximately 80 degrees of flexion, use of an exercise cycle without resistance is started on a daily basis and encouraged for home use.
   f. Partial weight-bearing ambulation is initiated, with or without a knee orthosis, about day 3 or 4, depending on the type of prosthesis, degree of leg control, pain, and other factors. The patient is progressed to independence on level surfaces and stairs prior to discharge. Patients are partial weight bearing for 6 weeks.
   g. ROM is limited by the soft tissue contracture, not by the prosthesis. Patients and therapists should not settle for 90-degree flexion. Gains are made after discharge. Outpatient physical therapy should be ordered for patients having difficulty achieving 90 degrees at discharge or who have difficulty on an exercise cycle.

h. The knee immobilizer is indicated for at least 1 to 3 months at night to maintain full extension. Usually the surgeon will have the patient wear the knee orthosis at least until the first outpatient visit. The orthosis is used only if the patient is having difficulty maintaining extension. At discharge patients should have at least 90 degrees of flexion and be able to walk independently with crutches and climb stairs. About 120 degrees of knee flexion is needed to climb reciprocal stairs independently and rise from a chair without use of hands.

Bilateral TKRs can be performed 1 to 2 weeks apart or simultaneously. Having both knees operated on at the same time is very hard on the patient and difficult for the therapist. These patients are likely to need placement in a rehabilitation facility upon discharge.

Postoperative Occupational Therapy

The most difficult task for patients following a TKR is lower extremity dressing and hygiene on the surgical extremity because of limited knee flexion. Patients with monoarticular arthritis are generally independent in functional activities by the second week, since they can substitute hip mobility for limited ROM. Patients with polyarticular involvement may need aids such as an extended shoe horn, sock donner, elastic shoe laces, and extended-handle sponge, to allow independence in these activities until full knee mobility is achieved. At the time of discharge, the patient should have at least 90 degrees of flexion.

When the patient begins ambulation, the following program is initiated.

1. Evaluation of lower extremity dressing skills; equipment issued as needed.
2. Review of methods for partial weight bearing during activities of daily living (ADL), particularly tub transfer, kitchen, and housework activities. Patient will be partial weight bearing for approximately 6 weeks.
3. Instruction in joint-protection methods.
4. Instruction in proper positioning at night and during leisure activities.

Ideally, the patient should be independent in ADL, with or without assistive devices, at the time of discharge.

REFERENCES

1. Cohen, LA, and Cohen, ML: Arthrokinetic reflex of the knee. Am J Physiol 184:433, 1956.
2. deAndrade, JR, Grant, C, and Dixon, A St J: Joint distention and reflex muscle inhibition in the knee. J Bone Joint Surg 47A:313, 1965.
3. Sledge, CB: Correction of arthritic deformities in the lower extremity and spine. In McCarthy, DJ (ed): Arthritis and Allied Conditions. Lea & Febiger, Philadelphia, 1978.
4. Insall, J: Reconstructive surgery and rehabilitation of the knee. In Kelley, WM et al (eds): Textbook of Rheumatology, 2nd ed. WB Saunders, Philadelphia, 1985.
5. Gschwend, N: Synovectomy. In Kelley, WM et al (eds): Textbook of Rheumatology, 2nd ed. WB Saunders, Philadelphia, 1985.
6. Zarins, B: Arthroscopy and arthroscopic surgery. Bull Rheum Dis 34(2):1–4, 1984.
7. Conventry, MB: Osteotomy of the upper portion of the tibia for degenerative arthritis of the knee: A preliminary report. J Bone Joint Surg 47A:984, 1965.
8. Laurin, CA et al: Long-term results of synovectomy of the knee in rheumatoid patients. J Bone Joint Surg 56(A):521, 1974.
9. Kettelkamp, DB, and Leach, RB (eds): Clinical Orthopaedics and Related Research: Symposium on Total Knee Replacement, 94:2, July–August 1973. (Review of all major knee replacement surgeries.)
10. Levy, RN, Volz, RG, Kaufer, H et al: Progress in arthritis surgery. Clin Ortho Rel Res 200:299–321, 1985.
11. Manske, PR, and Gleeson, P: Rehabilitation program following polycentric total knee arthroplasty. Phys Ther 57:915, 1977.
12. Rose, AH, Hood, RW, Otis, JC et al: Peroneal nerve palsy following total knee arthroplasty: A review of the Hospital for Special Surgery experience. J Bone Joint Surg 64A:347, 1982.
13. Thompson, FM, Hood, RW, and Install, J: Patellar fractures in total knee arthroplasty. Orthop Trans 5:490, 1981.
14. Coutts, RD, Kaita, J, Barr, R et al: The role of continuous passive motion in the postoperative rehabilitation of the total knee patient. Orthop Trans 6:277–278, 1982.
15. Salter, RB: Regeneration of articular cartilage through continuous passive motion—past, present and future. In Straub, R, and Wilson, PD (eds): Clinical Trends in Orthopedics. Thieme-Stratton, New York, 1982, pp 101–108.

ADDITIONAL SOURCES

Altman, RD, and Gray, R: Diagnostic and therapeutic uses of the arthroscope in rheumatoid arthritis and osteoarthritis. Am J Med 75(4B):50–55, October 31, 1983 (review).

Arden, GP: Surgical treatment of juvenile rheumatoid arthritis. Ann Chir Gynaecol 198:103–110, 1985.

Brumfield, RH Jr: Upper extremity assessment as it relates to lower extremity function in rheumatoid arthritis. Contemporary Orthopedics 2(6):455, 1980.

Buchanan, JR, Greer RB III, Bowman, LS, Shearer, A, and Gallaher, K: Clinical experience with variable axis total knee replacement. J Bone Joint Surg 64A(3):337–346, March 1982.

Dorr, LD (ed): Cementless total knee arthroplasty. Techniques in Orthopaedics 1(4), January 1987.

Garner, RW, Mowat, AG, and Hazleman, BL: Wound healing after operations on patients with rheumatoid arthritis. J Bone Joint Surg 55B:134, 1973.

Hecht, PJ, Bachmann, S, Booth, RE Jr, and Rothman, RH: Effects of thermal therapy on rehabilitation after total knee arthroplasty. A prospective randomized study. Clin Orthop (178):198–201, September 1983.

Hernigou, P, Medevielle, D, Debeyre, H, and Goutallier, D: Proximal tibial osteotomy for osteoarthritis with varus deformity. A ten to thirteen year follow-up study. J Bone Joint Surg 69A(3):332–354, 1987.

Insall, JN (ed): Surgery of the Knee. Churchill-Livingston, New York, 1984.

Lankhorst, GJ, Van de Stadt, RJ, and Van der Korst, JK: The relationships of functional capacity, pain, and isometric and isokinetic torque in osteoarthritis of the knee. Scand J Rehabil Med 17(4):167–172, 1985.

McGinty, JB: Arthroscopic removal of loose bodies. Orthop Clin North Am 13(2):313–328, April 1982.

Nordesijo, LO, Nordgren, B, Wigren, A et al: Isometric strength and endurance in patients with severe rheumatoid arthritis or osteoarthritis in the knee joints: A comparative study in healthy men and women. Scand J Rheumatol 12:152–156, 1983.

Scott, RD, Sarokhan, AJ, and Dalziel, R: Total hip and total knee arthroplasty in juvenile rheumatoid arthritis. Clin Orthop (182):90–98, January–February 1984.

Scott, WN (ed): Symposium on Total Knee Arthroplasty. Orthop Clin North Am 13:103, 1982.

Simon, SR, Trieshmann, HW, Burdett, RG, Ewald, FC, and Sledge, C: Quantitative gait analysis after total knee arthroplasty for monoarticular degenerative arthritis. J Bone Joint Surg 65A(5):605–613, June 1983.

Suman, RK, and Freeman, PA: Bilateral hip and knee replacement in rheumatoid arthritis. J Arthroplasty 1(4):237–240, 1986.

Wigren, A, Nordesjo, LO, Nordgren, C et al: Isometric muscle strength and endurance after knee arthroplasty with the modular knee in patients with osteoarthritis and rheumatoid arthritis. Scand J Rheumatol 12:145–151, 1983.

Chapter 35

Foot and Ankle Surgery

COMMON SURGERIES FOR FOREFOOT INVOLVEMENT
    MTP Resection Arthroplasty with Silastic Implant
    Metatarsal Osteotomy
    Hallux Valgus Correction
    Hallux Rigidus Correction
COMMON SURGERIES FOR HINDFOOT INVOLVEMENT
    Subtalar or Talonavicular Arthrodesis
    Triple Arthrodesis
COMMON SURGERIES FOR ANKLE INVOLVEMENT
    Total Ankle Replacement (TAR)

Rheumatoid arthritis (RA) involves the foot as frequently as it does the hand. It is common for RA to affect the metatarsophalangeal (MTP) and subtalar and talonavicular joints. Less frequently it may involve the true ankle joint. However, sometimes clinically this distribution is difficult to appreciate because patients unfamiliar with ankle anatomy mistakenly describe subtalar (hindfoot) synovitis as ankle pain.[1,2]

Initially synovitis creates swelling and pain in the MTP joints and possibly the distal digital joints. Patients often describe the pressure on the ball of the foot as "walking on marbles." During ambulation, particularly during the toe push-off phase, the MTP joints bear the full weight of the body in a dorsiflexed position. The kinematics of push off cause stretch of the plantar capsule and supporting ligaments, resulting in dorsal subluxation of the MTP joints.[2] Another dynamic force that occurs during the early phases of synovitis is spasm of the intrinsic muscles and the extrinsic digital flexor muscles.[1] All of these factors combine to create an imbalance deformity of the toes, referred to as **cock-up toe deformity.** The complete deformity consists of MTP dorsiflexion, proximal interphalangeal (PIP) flexion, and distal interphalangeal (DIP) hyperextension. Occasionally, patients do not develop hyperextension of the DIP joint and the deformity is referred to as a **hammer toe.** Additionally, chronic MTP joint synovitis stretches the transverse ligaments resulting in widening of the forefoot, referred to as **splayed forefoot.**[3]

The **hindfoot** includes the talus and calcaneus bones and the joints between these bones and the midtarsal bones. The **subtalar (talocalcaneal) joint** is the articulation between the talus and the calcaneus bones.[2,4] It is a critical joint and is responsible for inversion and eversion of the foot. (Flexion and extension take place in the ankle joint.) The signs and symptoms of subtalar joint synovitis and subluxation include: pain with passive inversion and eversion; greater than 5 degrees of valgus between the heel and tibia upon weight bearing, measured on the posterior surface (children with arthritis often develop varus deformity); and peroneal spasm elicited with brisk passive inversion, while the foot is dangling in mid air.[1]

When synovitis stretches the capsule and ligaments of the subtalar and talonavicular joints, the natural tendency of the talus to glide forward, downward, and medially is increased. Subsequent pressure on the calcaneus and plantar-calcaneonavicular (or spring) ligament typically results in hindfoot pronation and flattening of the longitudinal arch. Erosion of the sustentaculum tali (a process on the calcaneus that provides medial support to the talus) results in marked displacement of the talus and severe pronation of the foot.[1]

Ambulation with the hindfoot in pronation necessitates medial pressure against the large toe and contributes to a hallux valgus deformity of the first MTP joint and additionally alters the weight-bearing forces on the knee.[5]

Advances in foot orthotic materials and fabrication methods over the past decade have had a significant impact on management of the rheumatoid foot, helping to reduce the need for foot surgery. For adult RA, the most common foot surgeries are MTP resection arthroplasty and subtalar or talonavicular arthrodesis. Total ankle arthroplasty is seldom indicated because, as a rule, the main problem is in the hindfoot, or the ankle is grossly unstable, precluding this surgery! For primary OA the most common surgery is hallux valgus correction. Primary OA generally does not affect the ankle. For severe traumatic OA, arthrodesis of the joint or a total ankle replacement (TAR) may be indicated.

Surgery for rheumatoid foot involvement can be described by location: forefoot, hindfoot, and ankle. Treatment for midfoot synovitis is usually accomplished with conservative measures.[1]

COMMON SURGERIES FOR FOREFOOT INVOLVEMENT

MTP Resection Arthroplasty with Silastic Implant

This operation is for the first MTP joint and soft tissue correction of cock-up toe deformities. It combines several procedures and is the most common surgery for classic severe rheumatoid foot involvement.[2] This surgery relieves pain by eliminating the MTP joint and corrects hallux valgus and toe deformities, alleviating pressure areas on the dorsum of the PIP joints and plantar surface of the foot. The correction of de-

formities usually enables the patient to wear normal-style shoes. The main disadvantage of the surgery is that it shortens the toes and thus compromises the push-off ability of the toes. Frequently, the MTP joints dislocate, so they appear hyperextended. The first MTP implant preserves the length and stability of the first MTP for weight bearing.[1]

This operation is reserved for severe foot deformities and is often done on both feet during the same surgery.[1] Correction of toe contractures may require manipulation of the digits and Kirschner wire fixation.[1]

Postoperative Management

A hallux valgus orthosis, which maintains the first MTP in neutral, is used continuously for three weeks, and then at night for an additional three weeks.[1] Generally, commercial orthoses can be used or adapted. Occasionally, it is necessary to make custom hallux valgus orthoses.[3,6] The patient begins ambulation to tolerance on the second or third day following surgery and wears a wooden-sole postoperative sandal for approximately 6 weeks.[1] Plastazote liners can increase the comfort of these sandals. The average hospitalization for this surgery is about 4 to 5 days.

Metatarsal Osteotomy

When MTP subluxation results in a cock-up toe deformity that is easily reducible by pressing on the metatarsal head, the deformity can be corrected by a simple dorsal metatarsal osteotomy.[1] This is indicated for isolated MTP involvement in patients with nonerosive joint disease.[1] This surgery relieves pain from pressure on prominent MTP heads and associated callus is eliminated and prevents development of a fixed deformity.[1]

Hallux Valgus Correction

There are several operative procedures for this problem. The Keller procedure is widely used and involves resection of the proximal third of the proximal phalanx and the medial prominence of the metatarsal head.[1] Fusion of the first MTP in dorsiflexion is often advised to maintain the stability of the great toe for ambulation.[1] The postoperative orthotic program is the same as described under resection arthroplasty.

Hallux Rigidus Correction

Occasionally, osteophyte formation around the first MTP joint will block dorsiflexion, creating rigidity in the toe. This condition is painful, restricts the push-off ability of the foot, and causes compensatory stress to the IP joint of the great toe. This condition is most commonly seen in OA but can also occur in RA.[1]

For the younger active patient with OA, a simple débridement and removal of the spurs is the procedure of choice. For the patient with RA or the older patient with OA, an excision arthroplasty with Silastic implant is recommended.[1]

Postoperatively, active-assisted exercises are started as soon as symptoms permit. Ambulation is resumed to tolerance. Orthotic support is generally not indicated.[1]

COMMON SURGERIES FOR HINDFOOT INVOLVEMENT

Subtalar or Talonavicular Arthrodesis

In some patients, the subtalar or talonavicular joint may be the only joint in the hindfoot with significant involvement. For these patients, a single arthrodesis of the subtalar or talonavicular joint is recommended.[1]

Postoperative management includes immobilization in a posterior plaster splint for several days until swelling subsides, followed by cast immobilization for 10 to 12 weeks.[1]

Triple Arthrodesis

In the early stages, subtalar joint and hindfoot involvement can often be managed effectively with a heel cup orthosis, which restricts inversion and eversion of the foot.[1,6] If disability persists despite conservative measures or if the deformity cannot be reduced passively, a triple arthrodesis is often recommended.[1] This procedure effects a fusion between the talus and calcaneus, the calcaneus and cuboid, and the talus and navicular bones. When successful, this procedure provides a pain-free stable hindfoot; however, it is a difficult surgery in patients with RA because of the softness of the bone.[2] If there is severe ankle involvement, it may be necessary to perform a total ankle arthroplasty after the arthrodesis has healed, before pain-free functional ambulation is possible.[1]

Postoperative management involves 12 weeks of cast immobilization followed by use of a heel cup or foot–ankle molded orthosis for 6 to 12 weeks until the bone union is solid.[1]

COMMON SURGERIES FOR ANKLE INVOLVEMENT

The two operations commonly performed for arthritis of the ankle are arthrodesis and TAR.[1] Currently, the arthrodesis is recommended for the younger active patient with OA or traumatic arthritis who has sufficient mobility in the hindfoot to compensate for rigidity in the ankle, or patients with gross instability and uncorrectable hindfoot deformity. A total ankle arthroplasty is the procedure of choice for patients with limited mobility in the hindfoot either from ankylosis or arthrodesis; patients with RA, a stable ankle, and mild to moderate hindfoot involvement; and the older patient with OA with limited ambulation requirements.

Patients with a fused ankle often need a rocker sole and sach heel to facilitate ambulation. Patients should be assessed to determine if the fusion is limiting daily activities in any way.

Total Ankle Replacement (TAR)[4]

Indications
Cartilage damage to the talocrural joint. Persistent debilitating pain not responsive to conservative measures.

Occurrence
Traumatic arthritis, avascular necrosis, osteochondritis, RA.

Surgical and Functional Goals
1. Relief of pain.
2. Functional ROM (adequate for normal or near-normal gait).

Surgical Prerequisites
1. Ligamentous stability.
2. Balanced muscular function.
3. Intact joint sensation.
4. Stable hindfoot (hindfoot problems may be corrected first).
5. Absence of infection.

Surgical Procedure
1. Approach: Anterior lateral to midline.
2. Osteophytes and portion of the tibial and talar bone are excised.
3. Trial prosthesis is tested.
4. The tibial and talar components are cemented in with methylmethacrylate cement.
5. Drain is inserted.

Postoperative Physical Therapy
Average hospitalization: 3 to 7 days.

First day to discharge:

1. The foot is in a compression dressing and posterior cast or orthosis and elevated until swelling is decreased (about 2 to 3 days).
2. Isometric exercises of the gluteus maximus and quadriceps muscles are started. Some therapists do isotonic exercises to the contralateral ankle.
3. Toe flexion and extension exercises are started.
4. Instruction in transfer methods.
5. On about the fifth day, the dressing is reduced, and some surgeons replace it with an Ace wrap. Other surgeons prefer cast immobilization for 6 weeks.
6. Active ankle exercises are started.
7. Gait training on crutches with partial weight bearing to tolerance. Patient may be progressed to cane ambulation on an outpatient basis.

REFERENCES

1. Thomas, WH: Reconstructive surgery and rehabilitation of the ankle and foot. In Kelley, WM et al (eds): Textbook of Rheumatology. WB Saunders, Philadelphia, 1981.
2. Giannestras, N: Foot Disorders: Medical and Surgical Management, 3rd ed. Lea & Febiger, Philadelphia, 1980.
3. Wood, B: The painful foot. In Kelley, WM et al (eds): Textbook of Rheumatology. WB Saunders, Philadelphia, 1981.
4. Smith, CL: PT management of patients with total ankle replacement. Phys Ther 60(3):303–306, 1980.
5. Inman, VT: Hallux valgus: A review of etiologic factors. Orthop Clin North Am 5(1):59, 1974.
6. Inman, VT, and DuVries, HL: Surgery of the Foot, 3rd ed. CV Mosby, St Louis, 1973.

ADDITIONAL SOURCES

Buxbaum, FD: Surgical corrections of metatarsophalangeal joint dislocation and arthritic deformity: The partial head and plantar condylectomy. J Foot Surg 18(1):36–40, Spring 1979.
Coughlin, MJ: The rheumatoid foot. Pathophysiology and treatment of arthritic manifestations. Postgrad Med 75(5):207–216, 1984.
Dhanendran, M, Hutton, WC, Klenerman, L, Witemeyer, A, and Ansell, BM: Foot function in juvenile chronic arthritis. Rheum Rehab 19:20, 1980.
Dimonte, P, and Light, H: Pathomechanics, gait deviations, and treatment of the rheumatoid foot: A clinical report. Phys Ther 62(8):1148–1156. 1982.
Inman, VT: The Joints of the Ankle. Williams & Wilkins, Baltimore, 1976.
Jacobs, SR: Rehabilitation of the person with arthritis of the ankle and foot. Clin Podiatry 1(2):373–399, 1984.
Jahss, MH (ed): Disorders of the Foot. WB Saunders, Philadelphia, 1982.
Locke, M, Perry, J, Campbell, J, and Thomas, L: Ankle and subtalar motion during gait in arthritic patients. Phys Ther 64(4):504–509, 1984.
Mann, RA: Metatarsalgia. Common causes and conservative treatment. Postgrad Med 75(5):150–153, 156–158, 163–167, 1984.
Mann, RA: Biomechanical approach to the treatment of foot problems. Foot Ankle 2(4):205–212, 1982.
Miller, KS, and Hugar, DW: Foot surgery and the systemic lupus erythematosus patient. J Foot Surg 22(2):175–177, 1983 (review).
Moseley, HF: Traumatic Disorders of the Ankle and Foot. CIBA Symposium, Vol 17, No. 1, 1965. CIBA Pharmaceutical Co, Summit NJ 07901. (Presented 1980. Excellent resource for anatomical drawings of the foot.)
Newton, SE III: Total ankle arthroplasty: Clinical study of fifty cases. J Bone Joint Surg (Am), January 1982.
Park, C, and Craxford, AD: Surgical footwear in rheumatoid arthritis: A patient acceptability study. Prosthet Orthot Int 5(11):33–36, 1981.
Pullar, T, Anderson, M, Capell, HA, and Millar, A:

Comfort shoes—A cheaper alternative to surgical shoes in rheumatoid arthritis. Health Bull (Edinb) 41(5):258–262, 1983.

Spiegel, TM et al: Rheumatoid arthritis in the foot and ankle: Diagnosis, pathology, and treatment. The relationship between foot and ankle deformity and disease duration in 50 patients. Foot Ankle 2(6):318–324, 1982.

Tillmann, K: The Rheumatoid Foot: Diagnosis, Pathomechanics, and Treatment. PSG Publishing, Littleton, MA, 1979.

Woodman, RM, and Pare, L: Evaluation and treatment of soft tissue lesions of the ankle and forefoot using the Cyriax approach: A case report. Phys Ther 62(8):1144–1147, 1982.

Zamosky, I, and Licht, S: Shoes and their modification. Orthotics Etcetera, New Haven, 1966, pp 402–432.

APPENDICES

Appendix 1

Diagnostic Criteria for Rheumatoid Arthritis (Traditional Format)*

Criterion	Definition
1. Morning stiffness	Morning stiffness in and around the joints, lasting at least 1 hour before maximal improvement
2. Arthritis of 3 or more joint areas	At least 3 joint areas simultaneously have had soft tissue swelling or fluid (not bony overgrowth alone) observed by a physician. The 14 possible areas are right or left proximal interphalangeal (PIP), metacarpophalangeal (MCP), wrist, elbow, knee, ankle, and metatarsophalangeal (MTP) joints.
3. Arthritis of hand joints	At least 1 area swollen (as defined above) in a wrist, MCP, or PIP joint.
4. Symmetric arthritis	Simultaneous involvement of the same joint areas (as defined in 2, above) on both sides of the body (bilateral involvement of PIPs, MCPs, or MTPs is acceptable without absolute symmetry)
5. Rheumatoid nodules	Subcutaneous nodules, over bony prominences, or extensor surfaces, or in juxta-articular regions, observed by a physician
6. Serum rheumatoid factor	Demonstration of abnormal amounts of serum rheumatoid factor by any method for which the result has been positive in <5 percent of normal control subjects
7. Radiographic changes	Radiographic changes typical of rheumatoid arthritis on posteroanterior hand and wrist radiographs, which must include erosions or unequivocal bony decalcification localized in or most marked adjacent to the involved joints (osteoarthritic changes alone do not qualify)

*For classification purposes, a patient shall be said to have rheumatoid arthritis if he or she has satisfied at least 4 of these 7 criteria. Criteria 1 through 4 must have been present for at least 6 weeks. Patients with 2 clinical diagnoses are not excluded. Designation as classic, definite, or probable rheumatoid arthritis is *not* to be made.

Reference:
Arnett, FC, Edworthy, SM, Bloch, DA et al: The American Rheumatism Association 1987 revised criteria for the classification of rheumatoid arthritis. Arthritis Rheum 31(3):315–324, 1988.

Appendix 2

Classification of Progression of Rheumatoid Arthritis[1,2]

STAGE I, EARLY

*1. No destructive changes on roentgenographic examination.

2. Roentgenological evidence of osteoporosis may be present.

STAGE II, MODERATE

*1. Roentgenological evidence of osteoporosis, with or without slight subchondral bone destruction; slight cartilage destruction may be present.

*2. No joint deformities, although limitation of joint mobility may be present.

3. Adjacent muscle atrophy.

4. Extra-articular soft tissue lesions

---

*The criteria that must be present to permit classification of a patient in any particular stage or grade.

such as nodules and tenosynovitis may be present.

STAGE III, SEVERE

*1. Roentgenological evidence of cartilage and bone destruction in addition to osteoporosis.

*2. Joint deformity, such as subluxation, ulnar deviation, or hyperextension, without fibrous or bony ankylosis.

3. Extensive muscle atrophy.

4. Extra-articular soft tissue lesions such as nodules and tenosynovitis may be present.

STAGE IV, TERMINAL

*1. Fibrous or bony ankylosis.

2. Criteria of Stage III.

REFERENCES

1. Rodman, GP (ed): Primer on the Rheumatic Diseases. Prepared by a Committee of The American Rheumatism Association Section of the Arthritis Foundation, 1973.

2. Steinbrocker, O, Traeger, CG, and Batterman, RC: Therapeutic criteria in rheumatoid arthritis. JAMA 140:659, 1949.

Appendix 3

Polyethylene Gauntlet Splint (Manual Fabrication Method)

Important—Read the entire directions before beginning splint.

MATERIALS AND EQUIPMENT

1. Polyethylene (low density) ⅛- or ³⁄₃₂-inch thick. Can be purchased from most wholesale plastic distributors. It is very inexpensive compared with other thermoplastics.

2. Positive mold of the forearm (distal half) and hand with the thumb in palmar abduction, but mold only needs to extend to the end of the palm and middle of the thumb proximal phalanx. When making the negative mold be sure to form in the transverse arch. A rod should extend and should be centered in the shaft of the mold and extend out the proximal end for positioning in the vise. If a regular vise is used a wood stick ¾- by ¾-inch thick can be used. The stick should be positioned so the sides coincide with the anterior dorsal planes. If necessary use padding or additional plaster to build up the ulnar styloid or other bony prominences on the mold so the finished splint will form a bubble over those areas.

3. Oven 325°.

4. Piece of nylon tricot, 18 by 18 inches.

5. A flat cookie sheet, Teflon coated.

6. Stockinette, cotton.

7. 8-inch long, ¾-inch stay (as used in corsets).

8. Two asbestos oven mitts.

9. Electric grinder/sander that is shaped to fit inside curved edges, or a Dremel type hand grinder/sander.

10. Hack saw or other fine tooth saw.

METHOD

1. Preparation of the mold:

 a. With a hack saw cut a slit along the dorsum of the mold where the dorsal opening of the splint will be.

 b. Cover mold with stockinette.

 c. Pound or press the plastic stay into the dorsal slit (on top of the stockinette). This provides a guide for the final cutting.

2. Cut the polyethylene. Size: Length of the mold by 4 inches wider than the needed circumference. (This does not have to be precise as the material stretches and the excess can be cut off.)

3. Place mold rod in a vise so the wrist is horizontal with the volar aspect on top and the distal end toward the therapist. (Mold should be near oven if possible.)

4. Preparation of the polyethylene:

 a. Place the polyethylene on the nylon tricot on the cookie sheet. (The polyethylene becomes fluid and hot to handle. The tricot should be large enough so you can pick up the plastic, using the tricot, i.e., about 1 and ½ inches wider on the top and bottom, and 3 inches wider on the sides.) The tricot produces a flat finish on the outside of the orthosis; for a shiny finish, use a piece of Teflon cloth.

b. Heat the material for 10 minutes at 325° or until it just turns clear.

5. Making the orthosis (this is tricky and takes practice):

a. When the plastic is ready remove cookie sheet from oven and place near mold. (You have to work fast as the material cools rapidly.)

b. Lift the plastic using only the tricot and bring it over the mold. Flip it upside down and wrap and stretch it around the mold, pressing the edges along the stay and together. (It is okay if they seal together because you cut it later.) in other words, you seal up the mold (including the thumb area), but not the proximal and distal ends. Be sure to get a nice tight fit along the dorsal edge.

c. Take off the tricot.

d. Let the material cool slightly about 5 minutes, wrap with an Ace wrap, and let sit overnight. This allows the plastic to cool evenly.

e. Next day, take off Ace wrap. Position splint in the vise, dorsum of wrist up. Using a sharp mat knife, cut along the stay to make the dorsal opening of the splint. Cut the distal end as desired (see Chapter 25 regarding distal length of wrist stabilization orthoses). Cut thumb opening out, be careful not to cut it too large, about a ½-inch radial to the thenar crease. (You can always cut back later if necessary.)

6. Finishing. Take the orthosis off. Smooth down the edges with a Dremel type tool felt grinder attachment. With a drill make holes in a random pattern for ventilation (smooth hole edges).

7. Sew or rivet two or three Velcro closures, as desired.

Appendix 4

Diagnostic Exclusions for the Classification of Juvenile Rheumatoid Arthritis

The following conditions must be ruled out in order to make a diagnosis of juvenile rheumatoid arthritis.

1. **Acute rheumatic conditions**
   Acute rheumatic fever
   Henoch-Schönlein purpura
   Kawasaki disease (mucocutaneous lymph node syndrome)
   Erythema nodosum
   Serum sickness and drug reactions
   Mucha-Habermann disease
   Sweet's syndrome

2. **Chronic rheumatic conditions**
   Systemic lupus erythematosus
   Dermatomyositis/polymyositis
   Vasculitis (periarteritis nodosa, Wegener's granulomatosis, Churg-Strauss disease)
   Progressive systemic sclerosis (scleroderma)
   Mixed connective tissue disease
   Fibromyalgia

3. **Acute and chronic infections of the bones and joints**
   Acute hematogenous osteomyelitis
   Subacute osteomyelitis
   Bursitis
   Chronic osteomyelitis
   Iliac lymphadenitis and psoas abscess
   Tuberculosis
   Salmonellosis
   Cat scratch fever
   Acute septic arthritis (nongonococcal)
   The gonococcal arthritis-dermatitis-tenosynovitis syndrome
   Foreign body synovitis
   Fungal arthritis
   Syphilis
   Viral Arthritis
   Arthropod-borne arthritis
      Rocky Mountain spotted fever
      Lyme disease

4. **Inflammatory disorders**
   Inflammatory bowel disease with arthritis
   Familial Mediterranean fever
   Relapsing polychondritis
   Idiopathic periosteal hyperostosis (Goldbloom syndrome)
   Acute pancreatitis with arthritis
   Cortical hyperostosis (Caffey's disease)
   Sarcoid arthritis

5. **Hypertrophic osteoarthropathy**
   Secondary to pulmonary, cardiovascular, gastrointestinal, or endocrine disorders and neoplasms
   Cystic fibrosis
   Biliary atresia
   Primary hypertrophic osteoarthropathy

6. **Degenerative disorders**
   Avascular necrosis of bone
   Chondromalacia patella
   Osteochondritis dessicans
   Slipped capital femoral epiphysis

7. **Metabolic diseases**
   Diabetic cheiroarthropathy (hand involvement)
   Abnormalities of amino acid metabolism (alkaptonuria, homocystinuria, sulfite oxidase deficiency)
   Abnormalities of lipid metabolism (familial hyperlipoproteinemia, Fabry's disease, Farber's disease)
   Endocrinopathies (Cushing's syndrome, Addison's disease, thyroid disease, myxedema)
   Heavy metal (hemochromatosis)
   Hematological (hemoglobinopathies, hemophilia, deficiencies of complement, gamma globulin, and white cell killing ability)
   Bone metabolism (rickets, dysplasias, hyperparathyroidism, vitamin A and D poisoning, fluorisis)

8. **Heritable disorders with joint laxity**
   Marfan's syndrome
   Ehlers-Danlos syndrome
   Benign hypermobility

9. **Neoplasms**
   Benigh tumors of bone and cartilage (osteoid osteoma, hemangioma, villonodular synovitis)
   Malignant tumors of bone (synovial sarcoma, epithelioid sarcoma)
   Acute lymphoblastic leukemia
   Hodgkin's and non-Hodgkin's lymphoma
   Neuroblastoma

10. **Neuropsychiatric disorders**
    Psychogenic rheumatism
    Munchhausen's syndrome and factitious fever

11. **Miscellaneous**
    Acute chondrolysis of the hip
    Child abuse
    Congenital indifference to pain
    Frostbite
    Reflex sympathetic dystrophy
    Transient juvenile osteoporosis

Appendix 5

Procedure for Serial Casting of Contractures of Juvenile Rheumatoid Arthritis*

I. INDICATIONS
   A. Flexion contractures of knees and wrists (with radiographic evidence of some joint space)
   B. Varus or valgus contractures of feet
   C. Plantar flexion contractures of ankles

II. PROCEDURES PRIOR TO APPLICATIONS OF CASTS
   A. If muscle spasm of the flexor muscles is present:
      1. Apply a pack of crushed ice around the involved joint and extend it the length of the spasming muscles; maintain for 20–30 minutes.
      2. Concomitant facilitation of the extensor muscles of the involved joint (e.g., voluntary isometric contractions, low-amplitude electrical stimulation).
      3. Flourimethane spray may also be used over the spasming flexor muscles.
   B. If the joint is primarily stiff in a flexed position with no evidence of flexor muscle spasm:
      1. Gentle heat for 20–30 minutes (e.g., whirlpool, therapeutic pool, hotpacks, paraffin).
      2. For the knee, add gentle manual mobilization of the patella.

3. Active facilitation of the extensor muscles.

III. APPLICATION OF CASTS
   A. Position of child during casting procedure:
      1. For knee casts, place the child supine on a treatment table with a 1- to 2-inch pad under buttocks (to facilitate wrapping the plaster under the leg). Knee should be as straight as possible. Prone may be preferrable if more hamstring relaxation can be achieved.
      2. For wrist and foot casts, sitting on the treatment table with the knees over the edge has proved the easiest position.
   B. Stockinette lengths (use appropriate width for size of limb):
      1. Knee: ½ inch above buttocks crease to 1½ inches below malleoli (unless foot is to be included; then extend stockinette 1½ inches beyond toes).
      2. Wrist: Head of radius to proximal interphalangeal joints. (Make a small cut at the level of the base of thumb metacarpophalangeal joint for thumb hole.)
      3. Foot: Head of fibula to 1½ inches below toes.
   C. Wrap stockinette area with Webril (or other appropriate cast padding).

---

*Children's Hospital of Los Angeles Division of Physical and Occupational Therapy

547

For easiest wrapping, use 2-inch or 3-inch Webril on wrist and foot casts, 3-inch or 4-inch (rarely 6-inch) on leg casts. Make sure the Webril is wrapped smoothly and that all bony prominences and the superior edge of the patella are well padded.

D. Position the joint optimally—one person will usually need to maintain this position while the second person wraps the plaster of Paris.

Always position the joint with great care not to exert pressure that will subluxate the joint. Hold and position the joint immediately proximal and distal to the joint.

PRECAUTIONS
1. Do *not* put one hand under the foot or the distal end of the tibia to extend the knee. Place one hand at the medial side of the anterior knee surface and one underneath the proximal end of the tibia. Exert an upward pressure on the tibia and gentle downward pressure on the femur.
2. When casting the wrist, make sure you are *not* extending the carpometacarpal joints, but rather are holding immediately proximal and distal to the radial carpal joint. If the joint has already begun to subluxate, upward pressure to the carpals is essential prior to attempting increased extension of the joint.
3. The ankle and forefoot should be in a neutral position when casting varus or valgus contractures of the foot.

E. While the joint is held in optimal available position, the second person applies the plaster of Paris. (We have found the more "elastic" plasters such as Gypsona preferable to the "harder" plasters such as Zoroc.)
1. Suggested widths of plaster:
   a. 3 or 3 inches—wrist and/or foot casts
   b. 4 or 6 inches—knee and leg casts
2. Suggested amounts of plaster:
   a. 2 or 3 rolls—wrist casts
   b. 3 or 4 rolls—ankle and foot casts
   c. 3 to 5 rolls—knee and leg casts
3. Length of casts:
   a. Knee—½ inch below buttocks crease to 1½ inches above malleoli
   b. Wrist—2 inches below head of radius to distal palmar crease
   c. Foot—2 inches below head of fibula to ½ inch below metatarsophalangeals
4. Wet the plaster with cool water and wring out excess. Begin the casting using circular wraps around the wrist or foot and figure-of-8 wraps around the knee joint. Hold briefly in the desired position using only gentle pressure as described in 1 and 2, above. When applying the additional plaster, start distally using circular and figure-of-8 wraps. Before applying the last layer, the "extra" stockinette can be turned up as a cuff, thus providing a smooth edge to the cast.
5. Maintain support to optimal joint position for 3 to 5 minutes after last layer of plaster is applied.

F. Allow cast to dry non-weight bearing for 4 to 6 hours.
1. Once dry, children in knee casts begin intensive ambulation or weight bearing.
2. Once dry, children in wrist casts can use their hands for light activities.
3. Once dry, children casted for varus deformities of the feet can usually ambulate without adversely affecting the casting procedure. Children casted for valgus deformities often respond better if ambulation is limited for the period of casting.
4. Casts that include the foot often require reinforcement with fiberglass material on the foot portion of the cast to retard cast breakdown.

G. Casts are changed every 48 to 72 hours. As the gains made from the casts decrease in magnitude, the length of time the cast is on should be 72 hours. If marked flexor spasm continues to be a problem, increasing the length of time casted by another 24 hours has sometimes been of great benefit.
   1. The entire procedure of appropriate modality and exercise is repeated prior to each new cast.
   2. With marked flexor muscle spasm, the time out of the cast should be limited to the amount of time it takes to put on a new cast. Range of motion of joint with flexor muscle spasm should *never* be done during the casting procedure. We have found that flexion can be regained after extension in the optimal position is completed.

H. Diazepam (Valium) or other muscle relaxants may be necessary to allow a child adequate sleep at night while the casting procedures are being carried out. This is more often necessary when a marked amount of flexor muscle spasm is present.

Appendix 6

Roles and Functions of Occupational Therapy in the Management of Patients with Rheumatic Diseases

The role of occupational therapy in the management of patients with rheumatic diseases (Arthritis Foundation, 1983) has greatly expanded over the past few decades. The occupational therapist brings to this role an understanding of disease pathology and its effects on life tasks. Through assessment and treatment, occupational therapy personnel seek to improve the patient's ability to perform daily activities, prevent loss of function, and facilitate successful adaptation.

HISTORICAL PERSPECTIVE

Throughout their history, occupational therapy personnel have been concerned with the functional status of patients with chronic disabling conditions. During the growth of rehabilitation after World War II, the role of the occupational therapist in the treatment of rheumatic disease was concerned with patients severely disabled

by the deformities of rheumatoid arthritis and osteoarthritis (Cordery, 1965a). Research showing dynamic causes for some rheumatoid deformities led to the introduction in the 1960s of preventive management approaches early in the disease process. The principles of joint protection established a conceptual model that was pivotal in expanding the role of occupational therapy from restoration and maintenance to prevention (Cordery, 1962). Occupational therapy treatment programs included the education of the patient in modifying daily activities to facilitate joint protection, conserving energy at work and at home, and recognizing the importance of social roles and psychosocial factors (Cordery, 1965b). This coincided later with the development of community health education programs. The occupational therapist also became more active in community education, and intervention began to take place in the patient's home and workplace (Cordery, 1965b).

In the 1970s, occupational therapists began to specialize in working with patients with rheumatic diseases. The increase in early diagnosis of patients, the funding of multipurpose arthritis centers that required acceptance of the interdisciplinary approach to arthritis care, and advances in surgical techniques, including joint replace-

This roles and functions paper reflects the recommended practice in this area but is not binding. Occupational therapy personnel need to be informed about organization codes and policies; federal, state, and local laws; and professional licenses and regulations. Any of these codes or regulations may negate or revise the content of this paper.

ment, led to the development of comprehensive therapy programs by occupational therapists. Although the nature of the rheumatic diseases is such that it includes patients of all ages, the number of elderly affected is most significant and is increasing with increased longevity.

The Arthritis Foundation has always supported the role of occupational therapy, as evidenced in the 1950s by the publication of professional and patient education materials, in the 1962 sponsorship of an American Occupational Therapy Association (AOTA) Advisory Committee to the Arthritis Foundation, and in the 1965 establishment of its successor, the multi-disciplinary section of the Foundation. This eventually became the Arthritis Health Professions Association (AHPA). The annual national AHPA scientific conference, regional AHPA meetings, and AHPA fellowships and research grants have included major contributions by occupational therapists.

PHILOSOPHICAL BASE

The philosophical base of occupational therapy (AOTA, 1979) was adopted in 1979 by AOTA's Representative Assembly and was stated as follows:

> Man is an active being whose development is influenced by the use of purposeful activity. Using their capacity for intrinsic motivation, human beings are able to influence their physical and mental health and their social and physical environment through purposeful activity. Human life includes a process of continuous adaptation. Adaptation is a change in function that promotes survival and self-actualization. Biological, psychological, and environmental factors may interrupt the adaptation process at any time throughout the life cycle. Dysfunction may occur when adaptation is impaired. Purposeful activity facilitates the adaptive process.
>
> Occupational therapy is based on the belief that purposeful activity (occupation), including its interpersonal and environmental components, may be used to prevent and mediate dysfunction, and to elicit maximum adaptation. Activity as used by occupational therapy personnel includes both an intrinsic and a therapeutic purpose. (p 785)

The philosophical base of occupational therapy strongly supports the role of occupational therapy personnel in helping patients adapt successfully to the environment and to disruptions in their life-styles. The chronic nature of many rheumatic diseases indicates not only that patients will have to make an initial adaptation as a result of their disease, but that adaptations may be required throughout their life as the disease process varies and life tasks change. The person with a rheumatic disease finds that the disease process may affect his or her physical, social, and emotional well-being. Problems such as pain, fatigue, stiffness, loss of motion, muscle weakness, and deformity can interfere with an individual's ability to function at home, at work, and in leisure activities. By learning appropriate adaptations, the individual will be able to maintain the highest level of independent functioning possible. The occupational therapist treats the patient's physical and psychosocial dysfunction and helps the patient to develop the problem-solving skills needed to make adaptations throughout life.

OCCUPATIONAL THERAPY EDUCATION AND QUALIFICATION

The essentials for an educational program for an occupational therapist (AOTA, 1983a) require that course content include liberal and professional education. The biological, behavioral, and health sciences include courses in anatomy, physiology, kinesiology, human development throughout the life cycle, psychology, and the psychosocial aspects of disability and chronic disease, as well as the pathology and symptomatology of rheumatic diseases. Curriculum content of occupational therapy education includes human performance, activity analysis, the therapeutic use of activity, and therapeutic adaptation, including environmental adjustments, alternate methods of performing tasks, assistive devices, and orthotics. The therapeutic interventions related to daily living skills and health maintenance (including stress management, energy conservation, and joint protection) are also taught.

Occupational therapists who graduate

from an accredited professional curriculum and successfully complete the AOTA certification examination are qualified to treat patients with rheumatic diseases. Occupational therapy assistants who have graduated from an approved technical curriculum meeting the essentials for an educational program for the occupational therapy assistant (AOTA, 1983b) and have successfully completed their AOTA certification examination are qualified to assist in providing occupational therapy services.

Research in occupational therapy and the biomedical, social, and other sciences contribute to the expanding knowledge that forms the basis of clinical practice. Occupational therapy personnel should maintain and improve their knowledge and skills regarding the care of patients with rheumatic diseases through participation in continuing education and research. The selection of subject matter for continuing education is determined by practice settings, specific patient population, and individual needs. Participation in continuing education may be achieved by many methods such as workshops, seminars, conferences, clinical experiences, and independent study.

SCREENING AND REFERRAL

Screening is conducted to determine if a referral for occupational therapy is indicated. The occupational therapist responds to a request for services, which may come from various sources; the occupational therapy assistant enters at the request of the supervising registered occupational therapist (AOTA, 1980). The occupational therapist screens the patient by chart review, interview, observation, and administration of screening tests.

Patients are considered appropriate candidates for occupational therapy if they are at risk of losing function due to pain, fatigue, loss of strength and endurance, changes in joint range of motion, or loss of coping skills. These may interfere with self-care, work, and interpersonal, developmental, social, and leisure activities. Referral is also indicated when function may be improved through occupational therapy or, in the case of children, when the disease process may be interfering with normal growth and development.

Any member of the health care team, including the patient, may refer a patient for occupational therapy within the limits of existing regulations. State licensure laws, accrediting agency standards, reimbursement regulations, and the policies of the individual facility may require a physician's referral for assessment or treatment or both.

ASSESSMENT

Occupational therapy assessment refers to the process of determining the need for, and nature of, specific occupational therapy services for patients with rheumatic disease. The initial assessment consists of interview, observation, and objective testing to gather data necessary to determine the therapeutic goals and treatment plan for the patient. The assessment includes a review of medical history and the status of the specific rheumatic disease. Developmental milestones would also be assessed in the child. Manifestations of the disease such as muscle, tendon, joint, nerve, skin, and soft tissue involvement are identified. This is accomplished through range-of-motion evaluation, muscle testing, palpation of affected areas, and observation. The patient's report of pain, stiffness, and fatigue are obtained. The occupational therapist employs performance-based and self-reporting measures of function to evaluate the impact of the disease on daily living skills, including self-care, work, and leisure. The environments at home, school, and at work are evaluated for their influence on the patient's ability to function. The patient's psychological status, personal goals, interests, and expectations as well as the family and community resources are identified. The occupational therapist prepares written reports of the assessment results and recommendations for the patient's medical record and referring physician (Kielhofner, 1985; Melvin, 1982; Trombly & Scott, 1977).

INDIVIDUAL PROGRAM PLANNING

The results of the initial assessment are used to develop an occupational therapy program that identifies measurable and reasonable treatment goals, on which the patient and, if appropriate, the family, agree.

The patient's diagnosis and prognosis are fundamental to developing an appropriate treatment program. Program planning requires the occupational therapist to consider the complexity and diversity of individual needs. The program or treatment plan employs a comprehensive disease-specific and problem-oriented approach to the areas identified in the assessment. The treatment plan is developed within the context of the patient's life, environment, and community resources. Coordination of the total treatment plan and collaboration with other health professionals ensures comprehensive care for the patient with a rheumatic disease.

INDIVIDUAL PROGRAM IMPLEMENTATION

The nature and extent of treatment vary according to the stage of the disease process and the timing of the multiple interventions that may be needed during the patient's lifetime. In the early stages of the disease process, the occupational therapist focuses on helping the patient to develop the knowledge and skills to manage the disease. Education is an integral part of the program for the patient and family to learn about the patient's rheumatic disease and its impact on their lives.

Occupational therapy personnel teach management techniques and assist the patient in applying them to his or her daily life. Learning the principles of energy conservation, including organizing the environment and balancing rest and activity, allows the patient to accomplish daily activities while minimizing fatigue and effort. Teaching the principles of joint protection and adapting them to the patient's condition minimizes stress on joints, reduces pain in activity, and increases ease of accomplishment. Joint protection may include alternate techniques for performing activities, modification of the environment, and the use of adapted equipment. Techniques of stress management, such as relaxation, may be helpful skills for the patient whose pain and fatigue may be limiting physical performance.

An orthotics program may be necessary to reduce joint inflammation, prevent contractures, provide stability, reduce pain, and increase function. The occupational therapist analyzes the forces acting on the joints and the effects on the disease process and designs and fabricates appropriate splints. The patient is educated in splint use and its rationale. Because of the fluctuating nature of some rheumatic diseases, the occupational therapist monitors the orthotics program and makes changes as appropriate.

A therapeutic exercise program to maintain or increase muscle strength, endurance, and joint range of motion is considered by the multidisciplinary team. The role of occupational therapy personnel in implementing an exercise program may vary from setting to setting depending on the role delineation of the facility. The occupational therapist may identify a need for an exercise program when a potential loss of strength, endurance, or motion affects the patient's ability to carry out functional activities.

The exacerbations and remissions that characterize some chronic rheumatic diseases may mean repeated and intermittent occupational therapy interventions to respond to the changing needs of the patient. These changes may be in work, family, and community roles. As the work capacity of the patient changes, the occupational therapist may recommend modification of work tasks, explore alternate job sites, assess the appropriateness of job training, or evaluate disability. The occupational therapist counsels the patient in order to help in adjusting and achieving satisfaction in new family and community roles. Other changes experienced by the patient may result from a progressive disease process. When this results in deformities and significant loss of function, occupational therapy personnel train the patient in alternate methods of performing activities and may help to identify appropriate community resources.

Reconstructive surgery for rheumatic disease patients provides an opportunity to resume a more active and functional life. The role of the occupational therapist is to maximize the benefits of these surgical procedures by a pre- and postoperative program. The nature of the occupational therapy program will change with the surgery, but it can include positioning, orthotics, therapeutic activities, exercise, and training in daily living skills. Occupational therapy personnel continue to reinforce all the other aspects of the previous program, as appropriate.

For the child with a rheumatic disease, occupational therapy programs provide approaches consistent with the child's age and development. The activities of play and school, with family and friends, are analyzed, directed, and modified. Splints or assistive devices may be provided. Family education is undertaken. The relationship between the child and occupational therapy may be prolonged and span many of the normal developmental stages. The occupational therapist will be attentive to the need of the patient to take part in activities normally experienced by a growing child and will help the child to learn appropriate problem-solving and coping skills.

DISCONTINUATION OF SERVICE

The chronic nature of many rheumatic diseases is such that occupational therapy intervention may be needed at various times throughout the patient's life. As the patient's status changes, occupational therapy services may be intensified with exacerbation of the disease or surgery, or discontinued with remission of the disease or successful completion of the program. The discontinuation process is considered jointly by therapist, physician, patient, and family. When the patient demonstrates an increased knowledge and understanding of the disease process and when the therapy program has been completed, occupational therapy services may be discontinued. To successfully manage the chronic disease, the patient must be able to translate the program into skill, behavior, and attitudinal changes. The therapist may continue to be a resource in the future for the patient's program even though services have been discontinued.

INDIRECT SERVICES

To assure the quality and effectiveness of occupational therapy services, a system of quality assurance is required. Through quality assurance, problems are identified and studied, and solutions are implemented and monitored to improve the quality of care that patients are receiving. Management and supervision are needed to ensure that the delivery of occupational therapy services is both effective and cost-efficient. Occupational therapists have a responsibility to educate other health professionals and the consumer about the role of occupational therapy in the management of rheumatic disease patients. Consultation services may be provided to industry, schools, insurance companies, and community agencies.

LEGAL AND ETHICAL IMPLICATIONS

Providing care for patients with a rheumatic disease must be in accordance with state licensure laws, regulations of the facility, AOTA Standards of Practice, and the AOTA Code of Ethics (AOTA, 1983c; AOTA, 1984). Reports and patient records may not be released to anyone except the referring physician without a written release from the patient.

SUMMARY

Occupational therapy personnel make a major contribution to the management of patients with rheumatic diseases. Their unique skills include the ability to analyze activities, educate patients in alternate ways of performing these activities, and facilitate problem solving. The education and training of occupational therapy personnel in the physical, psychological, and social aspects of physical dysfunction make them valuable members of the health care team. The ultimate goal of occupational therapy is to help the patient gain the skills to achieve a maximum level of function in life tasks.

REFERENCES

American Occupational Therapy Association. (1979). [Minutes of the] 1979 Representative Assembly—59th Annual Conference. American Journal of Occupational Therapy, 33(11), 785.

American Occupational Therapy Association. (1980). Statement of occupational therapy referral. Rockville, MD: Author.

American Occupational Therapy Association. (1983a). Essentials of an accredited educational program for the occupational therapist. American Journal of Occupational Therapy, 37(12), 817–823.

American Occupational Therapy Association. (1983b). Essentials of an approved educational program for the occupational therapy assistant. American Journal of Occupational Therapy, 37(12), 824–830.

American Occupational Therapy Association. (1983c). Standards of practice for occupational therapy. American Journal of Occupational Therapy, 37(12), 802–804.

American Occupational Therapy Association. (1984). Principles of occupational therapy ethics. American Journal of Occupational Therapy, 38(12), 799–802.

Arthritis Foundation. (1983). Primer on the rheumatic diseases (8th ed.). Atlanta, GA: Author.

Cordery, J. C. (1962). The conservation of physical resources in the activities of patients with arthritis and the connective tissue disorders: Study Course III. Dynamic living for the long term patient. In [Proceedings of the] 3rd International Congress of the World Federation of Occupational Therapists. Dubuque, IA: Wm. Brown Co.

Cordery, J. C. (Ed.). (1965a). Rheumatic diseases, Part I [Special issue]. American Journal of Occupational Therapy, 19(3).

Cordery, J. C. (Ed.). (1965b). Rheumatic diseases, Part II [Special issue]. American Journal of Occupational Therapy, 19(5).

Kielhofner, G. A. (1985). A model of human occupation: Theory and application. Baltimore, MD: Williams & Wilkins.

Melvin, J. L. (1982). Rheumatic Disease, Occupational therapy and rehabilitation (2nd ed.). Philadelphia, PA: F. A. Davis.

Trombly, C. A., & Scott, A. D. (1977). Occupational therapy for physical dysfunction. Baltimore, MD: Williams & Wilkins.

Prepared by the AHPA Task Force (Lynn A. Caruso, MS, OTR, chair, and Joy Cordery, OTR, Peggy Thomas McKnight, BS, OTR, and Cynthia A. Stabenow, OTR, task force members) for the Commission on Practice (Esther Bell, MA, OTR, FAOTA, chair and project coordinator).

Approved by the Representative Assembly April 1986. Funded and approved by the Arthritis Health Professions Association.

GLOSSARY

This glossary defines specific terms used within this text and clinical rheumatological terms that are not defined in standard medical dictionaries.

Abduction pillow. Large triangular pillow used to position the legs in abduction following hip surgery.

Acromegaly. Enlargement of the hands, feet, and face, secondary to a pituitary gland tumor; may be associated with osteoarthritis and back deformity.

Acrosclerosis. Scleroderma and Raynaud's phenomenon confined to the hands.

Adhesive capsulitis (of the shoulder). Frozen shoulder, development of adhesions in the shoulder joint and in surrounding soft tissue.

Agglutination test, sheep cell. Method of testing for rheumatoid arthritis factor; less commonly used than the latex fixation text.

Air compression sleeves. Plastic sleeves that fit around the hand or arm and are intermittently filled with air to compress the enclosed body part; used to reduce edema.

Alopecia. Loss of hair; baldness.

Amyloidosis. Disease in which amyloid is deposited in tissues or in joints causing an arthritis; one of the causes of the carpal tunnel syndrome.

ANA. Antinuclear antibodies. Antibodies that react with nuclear antigens; found in the serum of nearly all patients with systemic lupus erythematosus and 20 percent of patients with rheumatoid arthritis, progressive systemic sclerosis, or polymyositis.

Analgesic. Medication or modality used to relieve pain.

Anaphylactoid purpura. Henoch-Schönlein purpura. (See Chapter 12.)

Anastomosis. A communication between two formerly separate structures.

Angiitis. Inflammation of blood vessels, including both arteries and veins.

Ankylosing spondylitis. Chronic bone and joint disease in which the inflammatory process has a predilection for the sacroiliac, spinal apophyseal, and sternal joints.

Ankylosis. Bony or fibrous fixation of a joint. (See Chapter 8.)

Anorexia. Lack or loss of appetite.

Anserine bursitis. Inflammation of the bursa beneath the distal aspect of the sartorius, gracilis, and semi-tendinosus muscles on the medial aspect of the proximal tibia.

Anteversion (e.g., of the femoral neck). A tipping forward of an organ as a whole, without bending.

Antinuclear antibodies. Antibodies that react with nuclear antigens; found in the serum of nearly all patients with systemic lupus erythematosus and 20 percent of patients with rheumatoid arthritis, progressive systemic sclerosis, or polymyositis.

Aortic arch arteritis. Arteritis of the large muscular arteries arising from the aortic arch. (See Chapter 12.)

Apophyseal. Pertaining to an apophysis, i.e., a projection, especially from a bone; an outgrowth without an independent center of ossification.

Architectural barriers (mobility barriers). Architectural structures (such as narrow doors, curbs, or telephones placed too high) that limit a person's ambulation, wheelchair mobility, or functional independence.

Arteritis. Inflammation of the arteries.

Arthralgia. Pain in a joint.

Arthrodesis. Surgical procedure designed to produce fusion of a join.

Arthropathy. Disease affecting a joint.

Arthroplasty. Any surgical procedure that reconstructs a joint; may or may not involve prosthetic replacement.

Arthroscope. Instrument for examining joint interiors. (The examination is called an *arthroscopy*.)

Arthrotomy. Surgical incision into a joint.

Articular. Of or pertaining to a joint.

Avascular necrosis. Necrosis of part of a bone secondary to ischemia; most commonly seen in the femoral or humeral head. Currently referred to as *osteonecrosis*.

Baker's cyst. Cystic swelling behind the knee in the popliteal space causing accumulation of fluid in various bursae.

Ballottement. A method for determining joint effusions by tapping or pressing on a joint; usually elicited in the knee by pressing on the patella.

Bamboo spine. Descriptive term for the radiographic appearance of the spine in ankylosing spondylitis.

Behçet's syndrome. Systemic disease of unknown etiological factors that presents with recurrent painful oral and genital ulcers and iritis; an inflammatory arthritis is present in most patients.

Bennett double ring splint. Slip-on metal finger splint to limit proximal interphalangeal joint hyperextension.

Blanching. Changing to white.

Bony spurs. A pointed projection of bone. (Syn: osteophyte)

Bouchard's nodes. Osteophyte formation around the proximal interphalangeal joint typical of osteoarthritis; similar to Heberden's nodes.

Boutonnière deformity. Finger deformity with flexion of the proximal interphalangeal joint and hyperextension of the distal interphalangeal joint.

Broach. Technique of preparing the intramedullary canal of a bone with a cutting instrument, usually for prosthetic replacement.

Buck's traction. Lower extremity traction unit, with adhesive skin attachment to the lower part of the leg.

Bunion. Hallux valgus with a painful bursitis over the medial aspect of the first metatarsophalangeal joint.

Burned-out phase. Chronic inactive phase of rheumatoid arthritis or other inflammatory joint disease.

Bursa. Closed sac, filled with fluid and lined with a synovial-like membrane; serves to facilitate motion between two structures.

Bursitis. Inflammation of a bursa, which can be due to frictional forces, trauma, or rheumatic diseases.

Calcific tendinitis. Inflammatory involvement of a tendon associated with calcium deposits; commonly affects the supraspinatus and biceps tendons in the shoulder.

Calcinosis. Pathological calcification of the soft tissues; occurs in a wide variety of systemic diseases.

Calcinosis circumscripta. Subcutaneous calcifications.

Capsulotomy. Incision through the joint capsule.

Carpal tunnel syndrome. Compression of the median nerve in the carpal flexor space; commonly seen in patients with flexor tenosynovitis. Initial symptoms are usually pain and tingling in the fingers, especially at night. Prolonged entrapment can lead to sensory loss and atrophy of the thenar muscles.

CARS. Canadian Arthritis and Rheumatism Society.

Causalgia. Burning pain accompanied by trophic skin lesions due to nerve injury.

C bar. Curved part of a hand splint that maintains the thumb web space.

Charcot's joint. See Neuropathic joint.

Chondrocalcinosis. Calcification of joint cartilage or menisci; may be seen in pseudo-gout, hyperparathyroidism, ochronosis, and other conditions.

Claudication, intermittent. Pain, tension, and weakness upon walking (not at rest) due to occlusive arterial disease.

Cock-up toe. Deformity with dorsiflexion of the metatarsophalangeal joint and flexion of the interphalangeal/distal interphalangeal joints.

Collagen. Protein molecule that provides the basic support for all connective tissue including fibrous tissue, cartilage, and bone.

Compression gloves. Any type of stretch glove designed to reduce edema such as Futuro Cotton-Stretch Glove and Jobst Custom Elastic Gloves.

Connective tissue. General term used to describe tissue that connects one part of the body to another; includes fibrous tissue, bone, cartilage, synovium, blood vessels, ligaments, tendons, and parts of muscle.

Cor pulmonale. Failure of the right side of the heart secondary to pulmonary disease.

Crepitation. A grating, crunching, or popping sensation (or sound) that occurs during joint or tendon motion.

CRST syndrome. Tetrad of symptoms consisting of calcinosis, Raynaud's phenomenon, sclerodactyly, and telangiectasia.

Cup (mold) arthroplasty. Arthroplasty that interposes a metal cup between the head of the femur and the acetabulum.

Cushingoid features. Characteristic physical changes with alterations in fat metabolism and the deposition of sucutaneous fat (1) in the face, producing moon facies or (2) at the dorsum of the neck called buffalo hump. Other features include obesity, purpura, and striae. This is a common side effect of long-term steroidal therapy.

Cyanosis. Bluish discoloration of the skin; used to describe the color of the hands in Raynaud's phenomenon or in other types of vascular insufficiencies.

Darrach procedure. Resection of the distal end of the ulna.

Degenerative joint disease. Noninflammatory slowly progressive disorder of joints caused by deterioration of articular cartilage with secondary bone formation.

Dermatomyositis. Variety of skin rashes that may accompany polymyositis.

de Quervain's disease. Stenosing tenosynovitis of the first dorsal compartment of the wrist involving the abductor pollicis longus and extensor pollicis brevis.

Diarthrodial joints. Synovial-lined joints.

Diathermy. A method of producing deep therapeutic heat by passing electronic or sound waves through tissue.

Discoid lupus. A disease of the skin presenting with well-demarcated erythematous scaly plaques. In later stages the skin becomes atrophic and scarred; although usually confined to the face, neck, ears, and scalp it may occur on the extremities. About 10 percent of patients will develop systemic lupus erythematosus.

Discogenic. A problem or symptom caused by derangement of an intervertebral disc.

Dislocation. Disruption of a joint charac-

terized by lack of contact between articular surfaces.

Dolorimeter. A device for quantitating the amount of external pressure a person can tolerate over a joint; used as an indicator of pain tolerance.

Dupuytren's contracture. Joint contracture secondary to shortening, thickening, and fibrosis of the palmar fascia; typically involves the fourth or fifth digits.

Dysphagia. Difficulty in swallowing. Frequently seen in progressive systemic sclerosis as a result of esophageal fibrosis and in polymyositis because of esophageal muscle weakness.

Eburnation, Eburnated. Changes in bone, causing it to become dense and hard like ivory.

Edema. Perceptible accumulation of excess fluid in the tissues.

Effusion. Excess fluid in the joint indicating irritation or inflammation of the synovium.

Enthesopathy. Inflammation of the end part of the tenon when it attaches to bone.

Erythema. Redness.

Erythema nodosum. Inflammatory rheumatic disease involving painful subcutaneous nodules in the legs; many patients have a self-limited arthritis.

Exacerbation. Increase of disease process either systemically or localized to a single joint; a flare-up.

Extension contracture. Fixed limitation of joint flexion.

Exostosis. Ossification of muscular or ligamentous attachments.

Felty's syndrome. A combination of rheumatoid arthritis, splenomegaly, anemia, and leukopenia.

Fibrosis. Deposition of fibrous tissue.

Fibrositis. Syndrome of pain, tenderness, and stiffness in deep tissue, such as muscle.

Finger ladder. Notched board positioned on a wall so that a person can "walk" each increment with the fingertips in a manner that increases shoulder flexion or abduction; it is an active-assisted exercise.

Flexion contracture. Fixed limitation of joint extension.

Fusiform swelling. Fusiform means spindle shaped and refers to the shape of the joint when there is synovitis. It is indicative of the inflammation being confined to the joint capsule.

GC. Gonorrhea (gonococci); can produce a secondary arthritis.

Ganglion. A cystic mass usually containing thick gelatinous material arising from or in close proximity to synovial-lined joints or tendon sheaths. Most commonly found over the dorsal and radio-volar aspects of the wrist.

Genu. The knee. Genu valgum: valgus deformity (knock knee); genu varum: varus deformity (bowleg).

Girdlestone procedure. Excisional arthroplasty of the femoral head and neck.

Gold therapy. Use of gold compound injections for treatment of rheumatoid arthritis.

Gout. Disease characterized by acute episodes of arthritis with the presence of sodium urate crystals in the synovial fluid or deposits of urate crystals in or about the joints and other tissues.

Hallux valgus. Valgus deformity (lateral deviation) at the first metatarsophalangeal joint.

Hashimoto's thyroiditis. Inflammatory disease of the thyroid that eventually leads to hypothyroidism; may be seen in association with systemic lupus erythematosus.

Heberden's nodes. Bony overgrowth or enlargement at the margin of the distal interphalangeal joint; characteristic of primary degenerative joint disease.

Henoch-Schönlein pupura. Self-limiting vasculitis that affects the small vessels of the skin, genitourinary tract, synovium, and kidneys.

HLA-B27. A genetically determined antigen associated with ankylosing spondylitis.

Honeycomb lung. Radiological appearance of the lung in pulmonary fibrosis.

Housemaid's knee. Prepatellar bursitis; a swelling between the skin and lower patella or patellar tendon that may result from frequent kneeling.

Hydrarthrosis. Noninflammatory effusion of a synovial-lined joint.

Hypersensitivity angiitis. A general term referring to inflammation of small vessels resulting from drug reactions, serum sickness, or other inciting factors.

Hypertrophic arthritis. Another term for degenerative joint disease.

Idiopathic. Pertaining to conditions without clear pathogenesis, or to disease without recognizable cause, as of spontaneous origin.

Intrinsic minus position. Extension or hyperextension of metacarpophalangeal joints with flexion of proximal and distal interphalangeal joints (claw deformity).

Intrinsic plus position. Flexion of the metacarpophalangeal joints and extension of the proximal and distal interphalangeal joints.

Iridocyclitis. Inflammation of iris and ciliary body.

Iritis. Inflammation of the iris and certain adjacent structures, typically seen in juvenile rheumatoid arthritis and the rheumatoid variants; can cause scarring and lead to visual loss.

Isometric exercise. Exercises involving maximal muscle contraction without joint motion.

Isotonic exercise. Exercises involving muscle contraction with joint motion.

Jaccoud's deformity. Development of metacarpophalangeal ulnar drift and proximal interphalangeal hyperextension without joint inflammation following rheumatic fever. (Syn: Jaccoud's polyarthritis, post-rheumatic fever arthritis)

Jog of motion. Minimal joint motion, usually less than 10 degrees excursion in any plane.

Joint mice (loose bodies). Small detached pieces of cartilage and bone found free in the joint which may be symptomatic if they get trapped between the joint surfaces; found in osteoarthritis and Charcot's joint.

Keratopathy, band. Calcium deposits in the superficial layer of the cornea and Bowman's membrane.

Knuckle bender splint. Dynamic hand orthosis that flexes the metacarpophalangeal joints and is used to correct metacarpophalangeal extension contractures.

Kyphosis. Forward curvature of the spine; e.g., humpback in the thoracic spine.

Lag. Difference between active and passive range of motion.

Latex fixation. Method of testing for rheumatoid arthritis factor; person may be described as Latex positive if factor is present and negative if it is absent.

LE Prep (preparation). Serological study to identify the lupus erythematosus cell;

one method of measuring antibodies to systemic lupus erythematosus nuclei seen in systemic lupus erythematosus.

Littler intrinsic release procedure. Excision of the oblique fibers of the extensor mechanism to overcome an intrinsic contracture.

Loose bodies. See Joint mice.

Lupus hair. Broken disorderly hairs about the forehead; seen in systemic lupus erythematosus patients.

Malabsorption. Inability to absorb foods; seen in progressive systemic sclerosis with severe intestinal fibrosis.

Malaise. Feeling of general discomfort or uneasiness; an out-of-sorts feeling.

Mallet finger deformity. Deformity involving only flexion of the distal interphalangeal joint; secondary to disruption of the insertion of the extensor tendon into the base of the distal phalanx.

Metatarsal bar. Ridge on the sole of the shoe to relieve metatarsal pressure and pain.

Metatarsal pad. Pad placed inside the shoe proximal to the metatarsal heads to relieve metatarsal pressure and pain.

Metatarsalgia. Pain over the metatarsal heads on the plantar aspect of the foot.

Micrognathia. Abnormal smallness of jaws, especially the lower jaw.

Moon facies. A rounding of the face due to fat deposition; a side effect of long-term steroid therapy.

Morning stiffness. This term describes the prolonged generalized stiffness that occurs in association with the inflammatory polyarthritides (especially RA and AS) upon awakening. The stiffness tends to be generalized and is indicative of systemic involvement. The duration of the stiffness correlates with the activity of the disease. This generalized stiffness is in contrast to the localized stiffness seen in osteoarthritis which results from inactivity.

Morphea. Localized scleroderma that may be a small circumscribed area or large diffuse patches; involves only the skin and subcutis.

Morton's neuroma. A neuroma of the plantar digital nerve caused by trauma to the nerve as it passes between the metatarsal heads; results in burning, numbness, tingling, or cramp-like pain of the forefoot.

May be due to wearing shoes with narrow toe width.

Muscle setting. Isometric exercise; usually used in reference to strengthening the quadriceps muscles (quad sets).

Muscular splinting. Protective reflex muscle spasm.

Mutilans deformity. Severe bony destruction and resorption in a diarthrodial joint. In the fingers it results in a telescoping shortening (opera glass hand).

Myalgia. Muscle pain.

Myositis. Inflammatory disease of striated muscle.

Myositis ossificans. (Heterotopic ossification). Ossification of muscles, soft tissues, fascia, and tendons; may be due to musculoskeletal trauma or repeated joint manipulations. The elbow is especially prone to this condition.

Neuropathic joint. Joint with severe destruction and disorganization caused by a disturbance of joint innervation; commonly seen in the knee with syphilitic tabes dorsalis, in the ankle with diabetic neuropathy, and in the shoulder with syringomyelia. (Syn: Charcot's joint)

Oligoarticular. Involvement of a few joints, usually three or less.

Orthosis. Any medical device applied to the body to provide support or increase function; includes splinting, bracing, and corsets.

Osteoarthritis. The most common term used for degenerative joint disease. (See Chapter 4.)

Osteonecrosis. This refers to the death of bone cells. It can be due to trauma to the blood supply (avascular osteonecrosis), or it can be idiopathic (aseptic necrosis). Osteonecrosis commonly occurs in the femoral and humeral heads. It can occur in other bones, including the carpal bones.

Osteophyte. Focal bone growth at joint margins occurring in response to joint destruction. (Syn: bony spurs)

Osteoporosis. Condition characterized by a loss of bone cells. It can be a primary condition or associated with other diseases, drug therapies (steroids), or disuse; can be improved or minimized with active motion and exercise.

Osteotomy. Surgical cutting of a bone.

Pannus. Excessive proliferation of synovial

and granulation tissue that invades the joint surfaces.

Palindromic rheumatism. Condition in which patient develops, within minutes, attacks of acute arthritis that last from several hours to several days without systemic signs or residual joint damage.

Pauciarticular. Involvement of a few joints.

Periarteritis nodosa. Same as polyarteritis. (See Chapter 12.)

Periarticular swelling. Diffuse swelling of the soft tissues surrounding the joint (extra-articular swelling).

Periostitis. Inflamed condition of periosteum, the membrane investing a bone.

Pes planus. Deformity of the foot characterized by loss of the longitudinal arch. (Syn: flatfoot)

Photosensitivity. Sensitivity to light, especially ultraviolet rays.

Polymyalgia rheumatica. Condition characterized by stiffness and pain of the shoulder muscles without weakness; affects older women and sometimes is accompanied by temporal arteritis.

Polyarteritis nodosa. Inflammatory disease of the medium-sized arteries producing diffuse musculoskeletal and neurological symptoms.

Polymyositis. Diffuse inflammatory disease of striated muscle that leads to muscle destruction and symmetric proximal muscle weakness.

Positive mold. It is the plaster replicate of the body part, e.g., of the wrist. A negative mold is the outer shell used to cast the positive mold.

Pott's disease. Tuberculosis of the spine.

Primary disease. A disease of unknown etiological factors.

Prodrome. Early symptom of a disease.

Prosthesis, joint. An artificial substitution for part or all of a joint. Examples are:
Austin-Moore. Metal femoral head and neck replacement.
Charnly-Mueller. Total hip replacement with a metal femoral component and plastic acetabular component.
MacIntosh. Metallic tibial plateau replacements.
Nibauer. Silastic finger implants covered with a Dacron mesh.
Swanson finger prosthesis. Silastic implants for the metacarpophalangeal and proximal interphalangeal joints.

Protrusio acetabulae. Condition in which the head of the femur pushes the acetabulum into the pelvic cavity.

Pseudogout (Articular chondrocalcinosis). Similar to gout clinically but a condition in which the synovitis is due to deposits of calcium pyrophosphate dehydrate crystals (instead of urate crystals).

Pulmonary osteoarthropathy (hypertrophic osteoarthropathy). Condition with clubbing of the distal interphalangeal joints, arthralgias, and effusion of other joints (knees, ankles, elbows, and metacarpophalangeal joints) as manifestations of various diseases, especially carcinoma of the lung.

Purpura. Condition characterized by hemorrhage into the skin.

Pyarthrosis. Pus in the cavity of a joint.

Raynaud's disease. Symptoms of digital paroxysmal vasospasm without an associated disease.

Raynaud's phenomenon. Paroxysmal vasospasm of the fingers in association with a disease; occurs in 90 percent of people with progressive systemic sclerosis and 50 percent with systemic lupus erythematosus. Vasospasm results in blanching, erythema, and cyanosis of the hands.

Reduction. Passive correction or realignment of a joint deformity or fracture.

Reefing. Surgical procedure for taking up the slack in an attenuated structure by folding the attenuated area back on itself and suturing it in place; e.g., radial side reefing of the extensor mechanism in the rheumatoid hand.

Reflex dystrophy (Sudeck's atrophy). Abnormal reflex sympathetic nerve involvement secondary to trauma, resulting in severe pain, edema, vasomotor instability, and atrophy of the bone, muscle, and skin.

Reflux esophagitis. Inflammation of the lower portion of the esophagus as a result of regurgitation of acid from the stomach.

Reiter's syndrome. Currently refers to arthritis associated with nongonococcal urethritis or dysentery; in classic cases conjunctivitis and skin lesions are also present. Typically the arthritis is limited to a single episode but it can become chronic.

Reposition. To replace or realign.

Resection arthroplasty. Removal of the articular ends of one or both bones forming a joint, e.g., Darrach procedure and girdle-stone procedure.

Rheumatism. Lay term used to refer to any type of muscle or joint pain or ache.

Rheumatoid arthritis. A systemic disease characterized by chronic inflammation of the synovium. (See Chapter 6.)

Rheumatoid factor (RF). A substance found in the blood of a high percentage of people with classic or definite rheumatoid arthritis. Alone, it does not indicate rheumatoid arthritis, but, with other rheumatoid arthritis features, can help lead to a diagnosis of rheumatoid arthritis. It may also occur in other diseases such as cirrhosis and tuberculosis. A person may be described as sero-negative or positive. A latex fixation or sheep cell agglutination test is used to determine if the factor is present.

Rheumatoid-like arthritis. A symmetric small-joint polyarticular arthritis that resembles rheumatoid arthritis but usually is not as severe. Typical of the arthritis found in systemic lupus erythematosus, polymyositis, and progressive systemic sclerosis.

Rheumatoid variants. A group of diseases characterized by (1) inflammatory joint disease of the spine and sacroiliac joints, (2) asymmetric peripheral arthritis, (3) iritis, and (4) presence of HLA-B27 antigen in a high percentage of patients. This disease classification includes ankylosing spondylitis, psoriatic arthritis, Reiter's syndrome, and the arthritis seen with ulcerative colitis, or regional enteritis.

Rocker sole. Shoe sole, curved at the toe to facilitate push off for limited ankle motion.

SI joint. Sacroiliac joint.

Sarcoidosis. Systemic disease of unknown etiological factors characterized by a reaction of neoplastic granulation tissue. It can affect almost any tissue; therefore, symptoms depend on the site. Associated arthropathy may include mild periarticular involvement, acute or chronic synovitis, or destruction of bone.

Sclerodactyly. Sclerosis and tapering of the fingers in progressive systemic sclerosis.

Sciatica. Vague term commonly used to refer to low back pain syndromes with involvement of the sciatic nerve.

Secondary disease. A disease in which the causal factor is known.

Sedimentation rate. The rate at which red blood cells sediment in serum; elevated in any inflammatory disease such as rheumatoid arthritis.

Shoulder-hand syndrome. Condition associated with reflex sympathetic dystrophy of the shoulder and hand secondary to pathology in the shoulder; pain, vasomotor disturbance, and diffuse swelling can lead to severe hand contractures and atrophy of tissues.

Sicca syndrome. A combination of lacrimal gland atrophy, resulting in insufficient tear production (keratoconjunctivitis sicca) and corneal changes, and salivary gland atrophy (xerostomia), resulting in a dry mouth. When associated with a rheumatic disease the triad is known as Sjögren's syndrome.

Sjögren's syndrome. Disease of the lacrimal and parotid glands, resulting in dry eyes and mouth; frequently occurs with rheumatoid arthritis, systemic lupus erythematosus, and systemic sclerosis.

Splayfoot. Transverse spreading of the forefoot.

Spondylitis. Inflammation of the spine involving the apophyseal (interfacet) and costoverterbral joints. Osteitis of the vertebral bodies, paravertebral ligaments, and muscles may be associated with spondylitis.

Spondylosis. Term applied nonspecifically to any lesion of the spine of a degenerative nature; reactive changes in the vertebral bodies about the interspace usually associated with discopathy.

Steinmann pin. A traction or fixation pin.

Still's disease. A variety of juvenile rheumatoid arthritis with severe systemic involvement and high spiking fevers.

Subluxation. Incomplete dislocation.

Swan-neck deformity. Finger deformity involving hyperextension of the proximal interphalangeal joint and flexion of the distal interphalangeal joint.

Symptom. Pathology that is felt or experienced. (A *sign* refers to pathology that is observable.)

Syncope. Fainting.

Synechiae. Adhesion of parts, especially adhesion of the iris to lens and cornea.

Synovectomy. Surgical procedure to remove the synovial lining of joints or tendon sheaths.

Synovium. Lining tissue in diarthrodial joints, tendon sheaths, and bursa. In the joint it produces fluid to lubricate the joint and is the part of the joint that becomes inflamed in inflammatory joint disease.

Synovitis. Inflammation of the synovium.

Systemic. A condition that affects the body as a whole.

Systemic lupus erythematosus. Systemic inflammatory disease characterized by small vessel vasculitis and a diverse clinical picture.

Tabes dorsalis. Tertiary form of syphilis characterized by neurological symptoms such as absent position and vibratory senses.

Telangiectasis. Chronic dilation of capillaries and small arterial branches which produces small reddish spots in the skin.

Tendinitis. Tendon inflammation.

Tendon ruptures. Sudden discontinuity in a tendon.

Tenosynovitis. Inflammation of the synovial lining of tendon sheaths.

Thermography. Method of photography that demonstrates the heat distribution in a body part.

Thrombocytopenia. Condition in which there is a reduced number of platelets in the circulating blood.

Tinnitus. Persistent ringing or buzzing sensations in the ear, used as an indicator of aspirin toxicity (aspirin levels are maintained just below the dosage that causes tinnitus).

Tophi. Deposits of uric acid crystals around the joints or in ear cartilage.

Torticollis. Stiff neck caused by spasmodic contraction of neck muscles drawing the head to one side with chin pointing to the other side.

Trigger finger (triggering). Inconsistent limitation of finger flexion or extension often caused by a nodule on a flexor tendon or stenosis of the tendon sheath.

UC-BL shoe insert. Plastic custom-molded shoe insert used for ankle or foot support.

Ulnar drift. Abnormal ulnar deviation of the fingers at the metacarpophalangeal joints.

Uveitis. Inflammation of the iris, ciliary body, and choroid, or of the entire uvea.

Venostasis. Pooling of blood in the lower legs because of poor circulation.

Wall walking. Walking the fingertips up a wall in a manner that increases shoulder flexion or abduction; method used in place of the finger ladder.

Weaver's bottom. Ischial bursitis, inflammation of the bursa separating the gluteus maximus from the underlying ischial tuberosity; usually resulting from prolonged sitting on hard surfaces. This can also occur with bicycling.

Wegener's granulomatosis. A destructive arteritis of the upper respiratory tract, lungs, and kidneys. It may have an associated joint pain.

Zig-zag effect. Ulnar drift at the metacarpophalangeal joints associated with radial deviation of the wrist.

INDEX

A page number in *italics* indicates a figure. A "t" following a page number indicates a table.

DATE DUE

NOV 1 3 1990			
NOV 6 1991			
PPF			
FE 09 '96			
Jan 2, 1997			
AP 28 '97			
DE 16 '97			
MAR 1 0 1998			
MR 8 '99			